IFMBE Proceedings

Volume 59

Series editor

James Goh

Deputy Editors

Fatimah Ibrahim
Igor Lacković
Piotr Ładyżyński
Emilio Sacristan Rock

The International Federation for Medical and Biological Engineering, IFMBE, is a federation of national and transnational organizations representing internationally the interests of medical and biological engineering and sciences. The IFMBE is a non-profit organization fostering the creation, dissemination and application of medical and biological engineering knowledge and the management of technology for improved health and quality of life. Its activities include participation in the formulation of public policy and the dissemination of information through publications and forums. Within the field of medical, clinical, and biological engineering, IFMBE's aims are to encourage research and the application of knowledge, and to disseminate information and promote collaboration. The objectives of the IFMBE are scientific, technological, literary, and educational.

The IFMBE is a WHO accredited NGO covering the full range of biomedical and clinical engineering, healthcare, healthcare technology and management. It is representing through its 60 member societies some 120.000 professionals involved in the various issues of improved health and health care delivery.

More information about this series at http://www.springer.com/series/7403

Simona Vlad · Nicolae Marius Roman (Eds.)

International Conference on Advancements of Medicine and Health Care through Technology; 12th – 15th October 2016 Cluj-Napoca, Romania

MEDITECH 2016

Springer

Editors
Simona Vlad
Faculty of Electrical Engineering
Technical University of Cluj-Napoca
Cluj-Napoca
Romania

Nicolae Marius Roman
Faculty of Electrical Engineering
Technical University of Cluj-Napoca
Cluj-Napoca
Romania

ISSN 1680-0737 ISSN 1433-9277 (electronic)
IFMBE Proceedings
ISBN 978-3-319-52874-8 ISBN 978-3-319-52875-5 (eBook)
DOI 10.1007/978-3-319-52875-5

Library of Congress Control Number: 2017930147

The IFMBE Proceedings is an Official Publication of the International Federation for Medical and Biological Engineering (IFMBE)

Printed on acid-free paper

This Springer imprint is published by Springer Nature
The registered company is Springer International Publishing AG
The registered company address is: Gewerbestrasse 11, 6330 Cham, Switzerland

Foreword

The 5th Conference on Advancements of Medicine and Health Care through Technology - MediTech2016 took place in Cluj-Napoca in October 12–15, 2016. The Conference aimed to provide opportunities for Romanian and foreign professionals involved in basic research, R&D, industry and medical applications to exchange their know-how and build up collaboration in one of the most important fields of science and technology - medical engineering.

MediTech is intended to be an international forum for researchers and practitioners interested in the advance in, and applications of biomedical engineering to exchange the latest research results and ideas in areas like hardware and software technologies, medical devices, biosignal and image processing, biomaterials, biomechanics, telemedicine, etc. The importance of this kind of scientific events was proven by the interest of the prestigious researchers from Romania and abroad who decided to take part in the 5th edition of MediTech. Moreover, we were honored to receive the visit of Prof. Kang-Ping Lin, Secretary General of IFMBE.

All papers submitted for presentation went through a review process and were evaluated by two reviewers. The papers chosen to be presented at the conference were accompanied by manuscripts to be published in these *Proceedings*.

We would like to kindly thank the members of the Scientific and Organizing Committees for their hard work and dedication and we hope that they will continue supporting MediTech.

MediTech2016 Conference Chair
Professor Nicolae Marius Roman

Organization

Organizer

Romanian National Society for Medical Engineering and Biological Technology

Endorsed by

International Federation for Medical and Biological Engineering

Partners

Technical University of Cluj-Napoca, Romania
"Iuliu Haţieganu" University of Medicine and Pharmacy Cluj-Napoca, Romania
Medical University of Vienna, Austria
The University of Sheffield, United Kingdom
"Dr. Constantin Papilian" Military Emergency Hospital, Cluj-Napoca, Romania

Conference Chair

Nicolae Marius Roman — Technical University of Cluj-Napoca, Romania

Honorary Chair

Radu Vasile Ciupa — Technical University of Cluj-Napoca, Romania

Scientific Advisory Committee

Laura Bacali (RO)
Doina Baltaru (RO)
Maria Beudean (RO)
Corina Botoca (RO)
Remus Brad (RO)
Simion Bran (RO)
Macarie Breazu (RO)
Lelia Ciontea (RO)
Radu Ciorap (RO)
Radu V. Ciupa (RO)
Hariton Costin (RO)
Cecilia Cristea (RO)
Vanessa Diaz-Zuccarini (UK)
Gabriele Dubini (IT)
Anca Galaction (RO)
Stefan Gergely (RO)
Zoltan German-Sallo (RO)
Laura Grindei (RO)
Flavius Gruian (SE)
Sorin Hintea (RO)
Rodica Holonec (RO)
Rod Hose (UK)
Adrian Iancu (RO)
Beriliu Ilie (RO)
Ioan Jivet (RO)
Mircea Leabu (RO)
Patricia Lawford (UK)
Angela Lungu (RO)
Eugen Lupu (RO)
Dan Mandru (RO)
Avram Manea (RO)
Alma Maniu (RO)
Raul Malutan (RO)
Winfried Mayr (A)

Local Organizing Committee

Invited Speakers

Kang-Ping Lin, IFMBE Secretary-General, Chung-Yuan Christian University, Taiwan
Heart, Heart Rate, & Heart Rate Variability with RSA Application

Helmut Hutten, Institute of Medical Engineering, Graz University of Technology, Austria
Innovations – From Good Ideas to Successful Products on the Market

Alessandro Pepino, University of Naples “Federico II”, Italy
The Discrete Event Simulation for Studying of Organizational Models in Health Care

Winfried Mayr, Medical University of Vienna, Austria
Interfacing neurons and muscles

Rod Hose - University of Sheffield, United Kingdom
ANSYS Healthcare Solutions

Lucio Tommaso De Paolis, University of Salento, Italy
Virtual Reality and Augmented Visualization in Medicine and Surgery

Mircea Gelu Buta, “Babeş-Bolyai” University of Cluj-Napoca, Romania
The Report between the Technics and Medical Clinic

Doru Ursuţiu, *“Transilvania” University of Braşov, Romania*
Online Technologies and Virtual Instrumentation in Sensing - Monitoring – Medicine. “Cloud Instrumentation and IoT

Mircea Leabu, University of Medicine and Pharmacy “Carol Davila” and “Victor Babeş” National Institute of Pathology, Bucharest, Romania
Half a Century for Jumping to Live Cell Studies at Nanolevel Resolution

Mihai Tărâţă, University of Medicine and Pharmacy of Craiova, Romania
Advantages of Frequency Domain Processing, in Monitoring the Neuro-muscular Fatigue

Radu George Ciorap, University of Medicine and Pharmacy “Grigore T. Popa”, Iaşi, Romania
Medical Device Testing – a Key Issue for Patient Safety

Doina Baltaru, “Dr. Constantin Papilian” Emergency Military Hospital of Cluj-Napoca, Romania
Aspects of Medical Technology in Military Medical System

Sponsors

Laitek Medical Software
Comelf SA, Avena Medica SRL, Tehno Industrial SA, Cefmur SA, Temco SRL, Constelatia Construct SRL

Contents

Part I
Clinical Engineering Assessment

Ultrasonographic Correlations and Challenges in Liver Hemangiomas

I. Grigorescu[1], Z. Sparchez[2], R. Badea[2], M. Dragoteanu[2], C.D.Piglesan[2] and D.L. Dumitrascu[1]

[1] 2nd Medical Department, „I.Hatieganu" University of Medicine and Pharmacology Cluj-Napoca, Romania
[2] „Octavian Fodor" Regional Institute for Gastroenterology and Hepatology Cluj-Napoca, Romania

Abstract- **OBJECTIVES. Gray-scale ultrasonography (US) represents the first method of detecting focal liver lesions. The aims of our study were to establish in liver hemangiomas possible correlations between tumoral and liver echogenicity; tumoral size and presence of chronic liver diseases (CLD); presence of peritumoral rim- tumoral and liver echogenicity, tumoral size and presence of CLD. MATERIAL AND METHODS. The study involved 352 liver masses in 270 patients with the presumptive diagnosis of benign liver tumor masses, established by ambulatory US, hospitalized at the Emergency Hospital "Prof. Dr. Octavian Fodor" and 2nd Medical Clinic Cluj-Napoca between 2006-2015. The final diagnosis was established based on the results of investigations such as US (gray-scale and color Doppler), SPECT, liver angioscintigraphy, CT, MRI, laparoscopy, histology, corroborated with clinical and biological examinations. RESULTS. The typical image of well-defined (94.81% of cases), hyperechoic mass (81.48% of cases), without Doppler signal (54.07% of cases), was detected in most hemangiomas. Presence of steatosis/nonalcoholic steatohepatitis (NASH) in 69 images from our study revealed the following patterns of hemangiomas: hypo- (16/69 cases), isoechoic (2/69 cases) and heterogeneous (51/69 cases). Fisher 's exact test shows that there exists moderate association between hyperechoic rim and hypoechoic hemangiomas; there were no other statistically significant associations found between: tumor-liver echogenicity, hypoechoic rim and tumor size-liver echogenicity. CONCLUSION. Classic US criteria of hemangioma was found in 81.85%. Hypo- and isoechoic hemangiomas moderately correlate with the presence of a hyperechoic rim. No statistical correlation was found between the underlying CLD and the hemangioma's echogenicity, nor with the presence of any tumoral rim.**

Keywords- **hemangioma, ultrasound, echogenicity**

I. Introduction

Gray-scale ultrasonography (US) is the first way of detecting focal liver lesions, but with lower specificity in establishing their etiology. Typical hemangiomas at US are hyperechoic, well defined masses, without peritumoral rim, without Doppler signal [1], but there exist also atypical forms (especially if the tumor is grafted on chronic liver disease-CLD): heterogeneous and/or hypoechogenicity hemangiomas, or with hyperechoic rim. Preoperative US, although sometimes their etiology is difficult to establish as gray-scale US has low specificity in characterizing liver tumors [2]; in such cases, complementary explorations like: liver scintigraphy, angioscintigraphy, contrast-enhanced CT and MR, or even invasive methods (puncture-biopsy, diagnostic laparoscopy) with histological examination, are mandatory. Although the typical aspect of hemangioma at US is of nodular hyperechoic, well defined mass, without peritumoral rim, without Doppler signal [1], there exist also atypical forms: heterogeneous and/or hypoechogenicity hemangiomas, or with hyperechoic rim [3].

The aims of our study were to establish in liver hemangiomas possible correlations between tumoral and liver echogenicity; tumoral size and presence of chronic liver diseases (CLD); presence of peritumoral rim- tumoral and liver echogenicity, tumoral size and presence of CLD.

II. Material and Methods

The study involved in the experiment group 270 patients (156 women, 114 men), aged 25-81 years, with the presumptive diagnosis of benign liver tumor masses, established by ambulatory US, hospitalized at the Emergency Hospital "Prof. Dr. Octavian Fodor" and 2nd Medical Clinic Cluj-Napoca between 2006-2015. There were found 352 liver masses in these 270 patients, 30 of them having concomitant other tumor tumors, and 52 being with multiple hemangiomas (hemangiomatosis).

The control group consisted of 60 patients (38 women, 22 men), aged 36-82 years with malignant hepatic tumors. Their diagnosis at admittance consisted of hepatocellular carcinoma (HCC) (12), metastasis (7), cholangiocarcinoma (3), hemangioma (2), hamartoma (1), tumor of unknown etiology (28) and the rest in other extra-hepatic pathologies.

Investigation of patients in this retrospective study was performed using ultrasonographs Logiq 7 (GE, USA), Si2000 Sonoline with transducers having 3,5MHz (for preoperative diagnosis) and 7,5MHz frequency (for intraoperative diagnosis), tomographic scintillation SPECT Orbiter Siemens camera, computed tomography (CT) and magnetic resonance imaging (MRI), along with clinical and biological examination.

All patients (both the experiment and the control group) underwent abdominal US examination in gray scale and color

S. Vlad and N.M. Roman (eds.), *International Conference on Advancements of Medicine and Health Care through Technology; 12th - 15th October 2016, Cluj-Napoca, Romania,*
IFMBE Proceedings 59,
DOI: 10.1007/978-3-319-52875-5_1

Doppler. Most of the patients (56%) underwent at least 2 types of imaging investigation in order to establish the final diagnosis. Planar liver scintigraphies and SPECT with sulphur-colloid (n=211), „*in vivo*" labeled-RBC scintigraphies (n=189) and liver angioscintigraphies (n=184) were performed. 72 patients underwent CT (1 native and 71 with contrast) and 28 MRI with contrast. Diagnostic laparoscopy was performed in 15 patients, surgical resection in 22, US-guided puncture-biopsies in 42 and histological examination in 69 patients. The final diagnosis was established based on the results of all these investigations corroborated with clinical and biological examinations.From the statistical point of view, in order to establish possible associations between echogenicity of the tumor and the liver, respectively tumor's size and the presence of liver diseases, we used the statistical software in order to obtain the Hi-square test and Fisher's exact test, coefficients of contingency and Cramer's coefficients; p values<0.05 were considered to have statistical significance. Estimation of possible association between the presence of hypo-/hyperechoic peritumoral rim and tumoral and liver echogenicity, tumoral size and the presence of CLD was done through the same tests and correlation coefficients mentioned above.

III. Results

US parameters in the 270 patients finally diagnosed with hemangioma revealed the features shown in Table 1.

There have been identified hemangiomas ranging in size from 0,3-24cm at US. Hemangiomas were located in the right lobe (298), left lobe (115), caudate lobe (4) and in both lobes (80).

As shown in Table 1, the presence of hyperechogenicity and homogeneous structure inside the tumor is not a universally valid criterion in the diagnosis of hemangioma.

The typical image of well-defined (94.81% of cases), hyperechoic mass (81.48% of cases), without Doppler signal (54.07% of cases), was detected in most hemangiomas (Fig.1). Hypoechoic masses (Fig.2) associated with the presence of a heterogeneous structure and hyperechoic rim raised problems of differential diagnosis in 7 cases, requiring supplementary investigations. Out of all 274 cases with US-presumption of hemangiomas, 270 patients proved to have finally hemangiomas, 3 HCC (and coexistence with one hemangioma in one case), 1 cholangiocarcinoma and coexistence with metastases (from gastric carcinoid); in 21 cases it was not possible to differentiate US from other tumors (1 lipoma, 1 pheochromocytoma, 1 area of calcification, 3 metastases, 2 regenerative nodules, 2 focal nodular hyperplasias, 3 patchy areas of steatosis, 6 HCC, 2 hemangiosarcomas). Coexistence with other masses was found in 30 (11.11%) patients: simple hepatic cysts (17), fatty-free areas (4), focal nodular hyperplasia (3), HCC (2), patchy areas of steatosis (2), hepatic hydatid cyst (1) and metastasis of gastric carcinoid (1).

Table 1 US parameters in hemangiomas

Echogenicity	
-high	220
-low	41
-isoechoic	6
-mixt	3
Echostructure	
-homogeneous	189
-heterogeneous	81
-calcifications	4
Delimitation	
-clear	256
-imprecise	3
-polycyclic	10
Peritumoral rim	
-hyperechoic	7
-hypoechoic	5
Doppler signal	
-absent	146
-weak	11
-present	26
-central	1
-peripheral	7
-central+ peripheral	1
-spotted-like	11
-arterial type	-
-venous type	6
-mixed type	6

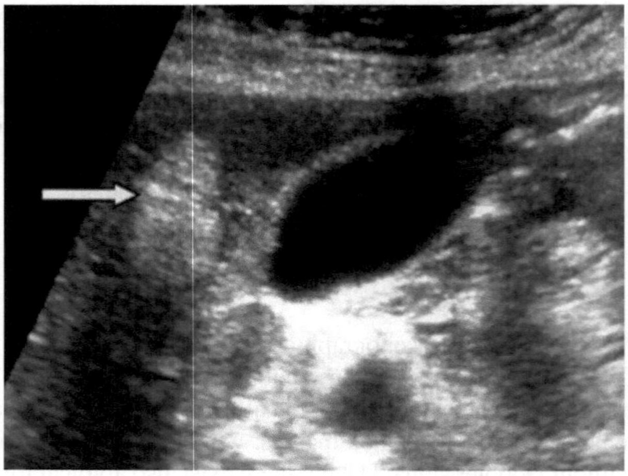

Fig.1 US: typical hemangioma

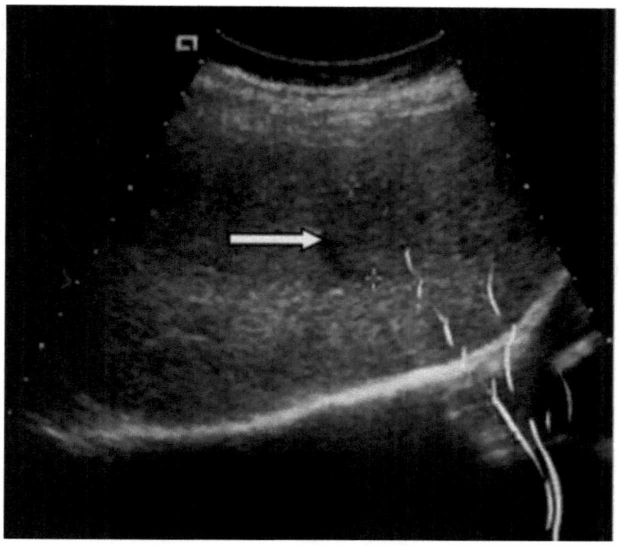

Fig.2 US: atypical hemangioma

Absence of Doppler signal (146/157), spotted presence (11/157) were identified in all hemangiomas located in the right lobe (157), the left lobe being difficult to explore due to artifacts produced by the cardiac cycle; in one case, exacerbated and tortuous vascularisation pattern (arterial and venous type) rose the suspicion of neoplasia, but puncture-biopsy confirmed the diagnosis of hemangioma.

There were identified multiple hemangiomas in 52 cases (19.25%), their increased echogenicity and multicentricity raising problems of differential diagnosis with liver metastases.

Table 2 US characteristics of hemangiomas grafted on normal liver and on different CLD

Hemangiomas on:	*normal liver*	*steatosis+ NASH +chronic hepatitis (alcoholic+ viral)*	*cirrhosis*
hyperechoic	126	45	28
hypoecoic	17	16	3
isoechoic	2	3	0
mixt	2	0	0
homogeneous	114	5	
inhomogeneous	38	65	
hypoechoic rim	2	2	1
hyperechoic rim	3	3	0

Legend: NASH- nonalcoholic steatohepatitis

Of all 17 cavernous hemangiomas, US described 14 (82.35%) as such, two of them being thrombosed, and in one case as atypical cavernous hemangioma.

Out of 270 patients explored by US, we detected 52 cases of hemangiomatosis, 17 cavernous hemangiomas, 213 hyperechoic masses (being grafted in descending order on: chronic hepatitis, cirrhosis, and normal liver, steatosis and NASH), 39 hypoechoic masses (with maximum percentage on: steatosis and NASH, followed by cirrhosis, normal liver, chronic hepatitis) and 5 isoechoic and 2 with mixed echogenicity (hypo- and hyperechoic) (Table 2).

When comparing echogenicity and echostructure of hemangiomas, we observed differences between the 2 groups of patients, namely those without liver disease and those with CLD. Also, the presence/absence of peritumoral and rim's echogenicity according to the size of hemangioma are shown in Table 3.

Diagnosis of hemangioma was suspected only in 93.70 % (253/270) cases of all patients with final diagnosis of hemangioma, the rest being diagnosed by US as: lipoma (1), metastasis (3), tumors of unknown etiology (5), regenerative nodule/HCC (1), steatosis, patchy steatosis (1), focal nodular hyperplasia (1), pheochromocytoma (1), benign tumor with arterial-venous shunt (1), malignancy (2), and in one case US did not detected any mass (isoechoic).

Table 3 Tumoral and rim's echogenicity according to the size of hemangioma

Hemangiomas:	*size≥2cm*	*size<2cm*
hyperechoic	136	77
hypoechoic	30	9
isoechoic	5	0
mixt	2	0
with hypoechoic rim	4	1
with hyperechoic rim	6	1

The presence of hypoechoic rim was described in 4/220 cases (0.018%) of histologically proven hemangiomas. The hyperechoic rim was present in 14.89% of the cases (representing 7/47 patients). There were no differences regarding the predominance of peritumoral hypoechoic rim in the two subgroups of hemangiomas grafted on normal liver and CLD (Table 4); the predominance of hyperechoic rim was observed in iso- and hypoechoic hemangiomas. The peritumoral rim depending on the size of the hemangioma was more commonly seen in hemangiomas ≥2 cm, but without any statistical significance.

Hi-square test of independence finds no association between tumor echogenicity and hypoechoic rim in patients with hemangiomas ($\chi2 = 1.125 < 7.81$, $p=0.650$); but it showed that there was only moderate association between hypoechoic rim and hyperechoic tumor in patients without hemangioma ($p=0.004$). Fisher 's exact test shows that there exists moderate association between hyperechoic rim and hypoechoic hemangiomas (Cramer coefficient=0.37, $p=0.001$) and between hyperechoic rim and isoechoic hemangiomas ($p<0.05$).

The association between the presence of the hypoechoic rim and hepatic echogenicity or tumor size is shown in Table 4.

Table 4 Correlation of hypo- and hyperechoic rim with hemangioma's echogenicity and size, echogenicity of liver and presence of CLD

Criteria:	hypoechoic rim	hyperechoic rim
Echogenity of hemangioma		
hyperechoic	5/270	1/270
isoechoic	0	3/270
hypoecoic	0	3/270
mixt	0	0
Echogenity of liver		
normal	4/270	5/270
increased	1/270	2/270
Size of hemangioma		
< 2cm	1/270	1/270
> 2cm	4/270	6/270
Presence of CLD		
yes	3/270	4
no	2/270	3

Legend: CLD- chronic liver diseases

Fisher's exact test shows no association between liver echogenicity and hypoechoic rim (p=0.205) or hyperechoic rim (p=0.273) of hemangiomas. Fisher's exact test shows no association between hemangioma size and hypoechoic (p=0.659) or hyperechoic rim (p=0.427) of hemangiomas.

Presence of steatosis/nonalcoholic steatohepatitis (NASH) in 69 images from our study revealed the following patterns of hemangiomas: hypo- (16/69 cases), isoechoic (2/69 cases) and heterogeneous (51/69 cases).

The association between the presence of the hyperechoic rim and tumoral size and the presence of CLD is shown in Table 4. Fisher's exact test shows no association between the presence of underlying CLD and hypoechoic (p=0.328) or hyperechoic (p=0,468) rim.Statistical parameters of the US method used in the diagnosis of hemangiomas are shown in Table 5.

Table 5 US sensitivity, specificity, positive and negative predictive laues in the diagnosis of hemangioma

	US diagnosis of hemangioma:			
	Presence of CLD		*Size of hemangioma*	
	No (n=155)	Yes (n=115)	<2cm (n=95)	≥2cm (n=175)
Se (%)	94.48 (90.08-97.75)	94.78 (88.99-98.06)	98.95 (94.27-99.97)	92.57 (87.63-95.99)
Sp (%)	94.12 (83.77-98.77)	84.21 (72.13-92.52)	94.87 (82.68-99.37)	85.51 (74.96-92.83)
PPV (%)	98 (94.27-99.59)	92.37 (86.01-96.45)	97.92 (92.68-99.75)	94.19 (89.57-97.18)
NPV (%)	85.71 (73.78-93.62)	88.89 (77.37-95.81)	97.37 (86.19-99.93)	81.94 (71.11-90.02)

Legend: Se-sensitivity, Sp-specificity, PPV-positive predictive value, NPV-negative predictive value, CLD- chronic liver diseases

US alone established the diagnosis of hemangioma in 44% cases and US together with scintigraphic methods in 36% cases; other imaging and invasive techniques (contrast-enhanced-US, computed tomography, magnetic resonance, puncture-biopsy, diagnostic laparoscopy, histology) were necessary to corroborate with the previous methods in the rest of 20% patients. Figure 3 shows the methods used in corroboration, being both imaging and invasive, that contributed to the final diagnosis of hemangioma.

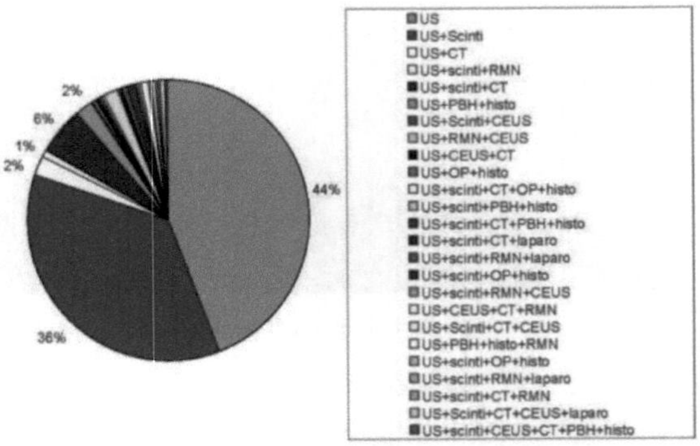

Fig.3 Imaging and invasive technics used in the diagnosis of hemangioma
Legend: Scinti-scintigraphy, RMN-MRI, PBH-punction biopsy, histo-histology, OP-surgery, laparo-diagnostic laparoscopy

IV. Discussion

The value of different US methods (pre- and intraoperatory), computed tomography (CT), magnetic resonance (MR), differ depending on etiology of the tumor. US represents the first method of detection of hemangiomas.

The issue of differential diagnosis of hyperechoic masses grafted on CLD is difficult, as far as it was shown that 15-50% of focal lesions grafted on cirrhosis initially interpreted as hemangiomas, are actually HCC [4, 5]. The chance of preexistence of a vascular malformation (hemangioma) grafted on CLD is about 50%, but it is always necessary to corroborate with complementary methods (CT, MR, „*in vivo*" labeled-RBC SPECT) in order to exclude a HCC. Transformation of hypoechoic nodule in a hyperechoic mass can be explained by necrosis and interstitial fibrosis; in these cases is not possible to differentiate from a typical small hyperechoic hemangioma [6].

Literature mentioned the typical "low-flow" hemangioma in cases of hyperechoic well defined masses, without peritumoral rim, and the "high-flow" hemangioma, which are commonly hypoechoic and with atypical aspect in gray-scale US [7]. There have been described both qualitative and quantitative differences regarding the presence of Doppler signal in color and Power Doppler, being cited both lack and presence of increased (especially peripheral, but also central) vascular signal, suggestive for the diagnosis of hemangioma [8].

Hemangioma occurs as hyperechoic masses, which sometimes presents central thrombi, cystic areas and intratumoral calcifications, due to the thrombotic formation in time, cystic degeneration and calcification, or intratumoral necrosis. These atypical features make difficult sometimes the differential diagnosis with malignant tumors [9, 10].

A special mention concerns the hemangiomas grafted on steatosis, showing various aspects of echogenicity (from hypo, to hyperechoic) and of CT density (hyperdense-native, isodense-arterial phase); in these cases MR and/or histological examination are mandatory, and sometimes fine needle aspiration biopsy is useful in order to clarify the diagnosis [9]. This might explain the 69 images from our study in patients with: *steatosis/nonalcoholic steatohepatitis (NASH)*, which were hypo- (16/70 cases), isoechoic (2/70 cases) and heterogeneous (91,66% cases); *cirrhosis* with 3/21 hypo- and 18/21 hyperechoic hemangiomas; *chronic viral and toxic hepatitis*, with 3/30 hypo- and 27/30 hyperechoic masses.

The attempt to establish an association between the tumor's echogenicity and presence of CLD, or tumor size has not shown any statistical significance; we found a good correlation ($p = 0.001$) between hyperechoic rim and hypo- and isoechoic hemangiomas.

Spotted presence of Doppler signal was identified in 7% (11/157) of our cases, the rest of the masses in the right lobe being without vascular signal. The model of the spotted mixed type of vascularisation (both arterial and venous) was encountered also in literature, but in a greater proportion (14 %) [11].

US is able to detect, within the 40% cases with hyperechoic rim in literature (where differential diagnosis with metastases from insulinomas is required), atypical forms as solid tumors with hypoechoic areas and with the described features in periphery [12].

We could establish the diagnosis of atypical hemangiomas in 19 of our cases, that would qualify as: *heterogeneous* (n=7), having hypoechoic inhomogeneous structure, hyperechoic rim, and size of 2,7-9cm (average 4,51cm); *hemangiomas with calcification* (n=4) and *multilocular cavernous hemangioma* (n=8).

Corroboration of US with dynamic CT and „*in vivo*" labeled-RBC SPECT have shown a high sensitivity, specificity, and high diagnostic accuracy [13], similar to the data in our study.

Limits of the study were: the impossibility of follow-up in all focal lesions and histopatological documentation for all, and the varying experience of the examiner.

V. Conclusion

Classic criteria of hyperechoic, well defined tumor and without Doppler signal was found in 81.85% hemangiomas, US proved to have increased specificity for masses <2 cm (94.87%) and grafted on normal liver (94.12%). Hypo- and isoechoic hemangiomas moderately correlate with the presence of a hyperechoic rim. No statistical correlation was found between the underlying CLD and the hemangioma's echogenicity, nor with the presence of any tumoral rim.

Presence of hemangiomas grafted on CLD is a challenge for the physician, as it is important for the differential diagnosis with HCC or even metastases, especially when atypical hemangiomas are hypoechoic. A good correlation of US parameters with other imaging methods (scintigraphy, CES), in case of atypical features, can avoid liver biopsy and enables to establish a correct positive diagnosis.

Conflict of Interest

The authors declare that they have no conflict of interest and there is no disagreement in this new approach of imaging assessment of hemangiomas.

Statement of Human rights

The procedures were in accordance with the ethical standards of the responsible local and national committee on human experimentation and with Helsinki Declaration of 2000.

References

1. Badea R. Ficatul. In: Badea R, Mircea PA, Dudea S, Stamatian F (2000)*Tratat de ultrasonografie clinică- vol.I Principii, abdomen, obstetrică şi ginecologie.* Ed. Medicală Bucureşti:105-175
2. Harvey CJ, Albrecht T (2001) Ultrasound of focal liver lesions. Eur Radiol 11:1578–1593
3. Farrell MA, Charboneau JW, Reading CC (2000) Sonographic pathologiccorrelation of the hyperechoic border ofan atypical hepatic hemangioma. J Ultrasound Med 20:169–170
4. Repiso A., Gomez Rodriguez, R., Gonzales de Frutos C. et al. (2007) Angioma like liver lesions in patients with chronic liver disease. Rev. esp. enferm. dig. 99(5): 259-263
5. Caturelli E, Pompili M, Bartolucci F et al. (2001) Hemangioma-like Lesions in Chronic Liver Disease: Diagnostic Evaluationin Patients1.Radiology 220:337–342
6. Sheu JC, Chen DS, Sung JL et al. (1985) Hepatocellular carcinoma: US evolution in the early stage. Radiology 155:463–467
7. Galanski M. Jördens S, Weidemann (2008) Diagnose und Differentialdiagnose benigner Lebertumoren und tumorähnlicher Läsionen. Chirurg 79:707-721
8. Choi BI, Kim TK, Han JK et al. (1996) Power versus Conventional Color Doppler Sonography: Comparison In the Depiction of Vasculature in Liver Tumors. Radiology 200:55-58

9. Vilgrain V, Boulous L, Vullierme MP et al. (2000) Imaging of atypical hemangiomas of the liver with pathological correlation. Radiographics 20: 379–397
10. Shimizu S, Tadatoshi T, Kosuge T et al. (1992) Benign tumors of the liver resected because of a diagnosis of malignancy. Surg Gynecol Obstet 174:403-407
11. Bartolotta TV, Midiri M, Quaia E (2005) Liver haemangiomas undetermined at grey-scale ultrasound: contrast-enhancement patterns with SonoVue and pulse-inversion US. Eur Radiol 15:685–693
12. Moody A, Wilson S (1993) Atypical hepatic hemangiomas: a suggestive sonographic morphology. Radiology 188:413-417
13. Weimann A, Ringe B, Klempnauer J et al. (1997) Benign liver tumors: differential diagnosis and indications for surgery. World J Surg 21:983-990

Author: Ioana Grigorescu
Institute: 2nd Medical Department, „Iuliu Hatieganu" University of Medicine and Pharmacology Cluj-Napoca, Romania
Street: Clinicilor Str. 2-4
City: Cluj-Napoca
Country: Romania
E-mail: ioanaducagrigorescu@gmail.com

Impact of Spectralis Optical Coherence Tomography in the Clinical Practice

S.D. Nicoară

"Iuliu Haţieganu" University of Medicine and Pharmacy/Ophthalmology, 8. V. Babes str., 400012, Cluj-Napoca, Romania

Abstract— **Optical Coherence Tomography (OCT) is a relatively new, high resolution, non-invasive imaging method which was applied for the first time in ophthalmology. It is rapid, easy to perform and analyze, very comfortable for the patients and it offers detailed information about the ocular structures, allowing early diagnosis and treatment in a variety of ocular conditions. The description of Spectral Domain OCT principle is followed by the presentation of the investigation capabilities, technical characteristics and examination modules belonging to the Spectralis device (Heidelberg Engineering). The contribution of this modern investigation tool in the clinical practice is illustrated with cases from the personal experience.**

Keywords— **Spectral Domain OCT, Age related Macular Degeneration, Vitreo-Macular Interface Syndrome, Diabetic Macular Edema.**

I. Introduction

Optical Coherence Tomography (OCT) is a high resolution, non-invasive imaging method that started to be used in the clinical practice in 1990s. The first application of OCT technology was in the field of ophthalmology and the images resembled the histological sections of the retina. However, the pictures depict the result of the scanned tissues' optical properties, not the tissues themselves [1].

OCT concept developed at Massachusetts Institute of Technology, at the beginning of 1990s. The first commercial device was made by Carl Zeiss (Jena, Germany) in 1996. The first OCT applications referred to quantitative and qualitative information about the peripapillary area of the retina and the coronary arteries [2].

OCT uses light, as opposed to ultrasonic biomicroscopy (UBM) that uses ultrasounds, with the aim to visualize eye structures. Light speed is 1 million times higher than sound speed. By consequence, resolutions lower than 10 μ microns are obtained in the posterior pole of the eye with OCT technology. For many years, UBM offered resolutions in the range of 150 μ. By using high frequencies, resolutions of 20 μ are possible with UBM technology. The ultrasound waves used in UBM are markedly attenuated by the biological tissues and therefore, are limited to the examination of anterior eye structures [3].

OCT exam is very comfortable for the patient, as it does not require the direct contact with the eye.

II. Description of the device

A. Overview

Spectralis is a multimodal platform that uses the confocal laser technology, in order to obtain color and spectral optical coherence tomography (OCT) images of the eye structure. Two different laser wavelengths catch simultaneously, the OCT and the fundus image of the eye [3].

The principle of Spectral Domain OCT (SD-OCT) is based on the Fourier equation, as compared to Time Domain OCT (TD-OCT) that developed on the ground of interferometry. In TD-OCT, an interferometer measures sequentially, the delay of light echoes that are reflected by the retinal microstructures. In SD-OCT, a spectrometer evaluates simultaneously, the light reflected by retinal microstructures. In TD-OCT, 6 radial scans are performed, whereas in SD-OCT, 65.000 scans are made within an area of 6 mm diameter. Acquisition time is about 60 times faster with SD-OCT devices and the axial resolution varies between 3 - 7 μ, as compared to TD-OCT (10 -15 μ) [3].

Eye tracking function is used to neutralize the errors induced by involuntary eye movements. Spectralis is able to detect changes within 1 - 2 microns, at the depth of 289 microns, and it is able to filtrate and select the high resolution images, in order to identify the finest details. The auto re-scan function is very important for the patient's follow-up, as it places the subsequent scans precisely at the initial examination site. The deep layers can be examined with the enhanced-depth OCT function (EDI-OCT) [3].

B. Investigation possibilities

Spectralis offers the following imaging possibilities for the eye: spectral domain OCT (SD-OCT), infrared (IR), red free, fundus autofluorescence (FAF), confocal multicolor 3D, wide field (55°), SD-OCT for the diagnosis and monitoring of glaucoma, anterior segment imaging [3].

C. Technical characteristics

Domain: Spectralis operates in the spectral domain OCT, based on the Fourier equation.

Minimal scan speed: 40000 A-scans /second

Laser light sources:

S. Vlad and N.M. Roman (eds.), *International Conference on Advancements of Medicine and Health Care through Technology; 12th - 15th October 2016, Cluj-Napoca, Romania,*
IFMBE Proceedings 59,
DOI: 10.1007/978-3-319-52875-5_2

A super luminescent diode λ 870 nm acquires the images.

IR light (λ 815 nm) allows the visualization of detailed images of the eye fundus.

A green laser (λ 518 nm) ensures the obtaining of confocal, 3D images of the retina, with multicolor technology.

A blue laser (λ 486 nm) is used for identifying fundus auto fluorescence (FAF) and obtaining the red free images. The blue light makes it possible to identify fundus auto fluorescence, based on the fluorescent properties of lipofuscin. With red free light, specific structures are visualized: nerve fiber layer, epiretinal membranes and retinal cysts.

The simultaneous, confocal, 3D collection of the imaging data with three different types of lasers (red, green and blue) allows to evaluate various retinal layers on a single image.

The device also offers the possibility to combine the above mentioned acquiring modalities, in various ways, according to the investigated retinal condition: IR and FAF, OCT and IR, OCT and FAF, OCT and red free, OCT and 3D multicolor confocal eye fundus examination [3].

D. Examination modules

Anterior segment: By the use of a high resolution 3D examination lens, images with 7 μ axial resolution and 30 μ lateral resolution can be obtained. The scanning depth in the tissue is of 1.9 mm.

Multicolor confocal 3D module: It allows the visualization of the 3D, color image of the eye fundus, simultaneously with the transverse section through the retina. Thus, different retinal structures are evaluated on one single image. Scanning with multiple laser wavelengths allows the detailed evaluation of the retinal structure: superficial, middle and deep retinal layers.

Wide field module: It makes possible to view the retinal periphery, by OCT and fundus image, using a non-contact, 55° lens. The high resolution visualization of the macula, optic nerve and retinal periphery is achieved in a single image. The scanning models are: radial 55° central and volume 55°x25° (for the diabetic patients) /55°x40° /25°x5 ° central.

Glaucoma module: It allows the complete analysis of glaucoma, with the evaluation of the neuro-retinal rim, retinal nerve fiber layer (RNFL) and asymmetry regarding the posterior pole and the ganglion cell layer.

The optic nerve head (ONH) analysis is made using the Bruch's membrane opening as the anatomical frontier for the rim. The neuro-retinal rim is measured between Bruch's membrane opening and the nearest point of the internal limiting membrane (ILM).

During scanning, the device lines up automatically, the fovea with the central axis of Bruch's membrane opening.

Future scans and sectors are placed exactly on the previous sites, which is very important for the accurate monitoring of the disease progression.

Various scans are available: 24° radial scan, circular scans with 3,5 mm/4,1 mm/4,6 mm diameter, volume scans of 30°x25°/30°x15° /15°x15 °, circular scan of the RNFL at 12°, with 768 analyzed points [3].

III. SPECTRALIS OCT IN THE DIAGNOSIS AND MONITORING OF MACULAR DISORDERS

Optical Coherence Tomography is widely used in the assessment and monitoring of macular diseases. We illustrate the contribution of Spectralis in the clinical practice with selected cases from our own experience. The patients were included in this study in accordance with the Helsinki Declaration of 1975, as revised in 2000 and 2008.

A. Age related Macular Degeneration (AMD)

AMD is one of the retinal conditions that benefited the most from the progress in of OCT technology. The main advantage of the OCT imaging is the quantification of the retinal thickness, allowing to monitor the anti-VEGF treatment efficacy in wet AMD. OCT is also able to identify the location of the fluid in neovascular AMD: intraretinal, subretinal or sub-Retinal Pigmented Epithelium (RPE) [4].

According to OCT imaging, the choroidal neovascular membranes (CNV) in wet AMD were classified into 3 types. In type 1 (occult neovascularization), CNV is located under the retinal pigmented epithelium (RPE), in type 2 (classic neovascularization), it is located above the RPE and in type 3, there is a retinal angiomatous proliferation (RAP). In large RPE detachments, breaks in the RPE layer can occur. The rupture of the RPE layer appears as a clearly demarcated region of RPE absence, adjacent to a region of RPE elevation. The reversed shadow effect is identified. Often, especially in type 2 CNVs, the interruption of the RPE layer is identified. In type 2 CNV, the neovascular membrane is located in the subretinal space and it penetrates through the RPE/Bruch's membrane complex. RAP is a rare form of wet AMD that originates in abnormal neovascular tissue from the deep retinal layers [5].

The response to anti-VEGF therapy is translated into the OCT imaging, by the diminishing/disappearance of the intra/sub-retinal fluid and by the decrease of the PEDs size and of the macular thickness [2].

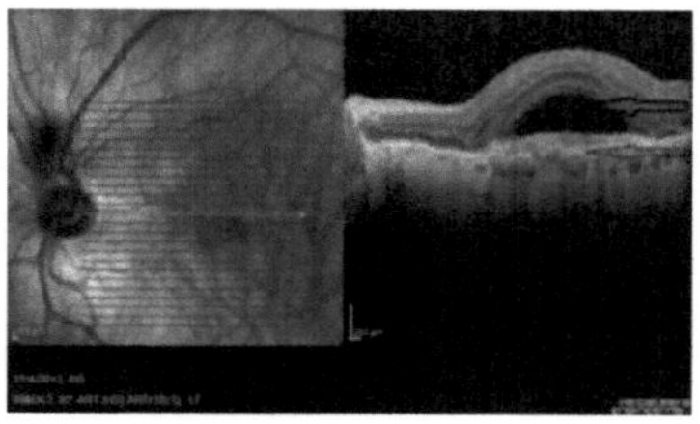

Fig. 1. Classic form of neovascular AMD

Figure 1 presents the combined IR-OCT image of the retina in a patient with wet age related macular degeneration (AMD). The neurosensitive retina is detached by fluid (superior arrow) originating in a fibro-vascular membrane under it (inferior arrow). The retinal pigmented epithelium (RPE) layer is irregular and disrupted in the area of lesion. The fluid has no reflectivity (it appears black on the black-white image). This aspect corresponds to the classic neovascular membrane which responds better to anti-VEGF therapy, as opposed to occult membranes which are located under the RPE. OCT has a major role in locating precisely the neovascular membrane in relationship with the RPE and the neurosensory retina.

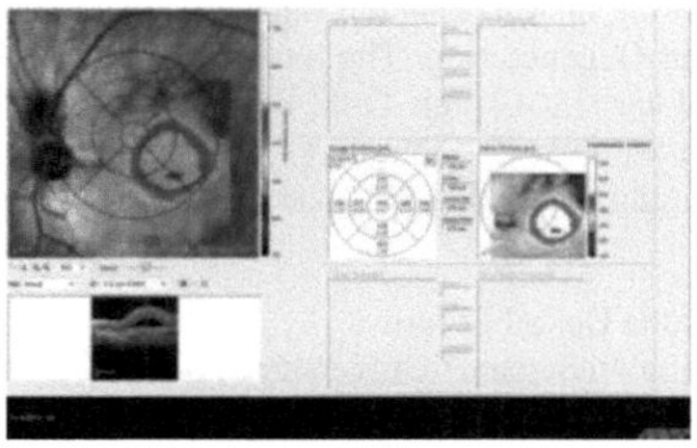

Fig. 2 RTM map in a patient with classic form of neovascular AMD

In figure 2, the retinal thickness map (RTM) in the same patient as in figure 1, is presented. The thickness of the macula is significantly increased in the macular area located infero-temporally from the fovea. This is signalized by white and red colors.

OCT is able to identify early stages of AMD, named drusen, as elevations and irregularities of the RPE line (figure 3).

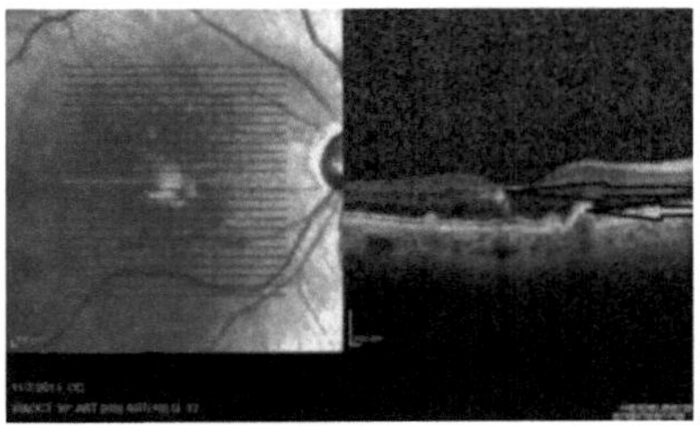

Fig.3. Drusen

B. Vitreo-macular interface disorders

Vitreo-macular interface disorders benefited from the advances in OCT technology, in terms of the diagnosis precision and surgical indication [3]. In figure 4, an advanced stage of vitreo-macular traction syndrome is presented. Along time, it led to the disorganization of the macular retina, which is dissected by liquid spaces and cysts. Therefore, the resistance of the retinal tissue is considerably diminished. In this situation, the dissection of the vitreo-macular interface, in order to relieve the traction, is risky, as it may lead to the break and detachment of the retina.

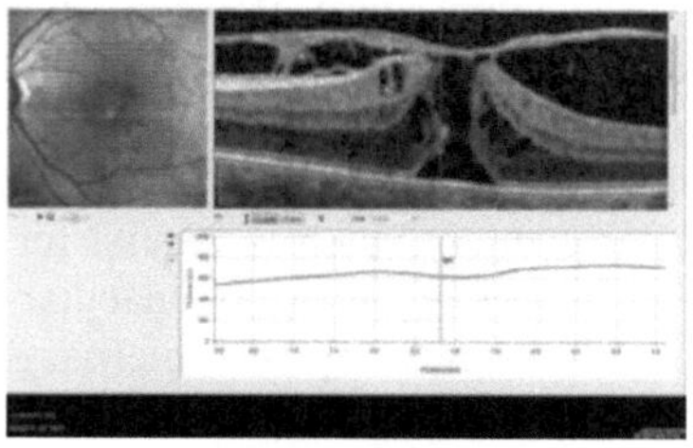

Fig. 4. Retinal disorganization following an advanced vitreo-macular interface syndrome

Figure 5 depicts the fellow eye of the same patient. Obviously, the vitreo-macular traction is less advanced, but there are modifications of the retinal structures: the macular thickness is increased and a hole within the retina is identified. Surgery in this situation is indicated, in order to prevent the progression of the disease.

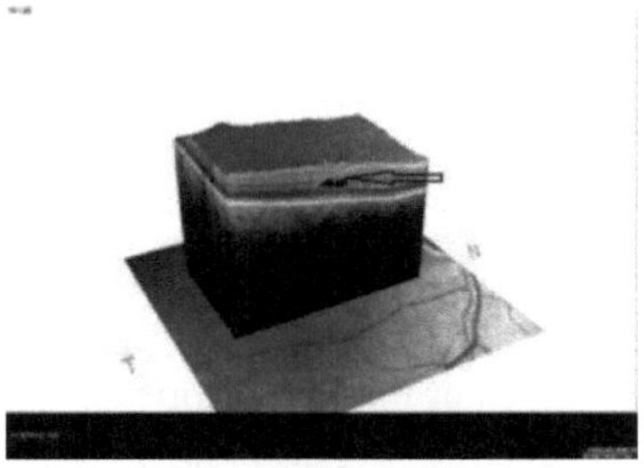

Fig. 5. Fellow eye in the same patient as in figure 3

RTM proves the increased macular thickness and offers precise values for this parameter, within the macular area (figure 6).

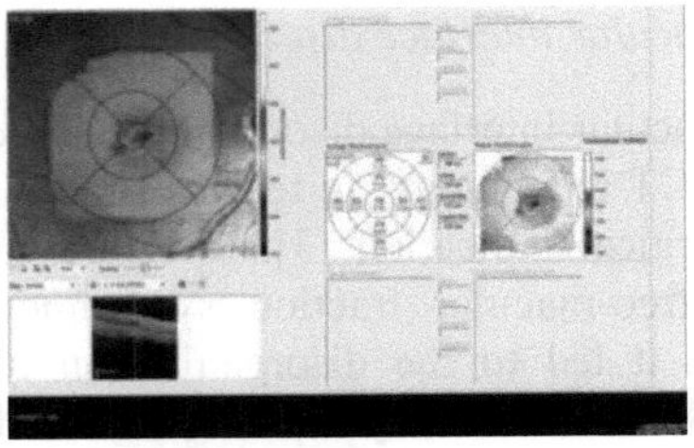

Fig. 6. RTM for the same eye as in figure

C. Diabetic maculopathy

Diabetes is the main cause of visual impairment in the group of working age population. Maculopathy is the main cause of vision decrease in the diabetic patients. Progress in OCT technology allows early diagnosis and treatment of diabetic macular edema, which is crucial for vision preservation [6]. The main mechanism of macular edema caused by diabetes is represented by the microangiopathy at the level of the retinal capillaries [3,6]. Figure 7 presents intraretinal microaneurysms (hyperreflective dots) that leak, as proved by the non-reflective material (liquid) elevating the neuro-sensory retina.

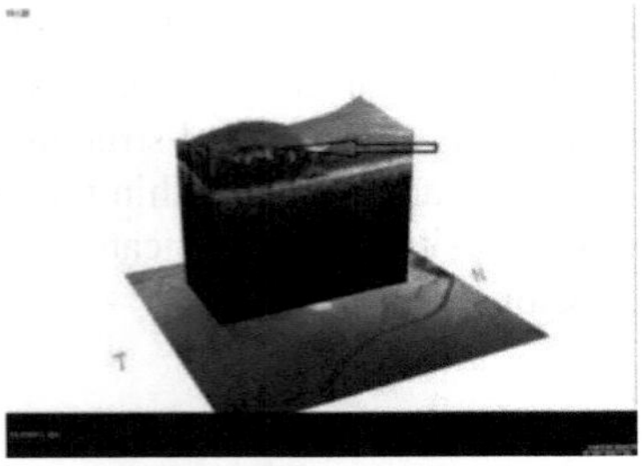

Fig. 7. Diabetic macular edema

The liquid within the neuro-sensory retina is responsible for the considerable macular thickening, as shown in figure 8 (the maximal macular thickness appears of 600 μ).

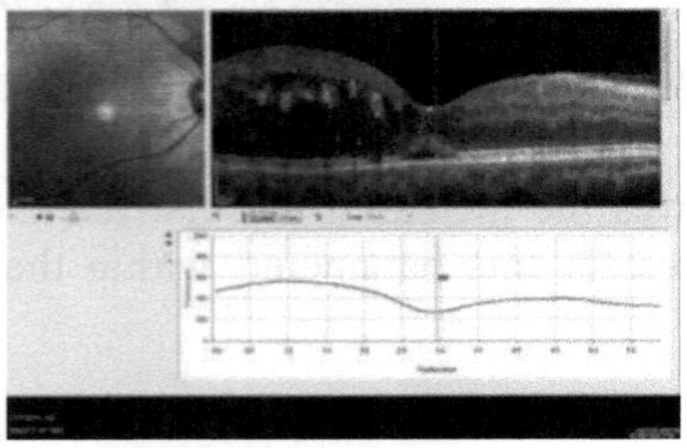

Fig. 8. Macular thickening in diabetes

IV. Conclusions

Spectralis is a very useful tool in the diagnosis and monitoring of macular diseases. A super luminescent diode (λ 870 nm) is used to acquire the OCT images. The simultaneous, confocal, 3D collection of the imaging data with three different types of lasers (red, green and blue) allows to evaluate the structure of various retinal layers on a single image.

Conflict of Interest

The authors declare that they have no conflict of interest.

References

1. Huang D, Swanson EA, Lin CP et al. (1991) Optical coherence tomography. Science, 22: 1178-1181
2. Simona- Delia Ţălu, New Insights into the Optical Coherence Tomography –Assessement and Follow-Up of Age-Related Macular Degeneration, in "Age-Related Macular Degeneration - Etiology, Diagnosis and Management - A Glance at the Future", (2013) InnTech, Rijeka, ed. Giuseppe Lo Giudice
3. Duker JS, Waheed NK, Goldman DR (2014) Handbook of retinal OCT, Elsevier, London
4. Lim LS, Mitchell P, Seddon JM et al. (2012) Age-related macular degeneration. Lancet, 379: 1728–38
5. Talu SD, Talu S, Use of OCT Imaging in the Diagnosis and Monitoring of Age Related Macular Degeneration, in Age Related Macular Degeneration. The recent advances in basic research and clinical care (2012) Inn Tech, Rijeka, ed. Gui-Shuang Ying.
6. Menke M, Lala C, Framme C, Wolf S. The Ever-Evolving Role of Imaging in DME Management (2012) Retin Physician, 9 (4): 24-32.

Author: Simona Delia Nicoara
Institute: "Iuliu Hatieganu" University of Medicine and Pharmacy
Street: 8, Victor Babes street, 400012
City: Cluj-Napoca
Country: Romania
Emai: simonanicoara1@gmail.com

Laparoscopic Repair of Morgagni Hernia – Transfascial Suturing with Extracorporeal Knotting

F. Graur[1, 2], E. Moiş[1, 2], N. Al-Momani[2] and N. Al-Hajjar[1, 2]

[1] University of Medicine and Pharmacy "Iuliu Hatieganu", Cluj-Napoca, Romania
[2] Regional Institute of Gastroenterology and Hepatology "Prof. O. Fodor", Surgery Department, Cluj-Napoca, Romania

Abstract — **Among the congenital diaphragmatic hernias, the Morgagni type lies in the anterior and medial aspect of the diaphragm, as a defect of fusion of the septum transversum. Even in asymptomatic cases a surgical repair is indicated because of potential complications. In this paper we report a 67 years old woman presented with an unclear symptomatology, but the CT scan shown a retrosternal diaphragmatic defect of 45 mm. The surgery performed was a laparoscopic repair with transfascial suturing with extracorporeal knotting. This report supports the laparoscopic repair of diaphragmatic defects and the particular technique presented is an easy and rapid procedure with excellent results.**

Keywords— **diaphragmatic hernia, laparoscopic repair, Morgagni hernia**

I. Introduction

The three principal types of congenital diaphragmatic hernias are Bochdalek, hiatal and Morgagni's, which is the rarest form. They were first described in medical literature in the early 18th century [1].

Generally, Morgagni's hernia, which is the topic of this case report, present early in life with respiratory symptoms. Adult presentations are less frequent, particularly symptomatic adult presentations [2]. Surgical repair is mandatory even in asymptomatic cases to avoid the risk of life-threatening complications, such as bowel prolapse and subsequent strangulation [3, 4]. Laparoscopic repair is the procedure of choice in uncomplicated cases [5].

In this report we present a case of a greatly successful laparoscopic repair by transfascial suturing with extracorporeal knot tying technique.

II. Case report

A 67-year-old female patient, known with ischemic heart disease, presented to the outpatient clinics at our Institute, in April 2015, with symptoms of intestinal subocclusion. About one year ago she start complain of intermittent, vague epigastric pain, which was aggravated mainly by heavy meals and associated with nausea and vomiting. She also noted that she'd lost 5 kg in the last 6 months. The patient reported no dysphagia, early satiety, dyspnea, sweating or palpitations. She denied any history of trauma as well.

Physical examination was unremarkable; her vital signs and lab tests were within normal limits. Cardiopulmonary and abdominal examinations were normal as well. Chest X-ray was normal, thus we performed a thoracic CT-scan with oral contrast that showed an anteromedial, retrosternal diaphragmatic defect of approximately 45mm (LL).

Furthermore, the transverse colon and part of the omentum were herniated into the thoracic cavity, and so the patient was diagnosed with Morgagni's Hernia. Routine preoperative investigations included complete blood count, liver function test, electrolytes levels, coagulation tests, ECG and an abdominal US, all of which were normal.

III. Surgical technique

The operation was performed under general anesthesia with endotracheal intubation, the patient was placed in a supine, 15 degrees, anti-Trendelenburg position and the lower limbs were in abduction. The operating surgeon stood between the patient's legs and the assisting surgeon on his left.

A 2 cm supraumbilical skin incision was made, Veress needle was used to create a CO_2 pneumoperitoneum of 12-14 mmHg under a 1/min flow rate. Then a 10 mm optic trocar was introduced in a closed technique at the supraumbilical skin incision as a camera port. Throughout inspection of the intraabdominal space, a 6x7 cm anteromedial diaphragmatic defect was detected and the hernia sac was empty as the abdominal contents were spontaneously reduced by the time of the operation (Figure 1). After that a 10 mm and a 5 mm trocars were inserted under direct camera visualization in the right and left hipochondriums, respectively, at the midclavicular lines. Thereafter we dissected and excised the hernia sac and sectioned the falciform ligament by electrocautery. Next, we performed 5 interrupted (1-0 silk) sutures in a U-shape manner using a Reverdin needle; meaning that we started inserting the suture extra-

S. Vlad and N.M. Roman (eds.), *International Conference on Advancements of Medicine and Health Care through Technology; 12th - 15th October 2016, Cluj-Napoca, Romania*,
IFMBE Proceedings 59,
DOI: 10.1007/978-3-319-52875-5_3

corporeally at a point on the skin going diagonally through the anterior abdominal wall and exiting at a point on the internal surface of the abdominal wall. Then we took the anterior edge of the defect and went back at another point alongside the first one on internal surface of the anterior abdominal wall but going out at the same point of skin entry (Figure 2).

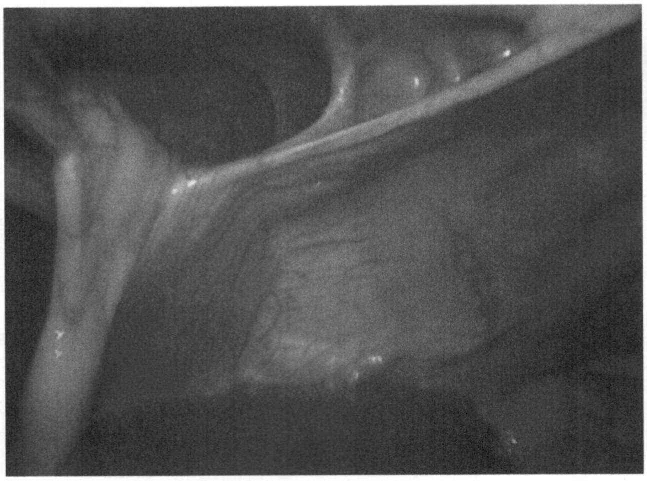

Fig. 1 - Intraoperatory aspect of Morgagni's Hernia

No knotting was made until all the sutures were in place, whilst the stitches were clamped with a grasper. The sutures were then manually tightened under videocamera visualization and tied at the subcutaneous level (Figure 3). A drainage tube was placed in the interhepatophrenic space. Postoperative evolution was uneventful and the patient was discharged on postoperative day one.

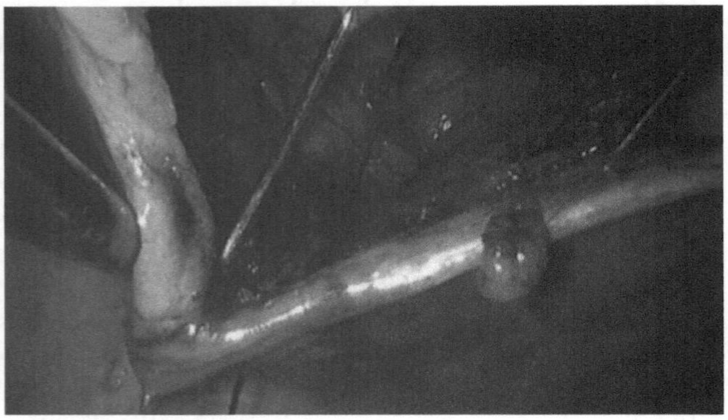

Fig. 2 - Insertion of the stitches with the Reverdin needle

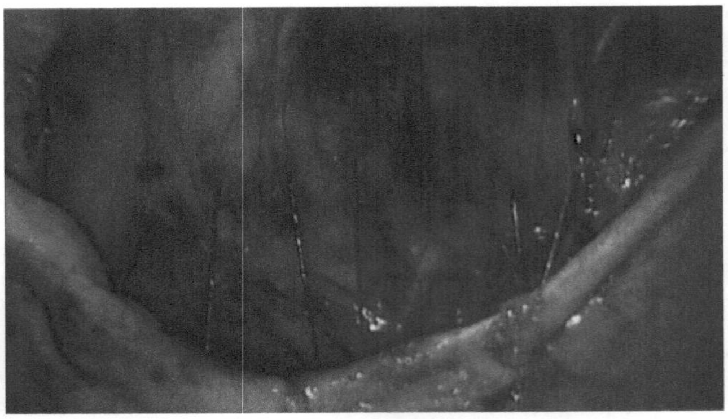

Fig. 3 - Stitches in place before knotting

IV. Discussion

Morgagni's hernia was first described by Giovanni-Battista Morgagni in 1761.[6] It is a rare type of congenital diaphragmatic hernias in which abdominal contents herniate into the thoracic cavity through a triangular retrosternal (anteromedial) diaphragmatic defect that results from failure of fusion of the pars costalis and pars sternalis of the septum transversum [7, 8].

Morgagni's hernia is frequently found on the right (91%), most probably because the heart and pericardial attachment would impede its occurrence on the left [9]. A well-formed peritoneal sac is usually found containing the transverse colon and the omentum in most cases and to a lesser extent, the liver, stomach and the small intestine [7].

When the defect is relatively large, significant visceral herniation and intrathoracic compression would lead to respiratory distress, strangulation, or even cardiac tamponade presenting early in life, otherwise, patients usually remain asymptomatic until later in life and are usually diagnosed incidentally by chest X-ray [10]. Acute life-threatening presentation is reported in adults as well, with strangulation and large bowel obstruction comprising most of the cases [11].

The gold standard for the diagnosis of diaphragmatic hernias is barium enema. A lateral CXR can demonstrate a gas pattern, haustrations and even the defect in the pericardiophrenic angle. CT scan and MRI may be needed in more vague cases to confirm the diagnosis [12]. Once the diagnosis is made, surgical repair is indispensable due to the risk of the life-threatening complications mentioned earlier [3, 4].

Generally, repair is performed through an abdominal or a thoracic approach. Laparotomy is more preferred in complicated cases with strangulation and intestinal obstruction, however, laparoscopic repair remains the optimal surgical approach in uncomplicated cases [5].

Numerous successful laparoscopic techniques were described in the literature, varying mainly in terms of placing a mesh, primary repair of the defect, knotting and the discussion of whether to remove the sac or not.

Intraoperatively we detected a retrosternal defect of approximately 6 cm in diameter, thus we chose to perform a primary repair with nonabsorbable silk (1-0) sutures placed in a U shape manner using Reverdin needle in a transfascial extracorporeal knotting technique.

Rau [13], Huntington [14], Del Castilo [15] and Bortul [16] used polypropylene mesh prosthesis. Their decision is mostly advocated to the relatively larger defect dimensions (6), (4x9), (12x15), (6x10) cm respectively. There is no established limit regarding the indication of a mesh placement, but when the defect is larger than 20-30 cm2, a mesh placement is substantially preferred [17].

Kuster [18], Vinard [11] and Fernandez [19] reported successful laparoscopic primary repairs with running sutures, in contrast, Newman [20], Orita [21] and Angrisani [22] choose to perform laparoscopic primary repairs with separate sutures. We preferred to do separate sutures because we believe and as other authors note it that separate suturing helps to avoid tissue tearing. Furthermore, intracorporeal knotting is rather challenging because of the defect location in a plane parallel to the instruments, aside from the scanty tissue to which the defect is supposed be sutured to [23].

Whether to remove the sac or not is genuinely controversial, systematic studies entailing complication risk assessment are lacking. The most serious complication related to sac removal is fatal pneumopericardium moreover injuries of the mediastinal and pericardial pleura were reported as well [24]. However, other authors stated that sac excision is a crucial step that can decrease the risk of recurrence if performed with supreme level of precision and accuracy avoiding pleural or pericardial injuries [25].

Rau [13], Newman [20] and Fernandez [19] excised the sac with no complications or recurrences reported. In our experience we decided to defy the risks with careful, confined dissection and excision of the sac with which we came through successfully.

Laparoscopic repairs using staples were implemented as well, Smith [26] performed a primary repair while Bortul [16] used a mesh. Regarding recurrence after laparoscopic repair, a valid estimation is unobtainable due to the lack of follow up figures. Our experience is quite recent, therefore follow up data is still unavailable.

V. Conclusion

Laparoscopic repair with transfascial sutures and extracorporeal knot tying is a distinct, durable, easy and efficient approach for the management of Morgagni's hernia. It offers a successful repair with less postoperative pain and hemorrhage, shorter hospital stay and recovery time, reduced risk of postoperative infections, rapid return to regular physical activity and overall it is cosmetically preferred. The transfascial suturing provides an easy, fast, durable and efficient repair of the defect without the need for a mesh placement. Likewise, the extracorporeal knotting is much easier to execute compared to intracorporeal knotting.

Acknowledgment

The authors are grateful for the financial support from the Romanian National Authority for Scientific Research UEFISCDI for project no. PN-II-RU-TE- 2014-4-0992 and Iuliu Hatieganu University of Medicine and Pharmacy, 3rd Department Of Surgery, Cluj-Napoca, Romania, internal grant no. 4945/14/08.03.2016.

Conflict of Interest

The authors declare that they have no conflict of interest.

References

1. Steinhorn RH (2014).Pediatric Congenital Diaphragmatic Hernia. www.medscape.com.
2. Loong TP,Kocher HM (2005) Clinical presentation and operative repair of hernia of Morgagni. Postgrad Med J. 81: p. 41-4.
3. Pairolero P, Trastek V, Payne W (1989) Esophagus and diaphragmatic hernias.In: Schwartz SI, editor. Principles of surgery. McGrawHil. New York. p. 1118–1132.
4. Kimmelstiel FM, Holgersen LO, Hilfer C (1987) Retrosternal (Morgagni) hernia with small bowel obstruction secondary to a Richter's incarceration. J Pediatr Surg. 22: p. 998-1000.
5. Pironi D, Palazzini G, Arcieri S et al. (2008) Laparoscopic diagnosis and treatment of diaphragmatic Morgagni hernia. Case report and review of the literature. Ann Ital Chir. 79: p. 29-36.
6. Morgagni GB. In: Millar A CT, eds. Seats and Causes of Diseases.London. 3: p. 1769:205.
7. Harris J, Super T, Kimura K (1993) Foramen of Morgagni hernia in identical twins: Is this an inheritable defect? . Fed Surg. . p. 28:177-178.
8. Sinclair L,Klein L (1993) Congenital diaphragmatic hernia—Morgagni Type. Emerg Med J. p. 11:163-165.
9. Horton JD, Hofmann LJ, Hetz SP (2008) Presentation and management of Morgagni hernias in adults: a review of 298 cases. Surg Endosc. 22: p. 1413-20.
10. Papia G, Gerstle J, Langer J (2004) Laparoscopic repair of Morgagni diaphragmatic hernia in children: technical challenges and results. Pediatric Endosurg Innovat Tech. p. 8:245–249.

11. Vinard J, Palayodan A, Collomb P (1997) Emergency laparoscopic treatment of a strangulated Morgagni hernia. Eur J Coeliosurg. p. 1:35-40.
12. Wolloch Y, Grunebaum M, Glanz I et al. (1974) Symptomatic retrosternal (Morgagni) hernia. Am J Surg. 127: p. 601-5.
13. Rau HG, Schardey HM, Lange V (1994) Laparoscopic repair of a Morgagni hernia. Surg Endosc. 8: p. 1439-42.
14. Huntington TR (1996) Laparoscopic transabdominal preperitoneal repair of a hernia of Morgagni. J Laparoendosc Surg. 6: p. 131-3.
15. Del Castillo D, Sanchez J, Hernandez M et al. (1998) Morgagni's hernia resolved by laparoscopic surgery. J Laparoendosc Adv Surg Tech A. 8: p. 105-8.
16. Bortul M CL, Gheller P (1998) Laparoscopic repair of a Morgagni-Larrey hernia. Laparoendosc Adv Surg Tech. p. 8(5):309-313.
17. Thoman DS, Hui T, Phillips EH (2002) Laparoscopic diaphragmatic hernia repair. Surg Endosc. 16: p. 1345-9.
18. Kuster GG, Kline LE, Garzo G (1992) Diaphragmatic hernia through the foramen of Morgagni: laparoscopic repair case report. J Laparoendosc Surg. 2: p. 93-100.
19. Fernandez-Cebrian JM,De Oteyza JP (1996) Laparoscopic repair of hernia of foramen of Morgagni: a new case report. J Laparoendosc Surg. 6: p. 61-4.
20. Newman L, 3rd, Eubanks S, Bridges WM, 2nd et al. (1995) Laparoscopic diagnosis and treatment of Morgagni hernia. Surg Laparosc Endosc. 5: p. 27-31.
21. Orita M OM, Yamashita K, Morita N, Esato K. (1997) Laparoscopic repair of a diaphragmatic hernia through the foramen of Morgagni. Surg Endosc. p. 11(6):668-670.
22. Angrisani L, Lorenzo M, Santoro T et al. (2000) Hernia of foramen of Morgagni in adult: case report of laparoscopic repair. JSLS. 4: p. 177-81.
23. Mallick MS,Alqahtani A (2009) Laparoscopic-assisted repair of Morgagni hernia in children. J Pediatr Surg. 44: p. 1621-4.
24. Pokorny WJ, McGill CW, Harberg FJ (1984) Morgagni hernias during infancy: presentation and associated anomalies. J Pediatr Surg. 19: p. 394-7.
25. Shah RS, Sharma PC, Bhandarkar DS (2015) Laparoscopic repair of Morgagni's hernia: An innovative Approach. Departments of Paediatric Surgery, and Minimal Access Surgery, P. D. Hinduja National Hospital and Medical Research Centre, Mahim, Mumbai, Maharashtra, India.
26. Smith J,Ghani A (1995) Morgagni hernia: incidental repair during laparoscopic cholecystectomy. J Laparoendosc Surg. 5: p. 123-5.

Author: Emil Mois
Institute: University of Medicine and Pharmacy "Iuliu Hatieganu", Cluj-Napoca, Romania
Street: Str. Victor Babeş Nr. 8, 400012 Cluj-Napoca
City: Cluj-Napoca
Country: Romania
Email: dr_emil_mois@yahoo.com

Ambulatory Heart Rate Variability Correlates with High-Sensitivity C - Reactive Protein in Type 2 Diabetes and Control Subjects

D.M. Ciobanu[1,2], A.E. Crăciun[1], I.A. Vereşiu[1,2], C. Bala[1,2] and G. Roman[1,2]

[1] "Iuliu Haţieganu" University of Medicine and Pharmacy, Cluj-Napoca, Romania
[2] Center of Diabetes, Nutrition and Metabolic Diseases, Cluj-Napoca, Romania

Abstract—**Type 2 diabetes mellitus has been associated with elevated high-sensitivity C-reactive protein (hsCRP), but the possible implication of ambulatory heart rate (HR) variability in enhancing chronic subclinical inflammation biomarkers remains to be elucidated. We aimed to evaluate the correlations between HR variability and coefficient of variance assessed during 24-hour ambulatory blood pressure monitoring (ABPM) and hsCRP in type 2 diabetes and control subjects. The observational study included type 2 diabetes (n=75) and control (n=11) subjects. HR variability was calculated as standard deviation of mean HR during daytime, nighttime and 24-hour periods. The coefficient of variation was calculated using standard deviation and mean HR. Nighttime HR dipping was calculated using daytime and nighttime HR variability. We found higher hsCRP in type 2 diabetes compared to controls. Also, we found that daytime, nighttime and 24-hour HR variability and coefficient of variance were lower in the type 2 diabetes group compared with the control group, while type 2 diabetes subjects receiving β-blockers had even lower ambulatory HR variability and coefficient of variance. Subjects with diabetic neuropathy, retinopathy and atherosclerotic cardiovascular disease had lower HR variability and coefficient of variance compared to their peers without disease. We observed that daytime and 24-hour HR variability inversely correlated with hsCRP, while all HR variability parameters inversely correlated with hypertension duration in the study population. Nighttime HR dipping inversely correlated with duration of type 2 diabetes and hypertension. Our results suggest that 24-hour ambulatory HR variability and coefficient of variance are significantly correlated with chronic inflammation evaluated using hsCRP in type 2 diabetes and control subjects, and these findings deserve further investigations.**

Keywords—**heart rate variability, high-sensitivity C-reactive protein, type 2 diabetes mellitus, ambulatory blood pressure monitoring.**

I. Introduction

Type 2 diabetes mellitus (T2DM) has been associated with abnormal cardiac autonomic function and elevated inflammatory markers. Heart rate (HR) variability is an established non-invasive measure of autonomic nervous function and, in subjects with diabetes, HR variability was able to discriminate cardiac autonomic neuropathy [1]. Decreased HR variability was described in T2DM [2] and was associated with increased risk for the development [3] and progression of cardiovascular disease [4].

The autonomic nervous system dysfunction affects the behavior of endothelial cell. HR variability was significantly inversely associated with CRP levels in healthy subjects [5], subjects with cardiovascular disease [6] and T2DM [7]. These evidences prove the relation of systemic inflammation with the function of autonomic nervous system.

There have been described many methods of assessing HR variability [6]. However, the possible implication of HR variability evaluated during 24-hour ambulatory blood pressure monitoring (ABPM), in modulating chronic inflammation biomarkers in subjects with diabetes remains to be elucidated. In our study, we aimed to evaluate the correlations between ambulatory HR variability and coefficient of variance and hsCRP in T2DM and control subjects.

II. Patients and Methods

The observational study included data from 86 persons. Consecutive T2DM subjects (n=75) were selected from Clinical Diabetes, Nutrition and Metabolic Diseases Centre, Cluj-Napoca, Romania, between July 2013 and February 2014. The control subjects (n=11) were selected from First Medical Clinic, Cluj-Napoca, Romania. The subjects fulfilled all the inclusion criteria: adults (men and women), Caucasian, previously diagnosed with T2DM and no diabetes and no hypertension for the control group. The subjects were not included in the study if they had: autoimmune diseases, estimated glomerular filtration rate <30ml/min/1.73m2, malignancies, major cardiac arrhythmias, unstable cardiovascular condition and secondary hypertension.

In accordance with the World Medical Association Declaration of Helsinki of 1975, as revised in 2000 and 2008, and with the ethical standards of the responsible committee on human experimentation (institutional and national), the study protocol was approved by the Ethical Committee of "Iuliu Haţieganu" University of Medicine and Pharmacy Cluj-Napoca, Romania. All participants were aware of the investigational nature of the study and agreed to participate after providing written informed consent.

S. Vlad and N.M. Roman (eds.), *International Conference on Advancements of Medicine and Health Care through Technology; 12th - 15th October 2016, Cluj-Napoca, Romania,*
IFMBE Proceedings 59,
DOI: 10.1007/978-3-319-52875-5_4

The study protocol, biochemical measurements and 24-hour ambulatory HR and blood pressure monitoring have been previously described [8]. T2DM and its complications (neuropathy, retinopathy and atherosclerotic cardiovascular disease) were diagnosed according to American Diabetes Association criteria [9]. Hypertension was diagnosed when two blood pressure measurements repeated at two visits were above 140 mmHg for systolic blood pressure or above 90 mmHg for diastolic, or the use of antihypertensive drugs [10]. The coefficient of variance (CV) was calculated using the formula [11]:$100 * \frac{HR\ standard\ deviation}{mean\ HR}$. HR variability was calculated as standard deviation of mean HR during daytime, nighttime and 24-hour periods. HR dipping index (%) was calculated using the formula: $(1 - \frac{nighttime\ HR}{daytime\ HR}) * 100$.

Statistical analyses were performed using R 2.15.1 and LibreOffice programs. The Kolmogorov–Smirnov test was used to assess the normality of all variables distribution. The continuous data were expressed as means +/− standard deviation when normally distributed or as median and inter-quartile range when not normally distributed. The categorical or dichotomous variables were expressed as percentages and absolute values. Group comparisons of variables were performed using ANOVA, chi-square and Kruskal-Wallis tests. The relationship between ambulatory HR and other variables were evaluated using Pearson or Spearman coefficient. Statistical significance threshold was considered $p<0.05$.

III. Results

The baseline characteristics of the study participants indicated significant differences in age, systolic blood pressure, body mass index and waist circumference between the two groups. Also, hsCRP was significantly higher in the T2DM group than in control group (Table 1). In the T2DM group, the duration of T2DM 8.0(3.0-13.0) years and the hypertension duration was 9.0(3.0-13.0) years.

Diabetic peripheral neuropathy was present in 50.7% of the T2DM subjects, while nephropathy and retinopathy were present in 34.7% and 33.3% of the T2DM subjects, respectively. Cardiovascular disease was present in 44% of the T2DM subjects, while hypertension was present in 88% of the T2DM subjects. In the T2DM group, 21.3% were receiving oral antidiabetic drugs and 78.7% were receiving insulin therapy. Treatment with β-blockers were receiving in 56% of the T2DM subjects, while 86.7% were receiving angiotensin-converting enzyme inhibitor or angiotensin receptor blockers, 30.6% were receiving calcium channel blockers and 64.0% were receiving diuretics.

Table 1 Baseline characteristics of the study groups

Variables	Control (n=11)	Type 2 diabetes (n=75)	p-value
Age (years)	54.1±8.0	59.6±7.3	0.027
Male Gender (n, %)	6(54.5%)	34 (45.3%)	0.57
Smoking status (yes, %)	5(45.5%)	13(17.3%)	0.032
Body mass index (kg/m^2)	27.3±3.7	31.5±4.4	0.004
Waist circumference (cm)	100±9.8	109.9±10.2	0.004
Office heart rate (beats/min)	75.6±10.2	75.9±12.1	0.93
Office systolic blood pressure (mmHg)	118.2±8.4	136.3±15.6	<0.001
Office diastolic blood pressure (mmHg)	76.9±6.7	81.7±10.6	0.15
HsCRP (mg/l)	0.48±0.15	0.71±0.35	0.015

We found no significant differences in mean daytime, nighttime and 24-hour HR between the two study groups. The daytime, nighttime and 24-hour HR variability were higher in control group compared with the T2DM group, but the statistical significance was reached only for 24-hour HR variability. When analyzing the CV, we observed that the T2DM group had lower levels compared to the control group, but the statistical significance was reached only for the 24-hour period. Nighttime HR dipping was significantly lower in the T2DM group compared with the control group (Table 2).

Table 2 The 24-hour ambulatory HR parameters of the study groups

Variables	Control (n=11)	Type 2 diabetes (n=75)	p- value
Mean daytime HR	75.6±5.7	73.9±8.8	0.54
Mean nighttime HR	62.7±6.6	66.1±8.1	0.19
Mean 24-hour HR	72.6±5.6	72.1±8.3	0.84
Daytime HR variability	9.0±2.3	7.7±2.8	0.13
Nighttime HR variability	5.9±2.3	5.2±2.1	0.36
24-hour HR variability	9.9±2.1	7.9±3.1	0.041
Daytime HR CV	11.9±2.9	10.4±3.5	0.16
Nighttime HR CV	8.7±3.1	7.5±3.0	0.19
24-hour HR CV	14.0±3.3	11.3±3.7	0.24
Nighttime HR dipping	17.0(11.4; 21.4)	11.4(6.1; 15.1)	0.005

When analyzing the T2DM group, we found that subjects receiving β-blockers (n=42) had significantly lower nighttime HR variability (4.3±1.7 *vs.* 5.8±2.1; p=0.001) and 24-hour HR variability (7.5±2.5 *vs.* 9.0±3.0; p=0.02), and lower daytime HR variability (7.1±2.3 *vs.* 8.3±3.1; p=0.06) compared with the T2DM subjects not receiving β-blockers (n=33). Also, T2DM receiving β-blockers had significantly lower nighttime HR CV (6.6.1±2.7 *vs.* 8.7±3.0; p=0.002), lower 24-hour HR CV (10.6±3.2 *vs.* 12.2±4.1; p=0.058) and lower daytime HR (9.9±2.9 *vs.* 10.9±4.0; p=0.188) compared with the T2DM subjects not receiving β-blockers.

The correlations of ambulatory HR variability in the study population are presented in Table 3. Daytime and 24-hour HR variability significantly and inversely correlated with hsCRP levels, even after adjustment for age, sex, smoking status, body mass index and diabetes duration. Similar results were observed when correlating daytime, nighttime and 24-hour CV of HR with hsCRP. Daytime (r= -0.23; p=0.040), nighttime (r= -0.23; p=0.040) and 24-hour HR variability (r= -0.30; p=0.008) significantly and inversely correlated with hypertension duration, even after adjustment for age, sex, smoking status, body mass index and diabetes duration. The CV of HR was not associated with hypertension duration. No significant results were obtained when assessing the correlation between mean ambulatory HR and hsCRP levels.

Table 3 Correlations of HR variability in the T2DM group

Variables	Daytime HR variability	Nighttime HR variability	24-hour HR variability
hsCRP	-0.23; p=0.030	-0.04; p=NS	-0.23; p=0.036

Nighttime HR dipping inversely correlated with T2DM duration (r= -0.27; p=0.013) and hypertension duration (r= -0.45; p< 0.001) in the study population, even after adjustment for age, sex, smoking status and body mass index.

In the study population, subjects with diabetic peripheral neuropathy had significantly lower daytime HR variability (7.0±2.1 *vs.* 8.6±3.0; p=0.006) and 24-hour HR variability (7.3±2.2 *vs.* 9.3±3.0; p=0.001) compared to subjects without neuropathy. Also, subjects with diabetic retinopathy had significantly lower daytime HR variability (6.6±1.9 *vs.* 8.3±2.9; p=0.007) and 24-hour HR variability (7.1±2.6 *vs.* 9.0±2.9; p=0.005) compared to subjects without retinopathy. Subjects with atherosclerotic cardiovascular disease had significantly lower daytime HR variability (7.1±2.2 *vs.* 8.3±3.0; p=0.05), nighttime HR variability (4.4±1.8 *vs.* 5.4±2.1; p=0.038) and 24-hour HR variability (7.4±2.3 *vs.* 9.0±3.0; p=0.007) compared to subjects without atherosclerotic cardiovascular disease. Similar results were observed when evaluating CV of HR in subjects with neuropathy, retinopathy and cardiovascular disease compared to subjects free of mentioned chronic diabetes complications.

IV. Discussion

HR variability is considered the earliest indicator of diabetic cardiovascular autonomic neuropathy [12]. We found that daytime, nighttime and 24-hour HR variability and CV were lower in T2DM group compared with the control group, while T2DM subjects receiving β-blockers had even lower ambulatory HR variability and CV. Similarly, Sucharita et al observed that T2DM subjects had lower HR variability using another method for assessing HR variability [2]. However, in a study evaluating type 1 diabetes subjects, the β-blockers proved a favorable effect on both autonomic function and inflammation by increasing HR variability and decreasing CRP [13]. The immunomodulatory effect of β-blockers, particularly on C-reactive protein, has been reported in coronary artery disease [14]. Our data on the direct relation between the use of β-blockers and decreased HR variability and CV, as shown by the reduction in standard deviation mean ambulatory HR confirm the HR decreasing effect of β-blockers.

Daytime and 24-hour HR variability negatively associated with hsCRP levels, even after adjustment for confounding factors. Our results agree with the findings of one study that described the inverse relationship between HR variability and inflammatory biomarkers in support to the role of autonomic nervous system in determining excessive inflammatory reactions [7]. Decreased daytime, nighttime and 24-hour HR variability associated with increased hypertension duration, suggesting that longer disease duration has a negative impact on autonomic system normal function. It is known that supine hypertension often coexists with orthostatic hypotension in autonomic dysfunction and it is associated with end-organ damage [15].

We found that nighttime HR dipping inversely correlated with duration of T2DM and hypertension in our study population, even after adjustment for confounders. Older age and longer diabetes and hypertension duration had lower nighttime HR dipping. The non-dipping pattern of the nighttime blood pressure was associated with increased risk for cardiovascular events [16] and related to longer diabetes [17] and hypertension duration. In addition, nighttime HR dipping was significantly lower in the T2DM group compared with the control group. The findings of the present study suggest the possible connection between HR non-dipping pattern and increase risk of cardiovascular events.

Autonomic neuropathy can coexist with peripheral neuropathy in subjects with diabetes. We found that the presence of diabetic peripheral neuropathy and retinopathy negatively correlated with daytime and 24-hour HR variability and CV. This finding suggests that the mechanisms involved in diabetic retinopathy development and progression might be similar to those involved in autonomic nervous system dysfunction. As previously described [4], the presence of atherosclerotic cardiovascular disease was negatively associated with daytime, nighttime and 24-hour HR variability and CV.

V. Conclusions

Our results suggest that 24-hour ambulatory HR variability and coefficient of variance are significantly correlated with chronic inflammation evaluated using hsCRP in type 2 diabetes and control subjects. Any speculation on cause/effect relationship of this two parameters is risky and beyond our intentions. Based on our results, we propose the use of 24-hour ABPM as a useful and reproducible method for assessing mean HR and HR variability when other more accurate methods are not available.

Acknowledgment

The work was supported by an internal grant (4994/3/08.03.2016) financed by the "Iuliu Haţieganu" University of Medicine and Pharmacy Cluj-Napoca.

Conflict of Interest

The authors declare that they have no conflict of interest.

References

1. França da Silva AK, Penachini da Costa de Rezende Barbosa M, Marques Vanderlei F et al. (2016) Application of Heart Rate Variability in Diagnosis and Prognosis of Individuals with Diabetes Mellitus: Systematic Review. Ann Noninvasive Electrocardiol 21(3):223-235 DOI:10.1111/anec.12372
2. Sucharita S, Bantwal G, Idiculla J et al. (2011) Autonomic nervous system function in type 2 diabetes using conventional clinical autonomic tests, heart rate and blood pressure variability measures. Indian J Endocrinol Metab 15(3):198-203 DOI:10.4103/2230-8210.83406
3. Ziegler D, Zentai CP, Perz S et al. (2008) Prediction of mortality using measures of cardiac autonomic dysfunction in the diabetic and nondiabetic population: the MONICA/KORA Augsburg Cohort Study. Diabetes Care 31(3):556-561 DOI:10.2337/dc07-1615
4. Yamaguchi Y, Wada M, Sato H et al. (2015) Impact of nocturnal heart rate variability on cerebral small-vessel disease progression: a longitudinal study in community-dwelling elderly Japanese. Hypertens Res 38(8):564-569 DOI:10.1038/hr.2015.38
5. Sloan RP, McCreath H, Tracey KJ et al. (2007) RR interval variability is inversely related to inflammatory markers: the CARDIA study. Mol Med 2007 13(3-4):178-184 DOI:10.2119/2006–00112.Sloan
6. Frasure-Smith N, Lespérance F, Irwin MR et al. (2009) The relationships among heart rate variability, inflammatory markers and depression in coronary heart disease patients. Brain Behav Immun 23(8):1140-1147 DOI:10.1016/j.bbi.2009.07.005
7. Aso Y, Wakabayashi S, Nakano T et al. (2006) High serum high-sensitivity C-reactive protein concentrations are associated with relative cardiac sympathetic overactivity during the early morning period in type 2 diabetic patients with metabolic syndrome. Metabolism 55(8):1014-1021 DOI:10.1016/j.metabol.2006.03.011
8. Ciobanu DM, Bala CG, Veresiu IA et al. (2016) High-sensitivity C-reactive protein is associated with 24-hour ambulatory blood pressure variability in type 2 diabetes and control subjects. Rev Rom Med Lab 24(1):65-73 DOI:10.1515/rrlm-2016-0013
9. American Diabetes Association. (2015) 2. Classification and Diagnosis of Diabetes. Diabetes Care 39(Suppl 1):S13-S22 DOI:10.2337/dc15-S005
10. Mancia G, Fagard R, Narkiewicz K et al. (2013) 2013 ESH/ESC guidelines for the management of arterial hypertension: the Task Force for the Management of Arterial Hypertension of the European Society of Hypertension (ESH) and of the European Society of Cardiology (ESC). Eur Heart J 34(28):2159-2219 DOI:10.1093/eurheartj/eht151
11. van den Berg MP, Haaksma J, Brouwer J et al. (1997) Heart rate variability in patients with atrial fibrillation is related to vagal tone. Circulation 96(4):1209-1216 DOI:10.1161/01.cir.96.4.1209
12. Vinik AI, Maser RE, Mitchell BD, Freeman R. (2003) Diabetic autonomic neuropathy. Diabetes Care 26(5):1553-1579 DOI:10.2337/diacare.26.5.1553
13. Lanza GA, Pitocco D, Navarese EP et al. (2007) Association between cardiac autonomic dysfunction and inflammation in type 1 diabetic patients: effect of beta-blockade. Eur Heart J 28(7):814-820 DOI:10.1093/eurheartj/ehm018
14. Jenkins NP, Keevil BG, Hutchinson IV, Brooks NH. (2002) Beta-blockers are associated with lower C-reactive protein concentrations in patients with coronary artery disease. Am J Med 112(4):269-74 DOI: 10.1016/S0002-9343(01)01115-9
15. Shannon J, Jordan J, Costa F et al. (1997) The hypertension of autonomic failure and its treatment. Hypertension 30(5):1062-1067 DOI: 10.1161/01.HYP.30.5.1062
16. Eguchi K, Pickering TG, Hoshide S et al. (2008) Ambulatory blood pressure is a better marker than clinic blood pressure in predicting cardiovascular events in patients with/without type 2 diabetes. Am J Hypertens 21(4):443-450 DOI:10.1038/ajh.2008.4
17. Ciobanu DM, Veresiu IA, Bala CG et al. (2015) Benefits of bedtime hypertension medication in type 2 diabetes demonstrated on ambulatory blood pressure monitoring. Proceedings of the 49th Annual Scientific Meeting of the European Society for Clinical Investigation. Medimond, Bologna, Italy, pp 107-112

Heart Rate Dynamics Study on the Impact of "Mirror Therapy" in Patients with Stroke

D. Andrițoi, C. Corciovă, C. Luca, D. Matei and R. Ciorap

University of Medicine and Pharmacy "Grigore T. Popa" Iasi, Department Biomedical Sciences, Iasi, Romania

Abstract— **Mirror therapy (MT) has been seen to provide encouraging results in hemiparesis treatment. For stroke there are evidence that MT, used like an additional intervention, improves recovery of arm function and a there are a few evidence regarding rehabilitation of lower limb function and pain after stroke. Firm conclusions could not be drawn yet, that's why the objective of this study is to evaluate the clinical aspects of mirror therapy (MT) interventions after stroke, which patients are likely to benefit most from MT, and how MT should preferably be applied. Co-monitoring blood pressure, HRV, respiratory rate and oxygen saturation can bring valuable information on cardiovascular reactivity in patients after stroke but also on the effectiveness of therapy, as MT. The study will attempt to correlate neurophysiological aspects and hemodynamic using both classical and modern methods of analysis based on nonlinear analysis, less used today. We used a series of additional tests of stimulation the sympathetic and parasympathetic system, to emphasize the influence of those two elements.**

Keywords— **mirror therapy (MT), stroke, Heart Rate Variability (HRV).**

I. Introduction

According to the World Health Organization, 15 million people suffer stroke worldwide each year. Of these, 5 million die and another 5 million are permanently disabled. High blood pressure contributes to more than 12.7 million strokes worldwide. More than 50% stroke patients remain vocationally impaired and about 30% need full support for activities of daily living [1].

Mirror therapy has been seen to provide encouraging results in treatment of hemiparesis. It seems likely that this illusion enhances activation of the premotor and motor cortex in a similar way to action observation or motor imagery as in Figure 1 [2]. For stroke there is a moderate quality of evidence that MT as an additional intervention improves recovery of arm function, and a low quality of evidence regarding lower limb function and pain after stroke [3][4]. Firm conclusions could not be drawn yet, that's why the objective of this study is to evaluate the clinical aspects of mirror therapy (MT) interventions after stroke, which patients are likely to benefit most from MT, and how MT should preferably be applied.

The novelty that will bring the study will attempt to correlate neurophysiological aspects and hemodynamic using both classical and modern methods of analysis based on nonlinear analysis, less used today.

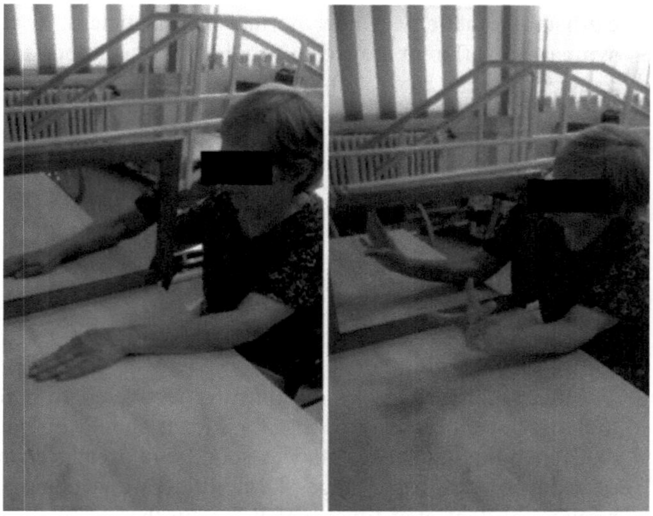

Fig1. Patient following mirror therapy

The paper aims to end acquisition, measurement and analysis parameters electrophysiology and hemodynamics using non-invasive methods in order to evaluate the clinical aspects of mirror therapy (MT) interventions after stroke. The complexity of the subject and the expertise and experience of the proposed team members, the project is interdisciplinary - medical and technical [5] [6].

II. Working methodology

The objective of this study is to evaluate the clinical aspects of mirror therapy (MT) interventions after stroke.

In subjects with cognitive impairment and post shock we analyzed blood pressure, heart rate variability, respiratory rate, oxygen saturation of peripheral, fasting and effort. Regulating autonomic processes in the cardiovascular system will be evaluated by the Ewing battery of tests (sample with slow deep breathing, active orthostatic test, Valsalva maneuver, BP response and BP response to standing and isometric contraction of the hand). Also it was also recorded

S. Vlad and N.M. Roman (eds.), *International Conference on Advancements of Medicine and Health Care through Technology; 12th - 15th October 2016, Cluj-Napoca, Romania,*
IFMBE Proceedings 59,
DOI: 10.1007/978-3-319-52875-5_5

and EEG at rest and the challenge will be detailed observations in other papers.

The concept of cardiovascular homeostasis is the tendency for the body to maintain a relatively regular heart rate (the amount of RR intervals varies within a relative range, as shown in Figure 2) and blood pressure regularly under variable environment. The heart rate is influenced, among others, by regulating autonomic (sympathetic and parasympathetic). Experimental sympathetic stimulation reduces ventricular refractory period, decreases ventricular fibrillation threshold, post-potential excitatory and stimulate cardiac automaticity. Vagal stimulation increases the refractory period, ventricular fibrillation threshold increases, decreases cardiac automaticity. Under normal circumstances, at rest, sympathetic efferent are weak; vagal activity is important, it reduces the heart rate to 60-70 / min.

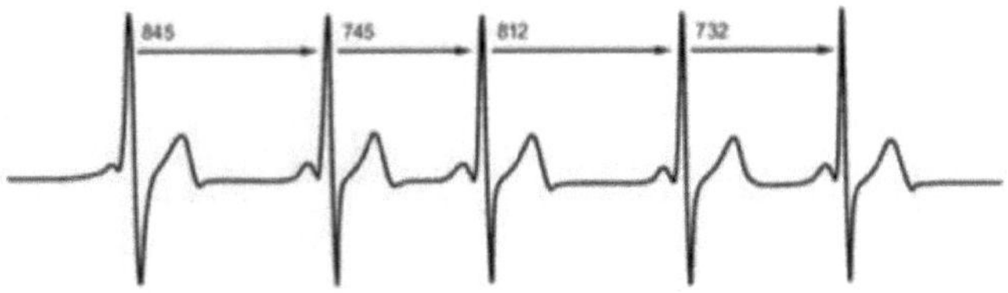

Fig.2. RR interval variation during recording

Most secondary stroke disability is recovered in a few months, but others may persist for life. It should be noted that rehabilitation should start as soon, so a greater chance of recovery this early stage. Disabilities are widening or remain constant over time, which is why the establishment of rehabilitation program has to be made as soon as possible.

The time needed for recovery after a stroke should not be underestimated. Studies have shown that if the recovery process is started and functions, the recovery of the patient is faster.

Methods of rehabilitation after a stroke vary from person to person, but the same purpose, namely:

- Acquiring a functional status that provide independence and minimal help from other people
- Accommodating of people with physical and mental changes caused by stroke
- Appropriate integration in family and community.

The experiment will try to evaluate changes in cardiovascular reactivity and response of the central nervous system and peripheral occurring disorders subsequent stroke. We achieved a correlation of various parameters obtained by non-invasive methods: neuropsychological tests, testing hemodynamic, neurophysiological, diagnostic algorithms to determine what can possibly lead to an early diagnosis followed by appropriate therapeutic sanctions.

Because a number of heart diseases may represent potential risk factors for stroke, interpretation of the ECG may show arrhythmias such as atrial fibrillation or may indicate acute ischemia. All patients with stroke should conduct an ECG as part of the initial assessment, and during the rehabilitation process.

In order to correlate hemodynamic and neurophysiological aspects we used both classical and modern methods of analysis based on nonlinear dynamics [7], [8].

RR series analysis is a standard method for estimating the heart rate a patient. Heart rate variability (HRV), as measured by ECG techniques, is used to assess vagal and sympathetic influences on the heart. A great variability in heart rate indicates that the mechanisms regulating normal cardiovascular functioning and decreases HRV indicates damage control mechanisms. Decreased HRV is a predictor of a cardiac event or death from cardiovascular causes.

Also in clinical trials were conducted all 5 tests within the "battery" Ewing, but in the present paper will refer only to the first 3 related to HRV.

The 3 tests referred to are:

1. Heart rate variability at controlled deep breathing;
2. Heart rate variability Valsalva maneuver;
3. Heart rate variability to standing (30/15).

In the first test HRV was measured during a 6 cycles of deep breathing. R-R interval difference between the longest (exhale) and the shortest R-R (inhale) is normally greater than 10 beats / minute. Reducing this gap signifies impaired parasympathetic component.

During Valsalva maneuver the patient expires, for 15-30 seconds in a chamber connected to a pressure gauge, a pressure of 40 mmHg, while the ECG is recorded. Valsalva ratio is calculated by dividing the interval R-R longest immediately following the test phase during bradycardia, the R-R interval soon noticed during the maneuver and reflecting tachycardia triggered by exertion. A Valsalva ratio greater than or equal to 1.21 is normal and if it is less than or equal to 1.10 is pathological.

In the last test, after 15 seconds of ECG recording supine subject is raised and recording continues until the 40th beat after assumption of the standing. R-R interval is measured from the 15th and 30th line. Shows a healthy subject at the 15th tachycardia and bradycardia beating the 30th, leading to a near 30/15 ratio R-R 1.2.

The other two tests of "battery" are related to measuring blood pressure and bring additional information in order to achieve the best possible image on the health of the subject as well as its evolution.

ECG signals were recorded using a data acquisition system data MP150 from BIOPAC Inc., which is comprised of a module amplifying electrocardiographic (ECG100C) represented by an instrumentation amplifier with a single channel, high gain, with differential input special designed to monitor the heart's electrical activity. As software tools were used Acknowledge ver. 4.2 (also developed by Biopac Inc.) for signal acquisition and processing, and analysis of HRV was performed using HRV Kubios.

III. HEART RATE VARIABILITY ANALISYS AND OBSERVATIONS

Heart rate variability was analyzed by statistical methods, linear and nonlinear.

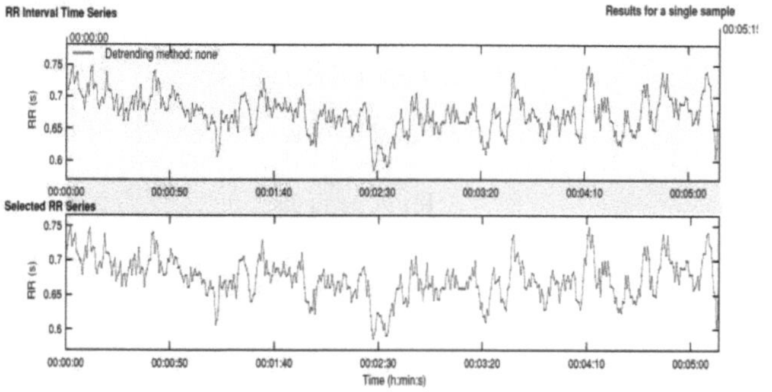

Fig.3. HRV time analysis result

The most important indicators of the time analysis are:

- Heart rate - average rate around 70 beats / minute. One person Normal heart rate is influenced by some of the vague nerve (parasympathetic) which has inhibitory effects on the other side of the sympathetic system that has stimulant effects. Regarding this parameter were observed major changes. There have been cases where that depending on laterality damage following treatment frequency decreased over time. In Figure 3 it can be seen a decrease in variability after the start of therapy.

- The standard deviation of all RR intervals (Standard deviation of the NN intervals - SDNN) shows the degree of homogeneity of values. SDNN was correlated with reducing dysfunction the left ventricle.

- SDNN index is the average standard deviation of all RR intervals for 5 min fragments of the ECG. SDNN index is considered primarily highlights autonomic nervous system influence on HRV.

- The root mean square of successive differences between normal beating of the heart (The square root of the mean of the squares of differences between adjacent NN intervals - RMSSD) estimates parasympathetic activity of the heart.

All parameters mentioned above have undergone changes illustrated in Figure 4, which may explain the effectiveness of therapy used.

Time–Domain Results

Variable	Units	Value
Mean RR*	(ms)	754.1
STD RR (SDNN)	(ms)	104.8
Mean HR*	(1/min)	81.28
STD HR	(1/min)	14.07
RMSSD	(ms)	59.8
NN50	(count)	82
pNN50	(%)	20.2
RR triangular index		17.696
TINN	(ms)	625.0

After

Variable	Units	Value
Mean RR*	(ms)	805.7
STD RR (SDNN)	(ms)	85.3
Mean HR*	(1/min)	75.26
STD HR	(1/min)	7.47
RMSSD	(ms)	54.9
NN50	(count)	95
pNN50	(%)	25.0
RR triangular index		18.143
TINN	(ms)	370.0

Fig.4. HRV time domain results before and after 6 weeks

Linear analysis - analyzing the frequency domain (PSD - power spectral density) allows an assessment of the autonomic nervous system at any time of registration. It uses Fast Fourier Transform and basic indices of spectral analysis of heart rate are:

- Total power spectrum (PT) fully reflect changing vegetative influences on heart rate,

- High-frequency spectral component (high frequency-HF) – 0.15-0.40Hz expressing parasympathetic innervation influence,

- Spectral component of low frequency (LF low-frequency) – 0.04-0.15Hz, characterizing maximum sympathetic activity,

- Spectral component, very low frequency (VLF-very low frequency) - 0.02-0.04 Hz, thermoregulatory mechanisms and influenced by the activity of the renin-angiotensin system.

- Coefficient sympathetic activity in relation to the parasympathetic expressed as LF / HF ratio sympathetic or parasympathetic predominance highlights.

As regarding the parameters obtained from the HRV frequency domain analysis, there were changes in their best condition outlined depending on the location and length of time since the manifestation of stroke, an example is shown in Figure 5.

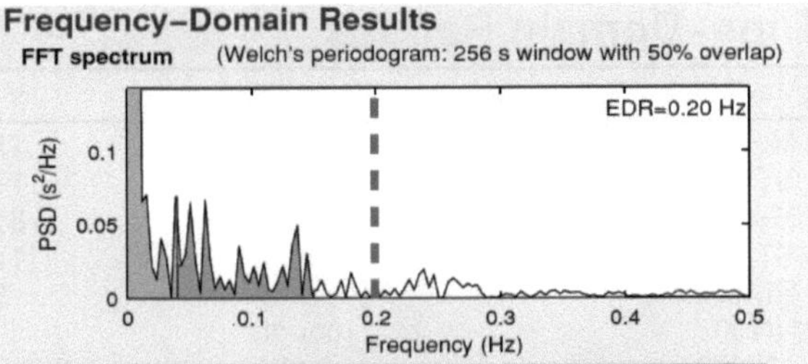

Frequency Band	Peak (Hz)	Power (ms^2)	Power (%)	Power (n.u.)
VLF (0–0.04 Hz)	0.0039	9019	71.7	
LF (0.04–0.15 Hz)	0.0625	2321	18.5	65.3
HF (0.15–0.4 Hz)	0.2383	1231	9.8	34.6
Total		12574		
LF/HF		1.886		

After

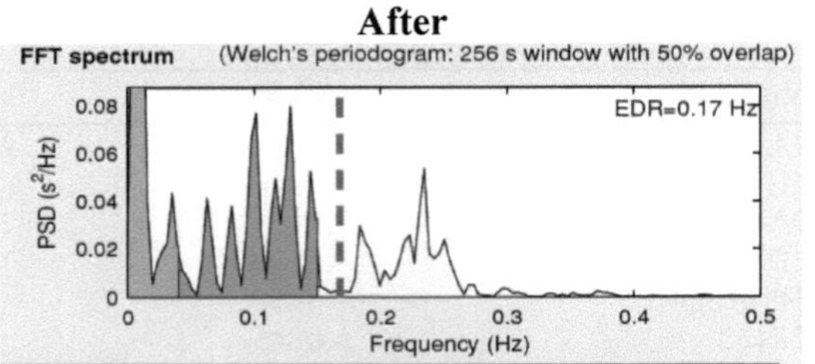

Frequency Band	Peak (Hz)	Power (ms^2)	Power (%)	Power (n.u.)
VLF (0–0.04 Hz)	0.0078	3385	41.0	
LF (0.04–0.15 Hz)	0.1289	3048	37.0	62.7
HF (0.15–0.4 Hz)	0.2344	1812	22.0	37.3
Total		8246		
LF/HF		1.682		

Fig.5. HRV frequency domain analysis result

IV. Conclusions

An important role in maintaining orthostatic homeostasis it has the autonomic nervous system. It is considered that under physiological conditions to lower blood pressure baroreceptors are activated, that initiate pressor reflex sympathetic influence of what is to increase the peripheral vessels, resulting in vasoconstriction and increased blood pressure respectively. This maintains adequate cerebral perfusion and avoids loss of consciousness. When these compensating mechanisms reach critical level, are inadequate to maintain continuous hemodynamic parameters (bradycardia, systemic hypotension) leading to decreased cerebral perfusion, frequently occurring after stroke. These patients also states restlessness, anxiety marked. Anxiety is associated with hyperventilation suggesting the role of the limbic system in the respiratory pattern. Hypocapnic hyperventilation that accompanies it can induce cerebral vasoconstriction exaggerated, increased peripheral vasodilation causing cerebral hypo perfusion and systemic hypotension. Co-monitoring blood pressure, HRV, respiratory rate and oxygen saturation can bring valuable information on cardiovascular reactivity in patients after stroke but also on the effectiveness of therapy, as MT.

Regarding the results, it has been shown that incorporating mirror therapy into the conventional stroke rehabilitation program during the early stages of treatment, but also in early chronic stroke and applying it for a sufficiently long period might generate a supplementary improvement of the patient. Evolution of motor parameters during our study was good all patients showing improvements of movements. There were changes in LF / HF ratio (HRV analysis in frequency domain), the vast majority of patients with increasing the number of sessions included in MT, but in the absence of correlation with information neurological we cannot draw certain conclusions.

Conflict of Interest

The authors declare that they have no conflict of interest.

References

1. Muzaffar T., Wadhwa RK, Borah D., Laisram N., Kothari SY. Evaluation of mirror therapy for upper limb rehabilitation in stroke. *IJPMR September 2013*; Vol 24(3): 63-9;
2. Fukumura K., *et al.* Influence of mirror therapy on human motor cortex. Int J Neurosci 2007; 117: 1039-48;
3. Andriţoi D, Matei D, Luca C, Corciova C, Ciorap R, (2015) Preliminary study of HR analysis on patients recovering after stroke, 9th International Symposium on Advanced Topics in Electrical Engineering (ATEE), 7-9 mai Bucureşti, p. 23-26;
4. Luca M. C., Matei D., Ignat B., Popescu C. D., (2015) Mirror therapy enhances upper extremity motor recovery in stroke patients, Acta Neurologica Belgica 2015, ISSN 0300-9009 Acta Neurol Belg DOI 10.1007/s13760-015-0465-5;
5. Pomazan V. M., Petcu L. C., Sintea S. R., Ciorap R., (2009) Active Data Transportation and Processing for Chronic Diseases Remote Monitoring, International Conference on Signal Processing Systems - ICSPS 2009, p.853 – 857, DOI: 10.1109/ICSPS.2009.120;
6. Andriţoi D., David V., Ciorap R., (2014) Dynamics Analysis of Heart Rate during Magneto-Therapy Session, International Conference and Exposition on Electrical and Power Engineering (EPE 2014), 16-18 October 2014, Iasi, Romania, p.514-517;
7. Munteanu M., Bechet P., Rusu C., Micu D.D., Munteanu R.A., Moga R., Amza C. (2014) Application of Virtual Instrumentation for Transmitting and Processing ECG Signals, IFMBE Proceedings of the 4 th International Conference on Advancements of Medicine and Health Care through Technology, Springer, 5th – 7th June 2014, Cluj-Napoca, Romania, p. 215-218;
8. Andriţoi D., David V., Ciorap R., Branzilă M., (2013) Recording and Processing ECG Signal During Magnetotherapy Procedures, ENVIRONMENTAL ENGINEERING AND MANAGEMENT JOURNAL, Volume: 12, Issue: 6, Pages:1231-1238 , Published: jun 2013.

Assessment of Nerve Fibers Dysfunction through Current Perception Threshold Measurement in Diabetic Peripheral Neuropathy

G.V. Inceu[1], G Roman[1 2] and I.A. Veresiu[1 2]

[1] "Iuliu Hatieganu" University of Medicine and Pharmacy, Cluj-Napoca, Romania
[2] Clinical Center of Diabetes, Nutrition, Metabolic Diseases, Cluj-Napoca, Romania

Abstract— **Diabetic neuropathy is a group of clinical syndromes that may occur separately or in various combinations and may affect various components of the nervous system. The involvement of different types of nerve fibers in the natural history of diabetic neuropathy is selective, being considered that the first affected in diabetic neuropathy are small unmyelinated nerve fibers and by measuring the current perceptions threshold (using the Neurometer®) we can quantify the status of three different types of nerve fibers. The aims of our study were to assess diabetic peripheral neuropathy (DPN) by measuring the rapid current perception threshold (R-CPT) using Neurometer, to estimate the prevalence of DPN using this method, and to analyze the possible correlation between R-CPT and clinical, biochemical and metabolic parameters.**

In our study, 52.6% of patients had abnormal (R-CPT) values to at least one of the three frequencies used (2000 Hz, 250 Hz, 5 Hz). Our results showed higher anthropometric parameters, higher values of glycated hemoglobin (p=0.004) and lipid fractions and higher percentage of diabetic retinopathy (p <0.001) and peripheral artery disease (p = 0.001) in patients with abnormal R-CPT values that in patients with normal values. Hyperesthesia was present in a higher percentage when frequency of 5Hz was applied compared with frequency of 250 Hz or 2000 Hz. We found higher R-CPT values in patients with higher diabetes duration and we obtained positive and significant correlation between duration of diabetes and R-CPT values for all three frequencies of alternative current.

The results of this study provide valuable information on the types of nerve fibers affected in DPN. The study highlighted a number of positive risk factors associated with the presence of DPN and demonstrated correlations between duration of diabetes and the subpopulation of nerve fibers affected.

Keywords— **rapid current perception threshold, Neurometer, neuropathy**

I. Introduction

Diabetes mellitus is one of the most common non-communicable chronic disease, becoming a public health problem and taking epidemic proportions globally [1, 2]. Due to its chronic and progressive feature, the severity of specific chronic complications that induces and not least, due to the financial means for proper management, diabetes is a costly disease not only for those affected and their families but also for the healthcare systems [3, 4, 5, 6].

Diabetic peripheral neuropathy is a common complication of diabetes, more than half of diabetic patients being affected during lifetime [7]. Diabetes can affect all structures of the nervous system, autonomic and somatic, central and peripheral, but the most frequent form of diabetic neuropathy, encountered in the vast majority of diabetic patients, is the typical diabetic peripheral neuropathy (DPN) or diabetic sensory-motor polyneuropathy (DSPN), according to the most recent definition and classifications proposed by the expert panels of the Diabetic Neuropathy Study Group of the European Association for the Study of Diabetes (NEURODIAB) [8]. According to this definition, DSPN is a "symmetrical, length-dependent sensorimotor polyneuropathy induced by the metabolic and microvessel alterations as a result of chronic hyperglycemia exposure". Diabetic peripheral neuropathy is a major risk factor for diabetic foot ulcerations [9, 10, 11], and foot ulcer is the most common single precursor to lower extremity amputation among persons with diabetes [12, 13]. So, there is a body growing of evidence that diabetes complications are commonly acknowledged as the leading cause of the global amputation burden and contribute to between 25% and 90% of all amputations [14, 15].

Consensus definitions for DSPN consistently recommend a combination of neuropathic symptoms and signs, in addition to specific abnormalities in nerve conduction studies (NCS), as criteria for diagnosis [16] Even though nerve conductions studies are considered the golden standard for the diagnosis of diabetic neuropathy, only large myelinated nerve fibers can be assessed using this method, while in diabetic neuropathy it was stated that small nerve fibers dysfunction precedes the involvement of large nerve fibers [17]. However, small fibers can be assessed objectively by quantifying intra-epidermal nerve fiber density (IENFD) in skin biopsies [18], which is an invasive procedure, or by corneal confocal microscopy [19, 20, 21].

Measurement of the current perception threshold (CPT) using the Neurometer® (Neurotron Inc., Baltimore, Maryland, USA) is a useful technique for assessing diabetic peripheral neuropathy [22, 23, 24, 25]. This method has the advantage to be able to quantify three different types of nerve fibers: Aβ, Aδ, and C fibers by using different electric stim-

S. Vlad and N.M. Roman (eds.), *International Conference on Advancements of Medicine and Health Care through Technology; 12th - 15th October 2016, Cluj-Napoca, Romania,*
IFMBE Proceedings 59,
DOI: 10.1007/978-3-319-52875-5_6

ulus frequencies (2,000, 250, and 5 Hz, respectively). Aβ fibers are large myelinated nerve fibers associated with touch and pressure sensation and C fibers play an important role in the autonomic nervous system and conduct impulses for temperature and pain.

II. OBJECTIVES

A. To assess diabetic peripheral neuropathy by measuring the current perception threshold using Neurometer
B. To estimate the prevalence of diabetic peripheral neuropathy by this method in the study group
C. To analyze the possible correlation between current perception threshold and clinical, biochemical and metabolic parameters

III. MATERIAL AND METHODS

In this observational cross-sectional study, were included 150 people with type 2 diabetes treated at Unirea Medical Center from Cluj-Napoca, between 2009-2011 and at Diabetes Clinical Center Cluj-Napoca between August-October 2012. Inform consent was obtained from all the participants. All the patients were evaluated in terms of anthropometric and metabolic measurement and were assessed for the rapid-current perception threshold (R-CPT) using the Neurometer®.

The Neurometer® generates an alternative current (AC) stimulus, which was applied at the right hallux using two golden plated electrodes, and the subject was instructed to press a button until a stimulus was detected at the site of the electrode and then to release the button. At each test site, three different frequencies of 2000, 250 and 5Hz of AC current were applied to stimulate large myelinated alpha beta fibers, small myelinated alpha delta fibers and small unmyelinated C fibers, respectively, and the Neurometer® generates R-CPT readings based on the minimal strength of (AC) stimulus that the patient can detect. For each frequency (2000, 250 and 5Hz), an R-CPT value was generated and ranged from 1 to 25. Values ranging from 6 to 13 were considered normal, values between 1 to 5 indicate hyperesthesia (increased sensation) while the values between 14 and 25 show hypoesthesia (decreased sensation). Both hyperesthesia and hypoesthesia reflect the presence of diabetic sensory neuropathy.

Statistical analysis was performed using SPSS 15.0 (SPSS Inc, Chicago, USA). The normality of variables distribution was evaluated using Kolmogorov–Smirnov test. Continuous data were expressed as means +/– standard deviation when normally distributed or as median for non-parametric data. Qualitative data were expressed as numbers and percentages. Group comparisons of all variables were performed using t-test for groups with normally distributed data, and Mann–Whitney test for groups with not normally distributed data. A ***p*** values less than 0.05 was considered statistically significant.

IV. RESULTS

The study group included 150 patients with type 2 diabetes who met the inclusion criteria. Of these, 50.7% (76) were female, and 49.3% (74) were males. The characteristics of the study group are presented in table 1.

Table 1 The characteristics of the study group

Parameter	Mean±SD	Minim	Maxim
Age (years)	58.8±10.71	21	82
Diabetes duration (years)	7.02±6.35	0	38
Weight (kg)	87.31±16.52	56	148
BMI (kg/m^2)	30.82±5.4	18.5	46.3
WC (cm)	107.81±13.31	76	150
HbA1c (%)	7.7±1.4	5.6	14.2
Total cholesterol (mg/dl)	179.78±40.77	52	314
HDL cholesterol (mg/dl)	44.82±11.69	12	100
Triglycerides (mg/dl)	164.42±85.59	34	691
LDL cholesterol (mg/dl)	102.07±35.03	14	195.8

HbA1c-glycated hemoglobin, BMI-body mass index, WC-waist circumference. Data are presented as means ± SD (standard deviation)

We divided the patients in two categories, depending on the R-CPT values, namely:
- Patients without DPN: R-CPT values between 6 and 13 (included) for all three AC frequencies
- Patients with DPN: R-CPT values between 1-5 (defining hyperesthesia) and between14-25 (defining hypoesthesia).

In our study 52.6% of patients had abnormal R-CPT to at least one of the AC frequency applied.

We noticed that, in patients with abnormal R-CPT values, diabetes duration, BMI, waist circumference, HbA1c, total cholesterol and LDL cholesterol were statistically significantly higher than in patients with normal R-CPT values (Mann-Whitney test). Clinical and biochemical parameters in the study groups are presented in table 2.

Patients with abnormal R-CPT values showed a statistically significant higher percentage of diabetic retinopathy ($p < 0.001$) and peripheral artery disease ($p = 0.001$) compared with patients normal R-CPT values (table 3).

We analyzed the patients in the study group based on the presence of hyper- and hypoesthesia when applying 2000Hz, 250Hz and 5Hz AC stimulus, and we noticed that hyperesthesia was present in a higher percentage (15.3%) when frequency of 5Hz was applied compared with frequency of 250 Hz (6%) or 2000 Hz (4%). The data are presented in table 4.

Table 2 Clinical and biochemical parameters in the study groups

Parameter	Patients with DPN	Patient without DPN	p-value
Age (years)	63(56-69)	57.28±11.13	0.085
Diabetes duration (years)	9(4-13)	6(4-10)	0.001
Weight (kg)	88.59±17.13	83(75-95)	0.301
BMI (kg/m²)	31.79±5.47	29.75±5.14	0.037
WC (cm)	110.65±13.31	104.65±12.68	0.01
HbA1c (%)	7.94±1.33	7.41±1.4	0.004
Total cholesterol (mg/dl)	175.3±43.21	184.75±37.54	0.045
HDL cholesterol (mg/dl)	42(37-48)	45(39-50)	0.034
Triglycerides (mg/dl)	172.06±95.82	155.92±72.28	0.352
LDL cholesterol (mg/dl)	97.01±36.96	107.7±32.08	0.041

HbA1c-glicated hemoglobin. Data are presented as mean or median ± SD

Table 3 The presence of comorbidities and chronic complications in the study groups

Parameter	DPN	No DPN	p	OR
Hypertension	83.5%	71.8%	0.084	1.99 95% IC (1.1 – 4.38)
Dyslipidemia	87.3%	80.3%	0.238	1.7 (95% IC 0.7 – 4.10)
Diabetic retinopathy	43%	9.9%	<0.001	7.11 (95% IC 2.87 – 17.57)
PAD	20.3%	2.8%	0.001	8.90 (95% IC 1.97 – 40.28)

DPN-diabetic peripheral neuropathy, PAD-peripheral artery disease, OR-odds ratio, IC-interval of confidence

Table 4 The presence of hypo- and hyperesthesia in the study group

AC Frequency	Normal R-CPT	Hyperesthesia	Hypoesthesia
2000 Hz	72.6	4	23.3
250 Hz	68	6	26
5 Hz	57.3	15.3	27.3

Data are presented as percent.

We decided the allocation of study patients in three categories, depending on diabetes duration: less than 5 years (66 patients), between 5 and 10 years (49 patients) and more than 10 years (35 patients).

We further analyzed the R-CPT values in the three groups of patients according to diabetes duration (table 5).

Table 5 The average values of R-CPT according to diabetes duration

	Diabetes duration (years)			
	<5	5-10	>10	p
2000 Hz	10.71±4.19	11.53±4.57	14.68±5.78	0.02
250 Hz	11±4.52	12.29±4.96	13.88±5.34	0.15
5 Hz	10.23±4.47	12.24±5.41	13.4±5.95	0.05

We obtained a R-CPT value significantly statistical higher (p = 0.02) when 2000 Hz stimulus was applied in patients with diabetes duration more than 10 years compared with patients with a lower diabetes duration.

R-CPT values were significantly lower in patients with a diabetes duration less than 5 years, compared with the patients from the other groups, when 5 Hz frequency AC stimulus was applied (p=0.05).

After calculating the Spearman correlation coefficient, we found a positive correlation between duration of diabetes and R-CPT values. The correlation was statistically significant for 2000 and 250 Hz frequencies (Spearman correlation coefficient 0.270 and 0.248) (table 6) and highly statistically significant for 5 Hz frequency (Spearman correlation coefficient 0.292) (figure 1).

Table 6 Correlations between diabetes duration and the three AC stimulus frequency (Spearman correlation coefficient)

AC frequency	Diabetes duration (Spearman Coefficient)
2000 Hz	.270(*)
250 Hz	.248(*)
5 Hz	.292(**)

** Highly significant correlation, p <0.001
* Significant correlation, p <0.05

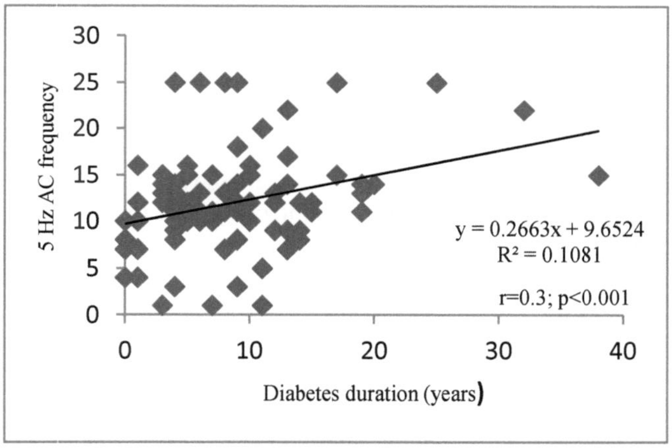

Fig. 1 Correlation between diabetes duration and 5 Hz AC frequency

Regarding the antihyperglycemic therapy, a statistically significant higher percentage of patients with DPN (62.1%, p = 0.002) were receiving insulin therapy (alone or in combination with oral antidiabetic agents), while more than half of patients without diabetic neuropathy were treated only with oral or noninsulin therapy (60.6%).

V. Discussions

In our study, 52.6% of patients had abnormal R-CPT values to at least one of the three frequencies used.

In the evolution of diabetic neuropathy, hyperesthesia is considered the first manifestation that appears, followed by hypoesthesia [26]. In our study, hyperesthesia was present in a much higher percentage (15.3%) when frequency of 5 Hz was applied compared with frequency of 250 Hz (6%) or 2000 Hz (4%), suggesting that the frequency of 5 Hz has a higher sensitivity in detecting abnormalities compared to the other two frequencies. This finding may suggest that impairment of small unmyelinated nerve fibers precedes the large myelinated nerve fibers damage, making it consistent with the existing evidence in the literature [18, 27].

Patients with abnormal R-CPT values presented in a higher percentage hypertension, dyslipidemia, diabetic retinopathy, peripheral artery disease, but the statistical significance was reached only for the last two conditions. In his work, Matsumoto and co analyzed the relationship between the CPT values obtained when 2000 Hz AC frequency was applied and severity of diabetic retinopathy, demonstrating that these values were significantly higher in patients with proliferative diabetic retinopathy compared with patients without diabetic retinopathy, suggesting that progression of diabetic neuropathy is accompanied by that of diabetic retinopathy [22]. The same results were also described by Koo Kyung Bo and co, showing a significant association between the presence of diabetic neuropathy and the severity of diabetic retinopathy [28]. Moulik and co [29] have shown in their study that 40 to 60% of patients with foot ulcers had also peripheral artery disease, a disorder which confers a high risk of amputation and mortality. In another study [30] conducted on 156 Swedes type 2 diabetic subjects, it was found that in patients with peripheral sensory neuropathy, peripheral artery disease was three times more common (52%) than in patients without diabetic neuropathy (16%, $p = 0.001$). In the same study it was demonstrated that the incidence of diabetic neuropathy increases with the severity of diabetic retinopathy. Regarding the association between diabetic neuropathy and hypertension, Jarmuzewska and co [31] have demonstrated a strong association, independent of other risk factors, between the two disorders in patients with type 2 diabetes, with a relatively short duration of diabetes.

Patient with abnormal R-CPT values had higher BMI and waist circumference compared with patients with normal R-CPT values. Wang and co [32] conducted a study on 552 type 2 diabetic patients from Saudi Arabia, aimed to assess the prevalence of diabetic neuropathy and the correlations between this microvascular complication and certain parameters. An important conclusion of this study was that duration of diabetes, abdominal obesity, blood glucose values, white blood cells and serum creatinine were associated with a higher risk of diabetic neuropathy. Also, Ziegler and co [33] in The MONICA / KORA Augsburg S2 and S3 Surveys have shown that, in the diabetic studied population, DPN was associated with age, waist circumference and peripheral artery disease, suggesting that abdominal obesity and peripheral artery disease could be important targets of the prevention strategies for diabetic neuropathy.

Another finding of our study was an unsatisfactory glycemic control, reflected by a mean glycated hemoglobin value of 7.94%, in patients with DPN, compared with patients without DPN (mean HbA1c=7.41%, p=0,004). Our results are consistent with the existing evidence. A study conducted on 141 diabetic patients who were admitted on a Neurology department, has shown that in patients with DPN, fasting blood glucose and HbA1c were significantly higher ($p < 0.05$) compared with patients without diabetic neuropathy [34]. The results of another study [35] involving 294 type 2 diabetic patients, demonstrated that age, a poor socioeconomic status, insulin therapy, a long duration of diabetes and poor glycemic control, were identified as risk factors for diabetic neuropathy.

When we applied 2000 Hz electrical stimulus, we obtained a mean R-CPT value significantly higher in patients with diabetes duration more than 10 years, compared with patients with a lower diabetes duration and the R-CPT values after application of 5 Hz frequency stimulus, were significantly lower in patients with a duration of diabetes less than 5 years. Consistent with our result, Young and co demonstrated in a multicenter cross-sectional study, which included 6487 patients with type 1 and type 2 diabetes, that the prevalence of diabetic neuropathy increases with age and duration of diabetes, being present in over half of patients over 60 years of age [36].

We noticed in our study that a significantly greater proportion of patients with abnormal R-CPT (62.1%, $p = 0.002$) were receiving insulin (alone or in combination with oral agents), while more than half of patients without diabetic neuropathy were treated only with non-insulin therapy (60.6%). Our results correlate with those obtained by Wang and co [32] in their study conducted on a population of 552 patients with diabetes, and the results showed that in insulin treated subjects, the risk of diabetic neuropathy was higher compared to patients treated with oral antidiabetic agents. Another study involving 294 subjects with type 2 diabetes demonstrated that insulin treatment is an independent risk factor for diabetic neuropathy [35].

VI. Conclusions

The results of this study provide valuable information on the types of nerve fibers affected in diabetic peripheral neuropathy. The study highlighted a number of positive risk factors associated with the presence of diabetic neuropathy and demonstrated correlations between duration of diabetes and the subpopulation of nerve fibers affected.

The involvement of nerve fibers in the evolution of diabetic neuropathy is selective, so it is important to be able to apply the proper technique in order to detect, in a non-invasively and quickly way, the exact nerve fiber type affected. And the Neurometer proved its ability to assess and quantify the functional status and integrity of the three nerve fibers types.

Conflict of Interest

The authors declare that they have no conflict of interest.

Statement of Human and Animal Rights

The procedures involving human subjects conducted in this study were in accordance with the ethical standards of the responsible committee on human experimentation (institutional and national) and with the Helsinki Declaration of 1975, as revised in 2000 and 2008.

References

1. Wild S, Roglic G, Green A et al. (2004) Global Prevalence of Diabetes: Estimates for the year 2000 and projections for 2030. Diabetes Care 27 (5):1047–1053
2. International Diabetes Federation (2015) IDF Diabetes Atlas, 7th edn. International Diabetes Federation. Available at: http://www.diabetesatlas.org/. Published 2015. Accessed august 30, 2016.
3. Seuring T, Archangelidi O and M. Suhrcke (2015) The Economic Costs of Type 2 Diabetes: A Global Systematic Review. Pharmacoeconomics 33 (8):811–831
4. American Diabetes Association (2008) Economic Costs of Diabetes in the U.S. in 2007. Diabetes Care 31 (3):596–615
5. American Diabetes Association (2013) Economic costs of diabetes in the U.S. in 2012. Diabetes Care 36 (4):1033–1046
6. Zhang P, Zhang X, Brown J et al.(2010) Global healthcare expenditure on diabetes for 2010 and 2030. Diabetes Res. Clin. Pract 87(3):293–301.
7. Boulton A J M, Vinik A I, Arezzo J C et al. (2005) Diabetic Neuropathies: A statement by the American Diabetes Association. Diabetes Care 28(4):956–962
8. Tesfaye S, Boulton A J M, Dyck P J et al. (2010) Diabetic neuropathies: Update on definitions, diagnostic criteria, estimation of severity, and treatments. Diabetes Care 33(10):2285-2293
9. Frykberg R G, Zgonis T, Armstrong D G, Driver V R et al. (2005) Diabetic foot disorders. A clinical practice guideline (2006 revision). J. Foot Ankle Surg 45(5):S1–66
10. Boulton A J M, Kirsner R S, L. Vileikyte (2004) Neuropathic Diabetic Foot Ulcers. N Engl J Med 351:48-55
11. Abbott C A, Carrington A L, Ashe H et al. (2002) The North-West Diabetes Foot Care Study: incidence of, and risk factors for, new diabetic foot ulceration in a community-based patient cohort. Diabet. Med 19(5):377–84
12. Lavery L A, Armstrong D G, Harkless L B (1996) Classification of diabetic foot wounds. J. Foot Ankle Surg 35(6):528–31
13. American Diabetes Association (1999) Consensus Development Conference on Diabetic Foot Wound Care: 7-8 April 1999, Boston, Massachusetts. American Diabetes Association. Diabetes Care 22(8): 354–60
14. Lazzarini P A, O'Rourke S R, Russell A W et al. (2012) What are the key conditions associated with lower limb amputations in a major Australian teaching hospital?. J. Foot Ankle Res 5(1):12
15. Ahmad N, Thomas G N, Gill P et al. (2016) The prevalence of major lower limb amputation in the diabetic and non-diabetic population of England 2003-2013. Diabetes Vasc. Dis. Res 13(5):348–353
16. Dyck P J, Albers J W, Andersen H (2011) Diabetic polyneuropathies: update on research definition, diagnostic criteria and estimation of severity. Diabetes. Metab. Res. Rev 27(7):620–628
17. Sumner C J, Sheth S, Griffin J W et al. (2003) The spectrum of neuropathy in diabetes and impaired glucose tolerance. Neurology 60(1):108–111
18. Umapathi T, Tan W L, Loke S C et al. (2007) Intraepidermal nerve fiber density as a marker of early diabetic neuropathy. Muscle Nerve 35(5):591–598
19. Tavakoli M, Petropoulos I N, Malik R A (2013) Corneal confocal microscopy to assess diabetic neuropathy: an eye on the foot. J. Diabetes Sci. Technol 7(5):1179–89
20. Tavakoli M, Marshall A, Pitceathly R et al. (2010) Corneal confocal microscopy: a novel means to detect nerve fibre damage in idiopathic small fibre neuropathy. Exp. Neurol 223(1):245–50
21. Inceu G, Demea H, Veresiu I A (2014) Corneal Confocal Microscopy – A Novel, Noninvasive Method to Assess Diabetic Peripheral Neuropathy. Rom. J. Diabetes Nutr. Metab. Dis 21(4):319–326
22. Matsutomo R, Takebayashi K, Aso Y (2005) Assessment of Peripheral Neuropathy Using Measurement of the Current Perception Threshold with the Neurometer(R) in Patients with Type 2 Diabetes Mellitus. J. Int. Med. Res.33(4):442–453
23. Nather A, Keng Lin W, Aziz Z et al. (2011) Assessment of sensory neuropathy in patients with diabetic foot problems. Diabet. Foot Ankle 2:6367
24. Nather A, Neo S H, Chionh S B et al. (2008) Assessment of sensory neuropathy in diabetic patients without diabetic foot problems. J. Diabetes Complications 22(2):126–131
25. Inceu G V, Veresiu I A (2015) Measurement of Current Perception Thresholds Using the Neurometer® – Applicability in Diabetic Neuropathy. Clujul Med 88(4):449-452
26. Takekuma K, Ando F, Niino N et al. (2002) Prevalence of hyperesthesia detected by current perception threshold test in subjects with glucose metabolic impairments in a community. Intern. Med 41(12):1124–9
27. Malik R A, Tesfaye S, Newrick P G et al. (2005) Sural nerve pathology in diabetic patients with minimal but progressive neuropathy. Diabetologia 48(3):578–85
28. Koo B K, Ohn J H, Kwak S et al. (2014) Assessment of Diabetic Polyneuropathy and Autonomic Neuropathy Using Current Perception Threshold in Korean Patients with Diabetes Mellitus. Diabetes Metab. J 38:285–293
29. Moulik K P, Tonga R M, Gill G V (2003) Amputation and Mortality in New-Onset Diabetic Foot Ulcers Stratified by

Etiology. Diabetes Care 26(11):3199-3200.
30. Kärvestedt L, Mårtensson E, Grill V et al. (2009) Peripheral Sensory Neuropathy Associates With Micro-or Macroangiopathy Results from a population-based study of type 2 diabetic patients in Sweden. Diabetes Care 32(2):317-322.
31. Jarmuzewska EA, Ghidoni A, Mangoni AA (2007) Hypertension and sensorimotor peripheral neuropathy in type 2 diabetes. Eur Neurol 57(2):91-95.
32. Wang DD, Bakhotmah BA, Hu FB et al. (2014) Prevalence and Correlates of Diabetic Peripheral Neuropathy in a Saudi Arabic Population: A Cross-Sectional Study. PLoS One 9(9):e106935. DOI 10.1371/journal.pone.0106935
33. Ziegler D, Rathmann W, Dickhaus T, Meisinger C et al. (2008) Prevalence of Polyneuropathy in Pre- Diabetes and Diabetes Is Associated With Abdominal Obesity and Macroangiopathy The MONICA/KORA Augsburg Surveys S2 and S3 FOR THE KORA STUDY GROUP. Diabetes Care 31:464-469
34. Suljic E, Kulasin I, Alibegovic V (2013) "Assessment of Diabetic Polyneuropathy in Inpatient Care: Fasting Blood Glucose, HbA1c, Electroneuromyography and Diabetes Risk Factors. Acta Inform Med 21(2):123–126
35. Mørkrid K, Ali L, Hussain A (2010) Risk factors and prevalence of diabetic peripheral neuropathy: A study of type 2 diabetic outpatients in Bangladesh. Int J Diabetes Dev Ctries 30(1):11-17.
36. Young M J, Boulton A J, MacLeod A F et al. (1993) A multicentre study of the prevalence of diabetic peripheral neuropathy in the United Kingdom hospital clinic population. Diabetologia 36(2):150–154

Author: Georgeta Victoria Inceu
Institute: "IULIU HATIEGANU" University of Medicine and Pharmacy
Street: 2-4 Clinicilor Street
City: Cluj-Napoca
Country: Romania
Email: georgetainceu@yahoo.com

Implantable Ports in Oncology

B. Micu[1], C. Micu[2], T-R. Pop[1] and N. Constantea[1]

[1] "Iuliu Hateganu" University of Medicine and Pharmacy/5th Surgical Department, Cluj-Napoca, Romania
[2] "Iuliu Hateganu" University of Medicine and Pharmacy/Department of Anatomy and Embryology, Cluj-Napoca, Romania

Abstract— **The paper analyze the method used by us in insertion of implantable ports for chemotherapy (port-a-cat/PAC) and to evaluate intra and postoperative complications. The authors conducted a prospective study in which we included patients operated at the Fifth Surgical Clinic of the Municipal Hospital Cluj-Napoca. Implantable chambers was installed in all cases, by ecoguided puncturing the internal jugular vein. Of the 250 patients included in the study, 97 patients (38.8%) had breast cancer, 26 (10.4%) lung cancer, 25 (10%) colorectal cancer, 22 patients (8.8%) neoplasms in ENT. Patients were aged between 19 and 74 years. 58% of patients were stage IV. The main intraoperative complications were incorrect puncturing / introduction of the catheter. Among postoperative complications were internal jugular vein thrombosis (1.2%), abscesses at the site of implantation (1.6%), extravasation of the port (2%). The method of insertion of implantable chamber through internal jugular vein, used by us, has very good results, the number of intra and postoperative complications is minimal, also avoiding catheter breakage, hemothorax and pneumothorax.**

Keywords— **implantabil ports, chemotherapy, venous access, surgery, postoperative complications**

I. Introduction

Implantable ports (or port-a-cath/PAC) are medical devices consisting of a port (reservoir compartment) and a catheter. The port is mounted subcutaneously and the catheter connects the port to a central vein. The port contains a special membrane that can be punctured over 3000 times. These devices are used to administer long-term injectable drug treatment or to deliver chemotherapy to cancer patients. The main advantages of implantable ports are the preservation of venous capital, the easier venous access, lower risk of extravasation of chemotherapeutic agents, the ability to inject irritants that can cause skin necrosis (cisplatin, epirubicin, paclitaxel) while allowing more comfort to both patients and medical staff [1]. Ports can be made of titanium, stainless steel or plastic and can be single chamber or dual chamber. The catheter can have different diameters and lengths and it is made of polyurethane or silicone [2]. It can be inserted into a central vein (subclavian vein, external and internal jugular vein, cephalic vein, basilica vein, femoral vein) by either open access or puncture: using the classic Seldinger technique or an ultrasound-guided method (ultrasound, fluoroscopy or electrocardiograpy) [1,3]. Regardless of the access path, the insertion of the port and catheter is performed in the operating room in aseptic and antiseptic conditions specific for vascular approach. Intraoperative and postoperative complications may occur due to the fact that this is a surgical procedure and it involves the introduction of a foreign body into the body (the port is implanted under the skin and the catheter is inserted into a vein). The main intraoperative complications may include: incorrect placement of the catheter, bleeding, cardiac rhythm disturbances, puncture of the carotid artery, pneumothorax, hemothorax, or even death. Among postoperative complications, the following can occur: infections of the skin and subcutaneous tissue, subcutaneous abscess, venous thrombosis, sepsis, pneumothorax, hemothorax, migration of the port, externalization of the port, rotation of the port, occlusion or migration of the catheter, catheter fracture, catheter disconnection, difficult removal of the catheter. Complications vary in type and frequency depending on the method used in mounting the port and the catheter. However, morbidity ranges from 8.6 to 31% with a mortality of up to 1.4% [1,2,3,4]. The method used in our clinic involves the insertion of the catheter into the internal jugular vein via ultrasound-guided puncture, and the placement of the port in the subcutaneous tissue in the anterior chest. The aim of our study was to analyze this method in delivering chemotherapy (port-a-cath/PAC) and to assess the likelihood of intraoperative and postoperative complications.

II. Materials and Methods

To achieve these objectives we conducted a prospective study which included cancer patients who underwent surgery at the Fifth Surgical Clinic of the Municipal Hospital in Cluj-Napoca between 2012 and 2015. Surgeries were performed by the same surgical team. Following local anesthesia, a lateral-cervical incision performed under ultrasound guidance will allow the puncture and cannulation of the internal jugular vein. The length of the inserted catheter was calculated using Czepizak's formula [5], which is based on patient height. After the longitudinal incision in the anterior pectoral region, the port is inserted into the subcutaneous tissue. The interventions lasted between 20 and 60 minutes. To check catheter placement, chest x-ray was per-

S. Vlad and N.M. Roman (eds.), *International Conference on Advancements of Medicine and Health Care through Technology; 12th - 15th October 2016, Cluj-Napoca, Romania,*
IFMBE Proceedings 59,
DOI: 10.1007/978-3-319-52875-5_7

formed in all patients 30-60 minutes after the surgical procedure. The correct positioning of the catheter was assessed in accordance with the criteria described by Petersen [6]. Postoperative follow-up of patients was performed for 6 months and consisted in a general clinical examination performed once every 30 days. Cervical ultrasound and chest X-ray were performed if there was a clinical suspicion of venous thrombosis or if patients experienced local pain, swelling, local edema or possible rupture or occlusion of the catheter or port. Complications were divided into: - intraoperative complications (failure, incorrect puncturing, puncturing of the carotid artery, arrhythmias, hemorrhage, pneumothorax or hemothorax) and - postoperative complications (thrombosis of the internal jugular vein, superior vena cava syndrome, abscesses at the implantation site, externalization, pneumothorax, local hematoma, hemothorax, downtime, extravasation, catheter rupture) [7].

Patient medical data was analyzed regarding the location of the primary tumor, disease stage, body mass index, oncologic history (preoperative chemotherapy, cervical-thoracic radiotherapy), duration of surgery, intra and postoperative complications that occurred, time until first use and the reasons and the incidence of premature removal (port removal program before the end of chemotherapy infusion). The results of parametric and nonparametric data were expressed as median values and range. Statistical analysis was performed using MedCalc version 14.8.1. and the significance level was $p \leq 0.05$

III. Results

Between 2012 and 2015, ports were implanted to deliver chemotherapy in 250 patients aged 19 to 74 years (median age 62) at the Fifth Surgical Clinic of Cluj-Napoca Municipal Hospital. Of these patients, 153 (61.2%) were women and 97 (38.8%) were men. Tumor location is presented in Table 1.

The catheter was inserted in the right internal jugular vein in 239 (95.4%) cases and in the left internal jugular vein in 11 (4.6%) cases. Of the 250 cancer patients, during implantation, 145 were in stage IV and 42% were in stages I-III. The main intraoperative complications that occurred in our study group were represented by: port implantation failure (4 cases / 1.6%), incorrect placement in the subclavian vein (2 cases / 0.8%), puncture of the common carotid artery (2 cases / 0.8%), occurrence of paroxysmal tachycardia during catheterisation (1 case / 0.4%). The presence of hemothorax or pneumothorax was not detected in any of the cases. In case of incorrect catheter placement (one intraoperative case and one case identified following chest x-ray) the catheter was repositioned immediately after the error was detected. In case of accidental carotid artery puncture (in both cases the problem was identified intraoperatively by the presence of red arterial blood at the injection site) the needle was quickly removed and mechanical compression was applied for about 5 minutes; after bleeding has stopped and the presence and size of the hematoma was identified (ultrasound), jugular vein puncture and correct placement of the catheter were resumed, ensuring 100% success rate.

Table 1. Location of primary tumor

Location of tumor	Number of patiens	Percentage (%)
Brest	97	38,8
Pulmonary	26	10,4
Colorectal	25	10
ENT	22	8,8
Ovary	16	6,4
Stomach	13	5,2
Esophagus	10	4
Sarcomas	10	4
Urogenital	9	3,6
Pancreas	6	2,4
Melanoma	4	1,6
Cervix	4	1,6
Leukemia	3	1,2
Peritoneum	2	0,8
Gallbladder	1	0,4
Limfoma	1	0,4
Eyes	1	0,4

These situations appeared when the normal anatomy of the region was affected by surgery in the laterocervical region (cancers of the head and neck). Cardiac arrhythmia (paroxysmal tachycardia) was identified in one patient (72 years old). In this case, when inserting the catheter, probably due to the introduction of the catheter over a much too long distance, it punctured the right atrium and led to the stimulation of the sinus node, which caused heart rhythm disorders. The catheter was removed and it was safely reinserted after the resumption of normal heart rhythm. Postoperative complications that occurred during the 6-month follow-up were the following: internal jugular vein thrombosis (2 cases / 0.8%), infection (8 cases / 3.2%), abscess at the implant site (4 cases / 1.6%), externalized port (5 cases / 2%), local hematoma (2 cases / 0.8%), non-functional implants (4 cases / 1.6%) with 2 cases of reimplantation, and extravasation (1 case / 0.4%).

In case of internal jugular vein thrombosis, patients accused localized pain in the right cervical region, accompanied by mild bulging and swelling of the region, three, respectively four months after surgery. The suspicion of thrombosis was confirmed by ultrasound. A CT angiography was also performed to exclude the presence of superior vena cava syndrome.

Abscesses at the implant site developed either by using the port in less than 7 days after the surgery or due to the immunosuppressive effects of preoperative chemotherapy or to locoregional radiotherapy performed preoperatively, tissues in these areas being extremely fragile. Externalization of the port occurred in five cases (three cases of pancreatic cancer, one case of stage IV colon cancer, one case of stage IV melanoma), 6 months postoperatively, probably because all these patients underwent home-based chemotherapy using elastomeric pumps, which add extra traction to the port and tissues, exerted continuously over 24 or 48 hours. In these cases, the port could not be preserved using surgical repositioning methods and had to be removed prematurely. Extravasation was detected in one case (stage IV gastric cancer), when chemotherapy was injected in the subcutaneous tissue around the port and due to its highly irritating effect, it caused necrosis of the tissue. Thus, we had to remove the port. The main causes for the premature removal of the port (before the end of chemotherapy) in our study group were represented by: externalization (5 cases), infection (12 cases), mechanical problems (4 cases), pain at the implantation site (3 cases), thrombosis (1 case), and extravasation (1 case). By analyzing the profile of patients with premature removal of the port, we noticed the presence of several predictive factors. Thus, the longer the duration of surgery, the higher the risk of obstruction (20%). Body mass index (BMI) also plays an important role in the occurrence of skin changes and mechanical problems.

A body mass index (BMI) greater than 32 causes a 15% incidence of skin changes and the percentage of mechanical port problems increases to 8%. Regarding patient history - ENT surgery caused skin changes in 10% of patients; cervical-thoracic radiation therapy resulted in a 10% increase in intraoperative complications and 14% increase in postoperative complications; preoperative chemotherapy determined a 10% increase in the incidence of complications (abscesses, hematomas). By analyzing the time until the first use of the port and the occurrence of complications, we noticed an increase in the number of complications when the port was used shortly after surgery (Table 2). The number of skin complications and infections decreases up to 0.7%, respectively 2.5%, when the port is first used 7 days after surgery.

Table 2. Time to first use

Time to first use (days)	0-3	4-7	>7
Skin modification	6,9%	4,1%	0,7%
Infection	8%	6,2%	2,5%

Data on premature removal and data regarding the first use of the port (Table 3) emphasize the fact that the incidence of premature port removal decreases if the port is only used for the first time 7 days after surgery (up to 1.9%; p = 0.05).

Table 3. Time to first use and premature withdrawal

	first use <7 days	first use>7days	p
Rate of premature withdrawal	3.5%	1,9%	0.05

IV. Discussions

The use of implantation ports to deliver chemotherapy by means of the ultrasound-guided catheterisation of the internal jugular vein did not result in the occurrence of intraoperative or postoperative complication such as pneumothorax or hemothorax. In the literature, there is a 2-4% frequency of pneumothorax, which is also influenced by the implantation method, directly associated with body mass index [2,8,9]. In our study, intraoperative complications were represented by the incorrect insertion of the catheter into the subclavian vein in 0.8% of cases and the accidental puncture of the common carotid artery in 0.8% of cases, while data in the literature indicate higher percentages for these complications, 7.6% and 4.3% [10]. Another type of intraoperative complication reported in the literature is the placement of the catheter in the right ventricle [11]. We used the right internal jugular vein approach more frequently than the left internal jugular vein approach because of the difficulties in left-side catheterization. The latter was only used when right-side approach was impossible to perform due to the lack of access (history of surgery with changes in local anatomy, right supraclavicular lymph nodes). The most common postoperative complications reported in the literature, occurring after port placement for chemotherapy are infections (0.7-7%) and venous thrombosis (1.5-13%) [7,10,12,13]. In our study, infections (4.8%) were associated with immunosuppression following chemotherapy performed preoperatively and short-timed, less than 7 days between surgery and the first use of the port. In these cases, the quick removal of the port is mandatory. Therefore, we recommend that the port is only implanted at least 14 days after the last chemotherapy session and WBC count should be greater than 3000 / mm^3 during surgery. We also suggest that the port should only be used 7 days after surgery. Internal jugular vein thrombosis occurred in two cases (0.8%) without subsequent superior vena cava syndrome. Patients responded well to anticoagulation therapy, without any requirements for the premature port removal, which only happened in one case when it was removed at the patient's request. We believe that internal jugular vein thrombosis does not require port removal if the patient does not develop superior vena cava syndrome and he/she responds well to anticoagulation therapy. In our study, the incidence of another postoperative complication – the externalization of the port (2%) – reached the upper limit of records from the literature [2,12,14], but it complied with the threshold recommended for this procedure by the Society of Interventional Radiology [14] . It occurred in 5 cases in which patients with home-based chemotherapy used elastomeric pumps continuously for 1-2 days. We recommend that the port should be implanted deeper and with additional and stronger fixation in these patients. Mechanical problems arising during the use of the implanted port were solved using conservative methods. In four cases, the port had to be removed prematurely (1.6%), but it was later repositioned using the same approach and the same vein, which is impossible when inserting the port into the cephalic vein [2,14]. Extravasation followed by necrosis occurred in only one case (0.8%). This type of complication has also been reported by other authors [12,14] and it required premature port removal.There was no evidence of catheter breakage or bending in our study. These complications have been reported in the literature, especially when using the Seldinger technique [2,14,]. Another important complication, the "pinch-off" syndrome (the catheter is compressed between the clavicle and the first rib), with 1.1-5% incidence in the literature [15], did not occur as a complication in any of the cases in our study.

V. Conclusions

To reduce the incidence of premature port removal it is necessary to reduce the incidence of infections and postoperative externalization. These objectives can be achieved by using the ultrasound-guided technique for internal jugular vein cannulation, which is also employed in our clinic. The use of this technique along with the avoidance of preoperative chemotherapy and preoperative cervical-thoracic radiotherapy, shorter duration of surgery and the first use of the port only seven days after surgery determine good results and reduce the number of intraoperative and postoperative complications, help avoid catheter breakage or the occurrence of pneumothorax / hemothorax, reduce the risk of infection and venous thrombosis, and thus improve quality of life in cancer patients undergoing chemotherapy.

Conflict of Interest

The authors declare that they have no conflicts of interest.

References

1. Ku YH, Kuo PH, Tsai YF, Huang WT, Lin MH, Tsao CJ. (2009) Port-A-Cath implantation using percutaneous puncture without guidance. Ann Surg Oncol. vol 16, no. 3, pp. 729-734.
2. Vandoni RE, Guerra A, Sanna P, Bogen M, Cavalli F, Gertsch P. (2009) Randomised comparison of complications from three different permanent central venous access systems. Swiss Med., pp. 313-316.
3. Biffi R, de Braud F, Orsi F, Pozzi S, Mauri S, Goldhirsch A, Nolè F, Andreoni B.(1998)Totally implantable central venous access ports for long- term chemotherapy. Ann Oncol., vol.9, no.7, pp. 767-773.
4. Marcy PY, Figl A (2010) Arm port implantation in cancer patients. Int J. of Clinical Oncology. vol.15, no.3, pp.328-330
5. Czepizak CA, O'Callaghan JM, Venus B. (1995) Evaluation of formulas for optimal positioning of central venous catheters. Chest, vol. 107, no. 6, pp.1662-1664.
6. Petersen J, Delaney JH, Brakstad MT, Rowbotham RK, Bagley CM Jr. (1999) Silicone venous access devices positioned with their tips high in the superior vena cava are more likely to malfunction.Am J Surg., vol.178, no. 1, pp. 38-41.
7. Walser (2012) Veous access ports: indications, technique, Cardiovasc Intervent Radiol., vol. 35, no. 4, pp. 751-764.
8. LaBella G, (2005) Port-A-Cath placement without the aid of fluoroscopy or localizing devices: a community hospital series. Cancer J., vol. 11, no.2, pp.157-159.
9. Shen-Gunther J, (2003) Outpatient implantation of a central venous access system in gynecologic oncology patients. J Reprod , vol 48, no.11, pp.875-881.
10. Rykov MY, (2016) Implantable venous ports in pediatric oncology. J Vasc Access.,vol.12, no.4, pp 345-347.
11. Wyles SM, Browne G, Gui GP. (2007) Pitfalls in Portacath location using the landmark technique: case report. Int Semin Surg Oncol.4:13
12. Aparna S, et all. (2015) Complications of chemoport in children with cancer: Experience of 54,100 catheter days from a tertiary cancer center of Southern India. South Asian J Cancer, vol. 4, pp.143-145
13. Binnebösel M, et all.(2009) Internal jugular vein thrombosis presenting as a painful neck mass due to a spontaneous dislocated subclavian port catheter as long-term complication. Cases J. 2:7991.
14. Gonda SJ, Li R. (2011) Principles of subcutaneous port placement. Tech Vasc Interv Radiol., vol. 14, no. 4, pp.:198-203
15. Ko SY, et all (2016) Spontaneous fracture and migration of catheter of a totally implantable venous access port via internal jugular vein--a case report. J Cardiothorac Surg., pp. 11-50.

Author: Micu Bogdan Vasile
Institute:Iuliu Hatieganu University of Medicine and Pharmacy, 5th surgical department
Street: Tabacarilor No. 11
City: Cluj-Napoca
Country: Romania
Email: micubogdan@yahoo.com

Robotic Splenectomy using the DaVinci Platform

B. Micu[1], C. Micu[2], T-R. Pop[1] and N. Constantea[1]

[1]"Iuliu Hateganu" University of Medicine and Pharmacy/5th Surgical Department, Cluj-Napoca, Romania
[2] "Iuliu Hateganu" University of Medicine and Pharmacy/Department of Anatomy and Embryology, Cluj-Napoca, Romania

Abstract— **The paper presents the assessment of the feasibility of *robot*-assisted *partial* and *total splenectomy* using the da Vinci surgical system. The authors conducted a retrospective study in which we included patients who underwent robotic surgery at the Fifth Surgical Clinic of Cluj-Napoca Municipal Hospital between 2010 and 2015. During this period, 15 robotic splenectomies had been performed, 8 women and 7 men, aged 9-69 years. Of these, 11 were total splenectomies and 4 partial splenectomies. There was only one case of conversion to open surgery and three cases of postoperative complications, two of which responded to conservative treatment. Robot-assisted splenectomy using the da Vinci surgical system is technically safe and feasible and represents an alternative to laparoscopic surgery, especially useful in difficult splenectomies.**

Keywords— **Robot, surgery, splenectomy, complications, hereditary spherocytosis**

I. .Introduction

Laparoscopic splenectomy is a minimally invasive intervention with a high degree of difficulty that has been used increasingly more often since its introduction in clinical practice in 1991, especially in hematological pathology. Subsequent studies have shown that laparoscopic splenectomy reduces morbidity, the length of hospital stay, postoperative pain, which in turn reduces the cost of hospital stay. It is today's gold standard in hematologic splenic pathology [1], indicated in: idiopathic thrombocytopenic purpura, hereditary spherocytosis, hemolytic anemia, autoimmune thrombocytopenic purpura, Hodgkin's lymphoma and non-Hodgkin lymphoma, chronic lymphocytic leukemia, hemangiomas, chronic idiopathic myelofibrosis , myelodysplastic syndrome, but also in non-hematologic disorders: abscesses, cysts or splenic tuberculosis, as well as in splenic trauma.

However, laparoscopic splenectomy has certain drawbacks, two-dimensional image and limited maneuverability of instruments, making surgery difficult sometimes, especially in case of splenomegaly, partial splenectomy and multiple adhesions.

The recent emergence of robotic surgery led to a reassessment of the indications of minimally invasive interventions for abdominal surgery [2]. The DaVinci robotic surgical system (Intuitive Surgical, Inc., Mountain View, CA) consists of: surgeon console, patient-side surgical cart with four robotic arms, 3-D vision system, and detachable instruments. By moving the console controls, the surgeon moves the instrument tips and guides the position of the video endoscope. The main technical advantages of this robotic surgical system are: high-quality three-dimensional image, increased handling of robotic surgical instruments, allows a safe and thorough dissections of vessels in the splenic hilum with mass ligature, helps preserve splenic tissue blood supply in partial splenectomy. The da Vinci equipment, the most widespread surgical robot nowadays, is in fact a computer-controlled telemanipulator, one that is capable of transmitting the finest movements of the operator to the surgical instruments, through *remote* human-computer interaction [3].

After the introduction of robotic surgery, urological and gynecological surgeries have gained ground and became fully accepted, while data on robotic splenectomy is limited and this type of procedure is performed on relatively small groups of patients. Our aim is to present the experience in robotic splenectomy of the Fifth Surgical Clinic in Cluj-Napoca, emphasizing: the indications, the technique, intraoperative and postoperative complications, as well as short-term results.

II. Materials and Methods

In order to achieve the objectives, we conducted a retrospective study in which we included patients who underwent surgery at the Fifth Surgical Clinic of Cluj-Napoca Municipal Hospital, Fifth Surgery Department of "Iuliu Hatieganu" University of Medicine and Pharmacy Cluj-Napoca. Between February 2010 and January 2015, a total number of 15 robot-assisted splenectomies were carried out in our unit; 8 women and 7 men aged between 9 and 69 years (median age 54). These interventions consisted of 11 (73.3%) total splenectomies and 4 partial splenectomies.

A database was created to include patient characteristics, diagnosis, intraoperative details, operative time, length of hospital stay, intraoperative and postoperative complica-

S. Vlad and N.M. Roman (eds.), *International Conference on Advancements of Medicine and Health Care through Technology; 12th - 15th October 2016, Cluj-Napoca, Romania,*
IFMBE Proceedings 59,
DOI: 10.1007/978-3-319-52875-5_8

tions and short-term evolution. The results of parametric and nonparametric data were expressed as median values and range. Statistical analysis was performed using MedCalc version 14.8.1. and the significance level was $p \leq 0.05$.

The operative technique for robotic total splenectomy. Following general anesthesia, the patient is positioned in 30-degree right lateral decubitus. Pneumoperitoneum is induced using Veress technique, and when the proper pressure is achieved, the trocars are placed: 12 mm endoscopic trocar in the left paraombilical region; 8 mm robotic trocar in the epigastrium, placed 8-12 cm from the endoscopic trocar; a second 8 mm robotic trocar in the left upper quadrant (subcostal), 8-12 cm from the endoscopic trocar; an additional 10 mm trocar in the left lumbar region (Figure 1).

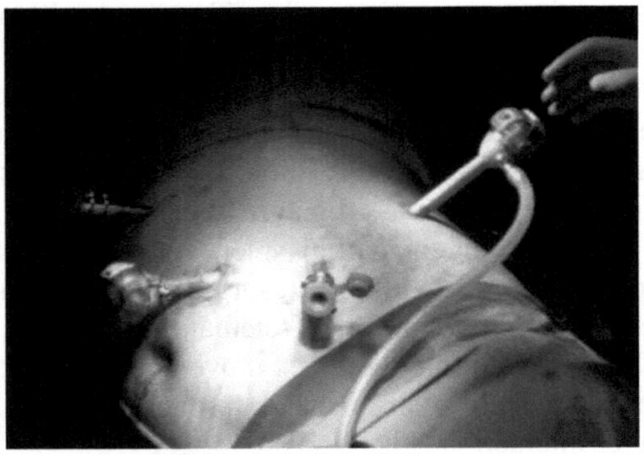

Fig. 1 Trocars position

Next, left lateral surgical robotic cart docking occurs, in an oblique position, at 45 degrees (Figure 2).

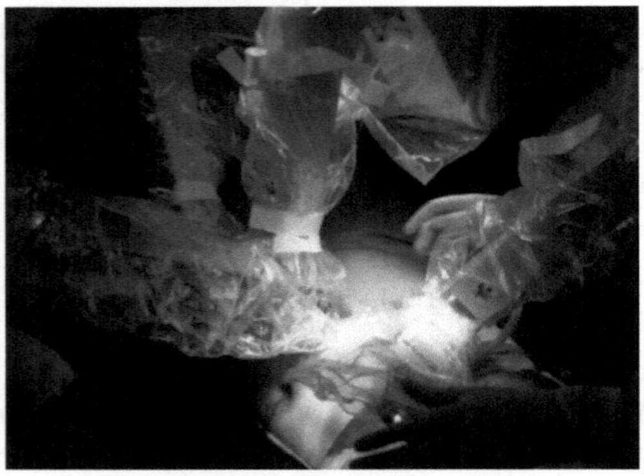

Fig. 2 Docking the robot

Specific tools for robotic surgery, such as Maryland dissector, end-gripping forceps, monopolar hook, bipolar forceps, dissecting scissors, needle holder, clip applicator, ultrasound-Harmonic scissors, are used in combination with instruments for laparoscopic surgery: LigaSure forceps, clip applicator, end-gripping forceps, retractors, laparoscopic staplers, vacuum grasper.

The procedure begins with the opening of the gastrocolic ligament and the sectioning of the short gastric arteries. The lower pole is mobilized by sectioning the splenocolic ligament. Splenic artery ligation (suprapancreatic caudal side) is performed using Prolene suture with intracorporeal knot-tying. Next, the splenorenal ligament is sectioned, followed by upper pole mobilization and sealing and sectioning of splenic pedicle vessels from the upper to the lower pole using LigaSure. After complete excision, the spleen is removed and placed into an endobag through a mini-laparotomy centered on the lateral part of the spleen or in case of a large spleen and benign splenic pathology a morcellator is used to place the spleen into the endobag. A drainage tube is placed in the splenic lodge and externalized through the left hypochondriac region. The surgery ends by withdrawing (undocking) the robotic cart, trocar extraction and suture of the mini-laparatomy and of cutaneous orifices of the trocars.

The operative technique for robot-assisted partial splenectomy. The surgical approach, that aims to preserve a fragment of splenic parenchyma, is achievable due to the anatomical characteristics of this organ, which is divided into different territories with different sources of blood supply. The terminal distribution of the splenic artery indicates anastomoses between the hilar, intraparenchymal and subcapsular arterial branches. Intraparenchymal anastomoses are of little importance and allow an effective hemostasis in a tissue section, even one as friable as the splenic tissue. Partial splenectomy, which achieves splenic arterial trunk ligation, preserves either short gastric arteries or the anastomotic branch between the left gastroepiploic artery and the inferior polar artery. For the best treatment it is necessary to assess the volume of splenic tissue to be removed and the tissue that needs to be preserved in order to maintain the phagocytic function and the formation of new tissue. We tried to preserve 15% of the spleen [4].

The objective of the surgery was to remove about 85% of the splenic tissue, preserving the upper pole of the spleen.

Initial operative time is identical to total splenectomy. After identifying the splenic artery, as distally as possible, the hilum of the spleen is dissected and all splenic arterial branches are identified for both superior and inferior poles. The blood supply of the superior pole is preserved to the level where the section will be performed. The branches of the inferior pole and the remaining tissue are sectioned using LigaSure or clips. Following ligation, the line of demarcation between the tissue to be preserved (vascular) and the remainder of the spleen is now visible. The spleen is cut using an Endo GIA roticulator™ blue cartridge stapler. Any bleeding in the transverse section is controlled using the electrocautery hook or LigaSure. The surgery ends when the excised splenic tissue is placed into the EndoBag, followed by the placement of a drainage tube.

III. Results

The daVinci Surgical System (Surgical Intiutive, Inc., Mountain View, CA) was used for all the procedures performed at the Fifth Surgical Clinic of Cluj-Napoca Municipal Hospital. Between February 2010 and January 2015, 15 patients underwent surgery (8 women and 7 men;median age54).The main patient characteristics are shown in Table 1.

Table 1 Patient characteristics

Gender	
Men	7 (53.3%)
Women	8 (46,7%)
Age	54 (median)
Range	9-69
BMI	28 (median)
Range	21-48

Robot-assisted total splenectomy was performed in 11 patients for: idiopathic thrombocytopenic purpura (4 cases), splenic lymphoma (3 cases), autoimmune hemolytic anemia (2 cases), subcapsular splenic hematoma (1 case), and chronic myelomonocytic leukemia (1 case). Robot-assisted partial splenectomy was performed in 4 patients for hereditary spherocytosis (4 cases) and splenic cyst (1 case) (Table 2).

Table 2. Indications for splenectomy

Indication for splenectomy	No. of cases
Total	11
Idiopathic thrombocytopenic purpura	4
Lymphomas	3
Autoimmune hemolytic anemia	2
Subcapsular splenic hematoma	1
Chronic myelomonocytic leukemia	1
Subtotal	4
Hereditary spherocytosis	3
Splenic cysts	1

The mean operative time was 110 ± 36 minutes. The difference in operative time between partial and total splenectomy is not statistically significant (198 vs. 101). Operative time also included docking time. Operative time decreased with the completion of the learning curve, both in terms of docking time and intraoperative time.

Conversion to open surgery was necessary in one case due to bleeding that could not be robotically controlled. In two cases, postoperative complications were represented by hematoma and seroma. One case required an additional intervention for the drainage of hematoma in the splenic lodge. In the other two cases, symptoms remitted under conservative treatment.

The mean length of hospital stay was 5 days (2-7). No death has been recorded in our patient group.

IV. Discussion

Of the four cases of partial splenectomy, three were performed for hereditary spherocytosis. Since 1993 when Tchernia et al. [5] first explained the benefits of partial splenectomy in hereditary spherocytosis, this technique has been increasingly accepted by surgeons and hematologists. The technique we practiced consisted in the preservation of the upper pole of the spleen, other authors presenting techniques for the preservation of the lower pole [6].

In what concerns the comparison between the laparoscopic approach and robot-assisted partial splenectomy, a meta-analysis by Balaphas et al. [7] concludes that robotic surgery is an attractive alternative, but further studies are needed on larger patient groups with a long-term postoperative follow-up.

Regarding the differences in intraoperative time between the two approaches, shorter time and lower costs were reported for laparoscopy [8], however, the robotic approach offers multiple advantages through improved visualization, more accurate control, meticulous dissection in tight spaces, which reduces the number of intraoperative and postoperative complications and the need for subsequent interventions [9], and it should only be used in difficult cases to get a good cost-benefit ratio [6].

In our study, there was one conversion to open surgery and three postoperative complications, one with subsequent laparoscopic intervention. In many previous studies, there were few or no cases of conversion and subsequent intervention due to rigorous selection criteria for robotic surgery [6-9], while the first cases are not reported, regarded as being part of the learning curve [9].

Some authors consider robotic surgery to also be useful in special anatomical conditions: short and multiple vessels in the splenic hilum; different anatomical positions of the tail of the pancreas; spleen volume and consistency [9].

The robotic approach would be indicated in partial splenectomy for a laborious dissection of the splenic hilum, with a better visualization the remaining tissue.

V. Conclusions

The introduction of robotic surgery into general practice aims to overcome the limitations of laparoscopic surgery.

The technical advantages of robot-assisted surgery in splenectomy are the more accurate dissection and hilar dissection safety, highly superior to laparoscopic surgery. We believe that robot-assisted splenectomy using the da Vinci Surgical System is technically feasible and safe, and may represent an alternative to laparoscopic surgery, especially difficult splenectomies for malignant hematopathies, splenomegaly or partial splenectomy, where it can reduce operative time, blood loss, the risk of postoperative bleeding, and may result in better outcomes for patients.

Conflict of Interest

The authors declare that they have no conflicts of interest.

References

1. Patriti A, Casciola L (2012) Robot-Assisted Splenectomy: Technique and Indications. Adv Robot Autom S1:002 http://dx.doi.org/10.4172/2168-9695.S1-002
2. Maeso S, Reza M, Mayol JA, Blasco JA, Guerra M, Andradas E, Plana MN. (2010) Efficacy of the Da Vinci surgical system in abdominal surgery compared with that of laparoscopy: a systematic review and meta-analysis. Ann Surg.vol. 252, no. 22, pp. 54-62.
3. Vasilescu C. (2009) Splenectomia robotica. Chirurgia vol.105, no.1, pp83-87
4. Vasilescu C, Stănciulea O, Coliţă A, Stoia R, Moicean A, Arion C. (2003) Splenectomia subtotala laparoscopica in tratamentul microsferocitozei ereditare. Chirurgia.vol. 98, no. 6, pp.571-576.
5. Tchernia G, Gauthier F, Mielot F, Dommergues JP, Yvart J, Chasis JA, Mohandas N. (1993) Initial assessment of the beneficial effect of partial splenectomy in hereditary spherocytosis. Blood. Vol. 81, no. 8, pp. 2014-2020.
6. Vasilescu C, Stanciulea O, Tudor S. (2012) Laparoscopic versus robotic subtotal splenectomy in hereditary spherocytosis. Potential advantages and limits of an expensive approach. Surg Endosc. Vol.26, no. 10, pp. 2802-2809.
7. Balaphas A, Buchs NC, Meyer J, Hagen ME, Morel P.(2015) Partial splenectomy in the era of minimally invasive surgery: the current laparoscopic and robotic experiences. Surg Endosc. Vol.29, no.12, pp.3618-3627.
8. Bodner J, Kafka-Ritsch R, Lucciarini P, Fish JH 3rd, Schmid T. (2005) A critical comparison of robotic versus conventional laparoscopic splenectomies. World J Surg. vol. 29, no. 8, pp. 982-985
9. Giulianotti PC, Buchs NC, Addeo P, Ayloo S, Bianco FM.(2011)Robot-assisted partial and total splenectomy. Int J Med Robot. Vol. 7, no. 4, pp.482-488.

Author: Micu Bogdan Vasile
Institute:Iuliu Hatieganu University of Medicine and Pharmacy, 5th su-Surgical Department
Street: Tabacarilor, No. 11
City: Cluj-Napoca
Country: Romania
Email: micubogdan@yahoo.com

Classical Chemometrics Methods Applied for Clinical Data Analysis

R.Bleiziffer[1], M. Culea[1], C. Sarbu[4], P. Podea[4], S.Suvar[1], A. Iordache[2] and C. Mesaros[3]

[1]Biomolecular Physics Department,"Babes-Bolyai" University, Cluj-Napoca, Romania
[2]National Institute R&D of Cryogenics and Isotopic Technologies – ICSI Rm. Valcea, Romania
[3]University of Medicine and Pharmacy, Târgu Mureş, Romania
[4]Department of Chemistry,"Babes-Bolyai" University, Cluj-Napoca, Romania

Abstract— **Two classical chemometrics methods namely Cluster Analysis and Principal Component Analysis have been applied to the evaluation of clinical data of several patients. A high correlation could be observed between some clinical parameters.**

Keywords— **Diagnosis, chemometrics, clinical data, Cluster Analysis, Principal Component Analysis.**

I. Introduction

Spectroscopic methods are powerful instruments used for the diagnosis of many diseases. Thus, IR, RAMAN, UV-VIS spectroscopy are used for the diagnosis by quantitative analyses of organic compounds from biological fluids [1-4]. There are a large number of publications regarding chemometric applications in clinical analytical data analyses [5-21]. These methods are very rapid and cheep.

The main goal of the present work was to perform a chemometric study of clinical data from analytical results by using Cluster Analysis and Principal Component Analysis methods and spectrophotometric techniques, for obtaining a method of disease identification, using data obtained from blood analysis of several patients.

II. Experimental

A number of 6 men (M) and 30 women (F) patients were studied. A spectrophotometric method was used, sample type: SER. The analytical clinical data are presented in Table 1 and Table 2. The investigated compounds in human blood samples were organic compounds of clinical interest (glucose, cholesterol, triglycerides, urea, creatinine;Table 1), inorganic compounds (Ca, Mg and Fe), enzymes (TGP-Transaminase) and ESR (erythrocyte sedimentation rate). (Table 2). The chemometric methods have been used in order to differentiate the patients (cases) according to their sex and age. The patients were separated more or less into two groups according to their sex and three groups according to their age in the score space defined by the first three principal components.

Table 1 Clinical Data studied

P	Sex	Age	Glu	Chol	Trigly	Urea	Creat
1	F	65	86.5	268	145		0.95
2	F	68		260	119		
3	M	65	91.5	165	136		0.95
4	F	12	83.1			42.44	0.41
5	F	14	97	145	62	25.1	0.65
6	F	81	109.6	160	116		0.83
7	M	69	98.5	207	73		1.07
8	M	33	95	230	101	36.84	0.81
9	F	58	**310**	266	225		1.22
10	F	73	131.1	221	57		0.54
11	F	71	100	194	128	38	1.08
12	F	60	107	353	219	25.93	0.84
13	F	49	88	273	134		0.58
14	F	76	88.5	217	86	30.39	0.95
15	F	54	92	250	117		0.78
16	F	45	85	199	132	11.23	0.91
17	F	21	74	177	36	28.18	0.82
18	M	48	94	262	191	22	1.24
19	F	65	123	256	62	22.69	0.77
20	F	54	94	201	124	39.11	0.82
21	M	56	109	165	42	26.04	0.82
22	F	72	145	179	94		0.8
23	F	25	78		41	22.65	0.88
24	F	50	83	195	48		0.87
25	F	54	101	220	227	65.64	1.32
26	F	51	86	276	191		0.92
27	F	74	84	230	57		0.71
28	F	29	72	142	49	14.85	0.82
29	F	60	89	259	116		0.97
30	F	49	95	168	125	29.67	0.84
31	F	87	101	187			1.1
32	F	53	82	293	69		0.84
33	F	27	81	175	73	18.95	0.86
34	F	76		213	70	29.42	0.99
35	F	41	78	194	45		0.67
36	M	61	84	170	92	27.87	0.93

S. Vlad and N.M. Roman (eds.), *International Conference on Advancements of Medicine and Health Care through Technology; 12th - 15th October 2016, Cluj-Napoca, Romania,*
IFMBE Proceedings 59,
DOI: 10.1007/978-3-319-52875-5_9

Normal blood values: Glucose(Glu): 60-110 mg / dL; Cholesterol(Chol): <200 mg / dL; high:> 240 mg / dL; Triglycerides(Trigly): Men (M): 40-160 mg / dL; Women (F): 36-135 mg / dL; Urea: 10-50 mg / dL; Creatinine (Creat): Men: 0.9-1.3 mg / dL; Women: 0,6-1.1 mg / dL;

Table 2 Clinical Data studied

P	Sex	Ac. uric	TGO	TGP	ESR	Ca	Mg	Fe
1	F	5.49	27	19	13			
2	F		30	38				
3	M	6.34	29	24	11			
4	F		28	14	5		2.25	87
5	F		25	17		9.27	2.11	
6	F	6.75	23	17				
7	M		32	23			2.36	98
8	M		49	66	5			
9	F	3.77	36	44	10			
10	F		20	18				
11	F		22	10	45	8.2	2.24	62
12	F		36	23	16	8.1	2.4	
13	F		24	26	6	9.57	2.35	94
14	F		27	18		9.31	2.29	
15	F	4.09	44	64	9	9.54		
16	F	4.11	23	16	13	8.63	2.19	74
17	F	3.32	30	13	5	9.17	2.18	102
18	M	11.1 2	53	70	5	9.49	2.32	123
19	F		28	22				
20	F		27	10	8		2.29	79
21	M	3.32	37	38				
22	F	4.66	25	27				
23	F	3.52	11	19		8.7	2.11	70
24	F	2.96	26	12	5			
25	F	7.05	27	18				138
26	F		28	22	12	8.25	2.3	87
27	F		27	16	6	8.35	2.31	69
28	F			16	5	8.94	2.25	108
29	F	4.95	22	19	5	8.79	2.46	123
30	F	3.06	34	56	15	8.93	2.27	
31	F		33	7	19	8.93	2.29	95
32	F		24	22	18	9.25	2.33	
33	F		43	46		8.73	2.06	
34	F		12	33		9.45		
35	F	3.23	15	29	5	8.86	2.56	128
36	M	5.92	57	61	18			68
		5.49	27	19	13			

Normal blood values Uric acid: Men: 3.4-7.0 mg / dL; Women: 2.4-5.7 mg / dL; TGO: 0-35 U / L; TGP: Men: 0-35 U / I; Women: 0-36 U / I; ESR: 2-12 mm / h Westergreen method, sample type: K3 EDTA whole blood; Calcium (Ca): 8.6-10.3 mg / dL; Magnesium (Mg): 1.6-2.5 mg / dL; Iron (Fe): Children: 50-120 mg / dL; Women: 60-160 mg / dL Men: 80-180 mg / dL.

III. Results And Discussion

The goal of the study was to find patterns of similarity, both between the patients and the clinical tests. Two classical chemometrics methods namely Cluster Analysis (CA) and Principal Component Analysis (PCA) have been applied to the evaluation of clinical data. These methods have been used in order to differentiate the patients (cases) according to their sex and age. Principal component analysis reduced the data set to a few representative activations, and cluster analysis measured the average dissimilarity [10].

The cluster analysis show the degree of relatedness by the values of ESR (VSH), Ca, Mg, uric acid, Creatinine, TGP, TGO, uree, Fe, triglyceride and cholesterol. There are similarity of samples from different patients. (Fig. 1). From cluster analysis we can observe a high correlation between magnesium and creatinine, fact observed also by others researchers. [19] Also calcium and uric acid proved to be high correlated. There are several studies which have found in a considerable percentage to oxalate patients, a high concentration of uric acid and also a hypercalciuria.[20] Cluster Analysis proved that ESR is correlated with Ca, uric acid, creatinine and Mg, which make ESR a good marker for renal diseases. This fact was also clinically proved.[21] Highly correlated are also TGP and TGO, liver transaminase enzymes, which can be found in amino acid metabolism and are direct correlated with urea concentration. The program showed a good correlation between transaminase enzymes, urea and ESR (VSH), Ca, Mg, uric acid, creatinine. A significant correlation was obtained between Fe and triglycerides and cholesterol.

The explanation of the clustering found is relevant and is based on the pattern of similarity like glucose level, enzyme level, liver function, kidney function. This classification help to optimize the performance of clinical data for patients and in patients diagnosis.

Fig. 2 presents the scatterplot of the clinical parameters considered in this study.

The patients separated into two groups according to their sex and three groups according to their age in the score space defined by the first three principal components showed a high correlation between some clinical parameters (Fig. 3 and Fig. 4).

By means of PCA, practically useful systematic information may be extracted from large sets of data, which is otherwise hardly interpretable in comprehensive physical terms. Such information can be of value for general prognosis and for making appropriate adjustments in treatment [14]. Further development of methods such as PCA may provide critical insights to drive advances in clinical care [15].

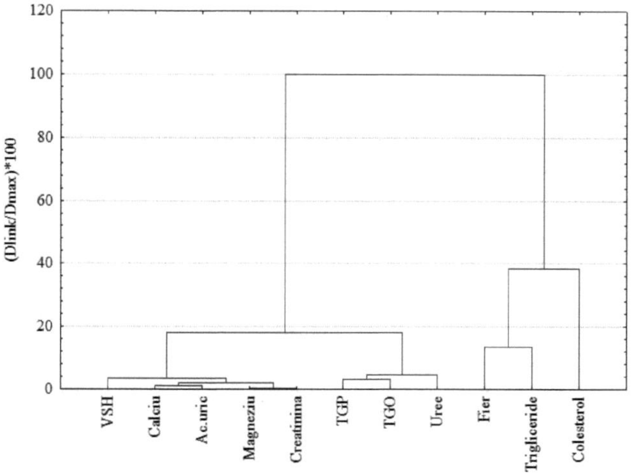

Fig. 1 Dendrogram corresponding to the clinical parameters considered in this study

Fig. 2 presents the scatterplot of the clinical parameters considered in this study.

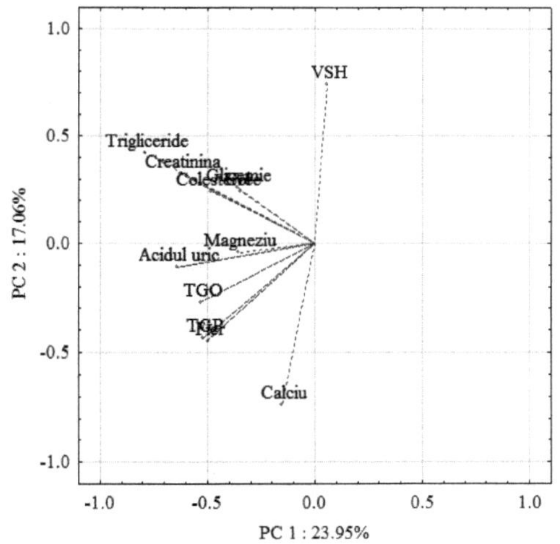

Fig. 2. Loadings scatterplot of the clinical parameters considered in this study

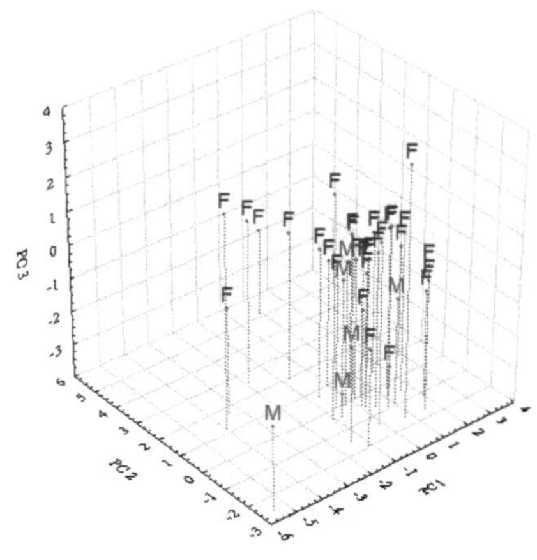

Fig. 3 Score scatterplot in the space defined by PC1, PC2 and PC3 (sex label).

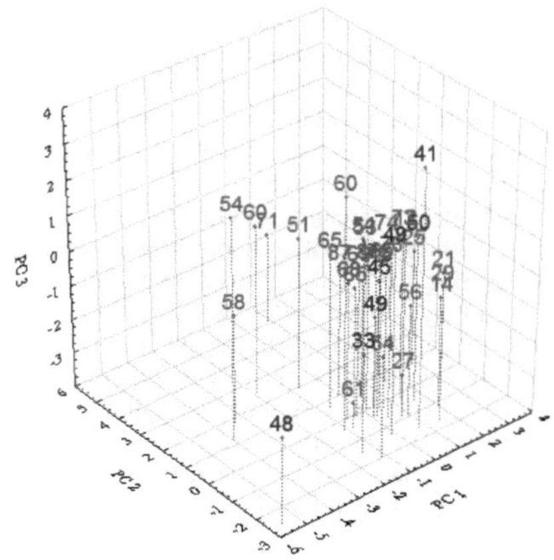

Fig. 4. Score scatterplot in the space defined by PC1, PC2 and PC3 (age label)

IV. Conclusions

Our results showed a high correlation between some clinical parameters (Fig. 1 and Fig. 2). The results confirm that clinical analysis combined with the chemometric methods are useful for disease correlations and interpretations. According to clinical analytical data concentration level the following deseases should be studied: hepatic diseases, lipid disorders, diabetes, renal disorders, etc [4].

Conflict of Interest

The authors declare that they have no conflict of interest.

References

1. Kourti T, MacGregor JF. (1995) Process analysis, monitoring and diagnosis using multivariate projection methods, Chemometr Intell Lab, 28:3-21.
2. Dang NA, Janssen HG, Kolk AH. (2013) Rapid diagnosis of TB using GC-MS and chemometrics. Bioanalysis. 5(24):3079-3097.
3. Madsen R, Lundstedt T, Trygg J. (2010) Chemometrics in metabolomics--a review in human disease diagnosis. Anal Chim Acta. 5;659(1-2):23-33. doi: 10.1016/j.aca.2009.11.042. Epub 2009 Nov 22.
4. Sârbu C, Pop H F, Elekes Rs, Covaci G. (2008) Intelligent Disease Identification based on Discriminant Analysis of Clinical Data, Rev Chimie, 59:1237-1241.
5. Geana I, Iordache A, Ionete R, Marinescu A, Ranca A, Culea M. (2013) Geographical origin identification of Romanian wines by ICP-MS elemental analysis. Food Chem. 13:1125–113
6. Beebe KR., Pell RJ, Seasholtz MB. (1998) Chemometrics: A Practica 1 Guide, John Wiley& Sons, New York.
7. Massart DL, Kaufman L.(1983) The interpretation of Cmemical Data By the Use of Cluster Analysis, John Wiley & Sons, New York.
8. Sârbu,C.. (2006) Fuzzy Clustering and its Applications in Chemistry in Chemometrics: Methods and Applications , D. Zuba, and A. Partczewski (eds.), Institute of Forensic Research Publishers, Kraków, , Chapt. 1, 17-47.
9. **Vyas** S, **Kumaranayake** L. (2006) Constructing socio-economic status indices: how to use principal components analysis, Health Policy Plan. 21 (6): 459-468.
10. Faes L, Nollo G, Kirchner M, Olivetti E, Gaita F, Riccardi R, Antolini R. (2001)Principal component analysis and cluster analysis for measuring the local organisation of human atrial fibrillation, Med Biol Eng Comput. 39(6):656-63.
11. Sih HJ, Zipes DP, Berbari EJ, Olgin JE. (1999): A high-temporal resolution algorithm for quantifying organization during atrial fibrillation,',IEEE Trans. Biomed. Eng.,46: 440–450.
12. Vandeginste B, Massart DL, Buydens L, De Long S, Lewi P, Smeyers-Verbeke J (1998) Handbook of Chemometrics and Qualimetrics, Elsevier, Amsterdam.
13. Stone M, Liu X, Chen H, Prince JL. A preliminary application of principal components and cluster analysis to internal tongue deformation patterns. Comput Methods Biomech Biomed Engin. 2010; 13(4): 493–503.
14. Buciński A, Bączek T, Waśniewski T, Stefanowicz M. (2005) Clinical data analysis with the use of artifi cial neural networks (ANN) and principal component analysis (PCA) of patients with endometrial carcinomaRep Pract Oncol Radiother. 10(5): 239-248.
15. Kutcher ME, Ferguson AR, Cohen MJ. (2013) A principal component analysis of coagulation after trauma, J Trauma Acute Care Surg. 74(5): 1223–1230. doi:10.1097/TA.0b013e31828b 7fa1.
16. Konishi T, (2015) Principal component analysis for designed experiments. BMC Bioinformatics201516(Suppl 18):S7 DOI: 10.1186/1471-2105-16-S18-S7
17. Denery JR, Nunes AAK, Hixon MS Tobin J. DickersonTJ, Janda KD. (2010) Metabolomics-Based Discovery of Diagnostic Biomarkers for Onchocerciasis,PLOS Negleted Tropical Diseases 4:e384:1-9.
18. Vinayavekhin N, Homan EA, Saghatelian A (2010) Exploring disease through metabolomics. ACS Chem Biol 5: 91–103
19. Cunningham J, Rodríguez M, Messa P. (2012) Magnesium in chronic kidney disease Stages 3 and 4 and in dialysis patients, Clin Kidney J, 5: i39–i51.
20. Coe F.L (1983) Uric acid and calcium oxalate nephrolithiasis, Kidney International, 24: 392-403
21. Stojan G, Fang H, Magder L, Petri M. (2013) Erythrocyte sedimentation rate is a predictor of renal and overall SLE disease activity. Lupus; 22:827-834.

Author: Ramona Bleiziffer
Institute: Biomolecular Physics Department,"Babes-Bolyai" University
Street: Mihail Kigalniceane, no 1
City: Cluj-Napoca
Country: Romania
Email: ramobleal@ yahoo.it

What do job adverts tell Higher Education about the 'shape' of Biomedical Engineering graduates?

A.E. Ward, B. Baruah, A. Gbadebo, and N.J. Jackson

Engineering Management Group, Department of Electronics, University of York, York, United Kingdom

Abstract— **Higher Education Institutions are required, at least in some Countries, to design their curricula taking into account the needs of relevant industry. Use of Industrial Advisory Committees is a common way of demonstrating this input. This paper explores an additional window to industry needs through the textual analysis of job advertisements. 36 internet published adverts using the "Biomedical Engineering" search phrase were downloaded and textually analysed to identify the mentioned technical skills, generic skills and the adjectives used to describe the required level of proficiency in them. Results of the analysis of these adverts, using qualitative research analysis software starts to reveal a relevant technical skills hierarchy that Higher Education can use to help inform curricular designed for this employment pathway. The analysis of the generic skills reveals those rated important by employers for different levels of jobs, again of potential use to curriculum designers. Finally the results reveal the adjectives used to show the level of ability employers seek of their graduates. Herein lies a significant difference across the supply and demand side of the first employment transition. The difference can be rationally explained but does not help in closing the gap between what Higher Education provides in terms of graduates and what Industry seeks. The paper concludes that dialogue between Industry and Higher Education could usefully focus on the way skills are defined and claims of ability warranted as a means of closing the "Higher Education is not gives us what employers want" claims.**

Keywords— **Skills Analysis, Skills hierarchy, Biomedical Skills, Graduate Skills, Employability.**

I. Introduction

Accredited academic programmes in the UK, in the areas of Electrical, Technology and Computer Science "... must be informed by current industrial practice" [1].

According to the IET 2015 Skills Survey [2] *"61% of industry find that graduates do not meet their "reasonable" expectations*". The greatest skills gaps being in Communication skills, ability to work across interdisciplinary teams, ability to work on own initiative, technical expertise, leadership and management skills, business acumen and practical skills.

The IET 2015 Skills Survey also found that "*28% of the employers reported that content of technical degrees does not meet their needs with 40% believing that courses are not up to date with industry; and 57% believing that courses do not develop practical skills.*" For IET accreditation the department must demonstrate that they seek industrial input throughout the design, development, delivery and review of the academic programmes. A common form of this input is through some form of Industrial Advisory Committee. Experience at the University of York is that it is reasonably easy to engage with staff from large employers as they often have University Liaison personnel or have the resources to enable them to engage with the Department in an active way. We have much greater difficulty in engaging with Small to Medium Sized Enterprises. Given that there are 5,389,450 businesses in the UK at the start of 2015 [3] of which only 6,965 had 250 or more employees, seeking the views of large employers is arguably not fully representative of the world of work. This is clearly a very broad-brush figure; in reality there are significant sectorial and regional variations. No suggestion is made in this paper that existing means of obtaining industrial input to academic programmes are in any way flawed, rather it explores and alternative window to employer needs – through an analysis of job advertisements.

II. Methodology

45 job advertisements were downloaded from the Internet from a single generic recruitment website [www.jobsite.co.uk]. The search used was "biomedical engineering" and the 45 adverts represent all those live on the search day.

The jobsite site acts as a collator of job descriptions and is not one that requires all job descriptions to follow a common homogeneous format. The sample was thereby considered essentially random in format and content.

A number of the adverts were direct duplicates indicating more than one identical position - these identical duplicates were removed from the sample selected for analysis. Of the 36 remaining jobs reviewed 34 were "permanent", one "full-time" and one unspecific in this aspect.

The text of each job advert was imported as "Internals" to NVivo, a qualitative research analysis software package. The adverts were coded in a number of different ways, by job titles, technical skills, generic skills and adjectives men-

S. Vlad and N.M. Roman (eds.), *International Conference on Advancements of Medicine and Health Care through Technology; 12th - 15th October 2016, Cluj-Napoca, Romania*,
IFMBE Proceedings 59,
DOI: 10.1007/978-3-319-52875-5_10

tioned in the advert text. The coding was essentially semantic with as little interpretation of meaning as could be achieved to minimize the potential for coder bias.

The approach to coding was a grounded theory approach based on the hypothesis that there is a hierarchical structure to skills and that there is a distinction between technical skills and generic skills. It was further based on the hypothesis that the competence level required for any particular skill is described by an adjective of some form.

A hierarchical node structure was then developed with the initial starting set being that used for a previous job advertisement analysis [4]. Matrix coding enquiries were then used to help in the analysis and understanding of the adverts.

III. The job adverts

The range of jobs offered within this sample is fairly broad, by their titles there are 21 Engineering posts, 5 with the Manager title, 2 with the Director title, 2 Scientist roles, 4 Specialist roles, 1 Software tester and 1 Technical Author, these were used as the job categories in the analysis presented herein.

IV. Technical skills

The job descriptions were reviewed for the requirement in technical skills using, as a starting point the skills hierarchy created in the analysis of job adverts from the Renewable Energies sector. There was limited overlap between the Renewable Energies and the Biomedical Engineering sector.

During coding recognition was given where the statement was a description of background experience required that implied ability in the skill. The skills were first listed randomly and then arranged into a draft hierarchy based on logical top-level category groupings. A matrix-coding query was used to show the occurrences of each technical skill by job category. In total 58 different technical skills were identified. These skills were grouped into 10 top-level categories as show in Table 1 which shows the number of sub-levels in the hierarchy and the total number of unique skills placed within that top-level node and all its sub-nodes. The table shows the breadth of skills mentioned in the adverts.

Table 1 show that Engineering roles are the most specifically defined in terms of technical skills followed by the Scientist and Specialist roles. There was only one each of Software Tester and Technical Author. Manager roles are the least technically defined, perhaps because the manager roles included in this study are mostly Business Development Managers with one Product Manager. The Director positions are back to being more specifically technically focused.

Table 2 shows the number of mentions of technical and generic skills by job category along with the number of adverts in each job category.

Table 1 Top level of the initial technical skills hierarchy

Top level	Sub levels	Total number of skills
Basic Science	0	1
Biomedical Skills	0	24
Chemistry	0	3
Equipment	1	5
Management	0	2
Mathematics	0	4
Product Development and Production Process	0	7
Sales and Marketing	0	1
Service	0	1
Software Design, Development & Testing	2	10

Table 2 Number of mentions of skills by Job Category

Job Category	Adverts	Technical	Generic
Engineer	21	54	33
Manager	5	2	5
Director	2	6	9
Scientist		37	13
Software Tester	1	12	8
Specialist		7	5
Technical Author	1	2	6

The frequency of occurrence of technical skills provides some information about the required content of curricula if HE is to provide employment graduates. It is unsurprising that for Biomedical Engineering jobs that Biomedical skills have the highest number of mentions. It is interesting to note that some understanding of Quality, Regulations and/or Standards relevant to the discipline is also sought. Service is seen in 6 adverts but this reflects the nature of these job adverts, service skills are not normally included in degree level programmes in the UK. This becomes a lot clearer in Table 3, which shows the number of times qualifications are mentioned in the job adverts by job category.

Table 3 shows that all of the service jobs require ONC or HNC qualification, the qualifications in the UK within which servicing equipment might be expected. The sample size which might explain why very few academic qualifications are required in Managerial jobs and an emphasis on higher-level qualifications for Director positions can be seen.

Table 3 Qualifications mentioned by Job Category

Job Category	ONC	HNC	HND	FCD	SCD	PhD
Director				1	1	2
Engineer	5	5	1	5	1	
Manager			1			
Scientist						2
Software Tester			1	1		
Specialist			3	3	1	
Field Service Engineer	5	4				

V. Generic skills

A total of 20 different generic skills were identified across the job adverts. Table 4 shows the mentions that have been coded as generic skills against the Engineer, Manager and Director job categories. Because there is a large difference in the number of adverts in each category the total number of mentions has been normalized to the number of adverts, as shown in the bottom row. This result, in conjunction with the results in Table 2 shows that when specifying jobs employers tend to place more of an emphasis on the generic skills for higher grade jobs. This has been seen in other studies [4].

An obvious challenge in this area is what is a generic skill and what might better described as a personal behavior or attitude, there is no clear consistency in this area at present. The naming of the generic skills here has been informed by the Tuning Methodology [5] and the comparative study of perceptions of students, academics and employers in the EIE-Surveyor Project [6] but it is accepted this is not an exact science.

The generic skills stated as being required by employers in job adverts, as in the case of the technical skills, provides information on what could usefully be included in academic programmes. That said there are some significant challenges in the area of generic skills, not least of which are the inconsistency in definition of their meaning, lack of any robust assessment methods (except in a few exceptions), a lack of means of stating a student's ability in a generic skill and the common argument of lack of time in the curricula. One exception to the lack of robust assessment method is in public speaking where steps are being taken on assessment [7]-[9].

There are examples of programmes where there is an emphasis on the development of generic skills alongside the technical content [10], pedagogies such as Problem Based Learning, Project Based Learning and Curiosity Based Learning are also methods of achieving this.

Table 4 Number of mentions of generic skills by Job Category

Job Category	Engineer	Manager	Director
Ability to get things done			1
Ability to work on own	2		
Analytical skills			1
Commercial Awareness/Acumen	1	1	
Communications	4		2
Customer focused or service	9		1
Entrepreneurial			1
Innovative/Creative	1		
Interpersonal skills	1	2	
Leadership	1		1
Management	1		
Personal Organization	5	1	
Problem solving			1
Team Working	8	1	
Work under pressure			1
Total	33	5	9
Number of adverts in category	21	5	2
Total / Number of adverts	1.6	1	4.5

Lack of clear definition of generic skills is made more difficult by the differences in which competence in them is specified. The following section explores this in the context of the job adverts analysed.

VI. Level of ability in generic skills

In the sample of job adverts 25 unique adjectives were identified, as shown in Table 4. These adjectives were variously used in the context of the persons: background; the company; the job; the offered package (salary, benefits, etc.); personal attributes and behaviours; and proficiency (as in the level of ability with reference to a technical or generic skill). The adjectives marked with a * are those which were used in the context of proficiency (they may or may not have also been used in the other contexts). The number of times the adjective was used in the proficiency context is shown in brackets.

To illustrate the way these adjectives are being used consider the following examples, the number in brackets indicates the number of instances across all job adverts:

"Adept" is found once in the job descriptions in relation to proficiency of a skill as in "You will be adept at reading and understanding technical diagrams".

"Basic" is used (3) to indicate the need for foundation level understanding, as in "Basic awareness of the SDLC (software development life-cycle)" and "Basic understanding of the role of a software tester, testing methodologies and tools".

Table 4 Adjectives identified in the sample of job adverts

Adjective	Adjective	Adjective
Adept* (1)	Fantastic	Proficient* (2)
Basic* (2)	Fluent* (3)	Proven* (1)
Effectively* (3)	Generous	Significant
Excellent/ce* (7)	Good* (8)	Solid* (1)
Exciting	Great* (1)	Strong* (24)
Experienced	High* (3)	Technical ability* (1)
Exposure to	Impeccable* (2)	Working with* (1)
Extensive	Outstanding	
Familiarity with* (4)	Passion	

"Effectively" is used in relation to communications/skill (1) as in "Effectively present information to a variety of people, including senior management, groups, and/or board of directors", personal effectiveness (1) as in "organise and prioritise effectively" and team working (1) as in "effectively managing a small team".

"Excellent or excellence" This adjective is used in three ways, firstly, and as one might expect in how the advert sells the role to the potential candidate (3), such as "Excellent opportunity to join a market leading supplier"; secondly in the description of what the job offers the potential applicant, such as "Excellent Opportunities for Career Advancement" (5) or in relation to the remuneration package (17) such as "excellent benefits package"; it is also used as a skills quality indicator (7), as in "Excellent communication skills", "Excellent interpersonal skills", "Excellent knowledge of all relevant regulations" and "Excellent laboratory practical skills particularly in the area of protein".

In Higher Education the student's performance transcript, the statement of their ability in the subjects they have been assessed, defines their overall ability and that in individual topics. The ability of a student to do any specific subject or assessed skill is indicated by either a mark, grade, or in some, less helpful cases, a qualitative descriptor (Excellent, good, etc.). The mark can be either a percentage or mark out of another defined figure. There are many different grading systems around the world including:

- Letter grades (usually A to F with A being top grade), can also have + and - to show finer gradations [11]
- Numerical grades, for example:
  - 10 (Excellent), 9 (Very good) , … 5 (sufficient), 4 (insufficient) .. 1 (academic dishonesty) as in Romania [12]
  - 5 (Excellent), 4 (Good) down to 1 (Very Poor) in Russia [13]
  - 10 (Excellent), 9 (Very good) ... 6 (Sufficient), to 0-5.9 (Insufficient/Failed) in Mexico [14]
- GP or GPA (Grade Point Average) which can be out of 4 (e.g. USA [15]) or 7 (e.g. Chile [16])
- Worded grades, for example:
  - First, upper second, lower second, etc. (e.g. UK [17]);
  - Excellent (85-100%), Very good or Distinct (75-84%), etc. as in Egypt [18];
  - High Distinction (85-100%), Distinction (75-84%) down to Fail (<50%) in some Australian Institutions[19].

In most academic cases a conversion from any statement to an equivalent percentage is usually provided. The percentage being the one measure that has global meaning.

Clearly there is a very great difference in the way the supply and demand sides of the first employment transition specify the level of ability and in part this is justifiable.

VII. Discussion

A number of questions fall out of the above discussions that apply equally to all graduates as they do to Biomedical Engineers, the main subject of this paper. Firstly, is it the academic's role, or that of any other staff member of the HEI to offer advice and guidance on interpreting the statements of need and helping the student demonstrate they meet the essential requirements to at least get them an interview? There is no doubt that calls for help are made by students to academic supervisors, friendly academics and career advisory staff. Given that the employment situations of graduates in general at a short time after graduation is one of the component measures in Higher Education league tables, it is important that students are given good advice in this respect. So academics, as well as the professional careers service staff in the institution need to be able to give informed advice in all aspects of the employment process including that of interpreting the needs of specific job adverts.

Secondly, is it HEI's responsibility to develop ability in the generic skills in students? Many argue that it is outside the scope of academic programmes and that there is insufficient time available to cover the technical aspects of the programme and that including generic skills development is a step too far. Other HEI's have rethought their pedagogy completely and now employ techniques that simultaneously develop technical and generic skills [20]-[23].

The third big question is how do we assess generic skills and warrant student ability in them in a way that is meaningful to all stakeholders (specifically HEIs and employers)? [8], [24], [25].

Finally, what is the objective of a job advert? It is to sell the company to prospective candidates but also to state the requirements of the job so that the company is not deluged by inappropriate applications. Therein lies a balance, making the advert too specific may mean there are none, or very few individuals who fit the job and hence applications may be low or zero, at the other end of the spectrum, an advert that is open or vague in terms of requirements is likely to attract too many applications. There is also a moral argument wherein if a candidate meets all the essential requirements should they not expect an interview? A negative answer to this would suggest the application reviewer is making some other judgment on the application – an area open to discrimination claims. This then is where the use of adjectives works for the employer – the requirement is stated, for example "Excellent communication skills", but the level qualifier, the adjective, allows applicants to be subjectively 'ranked' in that dimension and a line to be drawn for the number of candidates who can reasonably be taken to the next stage in the selection process.

In this way the adjective approach is possibly a more effective way of specifying a need.

Compliance with Ethical Requirements

There are no ethical issues in this research. No individuals are directly involved so there are no data protection issues or matters requiring informed consent.

VIII. Conclusions

In this paper a relatively small sample of job adverts in the general area of Biomedical Engineering have been textually analysed with the objective of extracting the specific and generic skills mentioned in each advert as part of an ongoing activity of exploring skills hierarchies. This type of analysis is argued to be an alternative window into industry needs at, in part, the student first employment transition. It can also inform the skills required for different career progression pathways.

In this study 45 job adverts were downloaded from a single job advertisement website, the adverts being all of those that were returned from a search of "Biomedical Engineering" on the search day. 36 of the adverts were used in the analysis. The NVivo qualitative research software package was used in the analysis and, using it, the text in the adverts was coded for role group, technical skills, generic skills and the adjectives used.

The results show the technical skills required of different types (and hierarchical levels) of jobs, which should be of interest to curriculum designers if their objective is to align curricula to employment areas. The analysis also shows the generic skills valued by employers – this is a more difficult area because skills are currently poorly defined and measurement and warranting ability is challenging.

The way employers define the level of ability required in skills is also very different to that used by academic institutions. Whilst this can be rationalized it does mean the gap between what Higher Education produces and what employers want is weakly correlatable and, given we frequently hear criticism from industry that HE is not producing the correctly 'shaped' graduates for their needs, perhaps there is a clue to the reason in this analysis.

What then can be done to close the gap? One solution lies in the communication between employers and the education system. A shift in discussion to the specifics of what skills mean and how they are measured along with a move to more common use of terminology could be beneficial, especially in the generic skills area.

This paper reports on the early findings of an ongoing project to explore job adverts and it is recognized tat the power of the findings will be greater with an increased number of adverts and adverts from multiple online sources. The intention of the authors is to expand the dataset so that meaningful recommendations for curricula developers can be derived.

Conflict of Interest

The author declares that they have no conflict of interest in the content of this paper.

References

1. "IET Academic Accreditation," 17-Apr-2015. [Online]. Available: www.theiet.org/academics/accreditation/policy-guidance/ahepguide.cfm?type=pdf. [Accessed: 16-Aug-2016].
2. "2015 IET skills survey," 20-Oct-2015. [Online]. Available: http://www.theiet.org/factfiles/education/skills2015-page.cfm. [Accessed: 16-Aug-2016].
3. "STATISTICAL RELEASE," 13-Oct-2015. [Online]. Available: https://www.gov.uk/government/uploads/system/uploads/attachment_data/file/467443/bpe_2015_statistical_release.pdf. [Accessed: 16-Aug-2016].
4. A. E. Ward, A. Gbadebo, and B. Baruah, "Using job advertisements to inform curricula design for the key global technical challenges," 2015, pp. 1–6. DOI:10.1109/ITHET.2015.7218042
5. J. Gonzalez and R. Wagenaar, "Tuning Educational Structures in Europe," Universidad de Deusto, Mar. 2003.

6. A. E. Ward, "The Alignment of Generic, Specific and Language Skills within the Electrical and Information Engineering Discipline," EIE-Surveyor Project, York, Dec. 2008.
7. T. Ward, "The Assessment of Public Speaking - a Pan-European view.," presented at the Information Technology based Higher Education and Training, Antalya, Turkey, 2013, pp. 1–2.
8. N. R. Jackson and A. E. Ward, "Assessing Public Speaking, A trial rubric to speed up and standardise feedback," presented at the 13th International Conference on Information Technology based Higher Education and Training (ITHET), York, England, 2014.
9. A. E. Ward, "The issues of certifying public speaking in technical subjects," in Project Work and Internship – Theory and Practice, N. Escudeiro, A. Klucznik-Toro, A. Pawelczyk, M. Carbonaro, S. Nanu, and T. welzer, Eds. The PRAXIS Project, 2013, pp. 199–216.
10. A. E. Ward and N. R. Jackson, "Simultaneous development of management skills and behaviours in taught academic programmes," presented at the 13th International Conference on Information Technology based Higher Education and Training (ITHET), York, England, 2014.
11. "Academic grading in Kenya." Wikipedia. [Accessed: 16-Aug-2016]
12. "Academic grading in Romania." Wikipedia. [Accessed: 16-Aug-2016]
13. "Academic grading in Russia." Wikipedia. [Accessed: 16-Aug-2016]
14. "Academic grading in Mexico." Wikipedia. [Accessed: 16-Aug-2016]
15. J. C. CARPER, "Education in the United States," The Educational Forum, vol. 47, no. 2. Wikipedia, pp. 135–149, 30-Jan-2008.
16. "Academic grading in Chile." Wikipedia. [Accessed: 16-Aug-2016]
17. "Academic grading in the United Kingdom." Wikipedia. [Accessed: 16-Aug-2016]
18. "Academic grading in Egypt." Wikipedia. [Accessed: 16-Aug-2016]
19. "Academic grading in Australia." Wikipedia. [Accessed: 16-Aug-2016]
20. A. Avramenko and A. Avramenko, "Enhancing students' employability through business simulation," Education + Training, vol. 54, no. 5, pp. 355–367, Jun. 2012. DOI: 10.1109/ITHET.2015.7218042
21. B. Sumrongthong, "Curiosity Based Learning," pp. 1–49, Sep. 2009.
22. N. R. Jackson and A. E. Ward, "Curiosity Based Learning: Impact Study in 1st Year Electronics Undergraduates," presented at the 11th International Conference on Information Technology based Higher Education and Training (ITHET), Istanbul, Turkey, 2012.
23. C. Hmelo-Silver, "Problem-based learning: What and how do students learn?," Educational Psychology Review, 2004.
24. B. Clayton, K. Blom, D. Meyers, and A. Bateman, Assessing and certifying generic skills:. National Centre for Vocational Education Research, 252 Kensington Road, Leabrook, South Australia 5068, Australia, 2003.
25. L. M. Schreiber, G. D. Paul, and L. R. Shibley, "The Development and Test of the Public Speaking Competence Rubric," Communication Education, vol. 61, no. 3, pp. 205–233, Jul. 2012. DOI: 10.1080/03634523.2012.670709

Ozone and Intense Electric Fields Applyance in Treating of External Wounds Become Overinfected

R.E. Suarasan [1], I. Suarasan[1], S.R. Budu[1], M.I. Suarasan[2], A. Maniu[2] and R. Morar[1]

[1] Technical University of Cluj-Napoca, Cluj-Napoca, Romania
[2] University of Medicine and Pharmacy of Cluj-Napoca, Romania

Abstract— **Paper presents the results of an interdisciplinary research, conducted at the Technical University of Cluj-Napoca upon the combined use of ozone and intense electric fields (IEF) in processing of gaseous and aqueous environments, used in order to treat overinfected external wounds. The proposed medical treatment in the present paper is complementary to medical conventional treatments. The advantages of increased speed and quality of healing, significantly reducing stress and time restraint - inactivation of patients and the medications used, and finally to increase their life expectancy, strongly recommends this treatment method. Authors experimental method presume treatments using ozonized air and distilled water in experimental cells. Based on the experience of authors were established requirements and criteria for ozone generation and processing of aqueous and gaseous environments in electric fields, and also procedures for their use for medical treating conditions. Preliminary studies can lead to innovative design of new treatment equipment used for treating varicose, opened ulcerations, skin burns, anaerobic infections, gangrenous, open and over infected ulcerations, bedsores, etc. Propose method recommends the use of this non-polluting and environmental friendly method in medicine.**

Keywords— **ozone, electric fields, ulcerations, treating**

I. Introduction

After fluorine, ozone is one of the best known oxidants, used ordinarilyin many industrial applications and an antiseptic and antibacterial gas too. The use of ozone is doubled by the fact that the resulted products are less toxic and are well suported by the living environments. Actually there are quite few studies on the use of ozone in medicine.

Ozone therapy treats the patients with a mixture of oxygen and ozone and is used as an auxiliary method to conventional therapies. Physical - chemical properties of ozone are very effective in order to reduce microbial infections in dental surgery [1], prosthetic hip surgery [2], also determines anti-apoptotic and anti-inflammatory potential at mice with acute renal ischemia [3], involves a rapid improvement of liver failure and jaundice detoxification patients [4].

Antimicrobial effects of ozone have been identified in necrotizing fascitis [5], osteonecrosis of the jaw, prostate surgery [6], at opened and/or infected ulcerations refractory to classic treatment [7]. Ozone therapy was applied in the form of extracorporal blood oxygenation too. Di Paolo N [7] had demonstrated therapeutic properties of ozone in controlling stress responses in different immune system dysfunctions and in some degenerative diseases.

Also has proven effects at patients with macular infections [8], refractory opened ulcerations [9], peritonitis [10].

Ozone treatment determines the decrease of mortality and infectious complications [11] patients in septic shock and sepsis.

Experimental results obtained at the Technical University of Cluj-Napoca using the combined use of ozone and intense electric fields in the treatment of biological environments, leads to inhibition of harmful processes and benefit (healing, antimicrobial and anti-inflammatory) biostimulative effects in the treated samples [12].

Based on these effects, authors had developed experimental equipment and methods for treatment of external overinfected wounds and diseases caused by chemical burns, varicose ulcers, bedsores, etc.[13].

Industrial ozone production method is known and applied, with the emergence of Siemens ozonizers equiped with ceramic-glass barriers determine significant increase of ozone concentrations [14].

Developing of inovative Corone discharge, performed directly on aqueous solutions leads to the production of smaller ozone quantities and ozone concentrations in comparison to Siemens ozonizers, but the effectiveness in treating medical conditions are comparable or, often, superior.

Also provides large amounts of free radicals, generated both in AC and DC, at different voltage polarities [15].

II. Equipments and Working Methods

Depending on the method of treating, the first using aqueous solutions processed with ozone, the second by use combined action of ozone and intense electric fields, upon the overinfected wounds, two different ozone generation equipments have been developed.

First of it, depicted in Figure 1, is the stand providing complex ozonization of aqueous solutions instalation.

The working methodology on this installation consists in connecting the stand to the single phase electric network,

S. Vlad and N.M. Roman (eds.), *International Conference on Advancements of Medicine and Health Care through Technology; 12th - 15th October 2016, Cluj-Napoca, Romania*,
IFMBE Proceedings 59,
DOI: 10.1007/978-3-319-52875-5_11

followed by introducing of the aqueous solution in the container 9, than in the bubbling vessel 6, until to the preset level (by actuating the valve 2.4), followed by the introduction of oxygen into the installation (valve 2.1), apressure regulator and flow meter 3 and 4, at the necesarily pressure and flow.

Further starts the ozonizer 5, followed by the required parameters adjustment; the ozone flow can be seen through the ozone bubbler 6, respectively in the vessel for ozone neutralisation 11, followed by evacuation of residual waste gases (12). Valves 2.2 and 2.4 are closed and valve 2.3 opened, the pump 8 and the ozonemeter 9 are switched on; when the concentration of ozone in the aqueous solution has reached the predetermined value, the entire equipment is set off from the network, all valves are closed, except valve 2.2, which will recover and stock the aqueous ozonized solution, which further is stored in the container 7. Further the solution is applyed to the wounds, in accordance with the medical methods and procedures.

Treatment of external overinfected wounds with aqueous ozonized solutions combined with exposure in intense electric fields (see the stand assumed according to figure 2), presume the presence of corone discharging cells, in which electrical discharges are produced directly on the liquid, through a dielectric barrier and only in the presence of oxygen.

The working methodology with the complex combined facility processing of aqueous ozone and intense electric fields consists in ozone neutralisation 11, followed by evacuation of residual waste gases (12). Valves 2.2 and 2.4 are closed and valve 2.3 opened, the pump 8 and the ozonemeter 9 are switched on; when the concentration of

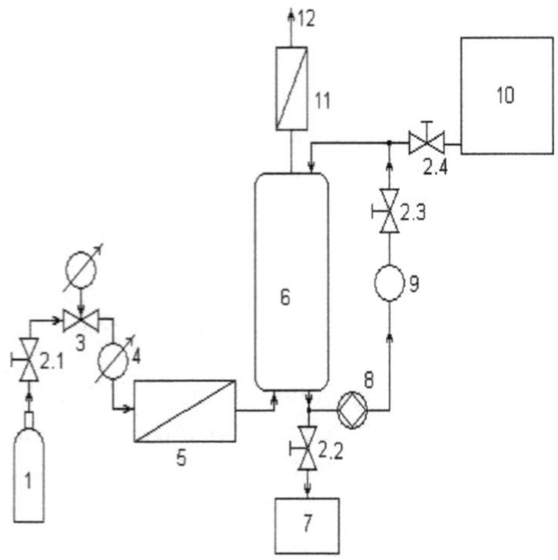

Fig. 1. Complex ozonization instalation for aqueos solution; 1 – oxygen cylinder; 2.1 ÷ 2.4 – valves; 3 – oxygen pressure regulator; 4 - flowmeter; 5 – ozonizer; 6 – barbotage vessel; 7 – ozonized solutions colecting vessel; 8 – pump; 9 – liquid phase ozonometer; 10 – treatment ready solutions vessel; 11 – ozone neutralizer; 12 – waste gases evacuation

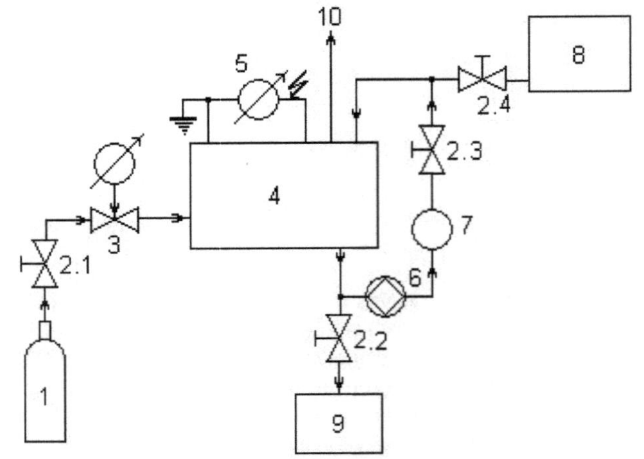

Figure 2. Complex aqueos solutions processing installation with ozone and intense electric fields; 1 – oxygen cylinder; 2.1 ÷ 2.4 – valves; 3 – oxygen pressure regulator; 4 – corone discharging cell for aqueos solutions processing; 5 – variable high voltage supply; 6 – pump; 7 – liquid phase ozonometer; 8- treatment ready solutions vessel; 9 – ozonized solutions colecting vessel;10 –waste gases evacuation.

ozone in the aqueous solution has reached the predetermined value, the entire equipment is set off from the network, all valves are closed, except valve 2.2, which will determine the recover and stock the aqueous ozonized solution, which further is stored in the container 9.

The aqueous solutions processed with ozone or ozone and the corone fields have been used to treat wounds become infected, following the procedures set out in a large number of clinic experiments on various kinds of diseases.

Using ozone and intense electric fields in treating external wounds become infected was applied to varicose ulcers, classic treatment refractory in skin burns with chemical agents and bedsores.

Adjustable high voltage supplies are used (pos. 5) were either dried source at main frequency of 50 Hz, output a.c. or d.c. with different polarities, or electronic sources providing adjustable voltage level, a.c. or d.c. output, with reversible polarity. The high voltage rise up to 25 kV and frequencies till 2 kHz.

A. Varicose ulcers treatment procedure

- thoroughly wash the wound with ulceration or plague with ozonized aqueous solution, daily, once in the morning. For the treatment of refractory ulcers, the method continues with the introduction of the affected area of ulceration (after cleaning with plenty of water treated) and its maintenance for 10-15 minutes in an enclosure containing strongly ozonized gas;

- applying sterile compresses and bandages, soaked with the processed aqueous solution all over the ulcer during a period of 20-30 min;

- simultaneously, implementation of medication based on antibiotics and steroids;
- applying a further 2 or 3 compresses soaked in sterile aqueous solution being processed, at periods determined by the state of eczematizate pericankerous area.

B. Method of treating skin burns

- applyance of sterile compresses and bandages, soaked with the aqueous solutions all over the burned areas; change compress every 2-3 hours to complete healing (4-5 days for first degree burns and 14-15 days for second degree burns);
- applyance of medication based on antibiotics and steroids.

The wounds become infected, reluctant to medicines, can be treated with aqueous solutions processed with ozone or ozone and electric fields, but sometimes also with ozonized air.

III. Results and Comments

Aqueous solution were used single or multiple distilled water experimental results are presented in Table 1 and Table 2 for ozonation and treating in corone electric fields with abundant ozone generation.

In all tested applications were obtained good results, but dependent on the particularities, the type, shape, size and stage of the ulcer, the residual ozone concentration in the processed solutions, presence of free radicals, frequencies and durations of treatment on the patient.

The most effective treatment is obtained by applying the ozonized aqueous solutions or the ozone combined intense electric fields immediately after processing. Good results are obtained after about 2 hours of processing aqueous solutions, and after about 8-10 hours, their efficacy drops sharply, even if kept sealed.

Storage temperature is a key factor of "preservation" properties acquired; at temperatures of about 4° C the characteristics after about 8 hours of storage are preserved.

The treatment methods indicates drastically shortens of the healing period; shortening is greater with use of air, oxygen or both, on processed aqueous solutions using proposed treatment devices.

With the shortened periods of healing, are removed the danger of microbial and fungal superinfection, without the patient requiring a preventive antibiotic treatment in general way.

Here is the record, particulary, varicose ulcers and pressure sores resulting from prolonged immobilization patient in bed when the peripheral circulation is poor.

Skin healing obtained for new treatments proposed are more aesthetic in comparison with classical treatments.

Table 1. Criteria and levels of ozonization of aqueous solutions

No crt	Solution type	The adjustment parameters of ozonizer				Exposure time [s]	Residual O_3 conc. of aqueous solution [mg/l]
		Oxygen		Ozone			
		Pressure [bar]	Flow [l/h]	Concentration [gO_3/m^3]	Amount [g/h]		
1.	Simple distilled water	0,1	10÷50	120,7÷41,8	1,21÷2,09	60 ÷ 300	5
2.	Double distilled water	0,1	10÷50	120,7÷41,8	1,21÷2,09	60 ÷ 300	3

Legend *- a – filiform electrodes with multiple corone discharge; - b – electrodes with multiple needle type corone discharge; - c – strainer corone discharge electrode ; - s – discharging gap; - p – distance between discharging elements of the electrodes

Table 2. Criteria and levels of ozonization and treatment procedure using aqueous solutions exposed to intense corone electric fields

Nr crt	Solution type	Electrical and constructive parameters of the treatment cells											Exposure time [s]	Residual O_3 conc. of aqueous solution [mg/l]
		Voltage levels, [kV]				Type of treatment cells *								
		c.a. 50Hz	c.a. 2kHz	c.c. +	c.c. -	With barrier	No barrier	s [mm]	p [mm]	a	b	c		
1.	Simple distilled water	5÷25	5÷25	5÷20	5÷25	x	x	10÷30	2,5÷10	x	x	x	60 ÷ 300	7
2.	Double distilled water	5÷25	5÷25	5÷20	5÷25	x	x	10÷30	2,5÷10	x	x	x	60 ÷ 300	4,5

IV. Conclusions

The ozone alone, or in combination with the free radicals generated by corona discharge performed on the aqueous solutions may have highly beneficial effects on patients who have external wounds superinfected and relates to:

-Drastic shortening healing time and reducing stress state of inactivation of the patient as a result of these long and difficult to cure diseases;

Elimination of the danger of microbial and fungal overinfection, generally without requiring a preventive antibiotic treatment;

Obtaining more aesthetic skin healing in comparison to conventional treatments;

Simplicity of the methods because do not interfere with anything to the patient, acting through oxidation in tissue, stimulating local, leukocytosis;

Achieving time, pain, costs savings by simplicityof the method, significant diminished duration of treatment and reducing the time medication of the patient.

The results obtained with complex ozonisation equipment can be matched, or even exceeded, using the processing equipment directly into intense electric fields, which is extremely simple and cheap.

Experiments can be conducted by ozone and type free radicals, eradicating microbial overinfected wound at first, followed by an apropriate amount of ozone and free radicals, or aerosols, generating sharp and fast recovery of damaged tissue ulceration.

Further research deserves to be channeled in this direction

Statement of human and animal rights

Procedures followed were in accordance with the ethical standards of the responsible committee on human experimentation (institutional and national) and with the Helsinki Declaration of 1975, as revised in 2000 and 2008.

Conflict of Interest

The authors declare that they have no conflict of interest.

References

1. Azarpazhooh A., Limeback H. - The application of ozone in dentistry: A systematic review of literature. Journal of Dentistry; 36:104-116, 2008.
2. Bialoszewski, D., Kowalewski, M. - Superficially, longer, intermittent ozone theraphy in the treatment of the chronic, infected wounds. Ortop.Traumatol.Rehabil.2003, 30; 5(5):652-8.
3. Chen H, Xing B, Liu X, Zhan B, Zhou J, Zhu H, Chen Z. - Ozone oxidative reconditioning inhibits inflammation and apoptosis in a rat model of renal ischemia / reperfusion injury. Eur. J. Pharmacol. 2007, Nov. 28.
4. Parkhisenko Iu.A, Bilchenko SV. - The ozone therapy in patients with mechanical jaundice of tumorous genesis. Vestn Khir Im I I Grek. 2003; 162(5):85-7.
5. Di Paolo N, Bocci V, Cappelletti F, Petrini G, Gaggiotti E. - Necrotizing fasciitis successfully treated with extracorporeal blood oxygenation and ozonization. Int. J. Artif. Organs. 2002. Dec; 25(12): 1194-8.
6. Mustafaev EM, Martov AG, et all., - The role of ozone therapy in prevention of pyoinflammatory complications after transurethral resection of prostatic adenoma. Urologiia. 2007 Jan-Feb; (1):18-23, 27.
7. Di Paolo N, Gaggiotti E, Galli F. - Extracorporeal blood oxygenation and ozonation: clinical and biological implications of ozone therapy. Redox Rep. 2005; 10(3):121-30.
8. Bocci V. - The case for oxygen-ozone therapy. Br. J.Biomed. Sci. 2007; 64(1):44-9.
9. Ozmen V, Thomas WO, Healy JT, Fish JM, Chambers R, Tacchi E, Nichols RL, Flint LM, Ferrara JJ. - Irrigation of the abdominal cavity in the treatment of experimentally induced microbial peritonitis: efficacy of ozonized saline. Am. Surg. 1993 May; 59 (5):297-303.
10. Vasiliev IT, Markov IN, et all. - The antibacterial and immune-corrective action of zone therapy in peritonitis. Vestn. Khir. Im. I I Grek. 1995; 154(3):56-60.
11. Parkhisenko Iu.A., Glukhov, A.A. - Use of ozone therapy and hydro-pressure technologies in complex intensive therapy of surgical sepsis. Khirurgiia (Mosk.), 2001; (4):55-8.
12. Suarasan, I., et all. - High Intense Electric Fields and Ozone – Inhibiting or Biostimulating Factors of the Seeds Treated and Food Security. IAO3 Conference and Exhibition Valencia, Spain - October 29-31, 2007.
13. Armando Figueroa, Hernández Juan, M. Salomón, Bacallao Alejandro, Díaz González - Ozone therapy on Otorhinolaryngology. A five-year study. MediSur. 2005; 3(3)53-57.
14. Suarasan, I., Ghizdavu Letiţia, Ghizdavu, I., Budu, S., Dăscălescu, L. - Experimental characterization of multi-point corone discharge devices for direct ozonization of liquids. Journal of Electrostatics. Vol. 54 (2002), pp. 207 – 214.
15. Suarasan, I., Mudura, M., Chira, R., Andrei, Gabriela, Muncelean, I., Morar, R. - A Novel Type Ozonizer for Wastewater Treatment. 2005. In: Journal of Electrostatics 63 (2005), pp. 831-

Comparative Analysis of Cardiovascular Risk Profile, Cardiac and Cervical Arterial Ultrasound in Patients with Chronic Coronary and Peripheral Arterial Ischemia

M.A. Stoia [1,2], A.D. Farcaş [1,2], F.P. Anton [1,2], A.I. Roman[3] and L.A.Vida -Simiti [1,2]

[1]"Iuliu Haţieganu" University of Medicine and Pharmacy, Cluj-Napoca, Romania
[2]Clinical Emergency County Hospital, Cardiology I Dept., Cluj-Napoca, Romania
[3] "Octavian Fodor" Regional Institute of Gastroenterology and Hepathology, Cluj Napoca, Romania

Abstract — **The aim of this study was to compare the cardiovascular ultrasound and risk factor profile in patients with peripheral arterial ischemia (PAD) and patients with stable angina pectoris (SA). We studied 55 patients with PAD and 22 patients with SA which were evaluated with cardiac and vascular ultrasound.We found the profile of cardiovascular risk factors, echocardiography and cervical artery ultrasound findings in patients with PAD and SA is relatively similar and the cardiovascular risk is relatively high for both types of patients. There are some specific therapeutic changes arising from the particular arterial territory involved.**

Keywords — **peripheral artery disease, chronic stable angina, cardiovascular risk profile, echocardiography, cervical arterial ultrasound.**

I. Introduction

Atherosclerosis (ATS) is an extensive and progressive arterial multisite disease that affects coronary, carotid and peripheral arteries. The impairment of a particular arterial sector varies and depends, in part, on the individual characteristics and the presence of cardiovascular (CV) risk (CVR) factors (CVRF) [1-3]. The patients with ischemic heart disease (or coronary artery disease – CAD) are considered to have a higher CVR than patients with peripheral artery disease (PAD). Also the patients with CAD benefit more often from the CV evaluation compared to patients with PAD. In terms of ultrasound assessment, the echocardiography is more used than arterial cervical echography. Despite the fact that are some registries [1-3] including patients with various ATS lesions (coronary, carotid, peripheral artery), there are no systematic studies comparing patients with chronic arterial ischemia and patients with stable coronary artery disease, regarding the cardiovascular ultrasound and risk factors profiles. A legitimate question then arises: what are the differences and the similarities between these two groups of patients, who had in common the same phenomenon (arterial ischemia), but located in different territories?

II. Material and Methods

The aim of this study was to compare the cardiovascular ultrasound and risk factor profile in patients with peripheral arterial ischemia (PAD) and patients with stable angina pectoris (SA). We tried to find what are the differences and the similarities between these two groups of patients regarding the cardiovascular risk factor, echocardiography aspects and arterial cervical ultrasound elements, in order to see if the CV clinic and imagistic profile of PAD patients is less or equal in term of significance with the CV clinic and imagistic profile of SA patients.

The study included 77 patients with chronic arterial ischemia: 55 patients with PAD without critical leg ischemia (CLI) and 22 patients with CAD and SA, hospitalized in Cardiology Department for complete cardiovascular evaluation, laboratory and ultrasound imaging assessment. All patients signed informed consent at enrollment. The study methodology was approved by the Ethical Committee and was in accordance with European ethical standards.

Review methodology included: clinical examination, ECG, echocardiogram and carotid-vertebral ultrasound. During echocardiography we measured standard sizes (Ao-aorta, LA-left atrium, LV-left ventricle, IVS interventricular septum, LVPW- LV posterior wall, EDDLV-end-diastolic diameter of LV, ESDLV- end-systolic diameter of LV), we evaluated the global and segmental LV parietal kinetics (highlighting segments with hypokinesia, akinesia and dyskinesia) and we quantified LV systolic function, based on ejection fraction (EF): LVEF = (EDVLV - ESVLV) / EDVLVx100, EDVLV - end-diastolic volume of LV, ESVLV - end-systolic volume of LV, calculated by the two-dimensional method. Normal values: Ao $\leq$ 40 mm, IVS $\leq$ 11 mm, LVPW $\leq$ 11 mm, EDDLV = 35-57 mm, ESDLV = 25-45 mm, LVEF $\geq$ 50%). We also assessed the LV diastolic performance (E and A waves amplitude, E/A ratio estimated by pulsed Doppler transmitral flow curve) [4-9].

We performed carotid and vertebral ultrasound and measured the thickness of the intima-media (IMT) in the common carotid artery, bilaterally (standard in the posterior-medial wall, 2 cm before the carotid bifurcation) (normal

S. Vlad and N.M. Roman (eds.), *International Conference on Advancements of Medicine and Health Care through Technology; 12th - 15th October 2016, Cluj-Napoca, Romania,*
IFMBE Proceedings 59,
DOI: 10.1007/978-3-319-52875-5_12

values <0.75 mm). We estimated the hemodynamic significance of carotid and vertebral stenoses by using the following criteria: morphological (cross-section Doppler color calculating the area of stenosis (%) by the formula: (Total vascular area - Permeable Doppler color area) / Total vascular area) and hemodynamic (intrastenotic Vmax- maximal systolic velocity, Ved-end-diastolic velocity and Vmax intra / prestenotic ratio). 50-70% stenoses are defined by Vmax = 1.2-2 m/s, Ved < 0.4 m/s, Vmax intra / prestenotic = 2-3 and the corresponding percent reduction in Doppler color functional area. Stenoses > 70% were defined by Vmax > 2 m/s, Ved > 0.4 m/s, Vmax intra/prestenotic > 3 and the corresponding percentage reduction in functional Doppler color area. [10-12].

Group comparison was done using Student test for continuous variables with normal distribution and Mann-Whitney U test for continuous variables with abnormal distribution and ordinal variables, while the chi-square test was used for categorial variables. SPSS 16 was used for statistical analysis, with a p value < 0.05 considered statistically significant.

III. Results

The prevalence of males and smokers was higher in PAD patients without CLI compared to CAD patients with SA. Among other CVRF, prevalence of hypertension (HT) was significantly higher in CAD patients with SA than in PAD patients without CLI. The prevalence of diabetes (DM) and dyslipidemia was relatively equal in the two groups. The most prevalent CVRF in patients with PAD without CLI, respectively in CAD patients with SA was hypercholesterolemia (HCst), followed by hypertriglyceridemia (HTgl) and DM. HTgl prevalence was highest in PAD patients without CLI, while DM prevalence was highest in CAD patients with SA.

We found a significantly higher prevalence of LV hypertrophy (LVH) and LV dilatation (LVD) in patients with SA than in PAD patients without CLI. The prevalence of septal hypertrophy (IVWH) was relatively similar in PAD patients without CLI and in CAD patients with SA, while the LVPW hypertrophy (LVPWH) was higher in CAD patients with SA compared with PAD patients without CLI. We found a statistically significant higher prevalence of diastolic dysfunction (DD) in CAD patients with SA compared to PAD patients without CLI (Table 1). Prevalence of segmental parietal kinetic disorders (SPKD) was moderately higher in CAD patients with SA (78%) than in PAD patients without CLI. The highest prevalence of SPKD in PAD patients without CLI was observed in the septum, followed (in descending order) by inferior-posterior, lateral and anterior walls. Septum wall SPKD prevalence was higher in CAD patients with SA compared with PAD patients without CLI. There was a moderately higher prevalence of the anterior and lateral walls SPKD in CAD patients with SA than in PAD patients without CLI. and a slightly higher prevalence of inferior-posterior wall SPKD in PAD patients without CLI than in CAD patients with SA (Table 1).

Table 1. Echocardiographic profile in PAD patients without CLI compared to CAD patients with SA (ns – not significant, s – significant

Parameter prevalence (values)	PAD without CLI	CAD with SA	Statistical significance
Concentric LVH	47%	72%	p < 0.001
IVSH	52%	64%	p < 0.1
(mm)	10.5±2.4	11.2±1.7	ns
LVPWH	51%	78%	p < 0.01
(mm)	10.2±2.2	11.2±2.7	ns
LVD	11%	22%	p < 0.01
EDDLV dilatation	20%	21%	ns
(mm)	48.48±8	50±9.9	ns
ESDLV dilatation	3%	21%	p < 0.001
(mm)	37±7.9	35.9±10.1	ns
Diastolic dysfunction	35%	90%	p < 0.001
Impaired systolic function	41%	43%	ns
LVEF	48.6±7.8%	47.8±7.8%	ns
LV SPKD	56%	78%	p <0.01
SPKD septum	35%	64%	p <0.001
SPKD inferior/posterior	29%	23%	p <0.1
SPKD lateral	19%	23%	ns
SPKD anterior	11%	28%	p <0.01

No statistically significant differences were found regarding carotid IMT in PAD patients without CLI compared with CAD patients with SA.

Table 2. Carotid and vertebral ultrasound profile in PAD patients without CLI compared with CAD patients with SA.

Parameter prevalence (values)	PAD without CLI	CAD with SA	Statistical significance
Carotid IMT (mm)	0.78±0.2	0.7±0,2	ns
>50% carotid and vertebral stenoses	29%	64%	p<0.001
>50% carotid stenoses	25%	50%	p<0.001
>50% vertebral stenoses	4%	14%	p<0.001
50-70% carotid and vertebral stenoses	15%	41%	p<0.001
>70% carotid and vertebral stenoses and thromboses	14%	24%	p<0.01

We found a higher statistically significant prevalence of cervical arterial, both carotid and vertebral stenoses >50% in CAD patients with SA than in PAD patients without CLI. The prevalence of 50-70% or >70% hemodynamic significance cervical arterial stenosis and thrombosis was equal in PAD patients without CLI, while in CAD patients with SA we found a significant higher prevalence of 50-70% cervical arterial stenoses than carotid and vertebral >70% stenoses and thromboses. The prevalence of 50-70% cervical arterial stenoses was significantly higher in CAD patients with SA than in PAD patients without CLI. Hemodynamically significant arterial cervical stenoses (>70%) and carotid-vertebral thromboses were found in a moderately greater proportion in CAD patients with SA compared with PAD patients without CLI (Table 2).

IV. Disscusion

In our study, HT as a CVRF was frequently found in both patient groups, mainly in CAD patients with SA, which indicates its involvement in the pathophysiology and progression of peripheral and coronary lesions, as shown in other studies [1-3]. Other CVRF such as male gender and smoking were found more frequently in PAD patients without CLI, whereas DM and dyslipidemia prevalence were similar between the two groups [1-3].

As expected, the high prevalence of HT in CAD patients with SA led to a significantly higher prevalence of LVH in these patients, both as septal and PW hypertrophy. These patients also had more frequent LVD. In PAD patients without CLI the prevalence of LVH was closer to the lowest intervals found in other studies [13-15]. The most likely cause for this finding was the evaluation methodology in our study, which included all criteria for hypertensive heart disease. While LVD in CAD patients with SA was caused both by EDDLV and ESDLV, in PAD without CLI patients it was caused mostly by EDDLV. However, the prevalence of dilated cardiomyopathy was low in PAD patients without CLI. The reasons for this particular echocardiographic pattern, specific to CAD patients with SA, are the long evolution of HT and frequent multi vessel coronary lesions on coronarography found in clinical and coronarography studies [16, 17]. It is possible for PAD patients without CLI to have multi truncal coronary vessels lesions as well [18]. Altered systolic performance was found with similar prevalence in the two patient groups, while diastolic dysfunction was present in most of CAD patients with SA. Published data show diastolic dysfunction in PAD patients has a prevalence of up to 62% [13, 19].Although SPKD was found in both patient groups, only the inferior-posterior SPKD was found with similar prevalence, (raising the possibility of a similar involvement of the right coronary artery) in both patient groups, while septal, anterior and lateral wall involvement was more frequent in CAD patients with SA.

Carotid IMT was marginally higher than normal in both patient groups but with no significant differences. We found similar values with published data for PAD without CLI (0.85 mm) [20, 21].

We found a significantly higher prevalence of cervical artery stenoses in CAD patients with SA compared to PAD without CLI, irrespective of the degree of stenosis and their location (carotid or vertebral). It is possible that long-term evolution of systemic ATS can lead to multiple lesions in the carotid and vertebral territories. Published data show the prevalence of carotid stenoses is lower than 60%, most of them being 50-70% and found in PAD patients without CLI [22, 23]. The higher prevalence of cervical artery stenoses found in our study can be explained by the inclusion of vertebral lesions (and not only carotid) as well. We found a significantly higher prevalence of >50% cervical stenoses (both carotid and vertebral) in CAD patients with SA compared to PAD patients without CLI. In PAD patients without CLI we found similar prevalence for 50-70% stenoses, >70% stenoses and thromboses, while in CAD patients with SA, we found a higher prevalence of 50-70% stenoses compared to >70% stenoses and thromboses. 50-70% stenoses were significantly more frequent in CAD patients with SA compared to PAD patients without CLI, whereas >70% stenoses and thromboses were more frequent in SA patients compared to PAD patients without CLI.

There is probably a relationship between a longer evolution of arterial ischemia both in the peripheral vascular and in the cervical territories and the prevalence of severe stenoses and thromboses in the carotid and vertebral arteries. On the contrary, patients with chronic ischemia in the coronary territory can have coronary thrombotic events that accelerate the clinical manifestations of the ATS process, thus making cervical stenoses being earlier diagnosed in a less severe stage of their evolution.

In our study we found that PAD patients had significant prevalence of CV (heart and arterial cervical) ATS lesions and their CV ultrasound and risk factors profile is comparable with the CV profile of CAD patients with SA. These CV pathological aspects are important for PAD patients in the perspective of a vascular interventional or surgical approaches, known that in the perioperative context there is a higher incidence of CV major events (myocardial infarction, stroke). Despite the fact that PAD patients are considered to have a lower CVR regarding CV major events, based on our results, we might suppose that CVR of PAD patients is relatively high, almost similar to the CVR of CAD patients with SA. Therefore, we consider that is important to make a thorough CV assessment of PAD patients, as complete as the CAD patient evaluation.

V. Conclusion

Patients with arterial or coronary chronic ischemia have a high incidence of major CVRF. HCst prevalence was higher in PAD patients without CLI and HT was more prevalent in patients with SA. PAD patients without CLI present significant cardiac and cervical arterial ultrasound spectrum changes, which are similar to patients with documented CAD and SA. The most significant echocardiographic aspects in PAD patients without CLI are the presence of LVH, the LVD mainly due to the increase EDDLV, the presence of DD, impaired systolic function by decreasing LVEF and the presence of SPKD, especially on the anterior and inferior-posterior walls. Both PAD patients without CLI and CAD patients with SA had similar carotid IMT, marker of endothelial dysfunction in both groups of patients. The prevalence of cervical arterial stenoses was greater in CAD patients with SA, both in carotid and vertebral arteries. In PAD patients without CLI we found moderate stenoses, severe cervical arterial stenoses and carotid and vertebral thromboses in equal proportion. In CAD patients with SA, we found moderate (50-70%) arterial cervical stenoses more frequently than severe (>70%) carotid and vertebral stenoses and arterial cervical thromboses. The PAD patients had a relatively high CVR, similar to CAD patients with SA.

Conflict of Interest

The authors declare that they have no conflict of interest.

References

1. Eraso LH and co. Peripheral arterial disease, prevalence and cumulative risk factor profile analysis. Eur J Prev Cardiol. 2014; 21(6):704-11
2. Valentijn TM and co. Lessons from REACH Registry in Europe. Current Vascular Pharmacology, 2012;10:725-727
3. Suarez C and co. Influence of polyvascular disease on cardiovascular event rates. Insights from REACH Registry. Vascular Medicine, 2015;15(4): 259-65
4. Ginghina C and co.. Esentialul in ecocardiografie, Editura medicala Antaneus, Bucuresti, 2005:24-28,39-43.
5. Otto CM. The cardiomyophaties, hipertensive heart disease, post-cardiac transplant patient and pulmonary heart disease in Textbook of Clinical Echocardiography, W.B. Saunders, Elsevier Science, Philadelphia, 2007:200-203.
6. Otto .M. Echocardiographic evaluation of ventricular diastolic filling and function in Textbook of Clinical Echocardiography, W.B. Saunders, Elsevier Science, Philadelphia, 2007:132-149.
7. Otto CM. Echocardiographic evaluation of left and right ventricular systolic function in Textbook of Clinical Echocardiography, W.B. Saunders, Elsevier Science, Philadelphia, 2007:100-120.
8. Otto CM. The utility of echocardiography in patients with ischemic cardiac disease in Textbook of Clinical Echocardiography, W.B. Saunders, Elsevier Science, Philadelphia, 2007:153-178.
9. Farcas AD. Evaluarea ecocardiografică a funcţiei ventriculare şi a pericardului în: Vida-Simiti L, Farcaş A, Stoia MA. Explorări nonivazive în bolile cardiovasculare. Indrumător pentru studenţi şi rezidenţi. Editura Medicală Universitară „Iuliu Haţieganu" Cluj Napoca, 2011: 149-164
10. Strandness E.D. Extracranial artery disease in Duplex scanning in Vascular Disease, Lippincott, Williamson and Wilkins, a Woter Kluver Company, Philadelphia, 2012;84-115
11. Dauzat M. L'examen ultrasonographique des axes carotidiens in Practique de l'ultrasonographie vasculaire par Dauzat M., Ed. Masson, Paris, 2002;96-177.
12. Stoia M. Ecografia arterelor periferice şi a sistemului arterial carotido-vertebral în: Vida-Simiti L, Stoia MA, Fărcaş AD.. Explorări nonivazive în bolile cardiovasculare. Indrumător pentru studenţi şi rezidenţi. Editura Medicală Universitară „Iuliu Haţieganu" Cluj Napoca, 2011:196-218
13. Ward RP, Min JK, McDonough KM, Lang RM. High prevalence of important cardiac findings in patients with peripheral arterial disease referred for echocardiography. J Am Soc Echocardiogr, 2005;18(8):844-9.
14. Brahimi M, Levy BI and co. Factors determining cardiac hypertrophy in hypertensive patients with or without peripheral vascular disease. Clinical Science,1998;95:241-67
15. Sukhija R and co. Prevalence of echocardiographic left ventricular hypertrophy in persons with systemic hypertension, coronary artery disease, and peripheral arterial disease and in persons with systemic hypertension, coronary artery disease and no peripheral arterial disease. Am J Cardiol. 2005; 96(6):825-6.
16. Maddox T.M.: Preoperative cardiovascular evaluation for noncardiac surgery. Mt Sinai J Med. 2005 May; 72 (3):185-92
17. Freeman WK, Gibbons RJ. Perioperative cardiovascular assessment of patients undergoing noncardiac surgery. Mayo Clin Proc. 2009; 84(1):79-90.
18. Poldermans D and co.. Preoperative risk assessement and risk reduction before surgery. JACC, vol51;No.20, 2008:1913-34
19. Van Kujik and co. Influence of left ventricular dysfunction (diastolic versus systolic) on long term prognosis in patients with or without diabetes mellitus having elective peripheral arterial surgery. Am J Cardiol, 2010;106(6):860-4
20. Cheng KS and co. Impaired carotid and femoral viscoelastic properties and elevated intima-media thickness in peripheral vascular disease. Atherosclerosis, 2002(1):113-20.
21. Mudrikova T, Szabova E, Tkac I. Carotid intima-media thickness in relation to macrovascular disease in patients with type 2 diabetes mellitus. Wien Klin Wochenschr. 2000 Oct 27; 112 (20): 887-91.
22. Arora V and co. Preoperative assessement of cardiac risk and perioperative cardiac management in noncardiac surgery. Int J Surg, 2011; 9:23-28.
23. Di Minno G and co. Systematic reviews and meta-analyses for more profitable strategies in peripheral arteries disease. Clinical perspectives and PAD research. Annals of Medicine, 2014;1-15

Author: FARCAŞ ANCA DANIELA
Institute: "Iuliu Haţieganu"University of Medicine and Pharmacy
Street: Victor Babeş street no 8
City: Cluj-Napoca
Country: Romania
Email: ancafarcas@yahoo.com

Cardiovascular Risk Profile, Cardiac and Cervical Artery Ultrasound in Patients with Peripheral Artery Disease

A.D. Farcaş[1, 2,] , M.A. Stoia[1, 2] , F.A. Anton[1, 2] , A.I. Roman[3] and L.A Vida-Simiti [1, 2]

[1]"Iuliu Haţieganu" University of Medicine and Pharmacy, Cluj-Napoca, Romania
[2]Clinical Emergency County Hospital, Cardiology I Department, Cluj-Napoca, Romania
[3] "Octavian Fodor" Regional Institute of Gastroenterology and Hepathology, Cluj Napoca, Romania

Abstract — **Patients with peripheral arterial present different hemodynamic significance of atherosclerotic lesions in the coronary and cervical arterial territories also, which are responsible for increased vital cardiovascular risk. The aim of this study was to assess the role of clinic and imagistic cardiac and carotid evaluation of PAD patients to estimate the cardiovascular risk in the perspective of perioperative therapeutic strategy revascularization. After clinical and imagistic evaluation we found that proving the polyarterial profile changes the medical and interventional therapy, prioritizing coronary and carotid arterial revascularization.**

Keywords—**peripheral arterial disease, polyarterial patient, arterial stenosis, heart disease, cardiovascular risk.**

I. Introduction

Atherosclerosis (ATS) is a pathological process of systemic, extensive and progressive nature affecting the circulation of coronary, cerebrovascular and peripheral arteries (PAD). PAD presence is an important predictive indicator of coronary and / or concomitant carotid disease existence, which increases the risk of mortality [1-3]. The presence of ATS lesions across multiple arterial territories deems the patient "polyarterial", even if one single arterial territory is symptomatic (e.g. peripheral arteries in case of PAD). Other coronary and / or carotid ATS lesions may be masked by the symptoms of PAD. A large proportion of patients are not diagnosed with PAD before presenting a major cardiovascular (CV) event, which limits the access towards using the evidence-based pharmacologic therapy recognized for CV risk (CVR) reduction [1-3].

II. Material and Method

The aim of this study was to assess the role of clinic and imagistic cardiac and carotid evaluation of PAD patients to estimate the cardiovascular risk in the perspective of perioperative therapeutic strategy revascularization. Beside the CVR factors profile, we tried to estimate how important and significant are the heart and arterial cervical lesions in PAD patients scheduled for vascular intervention

The study included 197 patients with PAD, hospitalized in the Cardiology Department for complete cardiovascular evaluation, laboratory and ultrasound imaging assessment. All patients signed informed consent at enrollment.

The study methodology was approved by the Ethical Committee and was in accordance with European ethical standards.

The evaluation methodology included: clinical examination, ECG, echocardiogram and carotid-vertebral ultrasound. Echocardiography measured standard parameters (Ao-aorta, LA-left atrium, LV-left ventricle, IVS interventricular septum, LVPW LV posterior wall, EDDLV-end-diastolic diameter of LV ESDLV-end-systolic diameter of LV), evaluated the global and segmental LV parietal kinetics (highlighting segments with hypokinesia, akinesia and dyskinesia) and quantified LV systolic function, based on ejection fraction (EF): LVEF = (EDVLV-ESVLV) / EDVLV x 100, EDVLV-end-diastolic volume of LV, ESVLV-end-systolic volume of LV, calculated by the two-dimensional method. Normal values: Ao $\leq$ 40 mm, LVIV $\leq$ 11 mm, LVPW $\leq$ 11 mm, EDDLV = 35-57 mm, ESDLV = 25-45 mm, EDVLV = 90-120 ml, ESVLV = 30-50 ml, LVEF $\geq$ 50%) and assessed the LV diastolic function (E and A waves amplitude, E/A ratio estimated by pulsed Doppler transmitral flow curve) [4-9].

We performed carotid and vertebral ultrasound and measured the intima-media thickness (IMT) in the common carotid artery (CCA) bilaterally (standard in the posterior-medial wall, at 2 cm before the carotid bifurcation) (normal values $\leq$ 0,75 mm). We estimated the hemodynamic significance of carotid and vertebral stenoses by using morphologic criteria: cross-section color Doppler exam calculating the percent of stenoses (%) as (Total vascular area - Permeable color Doppler area) / Total vascular area - and hemodynamic criteria: intrastenotic Vmax (maximal systolic velocity), Ved (end-diastolic velocity) and Vmax intra/prestenotic ratio). 50-70% stenoses were defined by Vmax = 1,2-2 m/s, Ved< 0.4 m/s, Vmax intra/prestenotic = 2-3 and the corresponding percent reduction in Doppler color functional area.

S. Vlad and N.M. Roman (eds.), *International Conference on Advancements of Medicine and Health Care through Technology; 12th - 15th October 2016, Cluj-Napoca, Romania,*
IFMBE Proceedings 59,
DOI: 10.1007/978-3-319-52875-5_13

Stenoses >70% were defined by Vmax> 2 m/s, Ved> 0.4 m/s, Vmax intra/prestenotic> 3 and the corresponding percentage reduction in functional area [10-12].

Group comparison was done using the chi-square test for categorial variables, Student test for continuous variables with normal distribution and Mann-Whitney U test for continuous variables with abnormal distribution and ordinal variables. Statistical analysis was performed with SPSS 16. The p value <0.05 was considered statistically significant.

III. Results

Most patients with PAD were male (87%) and elderly (60% were over 60 years, one of fourth of these patients were over 70 years). More than half of patients with PAD had almost all major CV risk factors. Of these, smoking had the highest prevalence (68%), followed by hypertension (HT) (66%), hypercholesterolemia (HCst) (52%), diabetes (DZ) (50%) and hypertriglyceridemia (Htgl) (47%). Regarding the associated CV diseases (CVD), 3% of patients with PAD had a previous diagnosis of hypertensive heart disease (HTD), 29% of ischemic heart disease (or coronary artery disease - CAD) and 2% of dilated cardiomyopathy (DCM) (of ischemic, hypertensive or ethanolic etiology). Dilated ascending aorta was found in 7% of patients with PAD. 51% of PAD patients presented symmetric or asymmetric concentric LV hypertrophy (LVH). 53% of patients had LVIVS hypertrophy and 41% of patients had LVPW hypertrophy. 12% of patients with PAD had LV cavity enlargement in both diameters (EDDLV and ESDLV), 14% of PAD patients had increased EDDLV and 7% of PAD patients had increased ESDLV. Diastolic dysfunction (DD) was found in 36% of PAD patients. The majority (75%) of PAD patients had stage I of DD (impaired relaxation pattern), while 25% of PAD patients had advanced DD (stage II with altered relaxation-compliance pattern and stage III restrictive pattern). Over 50% of PAD patients had segmental parietal kinetic disorders (SPKD), located in one or more LV walls. Most SPKD in patients with PAD were found in the inferior/posterior LV wall (34 %) and in the septum (33%), followed by SPKD in the lateral wall (26%) and in the anterior wall (17%); 2% of patients had post-infarction LV aneurysms. Impaired systolic function (LVEF ≤50%) was found in 51% of PAD patients (35% had FE between 40-50%, 12% between 30-40% and 4% between 20-30%).

At baseline, 34% of PAD patients had a known heart condition- 27% had CAD (silent myocardial ischemia on ECG, ST segment and/or T wave changes, previous infarction, known angina, atrial fibrillation or left bundle branch block), 3% had HTD and 2% had DCM. Following the complete CV evaluation during hospitalization, we found the prevalence of these comorbidities increased – with 29% for HTD (from 3% to 32%), with 22% for CAD (from 27% to 49%) and 17% for DCM (from 2% to 19%). We found that 17% of patients had both HTD and CAD.

After a complete CV evaluation (including clinical exam, ECG, echocardiography and coronary angiography) 68% of PAD patients were diagnosed with the following heart diseases: HTD in 29% of patients, CAD in 49% of patients and DCM in 19% of patients. Among patients with PAD and heart disease, the most prevalent was the HTD (43%), followed by CAD (32%) and DCM (25%). (Table 1).

Carotid and vertebral Doppler ultrasound evaluation found a significant increase in the IMT of the CCA in PAD patients (0,93 ± 0,25 mm). Over a third (34%) of PAD patients had >50% stenosis (28% carotid and 6% vertebral), 21% had 50-70% stenoses, while 13% had severe (>70%) stenoses and cervical artery thrombosis. (Table 2).

Table 1. Echocardiographic profile in PAD patients.

Parameter	Known heart disease	Newly diagnosed heart disease
Concentric LVH		51%
LVIVS hypertrophy		53%
LVPW hypertrophy		41%
LV dilatation		12
EDLVD dilatation		14%
ESLVD dilatation		6%
Diastolic dysfunction (DD)		36%
Decreased LVEF (<50%)		51%
SPKD LV		55%
SPKD inf/post		34%
SPKD sept		33%
SPKD lateral		26%
SPKD anterior		17%
Heart disease (total)	34%	68%
CAD	29%	49%
HTD	3%	32%
DCM	2%	19%

Table 2. Cervical arterial ultrasound profile in PAD patients with PAD

Parameter	Prevalence/value
Carotid IMT	0,93±0,25 mm
Carotid and vertebral stenosis>50%	34%
Carotid stenosis >50%	28%
Vertebral stenosis >50%	6%
Carotid and vertebral stenosis 50-70%	21%
Carotid and vertebral stenosis>70% and thrombosis	13%

IV. Discussion

Polyarterial (i.e. multisite arterial ATS lesions) patients with clinical signs of peripheral arterial ischemia (intermittent claudication, rest pain, trophic disorders) are patients with multiple major CV risk factors. HT, DZ and dyslipidemia are found in more than 50% of these patients. Similarly to other studies, PAD patients in our study were mostly older males and smokers [1]. However, unlike data from the REACH registry, we found a higher prevalence of HT, DZ and HCst [1-3].

Cardiac and vascular ultrasound evaluation has found not only significant peripheral arterial lesions (responsible for the clinical symptoms) but also significant cardiac changes and carotid lesions, although the patients were asymptomatic at admission and without known diseases in these territories [13-16]. A careful and complete clinical and echocardiographic evaluation has increased the diagnostic accuracy for the presence and type of cardiomyopathy, proven by the doubling in its prevalence at discharge. For example, CAD prevalence has doubled after non-invasive and invasive evaluation, in agreement with published data (30-60%, depending on the hemodynamic impact of coronary angiography lesions [1-3, 18, 19]. It is also possible that some previously diagnosed CAD patients had a dilated myopathic-type evolution before we evaluated them [4-8, 16, 17]. Besides, the leading cause of death in patients with peripheral artery ischemia is major coronary events [1-3, 18, 19]. HTD prevalence was also high, explained by a high prevalence of hypertension, in agreement with published data. We found both concentric and eccentric myocardial hypertrophy, mainly involving the septum [4-6, 18, 20]. Patients with PAD had significant prevalence of LVH (1/2 of patients) most likely related to pathophysiological direct presence in the high proportion of hypertension, as major CV risk factor [17, 18]. The diagnostic criteria of HTD (concentric LVH including LVIVS and LVPW hypertrophy) were present in 29% of patients with PAD. If is evolving an asymmetric hypertrophy, the LVIVS hypertrophy is prevalent, more commonly [4-6, 18, 21].

Diastolic function was altered with variable severity in approximately 1/3 of BAP patients in our study, both with HTD and CAD. In some cases, although LV diameters were normal we found noticeable parietal kinetic disorder that caused systolic dysfunction, by alteration of global systolic motion. We might have found some cases of dilated myopathic-type evolution of CAD [4, 5, 8, 9]. The high prevalence and multisegmentary distribution of SPKD found in our study group might be explained by and related to multi truncal vascular lesions identified at coronarography. The presence of multiple SPKD is correlated to decreased global parietal kinetic function and LV systolic dysfunction (EF <50%) [8, 9, 13].

The significant increase in carotid IMT (cIMT) is a strong and independent predictor for the presence of coronary lesions [21-25]. As a marker for extensive ATS, increased cIMT is logical in PAD patients [21-25]. The presence of cervical arterial lesions may be related to cerebrovascular events, which account for 10-15% of deaths in PAD patients [19, 20]. These patients have widespread ATS lesions, but only some of them have a hemodynamic impact (>50% stenoses) and some of them are symptomatic. Published data show a 20-40% prevalence of carotid lesions in polyarterial patients; similarly to the associated coronary lesions, this prevalence varies with the hemodynamic impact of carotid lesions [1-2, 19, 20]. More than one third of PAD patients had cervical artery stenoses, mostly carotid. The prevalence of 50-70% stenoses was a little higher than of severe (greater than 70%) stenoses and carotid-vertebral thromboses. The importance of cervical ATS lesion evaluation is related to the risk of stroke.

The CVR evaluation in patients with PAD is important in the context of interventional approaches and / or peripheral arterial surgery. Diagnosing a heart disease and / or significant cervical arterial lesions changes medical and interventional treatment strategy. Patients with PAD should receive drug therapy for plaque stabilization (statins, antiplatelet agents etc.), both before and after interventional and / or surgical treatment. In order to minimize the vital CV risk of patients with PAD, coronary and carotid intervention must precede peripheral arterial revascularization.

Our study demonstrates that in patients with PAD, the current CV evaluation - accessible in most of our county hospitals, but not routinely used - plays a major role in assessing the risk for coronary and cerebrovascular events, especially in the vascular perioperative context.

V. Conclusions

The polyarterial patient with PAD symptoms has a few features. CV risk factors present in more than half of PAD patients are: male gender, older age, smoking, dyslipidemic, hypertensive and diabetic.

The typical echocardiographic profile of more than half of PAD patients include: LV hypertrophy, decreased global parietal contractile function, segmental parietal kinetic disorder (especially in the interventricular septum – about 1/3 of patients, posterior and inferior wall – about 1/3 of patients) and decreased systolic performance – 1/2 of patients and diastolic function – more than 1/3 of patients.

Following a complete CV evaluation, PAD patients were diagnosed (with decreasing prevalence) with hypertensive, ischemic and dilative cardiomyopathy.

Cervical arterial ultrasound reveals that PAD patients have diffuse atherosclerosis (increased cIMT), mostly carotid stenoses – 1/3 of patients and more >50% stenoses than severe (>70%) stenoses and arterial thromboses.

Demonstrating the polyarterial profile (with significant ATS lesions in multiple artery territories - coronary and/or carotid) in a patient with PAD changes the orientation of the patient's therapy. In these cases, coronary and carotid arterial revascularization procedures must precede peripheral arterial revascularization intervention.

Conflict of Interest

The authors declare that they have no conflict of interest.

References

1. Eraso LH, Fukaya E, and co. Peripheral arterial disease, prevalence and cumulative risk factor profile analysis. Eur J Prev Cardiol. 2014; 21(6):704-11
2. Valentijn TM, Stolker RJ. Lessons from REACH Registry in Europe. Current Vascular Pharmacology, 2012;10:725-727
3. Suarez C and co. Influence of polyvascular disease on cardiovascular event rates. Insights from REACH Registry. Vascular Medicine, 2015;15(4): 259-65
4. Ginghina C, Popescu BA, Jurcut R. Esentialul in ecocardiografie, Editura MedicalaAntaneus, Bucuresti, 2005:24-28,39-43.
5. Otto CM. The cardiomyophaties, hipertensive heart disease, post-cardiac transplant patient and pulmonary heart disease in Textbook of Clinical Echocardiography, W.B. Saunders, Elsevier Science, Philadelphia, 2007:200-203.
6. Otto .M. Echocardiographic evaluation of ventricular diastolic filling and function in Textbook of Clinical Echocardiography, W.B. Saunders, Elsevier Science, Philadelphia, 2007:132-149.
7. Otto CM. Echocardiographic evaluation of left and right ventricular systolic function in Textbook of Clinical Echocardiography, W.B. Saunders, Elsevier Science, Philadelphia, 2007:100-120.
8. Otto CM. The utility of echocardiography in patients with ischemic cardiac disease in Textbook of Clinical Echocardiography, W.B. Saunders, Elsevier Science, Philadelphia, 2007:153-178.
9. Farcas AD. Evaluarea ecocardiografică a funcţiei ventriculare şi a pericardului în: Vida –Simiti L, Fărcaş A and co. Explorări nonivazive în bolile cardiovasculare. Indrumător pentru studenţi şi rezidenţi. Editura Medicală Universitară „Iuliu Haţieganu" Cluj Napoca, 2011: 149-164
10. Stoia M. Ecografia arterelor periferice şi a sistemului arterial carotido-vertebral în: Vida –Simiti LA, Stoia M and co. Explorărinonivazive în bolile cardiovasculare. Indrumător pentru studenţi şi rezidenţi. Editura Medicală Universitară „Iuliu Haţieganu" Cluj-Napoca, 2011:196-218
11. Strandness E.D: Extracranial artery disease in Duplex scanning in Vascular Disease, Lippincott, Williamson and Wilkins, a WoterKluver Company, Philadelphia, 2012;84-115
12. Dauzat M. L'examen ultrasonographique des axes carotidiens in Practique de l'ultrasonographie vasculaire par Dauzat M., Ed. Masson, Paris, 2002; 96-177.
13. Athyros V, Mikhailidis DP and co. Prevalence of atherosclerotic vascular disease among subjects with the metabolic syndrome with or without diabetes mellitus. The METSGREECE Multicentre Study Curr Med Res Opin. 2004; 20(11).
14. Ward RP, Min JK, and co. High prevalence of important cardiac findings in patients with peripheral arterial disease referred for echocardiography. J Am Soc Echocardiogr. 2005;18(8):844-9.
15. Brahimi M, Levy BI, et al. Factors determining cardiac hypertrophy in hypertensive patients with or without peripheral vascular disease. Clinical Science,1998;95:241-67
16. Sukhija R, Aronow WS, and co. Prevalence of echocardiographic left ventricular hypertrophy in persons with systemic hypertension, coronary artery disease, and peripheral arterial disease and in persons with systemic hypertension, coronary artery disease and no peripheral arterial disease. Am J Cardiol. 2005;96(6):825-6.
17. Cooper LL, Rong J, and co. Components of hemodynamic load and cardiovascular events; the Framingham Heart Study. Circulation, 2015;131(4):354-61
18. Raghava S, Velagaleti MD, and co: Left ventricular hypertrophy patterns and incidence of heart failure with preserved versus reduced ejection fraction. Am J Cardiol, 2014;113(1):1-16
19. Arora V, Velanovich V, and co. Preoperative assessement of cardiac risk and perioperative cardiac management in noncardiac surgery. Int J Surg, 2011;9:23-28.
20. Di Minno G, Spadarella G, Cafaro G and co. Systematic reviews and meta-analyses for more profitable strategies in peripheral arteries disease. Clinical perspectives and PAD research. Annals of Medicine, 2014;1-15
21. Hammill BG, Curtis LH, Bennett-Guerrero E, O'Connor CM, Jollis JG, Schulman KA, Hernandez AF. Impact of heart failure on patients undergoing major noncardiac surgery. Anesthesiology. 2008;108(4):559-67.
22. Bots ML, Sutton-Tyrrell K. Lessons from the past and promises for the future for carotid intima-media thickness. JAMA, 2012;60;17:1599-1604
23. Baldassarre D, Hamsten A and co. Measurement of carotid-media thickness and of interadventitia common carotid diameter improve prediction of cardiovascular events (results of the IMPROVE-Carotid Intima Media Thickness[IMT] and IMT-Progression as Predictors of Vascular Events in High Risk European Population) Study, J Am Coll Cardiol,2012;60;16:1489-99
24. Ruijter HM, Peters SAE and co. Common carotid intima-media thickness measurements in cardiovascular risk prediction-a meta-analysis, JAMA, 2012;308;8:796-803
25. Chironi G, Simon A. The prognostic of intima-media thickness revisited. Arch Cardiovasc Dis, 2013;106:1-3
26. Bots ML, den Ruijter HM. Variability in the intima-media thickness measurement as marker for cardiovascular risk? Not quite settled yet. Cardiovasc Diagn Ther, 2012;2(1):3-5

Author: STOIA MIRELA ANCA
Institute: "Iuliu Haţieganu" University of Medicine and Pharmacy
Street: V. Babeş street, no 8
City: Cluj-Napoca
Country: Romania
Email: mirelastoia @yahoo.com

Part II
Medical Devices, Measurements and Instrumentation

A Single-character Refreshable Braille Display with FPGA Control

M. C. Ignat[1], P. Faragó[1], S. Hintea[1], M. N. Roman[2] and S. Vlad[2]

[1] Bases of Electronics Department, Technical University of Cluj-Napoca, Cluj-Napoca, Romania
[2] Electrotechnics and Measurements Department, Technical University of Cluj-Napoca, Cluj-Napoca, Romania

Abstract— **Visual impairment, in terms of sight loss and blindness, affects 285 million people worldwide. While 80% of the cases are either treatable or preventable, the remainder require alternative means to compensate limitations in mobility, reading, communication, access technology, etc. For this purpose, braille is an alphabet used by the visually impaired for tactile reading. Refreshable braille displays are electromechanical devices used for the electronic display of braille characters. This paper presents a one-character refreshable braille display, implemented with electromagnetic relays and control logic implemented on a field programmable gate array (FPGA). The advantage of one-character braille display is that it enables static reading, which contributes to user comfort. From a technical point of view, one-character braille display requires a reduced number of electromechanical components. This allows a smaller size of the display device, as well as reduced costs. On the other hand, FPGA control exhibits several advantages in terms of ease of use and parallel processing. Experiments demonstrate the functionality of the proposed braille display device.**

Keywords— **Refreshable braille display, electromechanical relay, field programmable gate array**

I. INTRODUCTION

Visual impairment accounts for a reduced ability to perceive sight. While some forms of sight loss can be compensated by optical means, as for example glasses or contact lenses, some affections lead to severe visual impairment consisting in low vision and even blindness [1].

According to the World Health Organization, as reported in 2014, 285 million people worldwide suffer from some form of visual impairment, with 39 million suffering from blindness [2].

Visual impairment leads to limitations in mobility, reading, communication, access technology – such as access to computers, smartphones, etc. Up to 80% of the cases of visual impairment are either preventable or treatable [2]. In the remainder 20% however vision loss is permanent, and accordingly, require alternative methods for social integration. For exemplification, mobility is aided with instruments such as the white cane. Reading on the other hand is aided with audio books and the braille alphabet.

Braille is an alphabet used by the visually impaired for tactile reading [3]. A braille cell consists of six dots, arranged and numbered as illustrated in Fig. 1, and embossed on paper. The embossed pattern then encodes the characters.

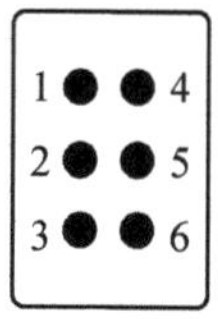

Fig. 1 The 6 dots of a braille character

Alternatively to braille written on paper, there are electro-mechanical devices which perform the display of braille characters. These devices are called refreshable braille displays. They come as a consistent aid for access technology. The most straightforward application is a tactile alternative to the e-book reader [4]. Similarly, braille display in conjunction with tactile graphics can be employed for the development of tactile displays for mobile phones and tablets [5].

Another exemplification of the employment of braille display in access technology is the development of web pages with tactile readability. For example, a platform for online shopping developed for the visually impaired was reported in [6].

To take matters a step further, refreshable braille display in conjunction with audio information and tactile graphics enables the development of virtual classrooms for e-learning environment [7].

Refreshable braille displays are indeed a very powerful tool for communication for the visually impaired. The limitation of these devices however consists mainly in size and costs. Indeed, refreshable braille displays are developed around electromechanical components, e.g. coils, piezoelectric devices, etc., which take up a rather large space. Consequently, the refreshable braille display results in a rather bulky device. In the same time, electro-mechanic devices increase the cost of the braille display cell, and consequently the price per character.

Another aspect to be considered with regard to refreshable braille displays is the braille cell driver. The refreshable braille display is usually driven by a microcontroller unit, which traditionally reads the contents of a source file which contains the information to be displayed, and drives each braille cell individually. Limitations from this point of view

S. Vlad and N.M. Roman (eds.), *International Conference on Advancements of Medicine and Health Care through Technology; 12th - 15th October 2016, Cluj-Napoca, Romania,*
IFMBE Proceedings 59,
DOI: 10.1007/978-3-319-52875-5_14

come from the number of characters that needs to be driven, i.e. the size of the display device, as well as the size and type of information which needs to be manipulated for display.

In this paper we propose a braille cell which is controlled by a field programmable gate array (FPGA). Our choice for a single-cell braille display is mainly motivated by size. In the same time, tactile reading on a single cell display will expectedly increase reading speed and user comfort.

The braille cell is built with six electromagnetic relays, which determine the elevation state of six pins for braille character display.

Our choice for an FPGA as the braille cell controller is mainly motivated by ease of use and parallelism. Indeed, FPGAs have direct access to each bit within the internal shift registers, in contrast to microcontroller which require bit-wise operations. Moreover, FPGAs enable parallel execution of several routines, in contrast to microcontrollers which execute routines serially. Accordingly, it is possible to further extend the proposed braille display cell with additional functionality, by deployment of motion and gesture analysis, monitoring, etc.

This article is organized as follows. Section II presents a review of refreshable braille display devices. Section III presents the implementation of the proposed braille cell with FPGA control. Section IV validates the proposed braille cell with experimental results. Some conclusions are finally drawn.

II. Related work

A first classification of the electronic braille display devices can be drawn considering the type of reading. Literature in the field differentiates among static reading and dynamic sweeping. Dynamic sweeping assumes the reader's finger moving over the braille characters in order to feel the elevation of the pins. Accordingly, refreshable braille displays meant for dynamic sweeping exhibit multiple braille cells for the simultaneous display of several characters, usually in-between 8 and 80 [8].

Traditionally, dynamic sweeping is most widely implemented using piezoelectric devices [9]. Accordingly, the height of the dots is controlled depending on the voltage applied across the piezoelectric devices. As another example, the solution reported in [10] for refreshable braille displays aimed for dynamic sweeping is based on piezoelectric linear motors. In this case, the piezoelectric principle is used for the actuation of a motor which in turn controls the elevation of the dots.

An alternative solution for the simultaneous display of multiple braille characters was reported in [11]. In this solution, selective elevation of the dots is controlled by the horizontal movement of some racks which exhibit variation of the rack width. Accordingly, sections of the rack with large width operate towards elevating the dots, while sections of the rack with smaller with will lower the dots. Horizontal movement of the racks is actuated by sprinkles attached to servomotors [11].

Static reading on the other hand assumes the reader's finger be laid on the braille cell and the finger stays immobile during the reading process. The user only senses the changes in the elevation of the dots without sweeping the braille cell. Accordingly, a single braille cell is required to be displayed for static reading.

The advantage of single braille cells for static reading is the reduced size and lower price, as only one character display needs to be implemented. For exemplification, the solution reported in [8] employs pulse width modulation (PWM) servomotors which actuate 6 needles to implement a single braille cell. Another very attractive solution for single braille cells is based on Microelectromechanical systems (MEMS) [12].

As far as driving the braille cells is concerned, most solutions are based on microcontrollers. Accordingly, the microcontroller reads a text file from a flash memory, e.g. SD card, pen drive, etc., or directly from a personal computer via serial communication, and applies the specific drive voltages to the braille cell. For example, the ATMEGA128 microcontroller is used in conjunction with a programmable logic device (PLD) in [10]. A PIC 18F2250 is used for the same purpose in [11]. To add some more flexibility to the braille display driver, an Arduino board is for driving the braille cell in [8].

III. Proposed braille display device

The solution proposed in this paper for a refreshable braille display is based on interfacing an FPGA with the electronic braille cell. The block diagram of the proposed system is illustrated in Fig. 2.

The text to be displayed is available in a text file on a personal computer. Binary encoding of the braille characters assumes six bits corresponding to the six dots, following the numbering presented in Fig. 1. Additionally, a two-bit prefix is added to the six bits as a delimiter for a new character, a new word, a new sentence, or as a text terminator respectively.

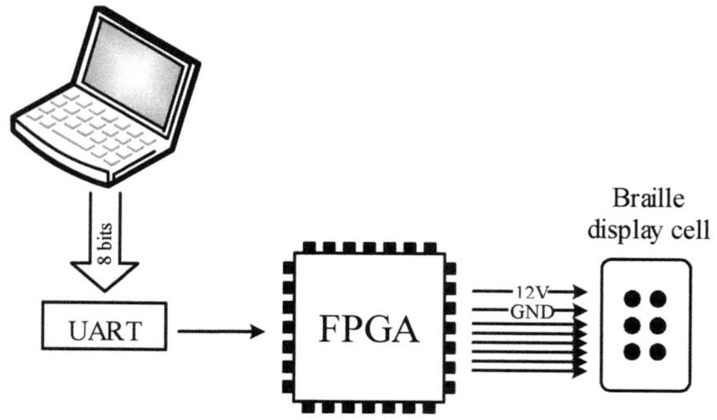

Fig. 1 Block diagram of the proposed refreshable braille display

The braille display driver was implemented on a Nexys4 FPGA board. The FPGA reads the text file from a personal computer over UART and delivers the corresponding signals to the relays. The needles of the braille cell are then elevated accordingly.

The FPGA decodes the most significant two bits into a delay in displaying the next character. Accordingly, a timing is imposed in-between successive character displays as follows. A character delimiter imposes a 1s delay, a word or sentence delimiter imposes a 2s delay, whereas the text terminator raises all braille dots to indicate end of text. The remainder six bits trigger the six dots of the braille display respectively.

The braille display cell is connected to the FPGA over an 8 line bus. Two lines are used for the 12V supply and ground respectively. The remainder six lines are applied directly to the braille pin drivers.

A braille dot driver is illustrated in Fig. 3. Each dot of the braille display cell is attached to a needle which is elevated by a LEG-5F electromagnetic relay. The relay is driven by a BD139 transistor. Accordingly, elevation of the needle is triggered by a 3.3V control signal V_{cmd}.

IV. Experimental results

The braille display, proposed and described in section III, was implemented practically and its operation was tested. The braille cell is illustrated in Fig. 4.

Figure 4 (a) shows a top view of the one-character braille display, illustrating the six dots of the cell. Next, Fig. 4 (b) shows a side view of the braille display, illustrating the circuitry of the cell made up by the 6 electromagnetic relays.

The braille cell circuit was deployed in-between two printed circuit board (PCB) plates. Holes in both top and bottom PCB operate towards maintaining the needles on the desired axis.

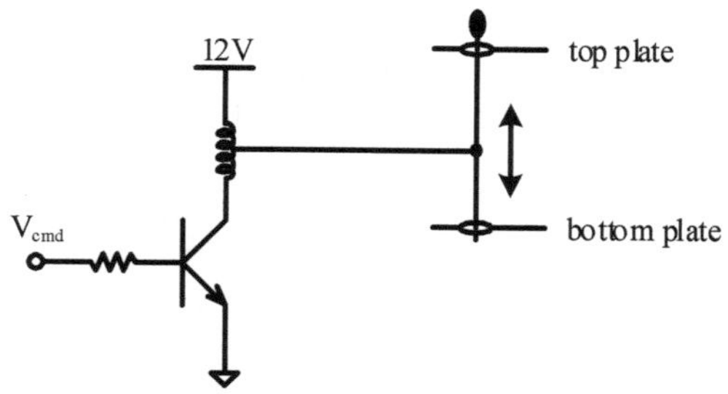

Fig. 2 The braille pin driver

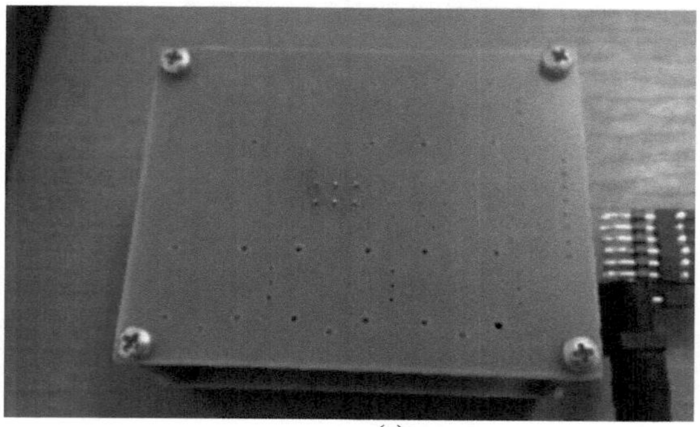

(a)

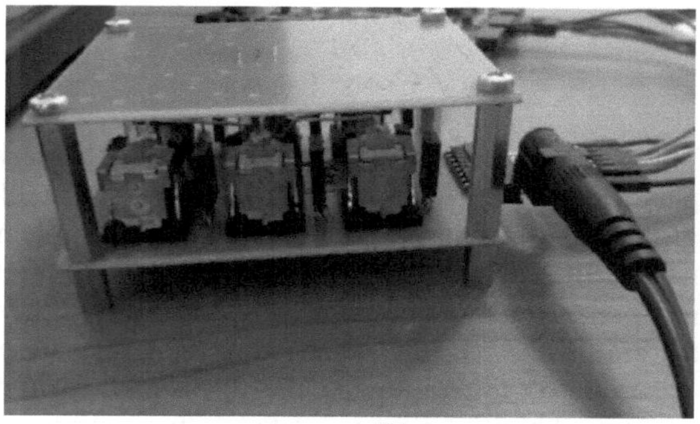

(b)

Fig. 3 The braille display: (a) top view and (b) side view

The braille display cell was supplied with a 12V supply able to deliver a 4A supply current. Spice simulation of one relay driver is plotted in Fig. 5.

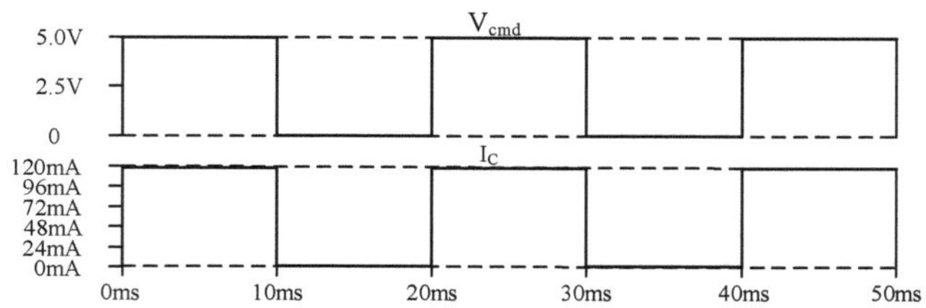

Fig. 4 The braille pin driver

The test bench of the braille display is illustrated in Fig. 6. For illustration purpose, the display of the test "Hello" in braille is shown in Fig. 7. To be noticed in Fig. 7 is that the first character indicates that the following character is capital, while the last character indicates termination of the text.

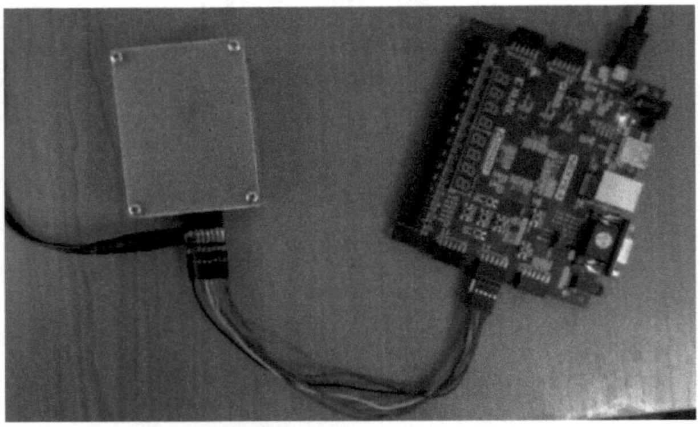

Fig. 5 The braille display test bench

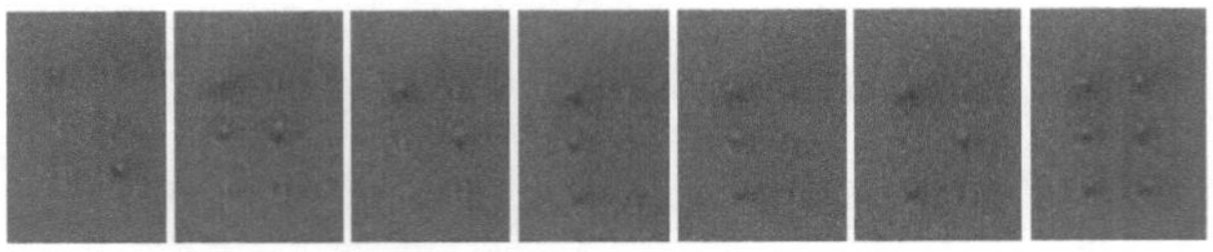

Fig. 6 Display of the word "Hello" in braille

V. Conclusions

This paper presented a one-character refreshable braille display. The braille cell was implemented using electromagnetic relays. Control of the braille cell was implemented using an FPGA. The FPGA reads the contents of a text file from a personal computer over UART, and drives the relays of the braille cell. Needles attached to the relays are elevated accordingly, thus allowing the display of desired text. The proposed braille cell is validated with experiments.

The control logic was implemented in this work using FPGA due to its advantages in terms of ease of use and parallel processing. As future work, we aim to make use of FPGA parallel processing and deploy the braille cell with additional functionality in terms of motion and gesture recognition. By this, we aim to improve user interaction with the braille display device, and this increase user comfort.

Conflict of Interest

The authors declare that they have no conflict of interest.

References

1. "Blindness and Vision Impairment", at http://www.cdc.gov/healthcommunication/ToolsTemplates/EntertainmentEd/Tips/Blindness.html
2. World Health Organization, "Visual impairment and blindness", at http://www.who.int/mediacentre/factsheets/fs282/en/
3. Pharmaceutical Braille, "The Braille Alphabet", at http://www.pharmabraille.com/pharmaceutical-braille/the-braille-alphabet/
4. Abhinav Kulkarni, Kishor Bhurchandi, (2015) "Low Cost E-Book Reading Device for Blind People", 2015 International Conference on Computing Communication Control and Automation (ICCUBEA), Pune, 26-27 Feb. 2015, pp. 516 - 520
5. M. Mohamed Iqbal, L. Padma Balaji , et al. (2014) "Virtual simulation and embedded module of mobile phone using modified Braille display", 2014 2nd International Conference on Devices, Circuits and Systems (ICDCS), 6-8 March 2014, pp. 1-6
6. Eu Jin Wong, Kian Meng Yap, et al. (2015), "HABOS: Towards a platform of haptic-audio based online shopping for the visually impaired", 2015 IEEE Confernece on Open Systems (ICOS), 24-26 Aug. 2015, pp. 62-67
7. Wiebke Köhlmann, Ulrike Lucke, (2015) "Alternative Concepts for Accessible Virtual Classrooms for Blind Users", 2015 IEEE 15th International Conference on Advanced Learning Technologies, pp. 413 – 417
8. Marcelo Bernart Schmidt, Luiz Gustavo, (2014) "Single Braille Cell",Biosignals and Biorobotics Conference (2014): Biosignals and Robotics for Better and Safer Living (BRC), 5th ISSNIP-IEEE, pp. 26-28
9. G. H. Yang, K. U. Kyung, et al. (2006) "Quantitative Tactile Display Device with Pin-Array Type Tactile Feedback and Thermal Feedback", Proc. IEEE Int. Conf on Robotics and Automation, Orlando, Florida, May, 2006, pp. 3917-3922
10. H. C., Cho, B. S. Kim, et al. (2006) Development Of A Braille Display Using Piezoelectric Linear Motors. International Joint Conference SICE-ICASE, October, 2006, pp. 1917-1921.
11. C. Guerra, D. Novillo, et al. (2015) "Electromechanical prototype used for physical deployment of Braille characters for digital documents", 2015 CHILEAN Conference on Electrical, Electronics Engineering, Information and Communication Technologies (CHILECON), Santiago, 28-30 Oct. 2015, pp. 191 - 198
12. Hira Arshad, Umar S. Khan et al. (2015) "MEMS based Braille system", 2015 IEEE 15th International Conference on Nanotechnology (IEEE-NANO) , Rome, Italy, 27-30 July 2015, pp. 1103 – 1106

Author: Paul FARAGÓ
Institute: Technical University of Cluj-Napoca, Faculty of electronics, Telecommunications and Information Technology, Bases of Electronics Department
Street: George Bariţiu, 26-28, 400027
City: Cluj-Napoca
Country: Romania
Email: paul.farago@bel.utcluj.ro

Assessing Microcirculation for Predictive Purposes with the Aim of Reducing the Amputation Rate in the Case of Patients with Critical Lower Limb Ischemia

O. Andercou[1], B. Stancu[1], A. Mironiuc[1] and H. Silaghi[2]

[1]University of Medicine and Pharmacy "Iuliu Hatieganu", 2nd Surgical Clinic, Cluj Napoca, Romania
[2]University of Medicine and Pharmacy "Iuliu Hatieganu", 5th Surgical Clinic, Cluj Napoca, Romania

Abstract - **The aim of the present study is to assess the role of the partial pressure of tissue oxygen with the purpose of having a prediction on the healing capacity of peripheral tissues affected by critical ischemia. As far as material and method are concerned, the study extended over a two-year period, broken up into three distinctive stages. A total of 198 patients diagnosed with critical ischemia in the lower limbs, in accordance with the TASC II definition, were enrolled and then divided into four groups: group 1: primary amputees; group 2: repeat amputees; group 3: revascularized patients; and group 4: unsuccessfully revascularized patients. Results: in the first stage, it was noted that the percentage of amputees was extremely high (75%), as compared to the percentage of revascularized patients (25%), and a large number of repeat amputees were also noted. The latter patient category is associated with a large number of days of hospitalization and high costs. By using the measurement of the partial pressure of tissue oxygen (TcPO2) as a matter of routine, it was possible to significantly lower the number of primary amputees (57%) and to raise the number of revascularized patients (43%), as compared to the first stage. Also, by assessing microcirculation, it was possible to use certain objective data on the healing capacity of the tissue, so that we no longer had any repeat amputees. Conclusion: Microcirculation is deeply affected in critical ischemia and the assessment thereof is important in raising the quality of life in the case of patients with critical ischemia.**

Keywords - **Critical limb ischaemia, microcirculation, amputation, partial pressure of oxygen**

I. Introduction

Peripheral arteriopathies are an important health and social problem worldwide. The frequency of this disease among the population is estimated to vary between 4 and 30% [1]. Atherosclerotic disease is associated with a high risk of mortality by acute myocardial infarction or stroke. Critical ischemia is the most advanced stage of the atherosclerotic disease [2].

The risk of a major amputation in the case of patients with critical ischemia is up to 40% over a 6 month period, with a mortality rate of 22-25% one year later. The definition of critical ischemia is based on clinical and paraclinical criteria and was established by the *Transatlantic Inter-Society Consensus* in the year 2000 [3]:

1) Chronic ischemic rest pain,
2) Opioid painkillers necessary ≥ 2 weeks,
3) Ulcerations or gangrenes of the lower limb or toes;
4) Ankle systolic pressure < 50 mm Hg,
5) Toe systolic pressure < 30 mm Hg
6) The absence of lower limb pulses in the case of diabetes patients,
7) Objectively proven occlusive arterial disease,
8) The necessity of a major amputation within the next 6 months – 1 year, in the absence of any significant hemodynamic improvement.

This definition was altered by the *European Working Group on Critical Limb Ischaemia* [4, 5]:

1) Ischemic rest pain,
2) Painkillers necessary ≥ 2 weeks
3) Ulcerations or gangrenes of the lower extremity,
4) Ankle systolic pressure < 50 mm Hg
5) Toe systolic pressure < 30 mm Hg.

II. Materials and Method

The study was conducted over a 2-year period, and it involved patients who were diagnosed with critical ischemia when they were admitted to hospital. The patients were included in this study in accordance with the Helsinki Declaration of 1975, as revised in 2000 and 2008. The patients were divided into four study groups: the first group comprised patients who underwent primary amputation (PA) as a first intention; the second group comprised patients who underwent repeated amputation during hospitalization (RA); the third group was made up of revascularized patients (R); and the fourth group included patients who were initially revascularized, but the procedure failed, so that eventually amputation was necessary (RF). The patient inclusion and exclusion criteria were defined. The inclusion criteria for this study were: patients with critical ischemia defined on the basis of clinical symptomatology: rest pain with painkillers required over a period exceeding 2 weeks or the presence of necroses or gangrenes; patients with critical ischemia defined on the basis of paraclinical examinations:

S. Vlad and N.M. Roman (eds.), *International Conference on Advancements of Medicine and Health Care through Technology; 12th - 15th October 2016, Cluj-Napoca, Romania,*
IFMBE Proceedings 59,
DOI: 10.1007/978-3-319-52875-5_15

ankle-arm index under 0.45, TcPO2 under 40 mm Hg, and age: over 50. The exclusion of patients from the study was carried out based on the following criteria: acute arterial occlusion, major surgery (including heart surgery) within the past 3 months, severe cardiopathy with an ejection fraction of under 25%, hepatic or renal insufficiency, anemia, coagulation disorders, acute or chronic infectious diseases, severe diseases (septicemia, HIV, type B or C hepatitis, lupus, multiple sclerosis).

The study had three distinctive stages. In the first stage, which extended over the first year, the patients who were treated in the usual manner were analyzed. The results obtained in the course of this stage indicated a high amputation rate, as compared to a low rate of revascularized patients. In the second stage, a more aggressive type of treatment was adopted, by extending the revascularization indication, as a result of which a significant drop in the percentage of amputated patients was achieved, corroborated with a significant increase in the number of revascularized patients. During this stage, complex equipment for the study of microcirculation (Perimed) was acquired. The equipment comprises 3 modules for measuring of partial pressure of oxygen in peripheral tissues (TCPO2), a module for measurement with the aid of laser-Doppler flowmetry, and a module for measuring toe systolic pressure. In the third stage, by using the acquired equipment as a matter of routine, we were able to completely eliminate repeated amputations.A complex study sheet was prepared for each patient and, in the end, a data base was created using Microsoft Excel. The purpose of this study was to achieve a drop in the rate of primary and repeated amputations in the case of critical atherosclerotic ischemia of the limbs. And the secondary purpose, derived from the main one, was to make profitable the cost – therapeutic efficiency ratio.

III. Results

The first stage of the study included a number of 96 patients, the second stage, 74 patients, and the last stage, 28 (Table 1).

The analysis of the patients' general data shows that the global average age of the patients was 65.7 years old, the minimum being 50 and the maximum, 87, and it is shown in detail in the 4 groups, with a much larger percentage of male patients as compared to female patients (Table 2).

The main risk factors identified are shown in Table 3. It is interesting to note that over half of the patients have dyslipidemia and almost 75% of the patients suffer from hypertension. Smoking was encountered in the case of only 33.5% of the patients, who were heavy smokers, in that they smoked over 1 pack of cigarettes per day.

Table 1. The total number of patients studied and their distribution by group.

	Result (1) 96 cases	**Result (2) 74 cases**	**Result (3) 28 cases**	**Global result 198 cases**
Primary amputees	52 (54.1%)	34 (45%)	12 (42.8%)	98 (49.5%)
Repeat amputees	21 (21.8%)	7 (12.5%)	0	28 (14.14%)
Revascularized patients	17 (17.7%)	28 (37.5%)	14 (50%)	59 (29.8%)
Unsuccessfully revascularized patients	6 (6.2%)	5 (5%)	2 (7.1%)	13 (6.5%)

Table 2. General data

		PA	**R**	**RF**	**RA**	**Total**
Age	Average	67.53	62.11	64	67.21	65.7
	min	51	50	51	54	50
	max	87	82	82	86	87
Sex	M	73	51	12	22	158
	F	25	8	1	6	40

PA – primary amputations – revascularized, RF – failed revascularization cases RA – repeated amputations

Table 3 Main risk factors

	PA	**R**	**RF**	**RA**	**Total**
Smoking	28	25	6	8	67(33.8%)
Diabetes meltitus	57	8	8	15	88(44.4%)
Arterial hypertension	75	48	4	20	147(74.24%
Dyslipidemia	53	35	7	17	112(56.56%)

Besides these risk factors, the presence of the following associated comorbidities was also noted (as shown in Table 4): cardiac (8.58%), renal (3%), respiratory (3.53%), and neurovascular (11.61%).

Table 4 Comorbidities

	PA	**R**	**RF**	**RA**	**Total**
Cardiac	12	4	1		17(8.58%)
Renal	5	1			6(3%)
Respiratory	6				7(3.53%)
Neurovascular	13				23(11.61%)

All patients underwent preoperative imagistic investigations. These were non-invasive (arterial Doppler scan) or invasive (digital subtraction aortic arteriography). Based on these investigations, the patients could be assigned to either one of the two stages of the Leriche classification, which correspond to the critical ischemia definition, namely stages III and IV. Following the examinations, it was observed that in over 75% of the cases the patients showed up in stage IV, which is the most advanced, when the possibilities of revascularization are greatly limited, the only surgical interventions being limited just to amputation, some of which were carried out with the purpose of saving the patient's life. Once the equipment for the assessment of microcirculation was acquired, we started using it on a regular basis, and the assessment was conducted in the case of all patients included in this study starting with the third stage (Table 5).

Table 5 Preoperative investigations and stages

	PA	R	RF	RA	Total
Stage III	5	33	4	3	45(22.72%)
Stage IV	93	24	9	25	151(76.26%)
TcPO2	16	0	1	13	30
Doppler scan	25	12	4	4	45
Arteriography	13	40	5	4	62

At the same time, an estimate was made for the length of the hospitalization of the patients in the four groups. It was noticed that the patients with repeated amputations and those with failed revascularization had the longest hospitalization periods (Table 6). Due to the extension of the hospitalization period, the risk for certain postoperative complications to occur is extremely high. A lengthy hospitalization period greatly raises the costs associated with these patients. The introduction of the new methods of investigation brought to zero the number of patients with repeated amputations, which also allowed costs to be significantly cut.

The analysis of primary amputations showed that the majority of these were major amputations (thigh) and the fact that the percentage of the minor (digit) amputations was lower (Table 7).

Table 6 Length of hospitalization period

		AP	R	RE	AI
	Average	3.71	4.67	6.61	4.03
Pre-op hospitalization	**Minimum**	1	1	1	1
	Maximum	16	12	**20**	9
	Average	11.61	11.7	**14.61**	**19.21**
Post-op hospitalization	**Minimum**	1	1	4	5
	Maximum	25	35	20	**60**
	Average	15.42	16.3	**21.23**	**23.21**
Total hospitalization	**Minimum**	2	8	9	8
	Maximum	24	39	48	64

Table 7 Primary amputations

Amputation type	**No.**	**%**
Toe	30	30.61%
Transmetatarsal	15	15.3%
Calf	3	3%
Thigh	50	51%
TOTAL	98	

As far as repeated amputations are concerned, these resulted in the end, in most of the cases, in a major thigh amputation (Table 8).

Table 8 Repeated amputations

Amputation type	**No.**	**%**
Toe	3	10.71%
Transmetatarsal	5	17.85%
Calf	5	17.85%
Thigh	15	53.57%
TOTAL	28	

IV. Discussion

Unlike the other methods, which investigate the hemodynamic changes, the measurement of transcutaneous oxygen pressure ($TCPO_2$) reflects the metabolic state of the tissues in the area where it is measured [6]. The measurement can in fact be conducted at any level; however, currently, the investigated areas are the instep, the anterior medial face of the calf 10 cm below the patella, and the anterior face of the thigh 10 cm above the patella.

The values measured depend on the metabolic activity of the tissue, cutaneous circulation, oxyhemoglobin dissociation, and tissue oxygen diffusion. Normally, a light progressive drop is reported in the $TCPO_2$ values from proximal segments toward distal ones, with age, as well as in an elevated position of the limb.

The measurement of $TCPO_2$ is extremely important in the appreciation of severe ischemia. Because the results are not affected by arterial calcifications, the test has as an election indication the assessment of the vascular state of diabetic patients. Two exhaustive studies conducted in 1984 show the normal and pathological $TCPO_2$ values in different localizations (Tables 9, 10) [7, 8]:

Table 9. :TCPO2 values at rest in different localizations (mm Hg)

Author	Normal			Claudication			Rest pain		
	Foot	Calf	Thigh	Foot	Calf	Thigh	Foot	Calf	Thigh
Cina (136)	64±4	64±4	-	46±5	55±4	-	17±4	42±6	-
Byrne (137)	60±7	63±8	66±8	56±4	59±5	66±7	4±4	29±2	50±1

Table 10. Foot $TCPO_2$ values at rest and after physical exercise

	Clino statism	Ortho statism	Orthostatism (during effort)	Clinostatism (after effort)
Normal	60±7	71±7	75±9	69±7
Claudication	37±12	58±12	49±18	23±20
Rest pain	4±4	25±20	26±26	5±7

The fact that microcirculation measurements were conducted on all patients as a matter of routine led to a significant decrease in primary amputations. The technique applied measures the tension of the oxygen in the skin capillary bed and is an indirect method for measuring skin perfusion. The application of the method is very useful especially in diabetes patients with non-compressible, calcified arteries, in whose case the circulation cannot be appreciated by determining the ankle-arm index [9]. It has very good predictability for the appreciation of the healing of ulcerations and it has the highest accuracy in the establishment of the optimum level of amputation with a predictability of over 87%. The measured tissue oxygen values of less than 20 mm Hg were associated with reduced tissue viability, confirmed by the intraoperative clinical criteria for establishing the optimum amputation level [10]. The intraoperative clinical criteria for the assessment of the viability of an amputation stump are: the appreciation of bleeding at the level of the cross-section cut, the macroscopic appearance of the muscular masses, the appearance of the sectioned vessels (the fact that they are loaded with atherosclerotic plaques, thromboses), the exteriorization of serous edema fluid, the intraoperative endovascular ultrasound scan, and the intraoperative angiography (if available). Other aspects are also appreciated: the presence of osteomyelitis, the existence of certain necrosis areas or purulent collections, and extended muscular necroses. The intermediate values larger than 20 mm Hg but less than 30 mm Hg correspond to the values of critical ischemia, tissue viability is at the limit, a revascularization intervention leads to an increase in local perfusion, and the chances of keeping the limb grow [11]. The studies showed that it is not recommended for TcPO2 measurement to be used as used as a primary diagnosis method; it should also be associated with other paraclinical examinations as well, but especially with a thorough clinical examination. The preoperative clinical criteria for the appreciation of the viability of an amputation stump are: the presence of gangrene and a possible associated infection, the state of the areas adjacent to the gangrene, the degree of arterial ischemia highlighted by imagistic investigations, and the duration and intensity of the pain. Last but not least, a complete assessment must be conducted of the general state of the patient and the presence of associated diseases: diabetes mellitus, the heart and renal function, arterial hypertension, and stroke [12].

On the other hand, value limits have not yet been accurately established, below which healing is no longer possible [13]. In our study there have also been cases in which the values measured were below those where tissue viability is very close to zero; however, the intraoperative clinical criteria showed good tissue viability with good postoperative healing. On the other hand, there were also patients with good tissue oxygenation values, but, intraoperatively, a more proximal amputation level was chosen, due to reduced tissue viability. These controversial results, encountered in a small number of cases, need to be elucidated by subsequent studies, on a larger number of patients. However, TcPO2 measurement is a useful method in the appreciation of the optimum level of amputation [14]. In fact, our study clearly showed that the introduction of this measurement brought the number of repeated amputations down to zero. Another advantage was the fact that amputations were performed at more distal levels [15, 16]. This was associated with much lower perioperative morbidity and mortality. On the other hand, it was easier to fit the patients with distal amputations with prostheses, and their social and professional reintegration went much faster. The questionnaires used in the case of these patients also showed a significant growth in their quality of life [17, 18].

V. Conclusions

The study has shown a correlation between the values measured and the healing of the amputation stump, although initially only a small number of patients were included. Another limitation was the expensive equipment and the necessity to have specially trained personnel to perform the measurements and to interpret the results. Moreover, the measurements themselves are time-consuming. However, TcPO2 assessment is a good predictive model on the healing capacity of the tissues. An amputation level that's as distal as possible is associated with better patient recovery and a greatly improved quality of life.

Acknowledgment

The results of this research were supported by University of Medicine and Pharmacy "Iuliu Hatieganu" Cluj-Napoca Internal Grant N° 27020/15.11.2011

Conflict of Interest

The authors declare that they have no conflict of interest.

References

1. Selvin E, Erlinger T (2004) Prevalence of and risk factors for peripheral arterial disease in the United States results from the national health and nutrition examination survey, 1999–2000. Circulation 110:738-74
2. Diehm C, Schuster A, Allenberg JR et al. (2004) High prevalence of peripheral arterial disease and comorbidity in 6880 primary care patients: cross-sectional study. Atherosclerosis 172: 95-105
3. Norgren L, Hiatt WR, Dormandy JA, Nehler MR, Harris KA, Fowkes FGR on behalf of the TASC II Working Group (2007) Inter-Society consensus for the management of peripheral arterial disease (TASC II). Eur J Vasc Endovasc Surg 33: S1-S70
4. Rutherford RB, Cronewett JL, Gloviczki P (2000) The textbook of vascular surgery. WB Saunders, Philadelphia
5. Hirsch AT, Haskal ZJ, Hertzer NR, Bakal CW, Creager MA, Alperin JL et al. (2006) ACC/AHA 2005 guidelines for the management of patients with peripheral arterial disease (lower extermity, renal, mesenteric, and abdominal aortic): executive summary a collaborative report from the American Association for Vascular Surgery/Society for Vascular Surgery, Society for Cardiovascular Angiography and Interventions, Society for Vascular Medicine and Biology, Society of Interventional Radiology, and the ACC/AHA Task Force on practice guidelines (writing committee to develop guidelines for the management of patients with peripheral arterial disease) endorsed by the American Association of Cardiovascular and Pulmonary Rehabilitation; National Heart, Lung, and Blood Institute; Society for Vascular Nursing; Trans-Atlantic Inter-Society Consensus; and Vascular Disease Foundation. J Am Coll Cardiol 47:1239-1312
6. Faglia E, Clerici G, Caminiti et al. (2006) Predictive values of transcutaneous oxygen tension for above-the-ankle amputation in diabetic patients with critical limb ischemia. Eur J Vasc Endovasc Surg 33:731-736
7. Cina C, Katsamouris A, Megerman J et al. (1984) Utility of transcutaneous oxygen tension mesurements in peripheral arterial occlusive disease. J Vasc Surg 1: 362
8. Byrne P, Provan JL, Ameli FM et al. (1984) The use of transcutaneous oxygen tension measurements in the diagnosis of peripheral vascular insufficiency. Ann Surg 200:159
9. Takkin L, Sample R, Moore P (2009) Prediction of wound healing outcome using skin perfusion pressure & transcutaneous oximetry. Wounds 21:310-316
10. Arsenault KA, Al-Otaibia A, Devereaux PJ (2012) The use of transcutaneous oximetry to predict healing complications of lower limb amputations: a systematic review and meta-analysis. European Journal of Vascular and Endovascular Surgery 43:329–336
11. Brown BJ, Attinger CE (2013) The below-knee amputation: to amputate or palliate? Adv Wound Care 2: 30–35
12. Fortington LV, Geertzena HB, van Netten JJ (2013) Short and long term mortality rates after a lower limb amputation. European Journal of Vascular and Endovascular Surgery 46:124–131
13. Fife CE, Smart DR, Sheffield PJ et al. (2009) Transcutaneous oximetry in clinical practice: consensus statements from an expert panel based on evidence. J Undersea and Hyp 36:43-53
14. Boulton JM, Armstrong DG, Albert SF (2008) Comprehensive foot examination and risk assessment. A report of the Task Force of the Foot Care Interest Group of the American Diabetes Association, with endorsement by the American Association of Clinical Endocrinologists. Diabetes Care 31:1679-1685

15. Kristensen MT, Holm G, Mollerb K et al. (2012) Very low survival rates after non-traumatic lower limb amputation in a consecutive series: what to do? Interactive Cardio Vascular and Thoracic Surgery 10:1-5
16. Singh RK, Prasad G (2015) Long-term mortality after lower-limb amputation. Prosthet Orthot Int 7:61-67
17. Schofield CJ, Libby G, Brennan MG (2006) Mortality and hospitalization in patients after amputation. A comparison between patients with and without diabetes. Diabetes Care 29:2252-2256
18. Tentolouris N, Al-Sabbagh S, Walker MG et al. (2004) Mortality in diabetic and non-diabetic patients after amputations performed from 1990 to 1995: a 5-year follow-up study. Diabetes Care 27:1598-1604

Author: Bogdan Stancu
Institution: University of Medicine and Pharmacy "Iuliu Hatieganu"
Street: Clinicilor str No. 4-6
City: Cluj Napoca
Country: Romania
Email:bstancu7@yahoo.com

An EIT Belt Reference Design with Active Electrodes and Digital Output

I. Jivet

Faculty of Electronics and Telecommunications, University Politehnica Timisoara, Romania

Abstract— **A reference design of an EIT (electrical impedance tomography) belt using the AFE4300 IC, with supplemental amplifying buffers, is presented. The experimental results are promising, recommending it for practical implementation. The paper also indicates the possibility to develop other EIT belts variants based on AFE4300, using multiple impedance measuring pairs, suitable for wireless wearable EIT belts. Lung function monitoring with tidal volume estimation using EIT, aims at the application area of sports medicine. The ECG sensor module of the AFE4300 was also explored as a supplementary bio sensor channel use-full in applications. In all, the reference design outlines a digital SPI bio-impedance and ECG sensing modules, with low total power and cost and ready of application in practice.**

Keywords— **EIT belt, AFE4300, monitoring lung function, wireless connection.**

I. INTRODUCTION

Although EIT (Electrical Impedance Tomography) research failed to deliver a cross sectional body imaging technique of X-ray resolution and quality, there are yet a number of specific application areas, where the technique is often preferred in practice. Pulmonary function monitoring in critically ill or new born are good examples [1], [2].

The impedance image of the cross section of the torso at the belt level is obtained by injecting currents into an electrode pair and measuring the voltage difference among the remaining pairs of electrodes around the belt [3].

The number of electrodes on the chest circumference is usually 16 or 32. This leads naturally to as many wires running from the electrodes to the measuring and imaging electronics. The currents and voltages at electrode pairs are used to generate a transversal plane impedance image [4].

The concept of 'active electrodes' refers to the idea of bringing the electronics of current generation and voltage measurement directly over the area of the electrodes. The harnessing of wires thus can be reduced, as well the power lines and noise from environment [5].

The main objectives of the work reported in the paper, is a generic design of a versatile EIT belt, using commercially available components.

The reference design for EIT thorax cross sectional monitoring, is based on the commercially available analog front end IC, AFE4300, from Texas Instruments [6]. The ASIC made available recently, was designed specifically for bio-impedance measurements, including multiple ports for both impressed currents and voltage measurements.

One obstacle found in using this IC for EIT belt realization was the different impedance range of the body mass composition target application and EIT applications. The device was designed to measure impedances on the order of 100 – 500 ohms, a factor of 10-50 times larger than impedance measured in EIT.

The sinusoidal impressed currents generated by the IC will be multiplexed directly to the belt electrodes in pairs. The voltage measurement electrode pairs will be supplemented with an amplifier to restore the collected signals range as in the original target application to maintain device resolution. In this way the AFE4300 16 bit precision of A/D convertor in the voltage measurement channels is preserved.

The weight measurement channel of the AFE4300 is used to sense the ECG signal from two electrodes placed across the torso parallel to standard ECG 'Lead I'.

One of the inconveniencies of an EIT impedance electrode belt is the need to have wires connected to it for power and to collect the measurement data.

The output of the AFE4300 is in digital format at an SPI (serial peripheral interface) port. The same port is used for configuration of the device. Therefore, measured values can be transferred to a computer using a standard SPI port. A Bluetooth, Wi-Fi or other proprietary wireless modules can be attached to the belt, transforming it into a wearable monitoring device.

II. BIOIMPEDANCE MEASUREMEMENT WITH AFE4300

AFE4300 ADC sampling frequency is limited to 860 samples per second by design, but since the nodes can do measurements almost simultaneously, we found that the acquisition of digital data frame rate is satisfactory for EIT applications.

S. Vlad and N.M. Roman (eds.), *International Conference on Advancements of Medicine and Health Care through Technology; 12th - 15th October 2016, Cluj-Napoca, Romania,*
IFMBE Proceedings 59,
DOI: 10.1007/978-3-319-52875-5_16

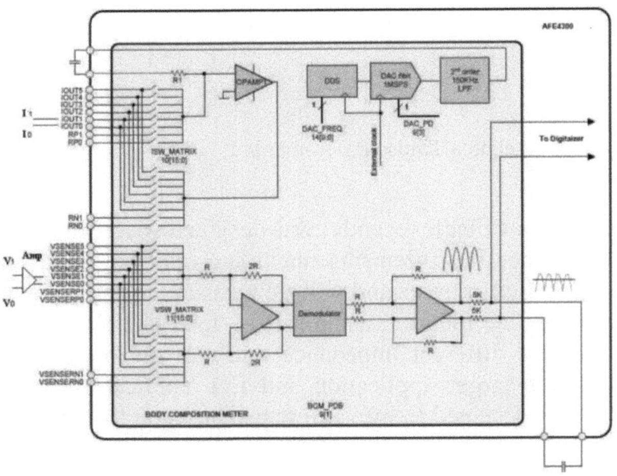

Fig. 1 Impedance sensing module with an external differential amplifier.

In order to gain in speed, the imaging digital computation part of a EIT system, is recently often implemented in H/W (FPGA technology) [7].

The presented reference design using the FEA3400 can generate data at a maxim of 10 image frame/s rate, but it does not exclude the digital processing in a FPGA for generating cross sectional impedance images at this rate. If image reconstruction can keep the speed the final system frame rate will be acceptable for a number of clinical applications in monitoring.

The impedance measurement module as presented in Fig.1 uses the bio-impedance measurement part of the AFE4300 supplemented with an external amplifier.

A modified band pass filter variation of a balanced differential amplifier is used similar to same purpose bio-amplifiers found in literature [8, 9].

The main requirement for the amplifier was to be symmetric in order to preserve the high CMRR (common mode rejection ratio) of the AFE4300 voltage input stage.

The gain of the amplifier was set to a fixed value of 40, determined experimentally as suitable, to preserve the device within the original design range of impressed current and measured voltages.

III. Presentation of EIT Belt Reference Design

The AFE4300 can measure, with internal multiplexing control, six pairs of differential voltage on the boundary of segments of the body. Although impressive and sufficient in a range of bio-impedance applications, for EIT cross sectional impedance imaging a larger number of voltage measuring pairs is necessary.

Even at a low area resolution the impedance image, representing anatomical regions within the thorax, important physiological parameters of the patient can be monitored.

T he two physiological parameters most frequently monitored by EIT are tidal volume and cardiac output [12]. Most of the recently published EIT systems designs use 16 electrodes quasi uniformly distributed around the thorax.

For a increased resolution of the impedance image, systems with 32 electrodes are also used. As depicted in fig. 3, with a 3/6 AFE4300 devices, all the electronics for currents generation and voltage measurement is covered for EIT systems with 16/32 electrodes.

Power, SPI ports select lines and the standard four SPI wires are all the necessary wires connecting the analog front end devices as a bus to wireless module for a complete wireless wearable belt.

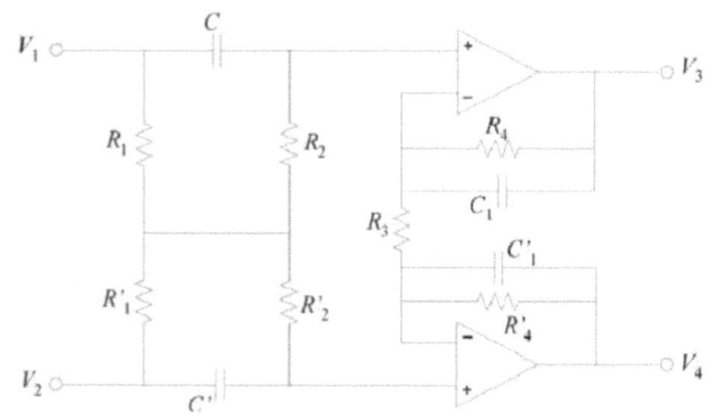

Fig. 2. The schematics of the symmetric AC voltage amplifier [8].

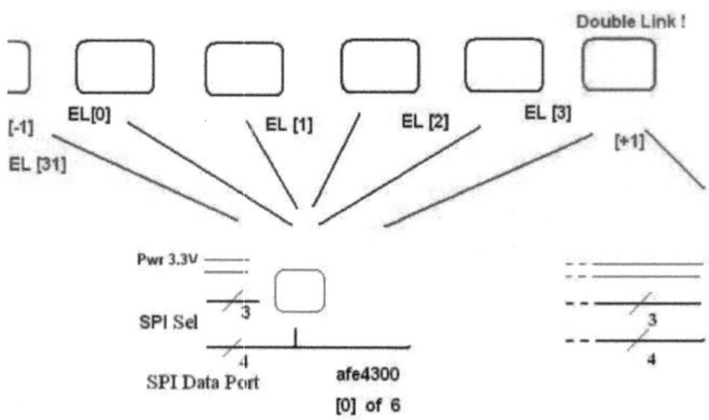

Fig. 3. The general architecture of the belt outlining resources and connections.

The power source for the whole assemble is 3.3 V at a total operating current of only a few miliampers. Given this power consumption a rechargeable battery with a capacity in excess of 100 mAh will cover continuous operation for a full day.

The wireless modules experimented with, for connection with AFE4300 modules has been: Olimex Wi-Fi and Nordic Semiconductor NRF24LE1 wireless modules.

The distance covered by both wireless modules is around 50 m in open space and 10-15 m inside buildings. No problems where encountered in connecting of the AFE4300 device with the wireless modules using the SPI port.

One important element of an EIT belt is the electrodes themselves. Lack of expertise in the domain led us to use regular (Ag-Ag chloride and contact gel) standard commercial ECG electrodes.

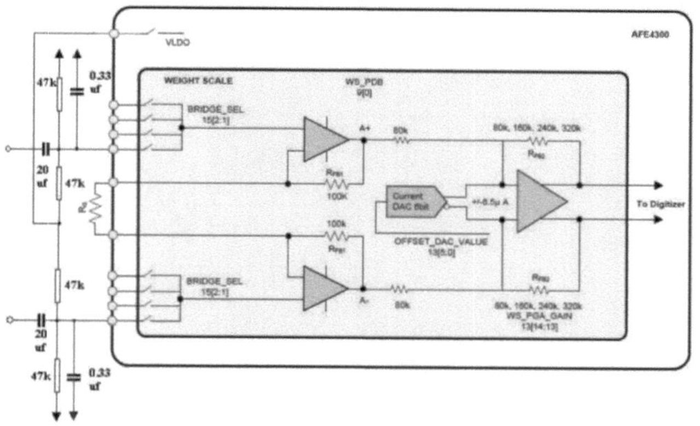

Fig. 4. The weight module of the AFE4300 used for ECG signal sensing similar to literature [10].

IV. Experimental results

The experimental results reported in this paper refer to the practical measurements on the body regions impedance using the AFE4300 supplemented with external amplifiers in front of the voltage measurement channels.

In Fig. 5 the original AFE kit with a pair of current and a pair of voltage measurement electrodes is shown. Standard ECG commercial electrodes have been used.

Measurements on the thorax at the heart level with electrode arrangements using the most commonly EIT style [3]. A data sample is presented in Fig. 6. The values measured have been one to two orders of magnitude smaller, compared to the device specifications (100 -500 ohms).

This problem was solved by adding an amplifier to each voltage measurement pair.

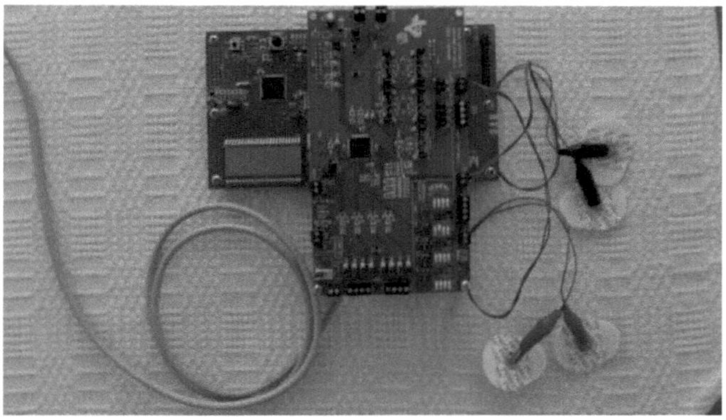

Fig. 5. The experimental kit used with current electrodes (black) and voltage electrodes (red).

Several sets of complete data to reconstruct the impedance image have been collected manually. The reason for this is a limitation of the demo software that comes with the original kit. Access to program the internal registers of the AFE4300 and configure the device is limited without modifications of both H/W and software.

The voltage values obtained following the addition of the amplifiers reached the specification range of the AFE4300.

A prototype is under development with configuration software in the wireless module MPU to collect real time data and then use a popular free EIT image reconstruction like EIDORS to get the cross section impedance image [11].

The speed of data collection will determine the maximum speed of image frames, assuming the ideal case in which computations for image reconstruction is faster.

Considering a data collection policy with one current generation pair and maxim number of electrodes minus the two, in pair combinations, one can estimate the image frame rate, possible to be obtained using the AFE4300 solution.

A general estimation leads to an imaging frame rate of 10/5 fps for a belt with 16/32 electrodes. The result was obtained taking in consideration that each AFE4300 device needs to multiplex in sending data from only its six measuring pairs, for a body cross section image. SPI speed at hundreds of thousands of bits per second is not a limiting factor.

According to the literature on EIT cross sectional impedance images show local variations depending both on lung function, breathing and heart blood pumping.

In order to monitor any of the above changes by impedance variation estimation the ECG sensing is also necessary. Fortunately the AFE4300 weight measuring channel can be used to sense the ECG voltage changes induces on the thorax surface [10].

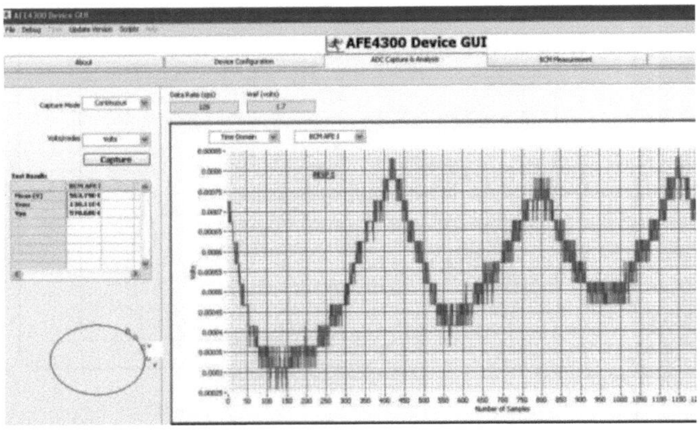

Fig. 6. Sample respiration data on the side of the thorax (with-ought amplification).

In Fig. 4 is presented the recommended band pass filter to be added to the AEF3400 weight measuring channel for ECG sensing. This channel measured voltages, share the same A/D conversion and SPI interface with the impedance channel.

The sensitivity of the surface measured voltage drops, to the lung breathing within the thorax, as can be seen from a measurement sample data set presented in Fig 6, are significant in value. The voltage sample rate was set to 128 samples per second and the instantaneous voltage displayed in volts.

Lung functioning, monitoring in critically ill or wearable tidal volume monitoring in sports medicine are thus justified by the capabilities inherent of the present design [12].

Simplified, with less electrode pairs variant of the belt presented, can be further developed.

The attained objective of the paper was to develop a reference design that can maximally cover a range of applications. Simplified and 'tuned' variants will follow as future objectives and work.

V. Conclusions

A reference design of an EIT belt, using the AFE4300 with supplemental amplifying buffers, is presented and shows promising results recommending a practical implementation.

The reduced sampling rate and other functional parameter of the proposed design, when compared with recently developed EIT belts found in the literature, is balanced by its SPI only digital interface, low total cost and practical feasibility.

The paper also indicates the possibility to develop an EIT belt with multiple impedance measuring pairs with low power consumption suitable for wireless wearable applications in monitoring body function.

Conflict of Interest

The authors declare that they have no conflict of interest.

References

1. De Vries P, What separates us from turning EIC and EIT into successful clinical bed-side instruments? Proc. of 13th Intern. Conference on Electrical Bioimpedance ICEBI07, Graz, Austria, pp. 3
2. Grimmes S and Martinsen O G Bioimpedance and Bioelectricity Basics 2008 (Amsterdam: Elsevier)
3. Barber D, Brown B, Applied potential tomography, J. Phys. E: Sci. Instrum. 1984,17, pp.723–733
4. R. Kusche et al. FPGA-Based Broadband EIT System for Complex Bioimpedance Measurements - Design and Performance Estimation, Electronics 2015, 4, pp.507-525
5. P. Gaggero et all. Electrical impedance tomography system based on active electrodes, Physiological Measurement 33(5):831-47 · May 2012
6. AFE4300 datasheet at http://www.ti.com/product/AFE4300.
7. J Wu, X. Chen, Z. Ding, Digital biomedical electrical impedance tomography based on FPGA, Journal of Biosciences and Medicines 01(02):14-18 · January 2013
8. R González-Landaeta, O Casas, R Pallŕs-Areny,Heart Rate Detection From Plantar Bioimpedance Measurements, IEEE Transactions on Biomedical Engineering, VOL. 55, NO. 3, March 2008, pp. 1163-1167
9. S Weyer, et all, Development of a real-time, semi-capacitive impedance phlebography device, Journal of Electrical Bioimpedance 6(1),2015,pp.2-9
10. Application Note at https://www.ti.com/cn/lit/pdf/tidu479
11. Free EIT software at : http:/ eidors3d.sourceforge.net/
12. V-P Seppa et all, Measuring Respirational Parameters with a Wearable Bioimpedance Device, in n book: IFMBE Proc. 13th Int Conf on Electrical Bioimpedance and 8th Conf on Electrical Impedance Tomography 2007. Graz, Austria., Editors: Scharfetter and Merwa, pp.663-666

Author: Ioan Jivet
Institute: University Politehnica Timisoara
Street: V Parvan 2
City: Timisoara
Country: Romania
Email: ioan.jivet@upt.ro

Age Simulation Suits for Training, Research and Development

H.L. Groza, S.B. Sebesi and D.S. Mandru

Technical University/ Faculty of Mechanics, Mechatronics Department, Cluj-Napoca, Romania

Abstract— **Simulation of old age can be a strong tool in providing information to researchers and developers for products that address to elderly people, and also for the disabled. Medical personal that is working with people that need care could be also users for an age simulator, with the purpose of understanding the needs of the ones they take care of. The benefits would be to provide better services and give empathy. In this paper technical solutions are proposed for development of age simulation suits, in order to identify different ways of integrating the physical functions.**

Keywords— **ageing suit, age simulator, elderly.**

I. Introduction

The importance of an age simulation suit is relevant thru the information that it provides to the users of this systems. So far we have identified a few areas of interest for this type of simulators: research and development; studies regarding elderly; development of assistive systems for elderly or the disabled; development of biomechanisms like exoskeletons; development of households for the elderly; development of vehicles; the use for life insurance companies; training of medical specialists.

There are different models of simulators that cover limitation for the limbs, back, neck and head, and also different sensorial losses like hearing and vision. The materials used for construction start from simple products like an elastic strap and can go up to virtual reality glasses to simulate vision deficiencies.

II. Ageing suits previously developed

A. AGNES

The Age Gain Now Empathy System also known as AGNES Fig. 1 is a suit developed by the MIT AgeLab researchers and it has been designed to simulate the motor, visual, flexibility, dexterity and strength of a person around 75 years old [1]. The main components of the suit are: a helmet- used to anchor the elastic straps attached to the belt; glasses to simulate eye related degradation; ear plugs to reduce hearing; a cervical collar to limit mobility at the cervical level; orthosis for the wrists to reduce mobility; gloves used to alter the tactile sense and reduce the hand mobility; a belt used as an anchor for the elastic straps; elastic straps connected between the belt and the helmet, belt and ankles, belt and wrists - they create a tension that creates difficulty in movement; orthosis for knees and elbows to reduce movement and induce fatigue; shoes made from foam to embrace the user.

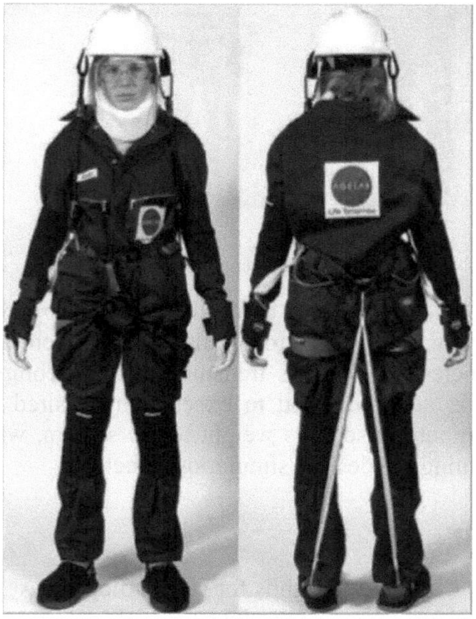

Fig. 1 AGNES Ageing Suit

B. Genworth R70i

The R70i suit, Fig. 2, produced by Applied Minds LLC for Genworth is considered to be the most evolved ageing simulator at this moment [2]. Latest technologies are combined to create a realistic feeling of old age.

The suit is made of an exoskeleton, controlled by a computer located in the back, and a virtual reality helmet. The helmet integrates a set of headphones, that simulate hearing disorders, and cameras combined with an augmented reality vision systems, that simulate age related vision disorders.

The exoskeleton is able to add force to the joints, in this way making movement difficult. This experience is highlighted to other participants by the LED-s installed and change color accordingly.

The augmented system simulate hearing impediments like hearing loss, tinnitus, aphasia, and vision deficiencies like glaucoma, cataracts, macular degeneration, and floaters.

S. Vlad and N.M. Roman (eds.), *International Conference on Advancements of Medicine and Health Care through Technology; 12th - 15th October 2016, Cluj-Napoca, Romania,*
IFMBE Proceedings 59,
DOI: 10.1007/978-3-319-52875-5_17

These technical elements have the role to disorient and weaken the user, in order to simulate the feelings of an elderly person. Due to the multitude of the stimulus it is not uncommon that the user would fall during utilization.

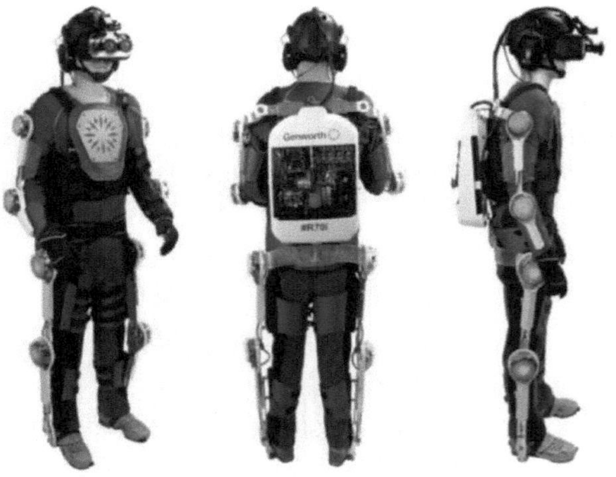

Fig. 2 R70i Genworth Ageing Suit

The whole system is controlled wireless by an operator that adjusts the settings to simulate the different age related deficiencies. The data is transmitted to the computer from the back, and processed to execute the desired functions. The computer also adds weight to the system, which helps in obtaining the desired simulation effect.

C. GERT system

GERT suit Fig. 3 stands for Gerontologic Test suit and is produced by company Produkt + Projekt Wolfgang Moll in Germany.

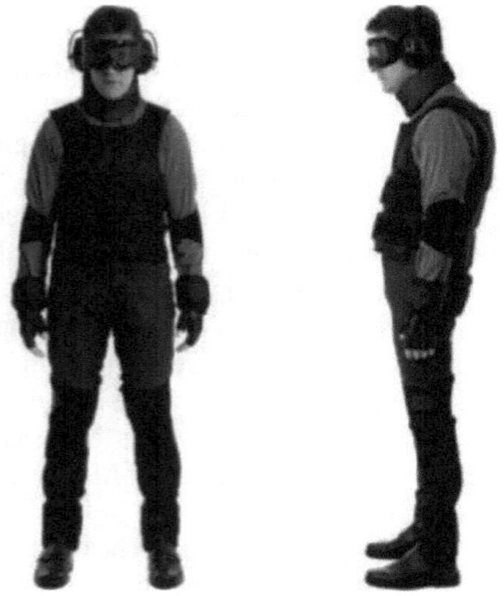

Fig. 3 GERT Ageing suit

GERT is a system that integrates different components into a suit to limit movement and sensorial capacities in order to create similar effects to the ones experienced by elderly people [3].

The different components are divided in modules. The head age simulation includes special goggles, hearing protection and a cervical collar. The torso age simulator includes a weight vest. The arms age simulation includes elbow wraps, weight cuffs and special gloves. The legs age simulation includes knee wraps, weight cuffs and special overshoes for unsteady walking.

Some special modules can be available to simulate: tremor, hearing loss and tinnitus, different eye diseases, hemiparesis simulator and a back pain simulator.

III. DEVELOPMENT OF AGE SIMULATION SUITS

A. Major components of an ageing suit

An ageing suit should integrate different devices or technological elements into a system that covers as much as possible all biological systems of the body, in order to simulate natural sensations of ageing. Of course all effects of the suit have to be reversible.

There have been identified 4 modules, as described in Fig. 4, which need to be integrated to obtain the ageing experience: the head module; torso module; arms module and legs module. Each module has to interact with the other ones so the simulation effect would as realistic as possible.

In the research and development step both sensorial and locomotion functions have to be taken into consideration. The loss of some sensorial functions, like taste for example, cannot be simulated in an immediate reversible way. Regarding motion related functions, we consider that most can be simulated.

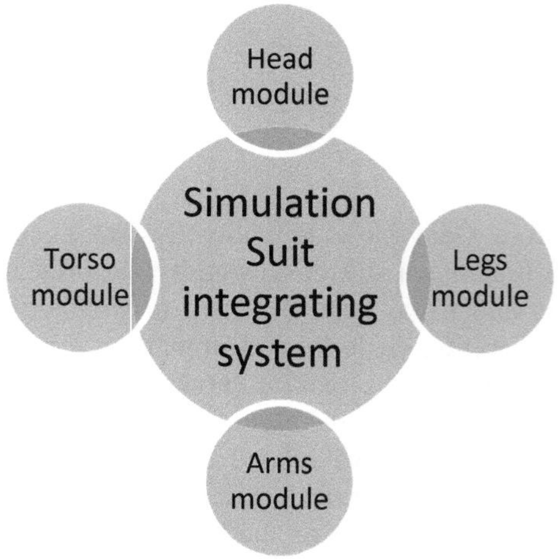

Fig. 4 Major components of an age simulation suit

Age related diseases are also a part of the project and will be taken into consideration. Affections like Parkinson disease can be a challenge in the project [4]. Physical disabilities like hemiparesis could be also simulated.

B. Module description

Each module can be divided in sub modules, and will be treated separately, having in mind the role in the integrating system. Both sensorial and motion functions have to be integrated. For each function more technical possibilities will be taken in consideration. The proposed technical solutions that have been identified could be extended and completed in the future.

The *head module* should include a vision module, hearing module and a neck mobility device. In the vision module special goggles that simulate eye disease could be used. A pair of headphones together with a sound playback device could be considered to be part of the hearing module. Affections like tinnitus or aphasia can be simulated. Headphones will also have the role of sound diminution. A cervical collar could be used to limit head movement. Some technical solutions for the physical functions diminution or loss are proposed in table 1.

Table.1 Head module proposed technical solutions

Physical function	Proposed technical solution
Vision	- Special glasses that simulate eye disease - Virtual reality system
Hearing	- Audio headphones with sound playback - Noise protection headset - Headphones with noise cancelation system
Neck mobility	- Cervical collar - Head torso fixation device - Exoskeleton

In the *torso module* a weight vest could be used to limit spine movement. The main role of the vest would be to reduce mobility in the spine and pelvis, grow the physical load and affect equilibrium. Adding weight to this part of the body would affect also breathing, by pressing the thorax. This would create in time fatigue for the user. A belt could be used in combination with the vest to attach elastic straps between the limbs and the belt. Table 2 describes the technical possibilities that could be used to limit the torso mobility functions.

Table.2 Torso module proposed technical solutions

Physical function	Proposed technical solution
Spine movement	- Vest with weight added - Backpack - Belt for connecting elastic straps - Exoskeleton

The *arms module* integrates sensorial diminution that could be simulated with a pair of gloves and movement limitation of the shoulder, elbow and wrist. The gloves have also the role of reducing mobility of the hand and the capability of grasping. A tremor simulator could be implemented using a functional electrical stimulation device. Reaching for objects and grasping capabilities are intended to be affected. In table 3 there have been identified some technical solution for physical function reduction.

Table.3 Arms module proposed technical solutions

Physical function	Proposed technical solution
Tactile sense	- Gloves - Fingers protections - Metallic exoskeleton - Tremor simulator
Shoulder, elbow and wrist movement	- Orthosis with elastic systems - Orthosis with braking systems - Elastic straps - Exoskeleton

In the *legs module* walking is affected by hip, knee and ankle restriction. Adding overshoes should affects stability and would give a better understanding for the user of using crouches and walking frames for example. Also by adding force to the joints, fatigue will be installed and the walking distances will be reduced. In table 4 the proposed technical solutions are displayed.

Table.4 Legs module proposed technical solutions

Physical function	Proposed technical solution
Hip, knee and ankle movement	- Orthosis with elastic systems - Orthosis with braking systems - Elastic straps - Exoskeleton
Foot movement	- Overshoes - Metallic plate - Exoskeleton

C. Simulation of physical disabilities

This type of suits could be also used to simulate different physical disabilities. Some physical handicaps could be easily simulated, but others would need more complex technical solutions. For example to simulate complete blindness, it would need just something to cover the eyes, but to simulate hemiparesis (Fig.5) more modules need to be adapted.

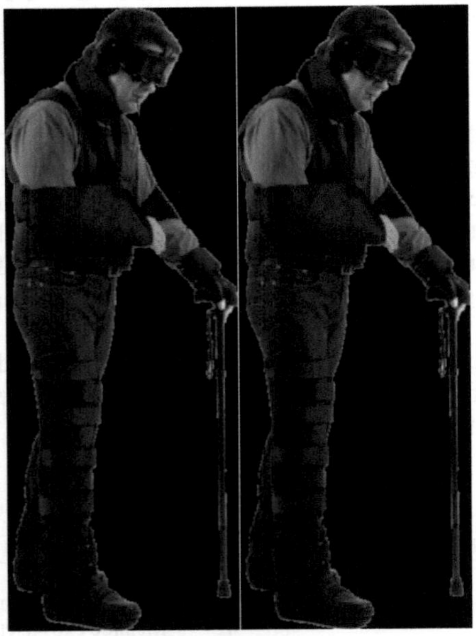

Fig. 5 Hemiparesis simulator

In a modular system this could be possible just by modifying the structure of the suit on the sub module that presents interest.

Better understanding the needs of a person that is in a wheelchair or is suffering of hemiparesis, could help designers develop products that would better fit the needs of the users. Smart homes integrate also devices and appliances addressed to the elderly and the disabled, in order to help them have a better life. Building homes for these social categories has always been a challenge, and simulating physical disabilities could help in better designs [5].

Training of the medical personal that is working with the physically disabled would be also a good possibility of better understanding the state of the patients that they are working with, and will create empathy for them [1].

IV. Conclusions

Ageing is associated progressively with chronic diseases that eventually would take the person to need special care or special devices adapted to their needs.

These simulation systems are willing to give a better understanding of ageing for young people especially for researchers, designers and medical personal.

The effects of these suits have to be reversible for the user, leaving behind an experience that could create empathy or even change a life style.

Simulating the motor effects represents just a part of the deficiencies accumulated by ageing. The loss of Sensorial capabilities represents also a reality, it this is very difficult to simulate the loss of all the sensorial receptors in a reversible way.

The ageing effects have to be taken into consideration when products are designed, and services are being given to the elderly or the disabled.

Acknowledgment

Research partially supported by PCCA Project 180/2012, "A Hybrid FES-Exoskeleton System to Rehabilitate the Upper Limb in Disabled People (EXOSLIM)".

Conflict of Interest

The authors declare that they have no conflict of interest.

References

1. MIT Age Lab, M. A. (n.d.). AGNES - Age Gain Now Empathy System. Oikonomou, T., Votis, K., Tzovaras, D., & Korn, P. (2009). An Open Source Tool for Simulating a Variety of Vision Impairments in Developing Swing Applications. Universal Access in Human-Computer Interaction. Addressing Diversity, 135–144.
2. Genworth R70i, http://www.digitaltrends.com/cool-tech/genworth-r70i-exoskeleton/
3. GERT Age simulation suit, www.age-simulation-suit.com
4. Boffi L., Fontana M., Rosati G., Milani M., Supporting the designers to build empathy with people with Parkinson's disease: the role of a hand tremor simulating device and of user research with end-users, 2013
5. Cardoso, C., & Clarkson, P. J. (2012). Simulation in user-centred design: helping designers to empathise with atypical users. Journal of Engineering Design, 23(1), 1–22.

Author: Groza Horatiu
Institute: Technical University Faculty of Mechanics
Street: Bulevardul Muncii 103-105
City: Cluj-Napoca
Country: Romania
Email: horatiu.groza@mdm.utcluj.ro

Low Cost Command and Control System for Automated Infusion Devices

B. Tebrean, S. Crisan, C. Muresan and T.E. Crisan

Electrical Engineering and Measurements Department, Technical University of Cluj-Napoca, Cluj-Napoca, Romania

Abstract— **The aim of this paper is to present a low cost system that can be adapted to different infusion devices. A laboratory test device is presented. The paper offers technical details about the sensor acquisition process using an ARDUINO UNO® board and the infusion process performed with a syringe actuation device. Several tests were carried out using a simple and adaptable virtual instrument created in LabVIEW®. Experiments involved a pulse sensor to test the viability of the solution. The applicability of this technical solution can be found in various fields of applications - medicine, engineering, chemistry, biology, food processing.**

Keywords — **infusion devices, virtual instrument, pulse monitoring.**

I. Introduction

The controlled delivery of a substance through automated infusion devices is an important area of research in various fields of engineering. The development of integrated medical systems used nowadays includes automated syringe pumps, controlled perfusion devices, peristaltic pumps or many other self-operated instruments that can ease the work of medical personnel. [1] [2]

A variety of sensors, electronic components, electric drivers and motors are integrant parts of the mentioned equipment. For that reason, in various cases, the real usage of the integrated medical device is reduced and the costs are high in respect with the real necessity of the product. [3]

The aim of this paper is to present a simple and low-cost method of monitoring and delivery a drug to patients through an automated syringe. The infusion device will be controlled with respect to the response from a pulse sensor, but the experimental device and the virtual instrument that controls and commands it can be easily adaptable to many other biomedical sensors or clinical situations besides the presented one.

II. Experimental device

A. Device configuration and working principle

The device that is subject to the present paper has the structure presented in figure 1.

The structure of the implemented application in based on two distinct levels:

- the signal acquisition and the actuation system;
- the measuring/processing unit and the actuation control.

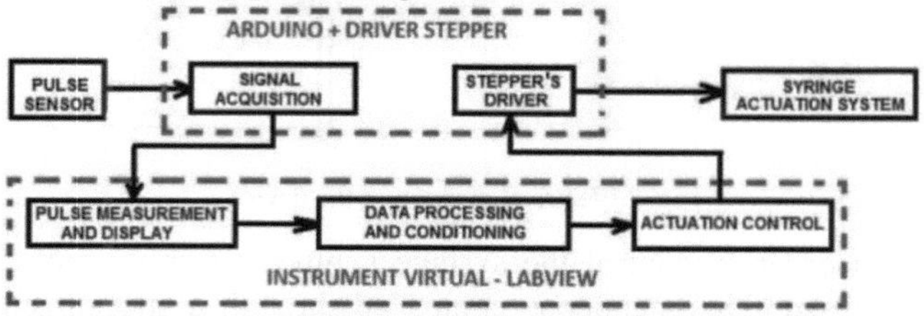

Fig. 1 The block diagram of the automated infusion device

Each element from this block diagram has a specific role in the functionality of the device:

- *the pulse sensor* – converts the patient pulse into a time dependent electrical signal;
- *the signal acquisition block* – using an analog input channel of an ARDUINO UNO® board, the electrical signal is acquired and converted to digital; [4]
- *the measurement and display block* – with the aid of a virtual instrument, created in a graphical programming software - LabVIEW®, the signal provided by previous structures is measured and displayed;
- *the data processing and conditioning block* – is used to compare the received information with certain limits and to correlate the decisions that will be sent to the actuation block in respect of the measured signal;
- *the actuation control block* – send the stepper's driver the digital code necessary to impose the speed and the direction of the stepper motor;
- *the stepper's driver block* – consist of a dedicated electronic driver for bipolar steppers - A4988 and the power circuits; [5]
- *the syringe actuation system* - through an electromechanical system that enables proper handling of syringes.

B. The device's components and electrical circuit

The electrical circuit and the components of the experimental device are presented in figure 2.

The main part of the electrical command and control circuit is an ARDUINO UNO® board. The properties of this platform allow for the measurement of the pulse provided from the sensor on channel A0 (analog input 0) and to give a 5V voltage to power-up the sensor.

S. Vlad and N.M. Roman (eds.), *International Conference on Advancements of Medicine and Health Care through Technology; 12th - 15th October 2016, Cluj-Napoca, Romania,*
IFMBE Proceedings 59,
DOI: 10.1007/978-3-319-52875-5_18

The pulse sensor is an open source hardware that measures the blood-oxygen concentration through an optical method. In the electrical diagram it is represented in the middle of the board, but in real situation it is placed on a finger or attached to the ear of the patient. [6]

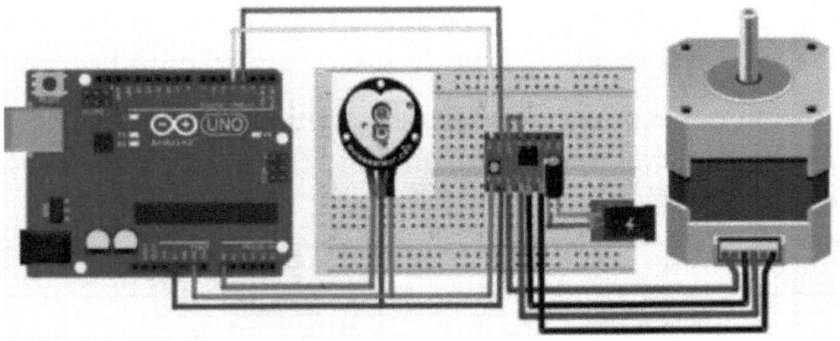

Fig. 2 Electrical diagram of the device

In order to control the syringe a bipolar stepper motor was used. This stepper is controlled through a specialized driver that generates the PWM used by it. The driver is also commanded by the ARDUINO UNO® board from two digital output channels, one used to select the rotation direction (digital-output 2) and one to set the speed (digital-output 3). The driver has its own power supply with 12V c.c. voltage that can provide a maximal current of 1A/phase for the stepper.

The syringe actuation system contains several components as it is shown in figure 3. This structure was adapted after a configuration created by the researchers from "Department of Materials Science & Engineering, Michigan Technological University, Houghton, USA as an "Open source syringe pump" [7] and builds on the work described in [8]

In our case, the structural parts ware built from high density PLA (polylactic acid) on a 3D printer. The material properties confer the mechanical resistance necessary in this situation.

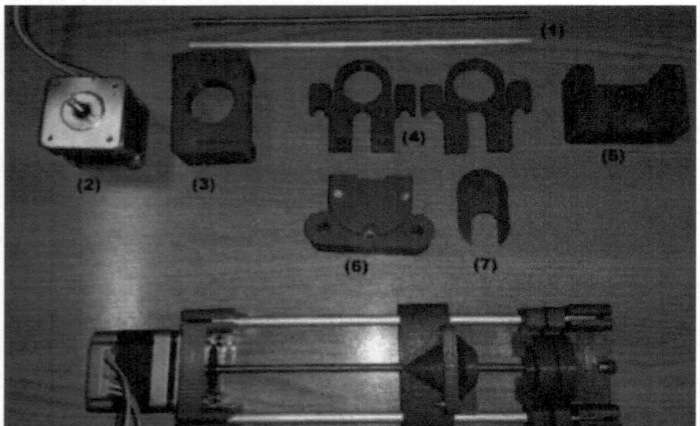

Fig. 3 The syringe actuation system

The components of the actuation system are:
- one steel threaded rod and two aluminum guide bars (1);
- the stepper motor NEMA 17 (2);
- the support for the stepper/guide bars (3);
- the syringe fixing elements (4);
- the end support for guide bars (5);
- the plunger holder (6) and the plunger fixing element (7).

III. EXPERIMENTAL RESULTS

In order to perform a set of tests, an experimental setup was implemented as it is shown in figure 4.

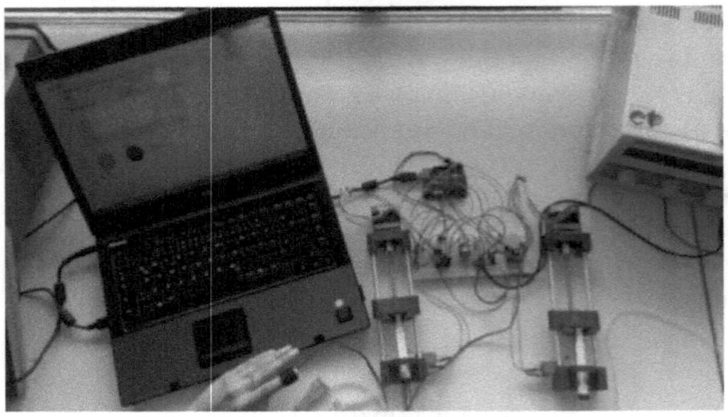

Fig. 4 The experimental implementation

For the control and the monitoring of the automated syringe, a virtual instrument was created with the aid of the graphical programming software - LabVIEW®. This software allows the user to visualize the signals through a frontal panel, to control the flowrate of the syringe or other critical parameters of the experimental setup.

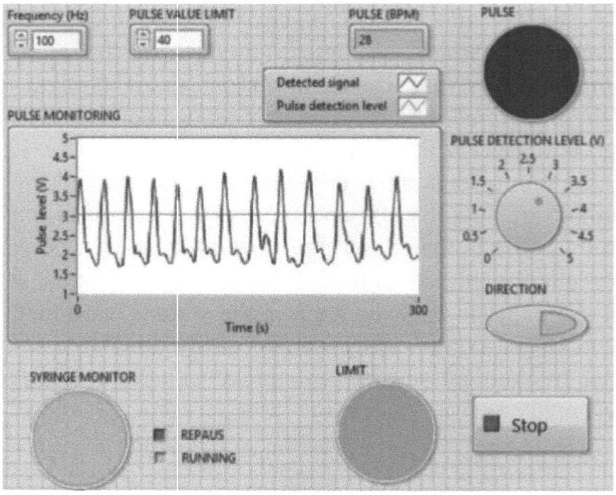

Fig. 5 The front panel of the virtual instrument

In the central part of the front panel it was disposed a waveform chart that presents the signal acquired from the pulse sensor. Also on this graph, the limit of detection is represented with a red line. This limit can be manually adjusted from the panel through a potentiometer, setting in this manner the triggering position with respect to the amplitude of the received signal. The snapshot of the application presented in figure 5 shows the case where the pulse was artificially decreased in order to trigger an infusion condition. The green led shows that the system is running as a response to the threshold limit of 40 bmp being reached.

The front panel can be easily modified in order to respond to various necessities of the user. In this situation just some of the features were used such as:

- frequency of the PWM signal – used to modify the speed of the stepper;
- direction switch – used to refill the syringe or to deliver the substance;
- pulse value indicators – display the numerical value of the pulse and a LED to show the presence of the pulse;
- operation and critical limit indicators – LEDs which show if the device is in normal operating process or some operational imposed limits have been reached.

The block diagram of the virtual instrument contains three different operational blocks, each of them having a precise purpose in the functionality of the experimental device:

- *the pulse measurement and display block (1);*
- *the data processing and conditioning block (2);*
- *the actuation control block (3).*

The first block of the diagram allows the initialization of the ARDUINO UNO® board and sets the serial port that operates, in this case COM 7. Using the function "Analog Read 1 Channel" prescribed on channel 0 – analog input - the signal from the pulse sensor is acquired. This signal is displayed on a graph together with the detection level.

The data processing and conditioning block receives the numerical data from the pulse sensor and stores it in a matrix on each iteration of the "While loop" with the aid of a "Shift Register". This operation is necessary in order to use the "Threshold Detector" function to count the number of times when the input signal is passing the detection level.

Using a timer function, the values given by the detector mentioned above will be introduced into another matrix that will hold, every 15 seconds, the number of pulses detected from the beginning of the program. In order to display the real values of the pulse, this array will be ordered descend-

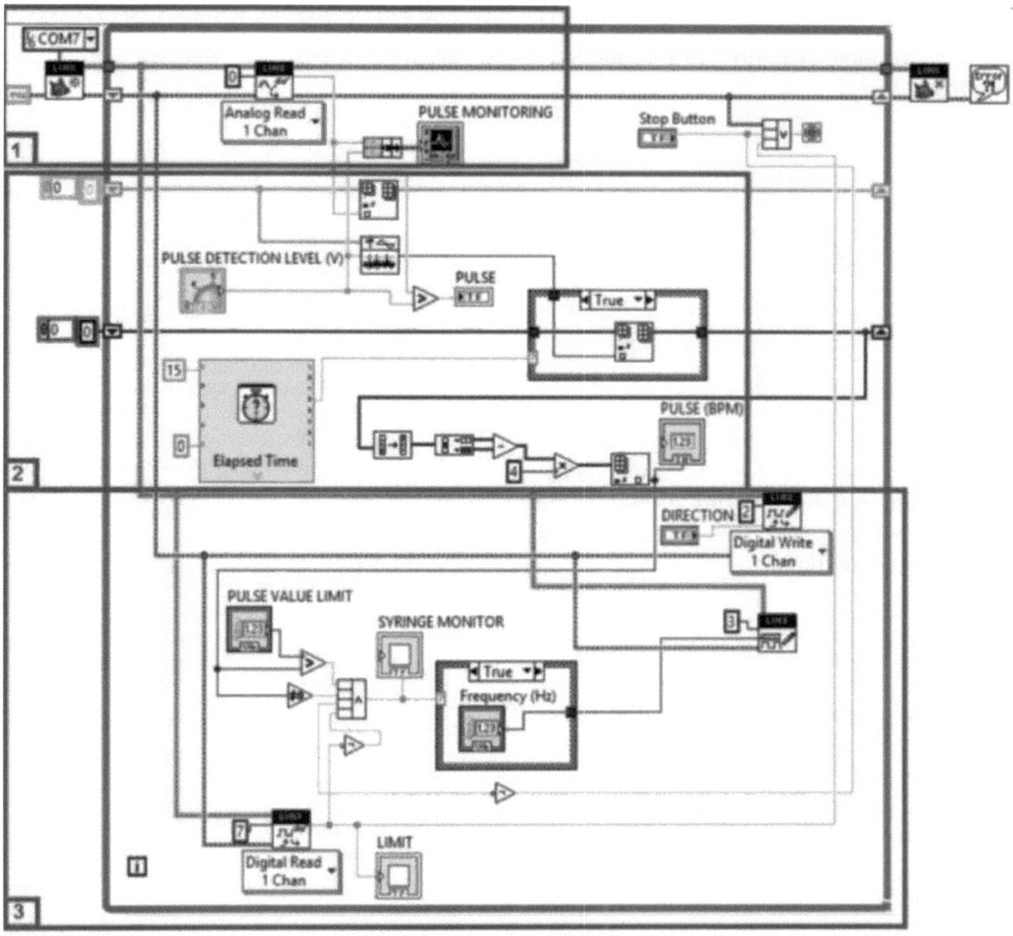

Fig. 6 The block diagram of the virtual instrument

ing and multiplying by four the difference between the last two values, the pulse rate in beats per minute is obtained.

In the actuation control block the pulse value is compared with a critical one and imposing the supplementary condition that the pulse is not zero, allows - through a “Case” structure - to select the frequency with which the control pulses will be sent on two digital channels of the ARDUINO UNO® board: the direction of rotation on channel 2 digital and the stepper speed on on digital channel 3. Those values can be modified from the frontal panel of the virtual instrument or included as constants in the block diagram. Also in this part of the block diagram, a signal provided by a switch sensor on digital input 7 channel is acquired, allowing the virtual instrument to stop the infusion process when the syringe has been completely emptied.

The flowrate of the infusion process (Q_{fi}) is proportional with the frequency of the PWM signal (f_{PWM}) that imposes the speed of the stepper. The equation is completed using several other terms such as: the pitch of the threaded rod (p_{Mj}), the step angle of the stepper motor (n) and the inner diameter of the syringe (d_{int}) as seen in equation 1.

$$Q_{fi} = d_{int} \cdot p_{Mj} \cdot \frac{f_{PWM} \cdot n}{360°} \quad (1)$$

For different syringe volumes, the flow rate of the system has been computed.

Table 1 Infusion flow rate on different values of PWM signal

Sringe volume (ml)	Inside diameter (mm)	Flowrate at different PWM frequences (ml/min)				
		100 Hz	200 Hz	300 Hz	400 Hz	500 Hz
1	4.69	0.07	0.14	0.21	0.28	0.35
3	9.65	0.15	0.29	0.43	0.58	0.72
5	12.45	0.19	0.37	0.56	0.75	0.93
10	20.05	0.30	0.60	0.90	1.20	1.50
20	22.9	0.34	0.69	1.03	1.37	1.72

Experiments have revealed that the current electromechanical construction of the device allows for a minimum resolution of 0.07 ml/min for the 1ml syringe – the syringe with the smallest volume - and 0.35 ml/min for the largest volume syringe tested of 20ml.

IV. Conclusions

The command and control system presented in this paper may represent a low-cost viable solution on various infusion automated devices. The applicability of this technical solution can be found in various fields of applications - medicine, engineering, chemistry, biology, food processing.

The virtual instrument can be easily adaptable to many types of sensors and the user interface can be modified without major effort in order to respond to different practical situations. The main advantage of this solution is that it allows a very fast modification of dosage of the substances, of the flowrate or the timing of the infusion process.

The device has been thoroughly tested under laboratory conditions. However, in order to implement such a device in a clinical trial further enhancements are needed.

From an economical point of view, the costs of such a system are relatively reduced in comparison with similar, classical solution used in practice.

Acknowledgment

This work was supported by a grant of the Romanian National Authority for Scientific Research and Innovation, CNCS-UEFISCDI, project number PN-II-RU-TE-2014-4-2196.

Conflict of Interest

The authors declare that they have no conflict of interest.

References

1. Roland A. Snijder, et al.(2016) Dosing errors in preterm neonates due to flow rate variability in multi-infusion syringe pump setups: An in vitro spectrophotometry study, European Journal of Pharmaceutical Sciences, http://dx.doi.org/10.1016/j.ejps.2016.07.019;
2. Martin Schmettow., et al.(2013) With how many users should you test a medical infusion pump? Sampling strategies for usability tests on high-risk systems, Journal of Biomedical Informatics 46, ISSN: 1532-0464;
3. Matthew Scanlon (2006) The Role of “Smart” Infusion Pumps in Patient Safety, Safety and Reliability in Pediatrics, http://dx.doi.org/10.1016/j.pcl.2012.08.005;
4. ***, “ARDUINO UNO – Technical specifications” https://www.arduino.cc/en/Main/ArduinoBoardUno;
5. ***, “A4988 Stepper Motor Driver Carrier” - https://www.pololu.com/product/1182
6. ***, “The Pulse Sensor – Techical article and specifications”, http://pulsesensor.com/pages/pulse-sensor-amped-arduino-v1dot1
7. Bas Wijnen, et al., (2014), Open-Source Syringe Pump Library, http://dx.doi.org/10.1371/journal.pone.0107216
8. Will Patrick, Taylor Levy (2013). Open source syringe pump. http://fab.cba.mit.edu/classes/863.13/people/wildebeest/projects/final/index.html

Author: Bogdan TEBREAN
Institute: Technical University of Cluj-Napoca
Street: Memorandumului no.28
City: Cluj-Napoca
Country: Romania
Email: bogdan.tebrean@ethm.utcluj.ro

Monitoring System for the Emotional States

M.Cenuşă, M. Poienar, L. D. Milici and S.D. Paţa

"Ştefan cel Mare" University, Suceava, Romania

Abstract— **The paper presents a developed system for monitoring emotional states, depending on different stress factors, based on electrodermal response. The system is based on e-Health Sensor Shield platform developed by the Libelium company. Parameters monitored in order to set off emotional states are: galvanic skin response and body temperature. The information is sent wirelessly to a computer and the precessed using a virtual instrument developed in LabView. The proposed system allows monitoring a maximum of 253 subjects simultaneously.**

At the end of the paper are presented the main conclusions related to the emotional states system development and implementation.

Keywords— **galvanic skin response, emotional states, LabView, sensor, Arduino**

I. Introduction

The emotional states represent an important parameter in the study of human being behavior and for introducing human factor in systems with artificial intelligence.

Encoding and interpreting the emotional states represent a challenge for researchers from various research centers, and were developed various solutions in this direction.

The systems developed for monitoring emotions are based on several parameters, including observable changes like face expressions, body postures, vocal tones, and physiological signal changes such as heart rate, temperature and respiration,skin response.

The skin is a conjunctive-vascular membranous integument that covers the entire body and that continues with the semi-mucous and mucous of the natural cavities, and it is composed by epidermis, dermis, hypodermis and skin annex: sebaceous and sweat glands [1], [2].

The last one presents a particular interest because its activity can be triggered by emotional stimuli, with its origin in the cerebral cortex.

The connection between emotional states and electrical phenomena of epidermis has been observed since 1880.

Subsequently, the electrically monitoring of the epidermis became one of the most used biosignals in psychophysiology. This was due to facile method of taking electrodermal response (EDR), whise intensity depends upon the psychological significance and intensity of the stimulus.

The term of electrodermal activity used to characterize all electrical phenomena on the skin and its annexes was introduced in 1966 of Jonson and Lubin.

Dermis parameter variation is due to changes induced by different stimulion sweat gland activitythrough the balance changing between the positive and negative ions in the fluid secreted on its level [3].

The electrodermal measurements can be achieved by applying an electrical current, direct or alternating, a method that is called exosomatic.

When it is applied direct current, the electrodermal response will be the skin conductance. For the case when it is applied, an alternating current theelectrodermal response will be the skin admittance.

The electrodermal activity measurement method without using a power source is called endodermal activity.

The latter is the most common method of measuring the electrodermal activity for the emotional states interpretation.

In this paper is presented a hardware solution for the electrodermal response measurement for monitoring the emotional states variation according to different stressors.

II. Systems developed within the "Stefan cel Mare " University

Within the "Stefan cel Mare" University were developed two variants of systems for assessing the emotional states. The first variant of the device is based on a resistive voltage divider which measures the skin conductance by using a DC voltage with an amplitude of 2,5 V, supplied by a source of reference voltage thermally compensated, performed with the circuit TL431. The voltage divider is made up of a fix resistor and the resistance of the skin segment placed between the contact electrodes [1].

The system has 4 acquisition channels and is calibrated to measure identically on each measurement channel available; the only differences in measuring will be those ones specific to the subjects connected (to the electrical characteristics of their skin). The potential difference recordes is measured with an 8- bit microcontroller "PIC18F458".

The data are transmitted to the PC by Bluetooth protocol and then are processed in a Labview application that displays them on individual graph and saves values on an .xls file. In Figure 1 is presented the block diagram of the device [1].

S. Vlad and N.M. Roman (eds.), *International Conference on Advancements of Medicine and Health Care through Technology; 12th - 15th October 2016, Cluj-Napoca, Romania,*
IFMBE Proceedings 59,
DOI: 10.1007/978-3-319-52875-5_19

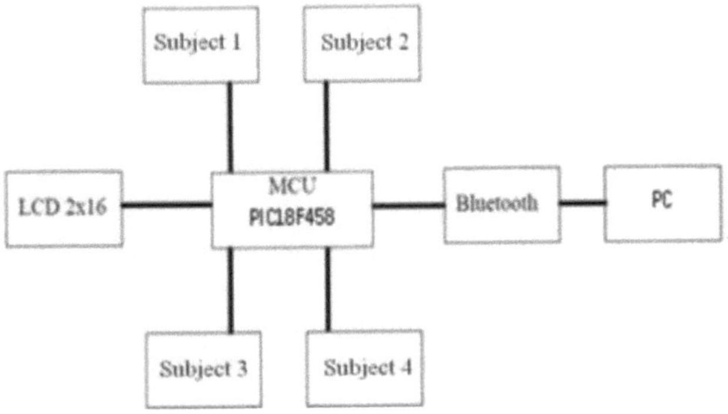

Fig.1 The block diagram of device for the first variant

The second variant of the acquisition system allows monitoring of a single subject, but increases the number of data taken. Can be used simultaneously more systems depending on the number of subjects monitored. The resistive voltage divider that measures the skin conductance by injecting a DC voltage with an amplitude of 2,5 V is powered by a source of reference voltage thermally compensated made with the circuit MAX6029. The voltage variation is then read by the analogical port of the microcontroller (Atmega328) that performs internally an average for 50 samples, then sends the value as characters by bluetooth to the virtual instrument, to be processed.

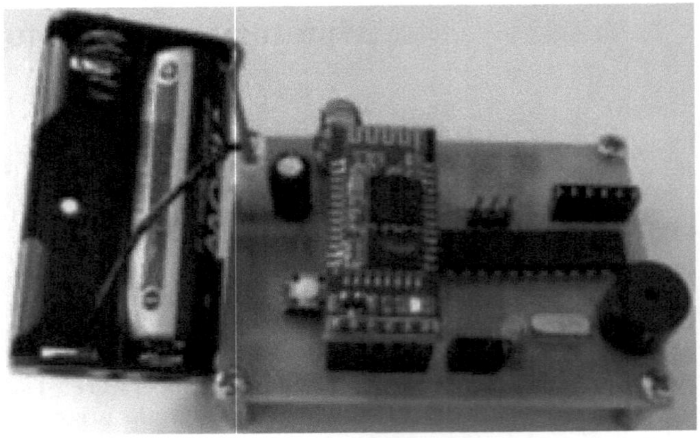

Fig. 2 The second variant of the system

In Figure 2 is presented the system for monitoring the emotional states [1].

In Figure 3 are shown graphically the skin resistance variation taken for 12 subjects when they were viewing a movie sequences chosen to transmit different feelings.

On the graphics are marked changes that occur in certain sequences of the film with the strong emotional charge. From the analysis can be observed that the measured values depend on the degree of involvement, reaction speed and attention of each subject [1].

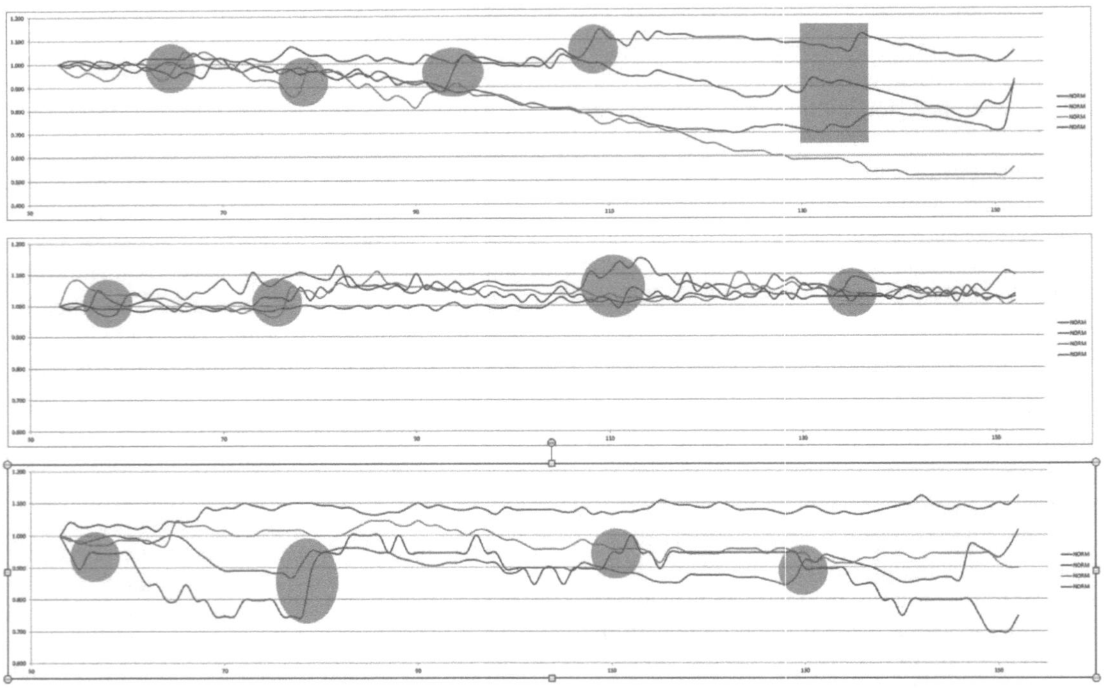

Fig. 3 Skin resistance variation for 12 subjects

III. Future development of systems for monitoring the emotional states

The system is based on e-Health Sensor Shield platform, produced by Libelium Company, that allow the real-time acquisition and measurement of multiple biomedical signals, as it is shown in Figure 4 [4].

Through it can be acquired the following signals:patient position sensor (accelerometer), glucometer sensor, body temperature sensor, blood pressure sensor (sphygmomanometer), pulse and oxygen in blood sensor, airflow sensor (breathing), galvanic skin response sensor (GSR - Sweating), electrocardiogram sensor (ECG), electromyography sensor (EMG).

Processing and transmission of the data taken by the e-Health Sensor Shield system is achieved through the Arduino Uno WiFi development board, as it is shown in Figure 5. The Arduino UNO WiFi board is based on the ATmega328 and it has an integrated ESP8266 WiFi Module.

The board can be powered via the USB connection or with an external power supply.

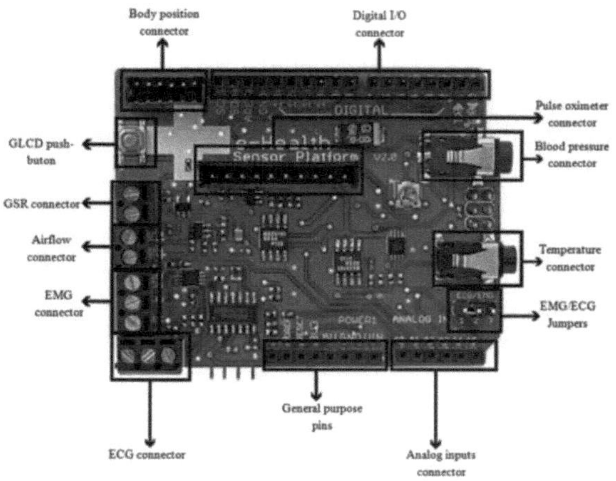

Fig. 4 Platforma e-Health Sensor Shied

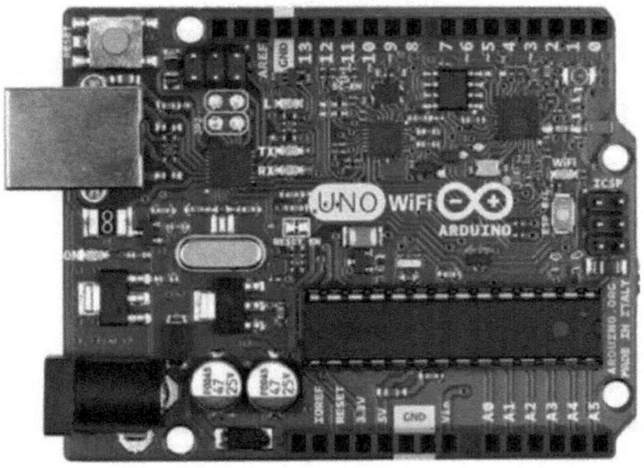

Fig. 5 Arduino Uno WiFI Sheld - front view

To highlight emotional states, a sensor for measuring skin resistance (galvanic skin response) and a body temperature sensor manufactured by Libelium are used. Also, the system aims to determine the influence of external environmental, humidity and temperature parameterson electrodermal measured resistance value [5]. To do this, a temperature and humidity sensor is used, which has as basis the SHT11integrated circuit.Information based on the external environmentalparameters is processed directly on the ArduinoUnoWiFi.

The device consisting of sensors, dedicated e-Health board and Arduino Uno board (Figure 6) transmitsevery 10 seconds wireless data acquired to a router and onto a central unit, which can simultaneouslyreceive data via the router and from up to 253 such devices (Figure 7). Data is processed and analysedin the central unit through an application developed in LabView programming environment.

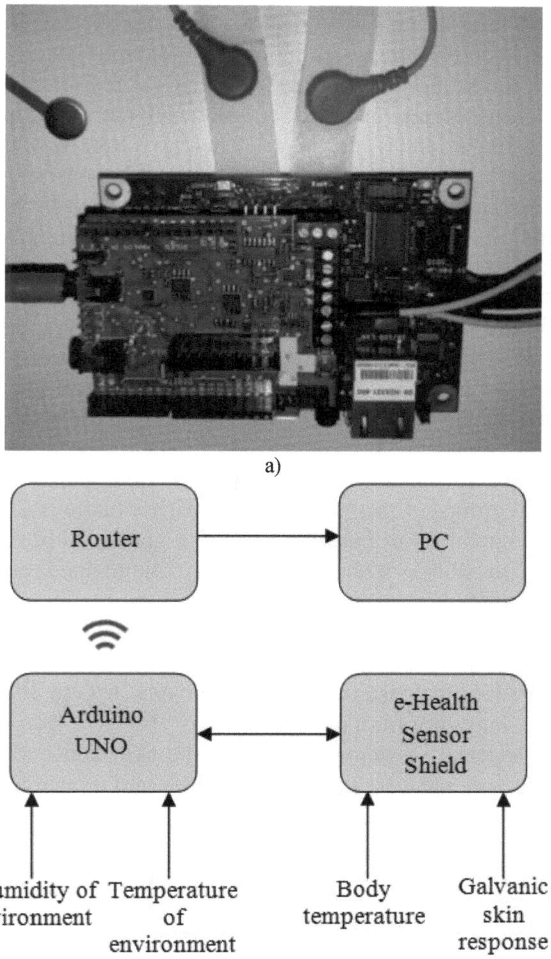

Fig. 6 System for electrodermal response measurement
a) prototype; b) block diagram

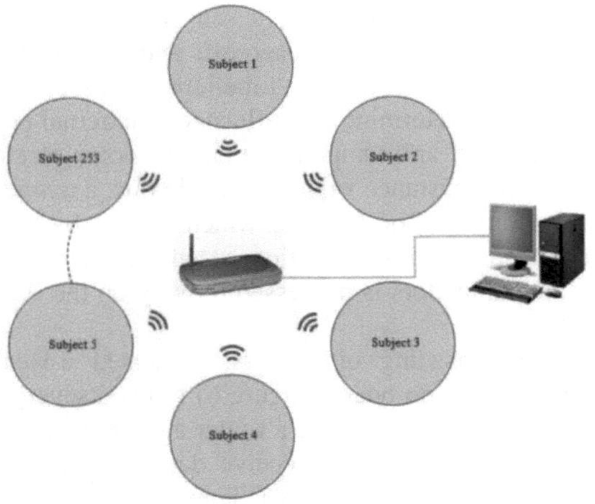

Fig. 7 Communication block diagram

The experiment will be performed on groups of 5 people, placed in a sitting position in a room equipped with video and air conditioning, with humidity and temperature control possibilities. For measuring the electrical resistance of the skin, sensors are installed on each subject, one on each index finger and ring finger. Their position was chosen considering that previous studies have demonstrated that this anatomical area is most suitable for measuring electrodermal response due to its numerous sweat glands (300 glands per cm^2). The temperature sensor is placed in the central area of the palm.

Before introducing the subjects, in the room the temperature will be set 16 C and the humidity will be set at 40%.

The screen will project a film with a lasting of two hours during which it will insert images, conversations or unexpected noises meant for anxiety induction and negative emotional reaction. The experiments were performed on several groups of people in the following situations:

- temperature in the room will rise gradually from 16°C to 30°C, with the humidity maintained constant (40%);
- temperature is maintained constant and the humidity will increase progressively up to 80%;
- gradual increase of temperature from 16°C to 30°C and humidity from 40% to 80%.

Electrical resistance values of the skin and body temperature are measured every 10 seconds and transmitted to a computer that runs an application in Labview which are processed and stored in a .xlx file.

Based on the results obtained is made a classification of subjects depending on the answer to stress, age, gender and occupation.In addition, parameters will determine the influence of ambient electrical resistance measurements on skin tests,and will be performed in different ambient environmental conditions.

IV. Conclusions

The paper presents two solutions for monitoring the emotional states. The measured values depend on the degree of involvement, reaction speed and attention of each subject.

The achieved systems are limited on the number of subjects that can retrieve data simultaneously.

The major advantage of the device proposed as a future development, is that it can take data from maximum 253subjects, that can be transmitted wireless on a PC, where can be analyzed.

Through the experiment is followed the influence of the environmental parameters (temperature, humidity), over the electrodermal response.

For this reason, the data collection is performed in an air-conditioned room, the temperature and humidity being controlled.

Acknowledgment

Infrastructure was partly supported by project Integrated Center for Research, Development and Innovation in Advanced Materials, Nanotechnologies, and Distributed Systems for Fabrication and Control, Contract No. 671/09.04.2015, Sectoral Operational Program for Increase of the Economic Competitiveness co-funded from the European Regional Development Fund.

Conflict of Interest

The authors declare that they have no conflict of interest.

References

1. Milici L D, Plăcintă V M, Bujor, L, Milici M R System for highlighting the emotional states, used in assessing the teaching methods, În: 9th International Symposium on Advanced Topics in Electrical Engineering, Bucharest, Romania, 7-9 May, 2015.
2. Boucsein W Electrodermal Activity, New York: Editura Oxford Springer, 2012.
3. Bronzino J D The Biomedical Engineering HandBook, Second Edition, Florida: CRC Press, 2000.
4. ***https://www.cooking-hacks.com/ehealth-sensors-complete-kit-biometric-medical-arduino-raspberry-pi, accessed in 08.08.2016.
5. ***https://www.robofun.ro/senzor-temperatura-umiditate-sht11, accessed in 12.08.2016.

Author: Cenuşă Mihai
Institute: "Ştefan cel Mare" University
Street: University Street
City: Suceava
Country: Romania
Email: mcenusa@yahoo.com

Low Cost Prototype for Viewing a Map of Vascularization

D. Iudean[1], R. Munteanu jr.[1], E.M. Bindea[1], D.F. Muresanu[2,3] and O. Selejan[3]

[1] Faculty of Electrical Engineering, Technical University of Cluj-Napoca, Romania
[2] Department of Clinical Neurosciences, "Iuliu Hatieganu"University of Medicine and Pharmacy, Cluj-Napoca, Romania
[3] "RoNeuro" Institute for Neurological Research and Diagnostic, Cluj-Napoca, Romania

Abstract— **Vascular access is the most common invasive medical procedure. Blood is a very good approach for a physician to assess the health of a patient. For obtaining blood samples, it is necessary to access the venous system. The overwhelming majority of vascular access procedures are performed without visualizing the venous system and instead rely on what specialists can see through the skin of the patient or the ability of the clinician to feel the vessel, which occurs practically by assumption and with hard work. This intervention can be quite traumatic, especially among children. Interest in the medical and scientific community to facilitate an intervention that reduces patient discomfort has been demonstrated by the development of devices that help visualize the vein map of the patient.**

To help solve this problem, a prototype based on infrared light is proposed. An infrared light source will be provided by 100 IR LEDs. Image acquisition of the patient's skin surface will be collected with a webcam that was modified in advance. The acquired images will be post-processed to ensure a better level of accuracy. This device will use infrared light to illuminate the patient's skin, thus revealing the veins under the skin like a map.

Due to the uniqueness of blood vessel networks, vein maps are often used in biometrics. They are also used to identify a person through a process similar to fingerprint-based identification.

Keywords— **prototype, vein, infrared, vascularization, image processing**

I. Introduction

Vascular access is the most common invasive medical procedure. Blood is a very good approach for a physician to assess the health of a patient. For obtaining blood samples, it is necessary to access the venous system. The overwhelming majority of vascular access procedures are performed without visualizing the venous system and just rely on what specialists can see through the skin of the patient or the ability of the clinician to feel the vessel, which occurs practically by assumption and with hard work. This procedure can be quite traumatic, especially among children. Interest in the medical and scientific community to facilitate an intervention that reduces patient discomfort has been demonstrated by the development of devices that help visualize the vein map of the patient. [1]

To help solve this problem, a prototype based on infrared light is proposed. An infrared light source will be provided by 100 IR LEDs (infrared). Image acquisition of the patient's skin surface will be collected with a webcam that was modified in advance. The acquired images will be post-processed to ensure a better level of accuracy. This device will use infrared light to illuminate the patient's skin and reveal veins under the skin like a map. [2]

Due to the uniqueness of blood vessel networks, vein maps are often used in biometrics. They are also used in security to identify a person through a process similar to fingerprint-based identification. [3]

II. Theory

The fact that IR light is associated with temperature makes it possible to use it in medicine. Human body temperature changes under the influence of certain aspects, such as inflammation, or other tissue abnormalities, including cancer. Fortunately, much of this variation in temperature can be detected with the help of an IR camera. To understand how the contrast of subcutaneous veins is improved, it is necessary to understand how energy is transferred from the veins to the infrared sensor. The human body in a neutral temperature environment loses approximately 60% of its energy through radiation, 25% by evaporation, 12% and 3% by convective conduction. This article will refer only to heat exchange by radiation. [4]

III. Optical Properties of Tissue and Blood

The human body radiates infrared light at an intensity of 10 mW/cm^2 in the range of 3,000-14,000 nm. [5]

The amplitude of the infrared energy emanating from the human body will vary depending on the spatial arrangement of blood vessels, veins and capillaries. The temperature varies due to a vein and the surrounding skin tissue, which also has a gradient for the skin. Together with the Stefan-Boltzmann law, the law of thermal radiation, thermal images can be generated according to equation (1): [6]

$$W = \varepsilon \cdot \sigma \cdot T4 \tag{1}$$

S. Vlad and N.M. Roman (eds.), *International Conference on Advancements of Medicine and Health Care through Technology; 12th - 15th October 2016, Cluj-Napoca, Romania,*
IFMBE Proceedings 59,
DOI: 10.1007/978-3-319-52875-5_20

- W - radiant emittance W/cm^2
- ε - emissivity, 0.98/0.99 to human skin
- σ - Boltzmann constant, $\sigma \cong 5.6705 \times 10^{-12}\ W/cm^2K^4$
- T - temperature at the skin surface, K

For individuals, ε is constant and σ is the only variable that intervenes and affects emissivity, and it reflects the temperature on the surface skin. Emissivity will be higher when it is measured at a point over a blood vessel than at a point between two blood vessels. Therefore, a model of a blood vessel can be captured by a detector that is sensitive to wavelengths above 3 pm and can be digitized in a thermal image. Quantitative differences in skin temperature will influence W and therefore significantly affect the thermal image quality and contrast. [7]

CCD sensors are more efficient than human vision and are sensitive to infrared light (which is invisible to the human eye) for wavelengths up to 1,100 nm. (Fig. 1) [8]

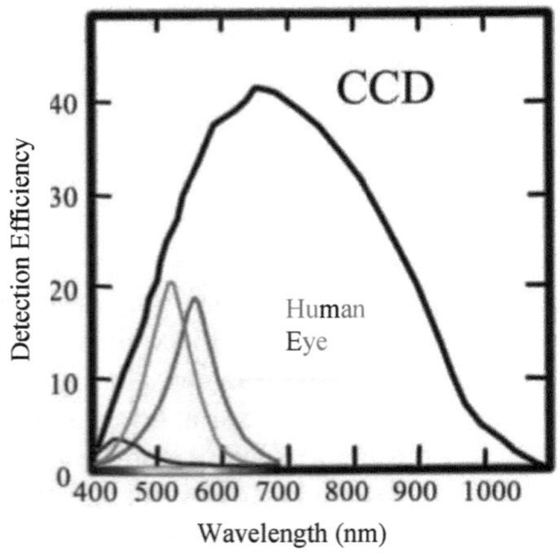

Fig. 1 The sensitivity spectrum of the human eye (efficiency of detection of light using the CCD compared to three types of cone cells (red, green, blue) and the components of the human eye)

IV. CCD and CMOS Sensors

CCD and CMOS image sensors can both be found in digital cameras. They are responsible for converting light into electronic signals. In the following sections, the differences between the two types of sensors and how they affect image quality will be discussed.

CMOS (Complementary Metal Oxide Semiconductor) are chips that use transistors at each pixel to move the charge through wires. This property provides flexibility because each pixel is treated individually, and the manufacturing processes used to create traditional CMOS sensors are similar to creating microchips. Because their production process is simple, CMOS are cheaper than CCD type sensors. Because CMOS technology followed CCD technology and is cheaper due to a more affordable manufacture process, CMOS sensors are the reason why the price of digital cameras fell. [9]

V. Hardware Configuration and IR Light Source

The hardware configuration has a significant importance for image acquisition. The camera used for this purpose must be sensitive to infrared light, and the IR light source to be strong enough to make the acquisition.

This prototype aimed to reduce or prevent discomfort caused by trying to properly access the vascular system for blood withdrawal or administration of various substances. Another goal would be to increase successful access in the first attempt because most often the first try is not successful, which requires a second or third attempt and often makes patients very uncomfortable.

This paper proposes enhancing the contrast of IR images of subcutaneous veins through optical means. While the main approach is similar to other practical studies, it differs in aspects of wavelength. This procedure produces a significant improvement in contrast and is harmless, effective and has a relatively low cost.

The system is based on transillumination. An NIR light source is placed over the area of interest, the image is captured by a camera specifically modified to be sensitive to IR, and then the image is displayed on a monitor.

A. Image Acquisition

The system consists of a compact low cost web camera with a CMOS sensor with a VGA (1280x960) resolution and adjustable focus. Prior to image acquisition, the webcam underwent some minor changes in which the filter was replaced by two layers of undeveloped film (35 mm). The film is used to block any source of visible light below 850 nm (Fig. 2, Fig. 3) (blocks most of visible light/allows NIR light to pass). The camera can be operated with one hand due to its small size.

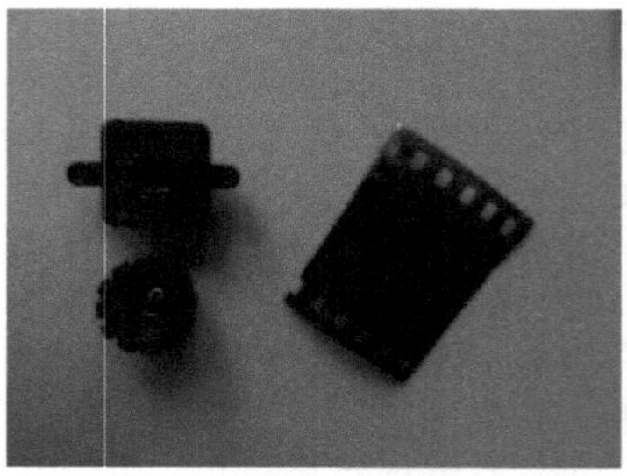

Fig. 2 The undeveloped film used to change the filter from the webcam

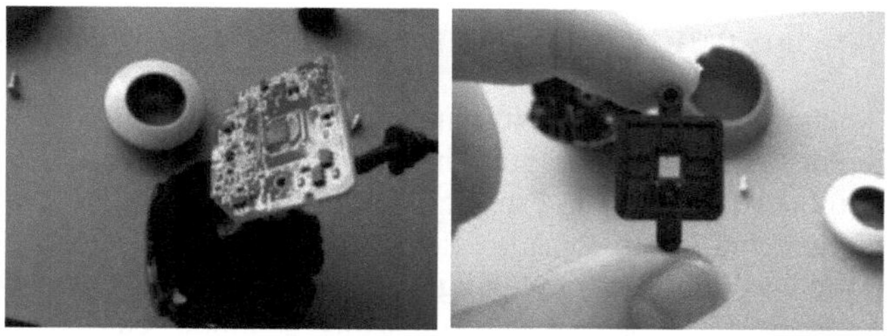

Fig. 3 Changing the optical filter with undeveloped film

B. DESIGN OF LIGHT SOURCE

Blood vessels, both venous and arterial, absorb IR and NIR light to a greater extent than the surrounding tissues. Therefore, when the body surface is illuminated, the tissue that is richest in blood will absorb more of this light, and other tissues will reflect this light. The analysis of this model allows veins to be visualized as localized reflections. [10]

To view the vein map using an IR sensitive camera, it is necessary to use an IR light source. This light will illuminate the area below the vascular system, and then it can be viewed on a monitor using the camera.

A strong light source was built using IR LEDs (OFL-5102). The characteristics of the light-emitting IR LEDs are described in Table 1 [11].

To create a light source powerful enough for detecting veins, 100 LEDs emitting IR light were chosen as the best solution after several tests.

Table 1 LED Characteristics

Characteristics	Values	Unit
Peak wavelength (λ)	940 nm	nm
Diode case style	5 mm	mm
No. of pins	2	
Operating temperature	- 25 - +85	°C
Reverse voltage	5	V
D.C forward current	50	mA
Medium wide emission angle	30	°
Chip material		AlGaAs

The best arrangement of the LEDs was determined to be a 10x10 matrix (Fig. 4), which can the area of interest where the vascular system map image acquisition will be performed. After positioning the LEDs, they were connected in a series of 20 LEDs. Additionally, they were linked to 5 resistors of 120 Ω each to prevent excessive current passing through the LEDs, which would ultimately require the LEDs to be replaced. To avoid overheating, the LEDs because they are placed directly on the circuit board, a second circuit board. This board was superimposed over the original board so the LEDs would have a greater distance between their base and the circuit itself.

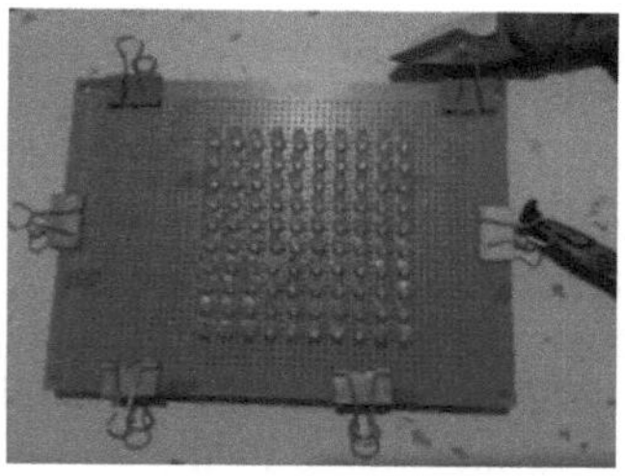

Fig. 4 Positioning the LEDs

An IR light emitting system was created, and it required a 32 V power supply.

Connecting the LEDs in a series was the best option because it was the most effective way to supply the LEDs from a constant current source. If they were connected in parallel, it might have led to problems of power distribution through each LED. Powering more LEDs that are connected in series also avoids uneven brightness due to variations in power supply. Thus, all LEDs have the same power to achieve the same level of brightness. The output voltage of the driver of LEDs will be equal to $Vout = VF\ x\ n$. So, for 5 LEDs, the voltage VF (rated operating voltage) equals 2 V when connected in a series, and the output voltage of the driver LEDs will be 10 V. Care should be taken to keep the limits of the input voltage nominal and not let them exceed output levels over the proper limit. When connecting LEDs in a series, the output current will be equal to: $Iout = IF$, where IF is the rated current of the LED, which is very important catalog data. [12]

Benefits of connecting LEDs in a series:

- Low Complexity of the Circuit
- Each LED will have the same current.
- High efficiency.

Disadvantages of connecting the LEDs in a series:

- The output voltage can become too large for LEDs connected in series.
- During the lifetime of the LEDs, the operation parameters can change unevenly, which leads to overcharging some LEDs and undercharging of others and causes a more rapid failure of the array of LEDs or uneven brightness.
- If an LED is faulty, it interrupts the brightness of the whole series. A shorted LED has little effect on the overall brightness of the circuit but can cause overvoltage in other LEDs from the series [12].

If an 8 V supply was used for the LED circuit, the production cost of this prototype would have increased considerably due to the limitation that the batteries provide. Although it would have created a more portable system, the lifetime of the supply provided by the 8 V batteries would have been much too short for the procedure that needed to be implemented. Therefore, a DC power source was used for the circuit power, and this source came from an old printer that could easily be connected to a normal 220 V outlet.

The input voltage of the source was 100-240 V, 50/60 Hz, it had a frequency as well as a current of 1300 mA, and the output characteristics of the voltage were 32 V, 325 mA.

Next-generation smart mobile phones have built-in a filter that enables visibility of the IR light in their photo camera. After connecting the source to the built circuit, it was powered from the outlet and tested with the camera of a mobile phone to check if its working properly. The result can be observed in (Fig. 5).

After mentioning the functionality of camera mobile phone in IR domain, a series of questions was raised, including the following: Why not chose to implement the prototype using a telephone that is within reach of anyone? Why was the prototype complicated with modification of the webcam? Initially, that was the plan: to design a system to show the venous map using a smart mobile phone camera.

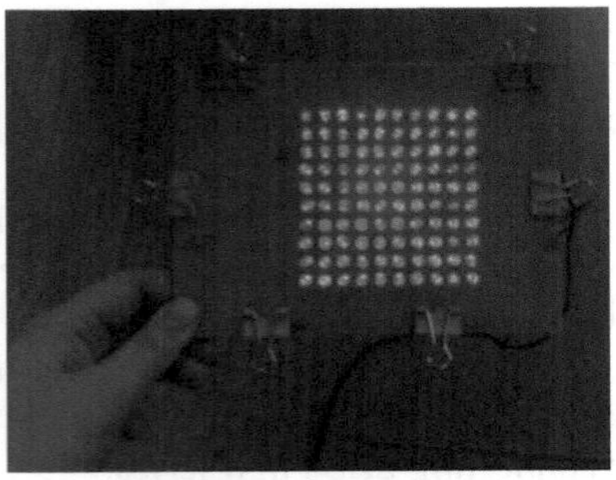

Fig. 5 Powering the IR light source

After the IR light source was functioning, acquisition of images was attempted with the mobile phone camera. As observed in (Fig. 6), other light sources can interfere with the IR light source, and positioning the source on the surface of the hand did not lead to any satisfying results.

On the hand, only a purple spot could be distinguished from IR LEDs without being able to see a high contrast image of the hand vascularization. The hand of the subject was isolated from any disruptive light source, and a new image was acquired. This time, the result was not satisfactory either because the camera on the phone does not distinguish between the hand of the subject and the environment, which made the captured image unintelligible.

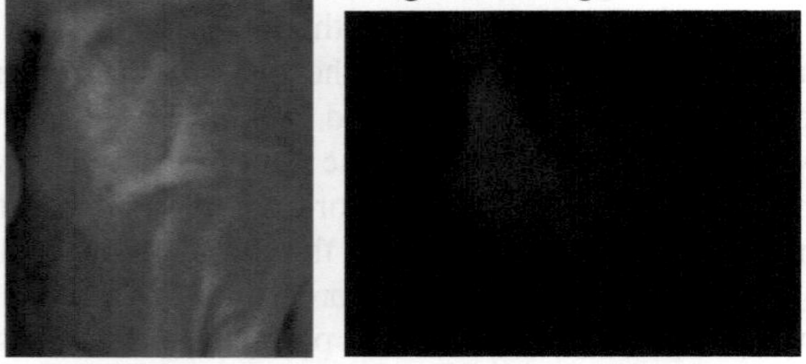

Fig. 6 Image acquisition with the mobile phone camera

VI. The Actual Implementation of the Prototype

The previous test, which included eliminating any interference of light, was a great help later on, when it was determined that the same principle could be applied to the implementation of the modified web camera. Therefore, a stand was built for both the light source and the IR sensitive webcam. The stand was made using a simple cardboard box.

On the sides of the box, a portion of approximately 8x12 cm was cut so that the subject could insert their hand. To ensure that the system was sufficiently contained and not penetrated by disturbing light sources, a dark colored fabric was used to minimize noise in the acquired images. (Fig. 7)

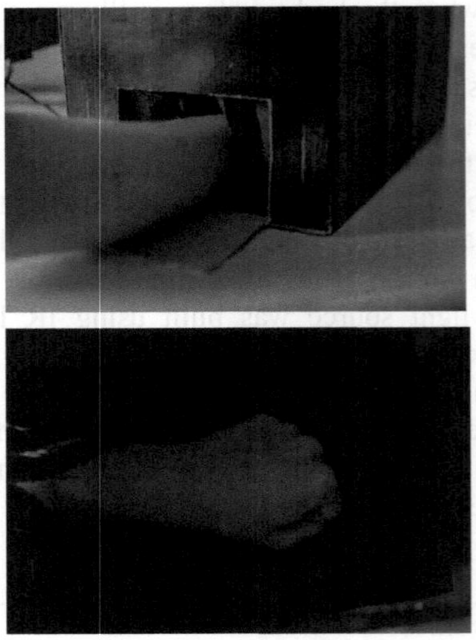

Fig. 7 View inside the acquisition environment

Parts of the box cover were cut for positioning the IR light source and the webcam. Once they were in place, acquisition of a new image without any disruptive sources of light was attempted, but another obstacle arose. Because the space was too small and the light too strong, the acquired images were completely burned, which were displayed as entirely white. After the study of several references and patents in this area, it was considered necessary to use a filter that could diffuse this light. To diffuse the light, 4 pieces of tracing paper were used, which is a translucent paper obtained by finely grinding pulp.

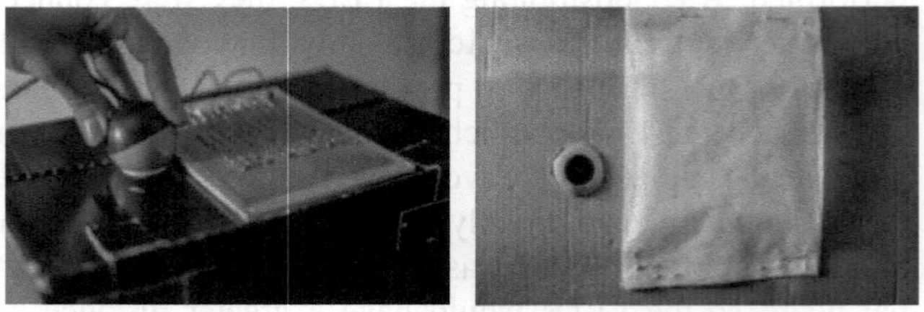

Fig. 8 Positioning of the light source and the camera for image acquisition

To enhance contrast and the quality of the acquired image, a black background was used (Fig. 8). Because blood vessels are visible as dark lines on the display, the black background helped to determine the differences between the surrounding tissue, the blood vessels and the initial background of the acquisition environment.

The hand of the subject was inserted into the box, and with the camera that was connected to a laptop to communicate with its associated software, the focus of the camera could be adjusted in real-time while positioning the hand to optimize the results. For better experimental results, it is recommended that hands be kept still during image acquisition. The thumb was placed inside the palm, and fingers are tightly held in a fist to apply pressure and increase the visibility of venous structures.

The images that were acquired by the webcam had a size of 1280x960 px. Using a photo editing program that required minimal knowledge of the photo-editing field, the image size was reduced to 25% of its original size. Then, the images from the tests had a dimension of 320x240 px. This minimum image-processing operation increased the contrast and visibility of veins.

All of these adjustments were conducted during a series of tests on subjects of various ages, weights and skin pigments. (Fig. 9, Fig. 10)

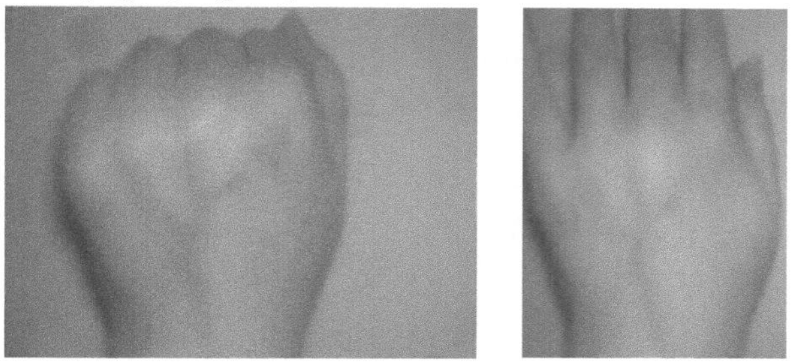

Fig. 9 Image acquisition of a 23 year-old overweight female subject

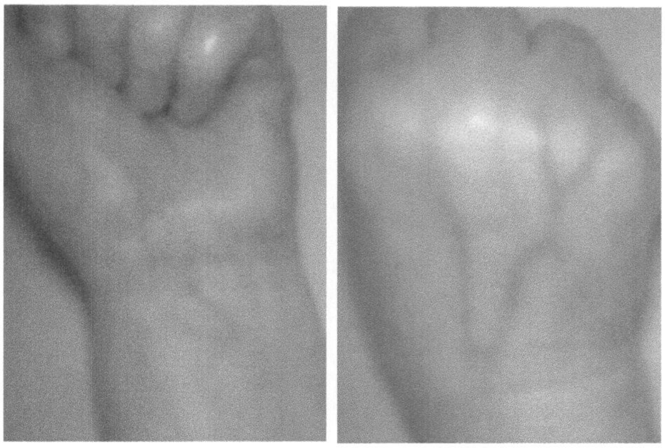

Fig. 10 Image acquisition of a 62 year-old, darker-skinned female (acquisition was made on the wrist and hand)

VII. Conclusions

At one point in our lives, every individual must go to a medical center to undergo some tests, routine tests or check-ups after some medical intervention.

The best way for a physician to assess the health of a patient or the development of pathological conditions is through analysis of blood.

Gaining access to the blood vessels can be difficult, especially in children. Viewing a real time map of the subcutaneous blood vessels may be a solution.

To advance the solution for this frequently encountered problem in the medical field, this study provides another step towards extensive field research using the infrared light spectrum.

A compact prototype with a strong light source in infrared (IR) wavelength was constructed, and the IR source is formed by 100 IR LEDs connected in series and a commercial web camera was used for image acquisition. The importance of the webcam in implementing this prototype was determined by the modifications that were made to enhance the sensitivity of the camera to infrared light.

Using this prototype in healthcare can increase the percentage of successful attempts to access the vascular system. Failure of such interventions could lead to a great deal of patient discomfort, especially for children.

Future work should focus on finding new applications for this prototype or attempt 3D remodeling of vascularity to implement this system, which is a more affordable approach to Doppler Ultrasound.

Conflict of Interest

The authors declare that they have no conflicts of interest.

References

1. R. Munteanu jr., C. Mureşan, D. Iudean, M. Munteanu, B. Amza "*Didactic Application for Monitoring Biomedical Parameters and Data Transfer Over the Network Using Virtual Instrumentation*", IFMBE Conference, MediTech 2014, Advancements of Medicine and Health Care Through Technology, June 5-7, 2014, Cluj-Napoca, Romania, Proceedings 44, pg.87-92, DOI: 10.1007/978-3-319-07653-9_18, Springer International Publishing Switzerland 2014, ISSN 1680-0737 ISSN 1433-9277 (electronic), ISBN 978-3-319-07652-2 ISBN 978-3-319-07653-9 (eBook), DOI 10.1007/978-3-319-07653-9, Springer Cham Heidelberg New York
2. D. Iudean, R. Munteanu jr., P. Bechet, C. Muresan, A. Creţu „Reliability Indicators and a Failure Mode and Effect Analysis Calculation for a Holter Recorder", IFMBE Conference, MediTech 2014, Advancements of Medicine and Health Care Through Technology, June 5-7, 2014, Cluj-Napoca, Romania,

Proceedings 44, pg.113-118, DOI: 10.1007/978-3-319-07653-9_23, Springer International Publishing Switzerland 2014, ISSN 1680-0737 ISSN 1433-9277 (electronic), ISBN 978-3-319-07652-2 ISBN 978-3-319-07653-9 (eBook), DOI 10.1007/978-3-319-07653-9, Springer Cham Heidelberg New York Dordrecht London, Library of Congress Control Number: 2014939994
3. Dan Iudean, Radu Munteanu jr., Florentina-Ancuta Cadar, Petru-Marius Maier, Alexandru Bogdan Amza, "Reliability calculus for an experimental device performing quantitative analysis of alcohol vapors from exhaled air", The 5th IEEE International Conference on E-Health and Bioengineering - EHB 2015, Grigore T. Popa University of Medicine and Pharmacy, Iaşi, Romania, November 19-21, 2015, ISBN 978-1-4673-7545-0/15/$31.00 ©2015 IEEE
4. Contrast enhancement of mid and far infrared images of subcutaneous veins Carlos Villasen˜or-Mora a, Francisco J. Sanchez-Marin a,*, Maria E. Garay-Sevilla
5. Godik, E. E. and Gulyaev, Y. V. (1991) Functional imaging of the human body. IEEE Engineering in Medicine and Biology Magazine 10, 21-29
6. Lin, C.-L. and Fan, K.-C. (2004) Biometric Verification Using Thermal Images of Palm-Dorsa Vein Patterns. IEEE Transactions on ciruits and systems for video technology 14, 199 – 213
7. Willmore, M. R. (1994) Infra-red imaging and pattern recognition system. United States USPatent #5351303
8. Treiman,A.(2005):http://www.lpi.usra.edu/education/fieldtrips/2005/activities/ir_spectrum/ Life at the Limits: Earth, Mars, and Beyond "Seeing" Infrared Light
9. http://www.adelaida.ro/led-emitator-infrarosu-940 nm-100 ma-890 nm-160 mw-vishay-clone.html
10. Feature extraction of finger-vein patterns based on repeated line tracking and its application to personal identification Naoto Miura, Akio Nagasaka , Takafumi Miyatake, Machine Vision and Applications, October 2004, Volume 15, Issue 4, pp 194–203
11. http://www.steves-digicams.com/knowledge-center/how-tos/digital-camera-operation/ccd-vs-cmos-whats-the-difference.html#b
12. http://www.tehniumazi.ro/page/articole_articles/_/articles/notiuni-teoretice-din-electronica/led-uri-si-montaje-cu-led-uri-r39

Author: Dan IUDEAN
Institute: Technical University of Cluj-Napoca
Street: 26-28, George Baritiu
City: Cluj-Napoca
Country: Romania
Email: dan.iudean@ethm.utcluj.ro

Modular Multi-channel Real-time Bio-signal Acquisition System

C. Kast[1,3], M. Krenn[1,2], W. Aramphianlert[1,3], C. Hofer[3,4], O.C. Aszmann[3] and W. Mayr[1,3]

[1]Center for Medical Physics and Biomedical Engineering, Medical University of Vienna, Vienna, Austria
[2]Institute of Electrodynamics, Microwave and Circuit Engineering, Vienna University of Technology, Vienna, Austria
[3]Christian Doppler Laboratory for Restoration of Extremity Function, Division of Plastic and Reconstructive Surgery, Department of Surgery, Medical University of Vienna, Vienna, Austria
[4]Otto Bock Healthcare Products GmbH, Vienna, Austria

Abstract— **Here, we present a multi-channel data acquisition system designed to record bio-electrical signals. The hardware concept is modular and consists of front-end acquisition modules and a synchronization module. The raw data streams are analyzed and stored on a personal computer or a single-board computer, which enables complex decisions and control algorithms even in real-time applications.**

The system is capable of combining up to eight front-end acquisition modules, each using a separated universal serial bus data-link to the computer. Therefore, it is important to ensure a reliable synchronization of all acquired signals. Hence, the modules are synchronized by an external clock module, which provides the time-base for the microcontrollers and generates repetitive trigger pulses. The developed system ensures a synchronization error smaller than 10 µs which meets the requirements for real-time analysis of movements. The analog front-end circuit is based on the high integrated chip ADS1299 (Texas Instruments Inc., Dallas, TX, USA), which incorporates analog filters and simultaneous digitalization of eight bipolar channels. The hardware is designed to suit transcutaneous recording of bio-electrical signals, like electromyogram, electrocardiogram, and electroencephalogram. Nevertheless, the device is also capable of acquiring sensor and other bioelectrical signals.

The advantage of the system is a flexible design which supports real-time recordings up to 64 bipolar channels. The modular design reduces the front-end complexity and enables simple integration in complex acquisition systems.

Keywords— **electromyography, bio-electric signal, analog front-end circuit, bio-signal amplifier, ADS1299**

I. Introduction

In biomedical applications, EMG recordings are widely used [1] and there are different concepts for data acquisition systems for EMG signal detection [2], [3]. However, most of them do not offer the possibility to record as much as 64 channels or lack synchronization.

One main benefit of multiple channels, EMG electrode arrays and multi-channel data acquisition systems is that it can replace the need of invasive needle electrode techniques and calculate single motor unit activities from multiple projections in certain cases [4]. Another useful application is the use of array based multi-channel EMG recordings to identify optimal electrode positions without multiple repositioning of skin attached electrodes by applying quantitative selection algorithms [5].

Our hardware design is based on an eight-channel recording module and a synchronization module. The system is capable of combining up to eight acquisition modules via universal serial bus (USB) data link. In addition to EMG measurements, the device is capable of recording various sensor or bio-electrical signals like electroencephalogram (EEG) or electrooculogram (EOG). A computer processes the input data and offers data management like filtering, storage or visual feedback.

Finally, the system should be comfortably wearable. Therefore, it has to be lightweight, compact, and battery-powered. For real-time signal analysis, the system requires high computing capacity which will be solved by integrating a compact single-board computer.

II. Implementation of the System

We designed a modular system for data acquisition (DAQ) which integrates recordings of multiple EMG devices. The recorded data should be processed using customized algorithms.

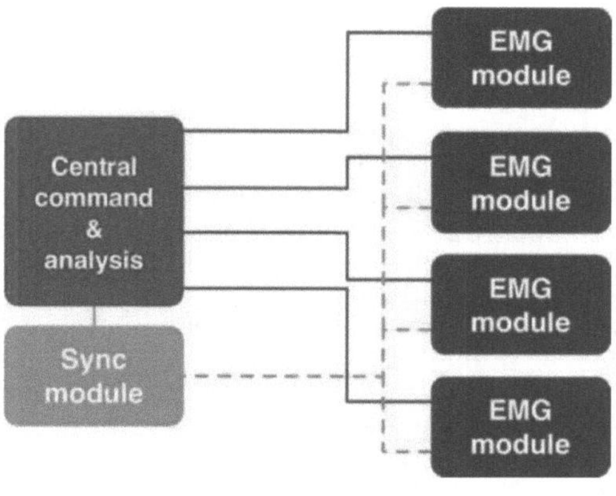

Fig. 1 This system configuration contains four recording units for electromyography (EMG module). These units are synchronized with a separate module (Sync module). A personal computer (PC) or a Raspberry Pi 3 analyzes and manages the input data.

S. Vlad and N.M. Roman (eds.), *International Conference on Advancements of Medicine and Health Care through Technology; 12th - 15th October 2016, Cluj-Napoca, Romania,*
IFMBE Proceedings 59,
DOI: 10.1007/978-3-319-52875-5_21

The modules are interconnected with the USB-interface that allows simple plug and play solutions. Reliable synchronization of all acquired signals is necessary for precise data analysis. The main drawback of comparable commercial devices is the limited access to the raw data.

The designed system consists of one or more EMG modules that are connected to the participant via surface electrodes to acquire the input control signals. The USB port powers the modules and transmits the measured data to a personal computer (PC) or a single-board computer (Raspberry Pi 3, Raspberry Pi Foundation, Caldecote, United Kingdom). The synchronization module is also directly connected to the computer, to set up the clock rate and trigger outputs. Additionally, the computer provides the power supply for the module.

III. Hardware Design

The EMG module (Fig. 2, Fig. 3) is based on an ADS1299 analog-to-digital converter (Texas Instruments Inc., Dallas, TX, USA) and is applicable for various electrical biosignals. The ADS1299 is capable of simultaneous sampling of eight channels with an overall sampling rate of 16 000 samples per second (SPS) and a resolution of 24-bits. The amplifier gain is programmable up to 24. The microcontroller (PIC32MX250F128D, Microchip Technology Inc., Chandler AZ, USA) is used for controlling the data stream. The clock frequency is up to 50 MHz, which allows a high recording rate. The integrated 64 KB memory is used to buffer the data which is received from the ADS1299. The microcontroller provides a USB 2.0 compliant full speed interface.

Because of the fact, that the device will be used in medical applications an electrical isolation barrier is mandatory. An ADuM4160 (Analog Devices Inc., Norwood MA, USA), which is suitable for this purpose, is implemented and offers 5 kV isolation.

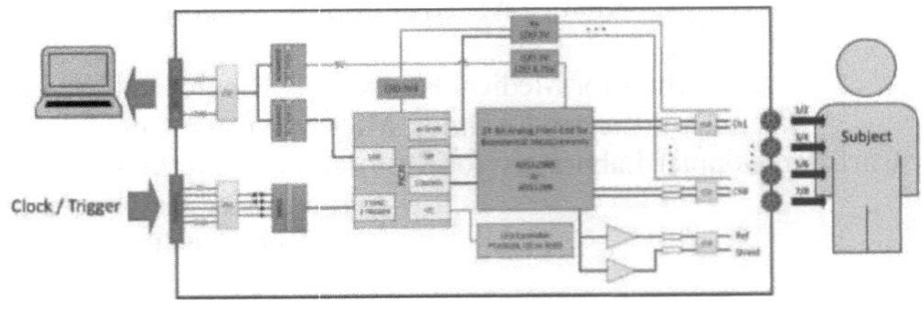

Fig. 3 Schematic representation of the EMG module.

The EMG module can be used as a standalone device with eight bipolar recording channels or integrated in a cascaded system of multiple modules interconnected by an additional USB cable for receiving clock trigger impulses from the synchronization module.

To synchronize data from up to 64 inputs, another USB module was developed that acts as a clock distributor, which provides the time base for the microcontrollers and delivers trigger signals to reset the timestamp of the data packets. The developed system ensures a synchronization error smaller than 10 μs within 10 s for simultaneous signal recording. A microcontroller generates a reliable clock source that is distributed to up to eight different modules. The low-voltage differential signaling (LVDS) standard was used to distribute the high frequency clock signal to all peripheral modules.

The central element of the system is a computer (PC or Raspberry Pi 3), which is used to process the data and, in the case of the Raspberry Pi 3, makes the system portable.

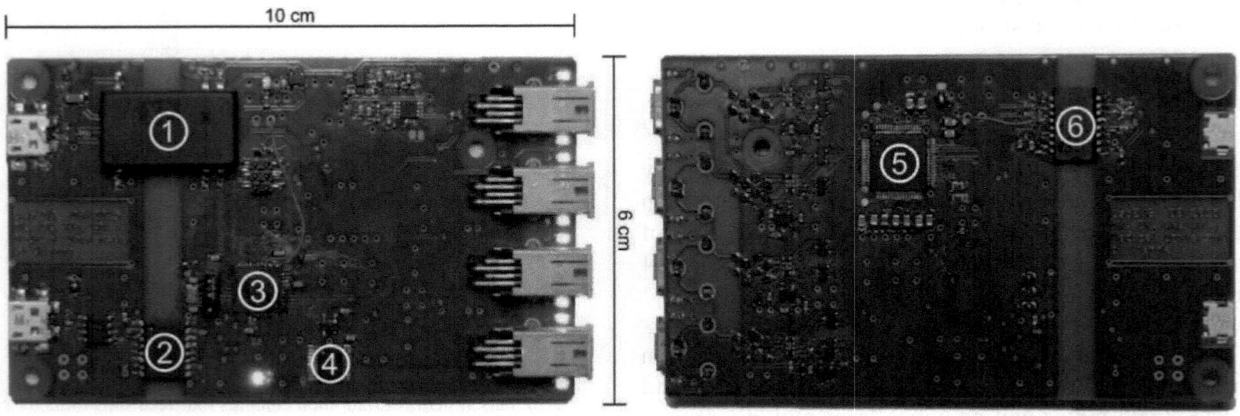

Fig. 2 Eight channel EMG module (usbEMG). 1 – isolated DC/DC converter; 2 – digital isolator for clock and trigger signals; 3 –microcontroller (PIC32MX250F128D); 4 – LED driver; 5 – analog frontend (ADS1299); 6 – USB port isolator.

IV. Firmware

The firmware of the PIC32MX-microcontroller is programmed with MPLABX an IDE (Microchip Technology Inc.) which includes an assembler, software simulator, and a debugger. The MPLAB Harmony Integrated Software Framework (Microchip Technology Inc.) offers a flexible, abstracted, fully integrated firmware development platform for PIC32 microcontrollers.

The communication between ADS1299 and the microcontroller is realized via serial peripheral interface (SPI). It offers data rates up to 25 Mbps. To ensure fast and safe data transfer the direct memory access (DMA) module is used to reduce CPU workload.

Using all eight channels and having a sampling rate of 8 kSPS the ADS1299 is producing 216 kB/s, which is within the USB bulk transfer limit of about 1245 kB/s.

It is not possible to transfer the data in real time via USB, therefore, a buffer is needed. Ideally, this is realized with a ring buffer, to ensure data consistency. The ADS1299 writes data in blocks of 27 Bytes but the USB is reading 64 Bytes at once. Therefore, the smallest possible ring buffer size is the least common multiple which is in that case 1728 Bytes. To get the best results, the ring buffer was chosen to be as big as possible. The PIC32MX offers 64 kB RAM, with the space occupied by the program itself, the resulting ring buffer size is around 55 kBytes.

V. Software

A C# program was developed to process the data packets. It allows digital filtering and visualizes the recorded signals per channel. The software detects all connected modules and offers the possibility to trace every channel per device. It is also possible to set the configuration of each module, i.e. sampling rate, gain, and other registers of the ADS1299. Furthermore, the data can be recorded and saved in the common Hierarchical Data Format (HDF5), which is particularly useful for managing large amounts of data. It is supported by many commercial and non-commercial software platforms including C#, Java, MATLAB. Data compression is necessary because of a large amount of data. Eight channels sampled with 8 kSPS generate about 13 MB data per minute. Using eight modules, this would produce more than 100 MB per minute. So structured data and especially compression are essential.

VI. Evaluation of the System

A. EMG during voluntary motor task

In a preliminary evaluation, we recorded an input signal of the biceps brachii in a human subject. Figure 4 shows the myoelectric signal during a contraction of the biceps brachii muscles, software filtered in a range from 20 to 300 Hz.

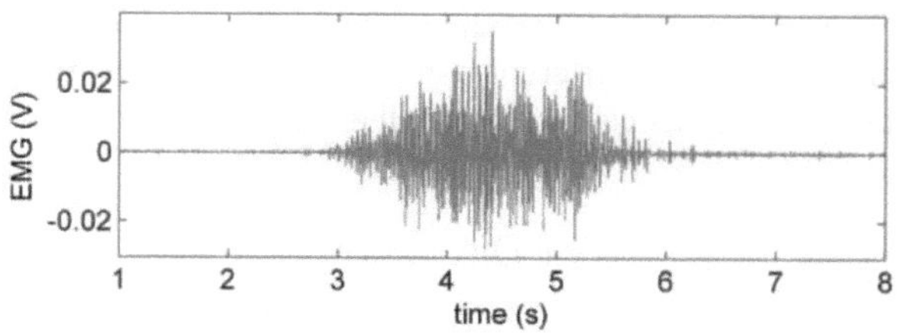

Fig. 4 Exemplary control input based on a myoelectric signal during a biceps brachii contraction. The EMG signal is filtered in a range from 20 to 300 Hz. Sampling rate: 8 kSPS; Gain: 6; Resolution 24-bit

B. Evoked myoelectric signal

Short Methods: Surface stimulation of quadriceps, bipolar stimulation, large electrodes (8x13cm), electrodes 5-10 cm apart. EMG sensor electrodes centrally to the stimulation electrodes.

Results: Figure 5 shows five superimposed responses at different stimulation intensities. At time zero stimulation artifact. CMAP is 3 ms after stimulation.

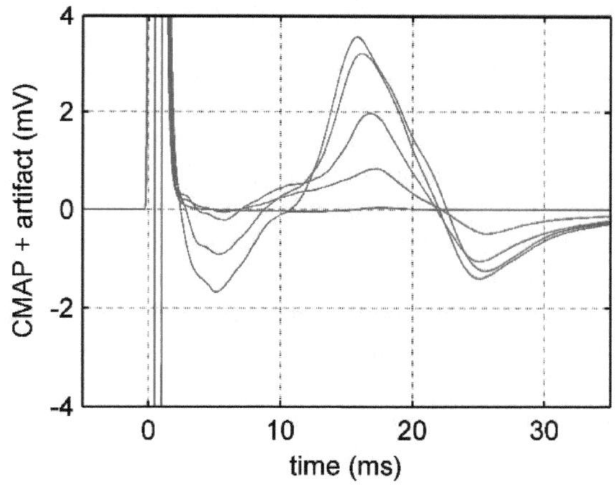

Fig. 5 Compound muscle action potential (CMAP) at different biphasic stimulation amplitudes (±10V, ±15V, ±20V, ±25V and ±30V), pulse width: 2x500µs. Sampling rate: 8 kSPS, gain: 12; Adapted from [6]

Healthy subjects received electrical stimulation of the anterior thigh muscle group. Single biphasic, charge balanced stimulation impulses with a width of 2x500 µs were used to evoke muscle twitch and related M-wave response. The evoked myoelectric signal was measured at the rectus femoris with EMG electrodes. Those electrodes were placed between the stimulation electrodes, transversally oriented in respect to the stimulation electrodes and the fiber orientation of the rectus femoris muscle to minimize stimulation artifacts [6].

The presented EMG module is not only capable of measuring M-waves at different stimulation amplitudes, but also evoked potentials caused by small activation levels.

VII. Discussion

The advantage of the system is a flexible design which supports real-time recordings of up to 64 channels. The modules are compact enough to be carried e.g. on a belt as a light weight and small experimental recording unit. We intend to use the system wirelessly, so power consumption is essential. The estimated supply current of the acquisition system is below 1 A. Because we use the USB standard for all our devices, it is possible to use commercially available powerbanks. By using only one core of the Raspberry Pi 3 the power consumption halves [7].

Due to the high resolution of the ADS1299 it is possible to abstain from high-pass filters. This again results in a beneficial design for measuring evoked potentials.

Additionally, the signals measured with the EMG module can be used as control inputs for a custom-built prosthesis prototype, developed at the Center for Medical Physics and Biomedical Engineering, Medical University of Vienna. By calculating the envelope of the EMG signal, the muscle activity intensity can be measured. One of the most widely used methods is the root mean square (RMS) [8]. Using this envelope signal, it is not only possible to calculate an on/off signal, but also to control the speed of the actuators based on the intensity of the muscle contraction.

The presented front-end device, ADS1299, is a versatile component for EMG acquisition. The small size of the chip, the low supply voltage, and low power consumption make it especially suitable for small, battery-powered, portable solutions.

Acknowledgment

Collaboration with the Christian Doppler Laboratory for Bionic Reconstruction sponsored by the Christian Doppler Gesellschaft, Austria.

Conflict of Interest

The authors declare that they have no conflict of interest.

References

1. M. B. I. Reaz, M. S. Hussain, and F. Mohd-Yasin, "Techniques of EMG signal analysis: detection, processing, classification and applications.," Biol. Proced. Online, vol. 8, no. 1, p. 163, 2006.
2. S. Boukhenous, N. Meziane, M. Attari, and Y. Remram, "A USB based data acquisition system for EMG signal recording," 2013 8th Int. Work. Syst. Signal Process. Their Appl. WoSSPA 2013, pp. 230–232, 2013.
3. A. Ruvalcaba, A. Altamirano, C. Toledo, R. Muñoz, A. Vera, and L. Leija, "Multichannel EMG acquisition system for arm and forearm signal detection," Conf. Rec. - IEEE Instrum. Meas. Technol. Conf., pp. 1075–1078, 2014.
4. B. U. Kleine, J. H. Blok, R. Oostenveld, P. Praamstra, and D. F. Stegeman, "Magnetic stimulation-induced modulations of motor unit firings extracted from multi-channel surface EMG," Muscle and Nerve, vol. 23, no. 7, pp. 1005–1015, 2000.
5. D. Farina, P. Madeleine, T. Graven-Nielsen, R. Merletti, and L. Arendt-Nielsen, "Standardising surface electromyogram recordings for assessment of activity and fatigue in the human upper trapezius muscle," Eur. J. Appl. Physiol., vol. 86, no. 6, pp. 469–478, 2002.
6. M. Haller, M. Krenn, K. Lezak, W. Mayr, D. Rafolt, and M. Bijak, "High integrated analog front-end device for measurement of evoked myoelectric signals during electrical stimulation," in 16th Annual Conference of the International Functional Electrical Stimulation Society, 2011, p. 23.
7. S. Macdonald, "Raspberry Pi 3 - First Look," *Piratical Tales From Pimoroni*, 2016. .
8. M. Polisiero, P. Bifulco, A. Liccardo, M. Cesarelli, M. Romano, G. D. Gargiulo, A. L. McEwan, and M. D'Apuzzo, "Design and assessment of a low-cost, electromyographically controlled, prosthetic hand," Med. Devices Evid. Res., vol. 6, no. 1, pp. 97–104, 2013.

Author: Christoph Kast
Institute: Center for Medical Physics and Biomedical Engineering, Medical University of Vienna
Street: Währinger Gürtel 18-20
City: Vienna
Country: Austria
Email: christoph.kast@meduniwien.ac.at

An ECG Front-End Device based on ADS1298 Converter

C.M. Fort, A.M. Ciupe and S. Vlad

Technical University of Cluj-Napoca/Department of Electrotechnics and Measurements, Biomedical Engineering, Cluj-Napoca, Romania

Abstract— **In cardiac diseases, the real-time electrocardiogram (ECG) signal acquisition using portable devices is very important for the patient's survival. The aim of this paper is to presents our research regarding the design and the development of a bio-signal acquisition device based on the ADS1298 circuit which is miniaturized and capable of extracting a high quality ECG signal. At the beginning our study was made on an ADS1298 ECG-FE model from Texas Instruments. Later we design a new front-end module of small size and low power consumption. Due to its architecture the proposed device is versatile and it can be used for other bio-signals acquisition like electromyogram (EMG) or electroencephalogram (EEG) signals.**

Keywords— **ECG, ADS1298, Serial Peripheral Interface (SPI), bio-signal acquisition, delta-sigma converter**

I. Introduction

The electrocardiogram (ECG) is one of the most analyzed bio-signals in the world. This signal is a favorite among specialists because it can give information regarding heart related pathologies.

It is important to know that such an investigation is non-invasive, painless, without any undesirable effects, which means that the patient should not have anxiety or be reticent in any way to do this investigation.

There are no risks in using this investigation. The ECG is a very reliable test. The electrodes detect just the impulses from the heart. Through the body there is no electrical current caused by the device, so there is no risk of an electrical shock.

The ADS1298 is an analog-digital delta-sigma circuit, on 24 bits, with electromagnetic (EMI) protection, simultaneous sampling and that can function on multiple channels; it contains programmable amplifiers, internal reference and an oscillator [1] [2].

This circuit contains all the necessary characteristics necessary for medical applications (ECG and EEG). The communication with a microcontroller can be done with the help of the serial peripheral interface (SPI), and with a computer through the SPI/USB. It can be used in different reference configurations and differential inputs, like passive ground module or right leg drive (RLD) [1] [2].

The ADS1298 can be operated from unipolar or bipolar supplies. The capabilities used for decoupling can be assembled on the surface, with low cost ceramic capacitors, but in systems where the board is subjected to low or high frequencies, it is recommended to use non-ferroelectric capacitors.

Texas Instruments [3] has projected a testing module that can simulate and acquire the ECG signal on an interface that uses the ADS1298 circuit. The disadvantages of this module are its dimension and dependency of an AC external power supply.

The aim of this paper was to design and develop another device based on the ADS1298 circuit. The proposed solution finally derived to a miniaturized module capable of extracting a clean ECG signal from the patient. Due to the battery power supply, the developed system respects the conditions for a portable device.

II. Testing ADS1298 ECG-FE Device in ECG Signal Aquisition

We have used the module given by Texas Instruments [3] in order to make some experimental tests to verify the utility of this converter.

The ADS1298 circuit can be programmed with the help of the user graphical interface. The ECG data captured are later post-processed by using high-pass, low-pass and notch filters of 50/60 Hz.

The software delivered ensures complete control over the ADS1298ECG-FE board. By means of the user interface, the control registers can be programmed to evaluate the functioning options of the device. This interface contains the user menu, some control elements to obtain the signal and different tabs like "About", "ADS register", "Analysis" and "Save".

In vivo tests were made on three subjects (Fig. 1, Fig. 2 and Fig. 3), a 29 year old female, a 60 year old male and a 65 year old male.

In vitro test were made with an ECG simulator, with ten ECG waveforms. The ECG electrodes were fixed in the standard leads I, II and III (Einthoven), aVL, aVF, aVR (Goldberger) and chest leads V1-V6 (Wilson).

Some of the most common applications that this module can be configured for are: unipolar and bipolar supply operations, direct and alternative current inputs, 12-channel

S. Vlad and N.M. Roman (eds.), *International Conference on Advancements of Medicine and Health Care through Technology; 12th - 15th October 2016, Cluj-Napoca, Romania*,
IFMBE Proceedings 59,
DOI: 10.1007/978-3-319-52875-5_22

ECG, Right-Leg Drive(RLD) reference circuit, external voltage for Wilson configuration, etc. [4].

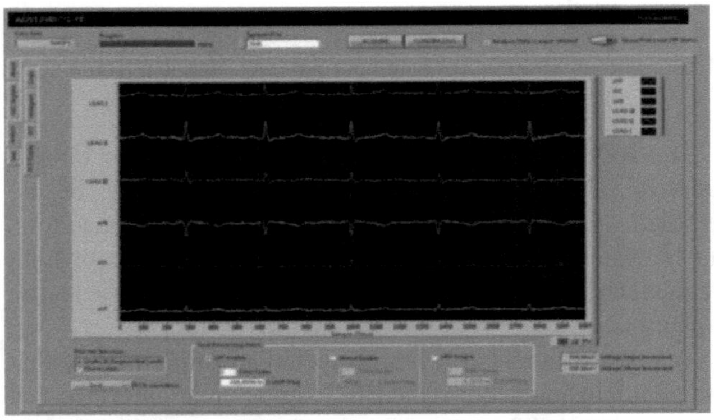

Fig. 1 Eindhoven and Golberger Leads of a normal ECG (29 year old woman)

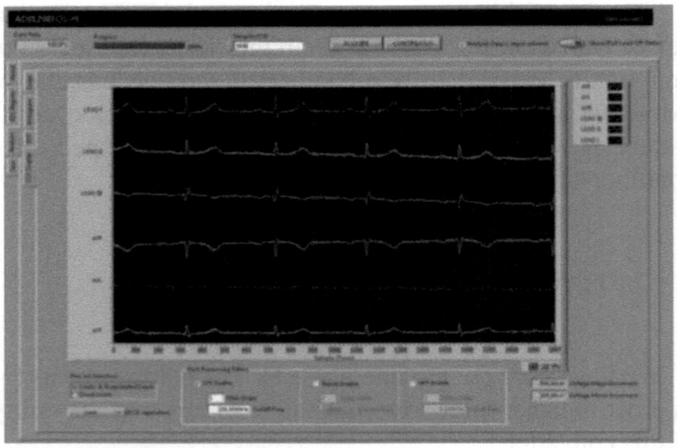

Fig. 2 Eindhoven and Golberger Leads of a normal ECG (60 years old male)

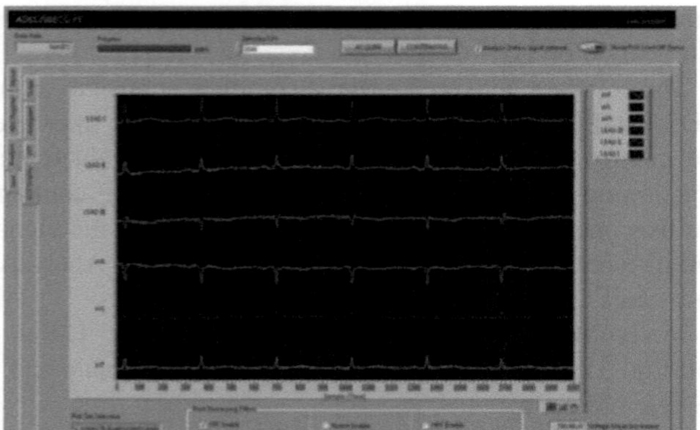

Fig. 3 Eindhoven and Goldberger Leads of a normal ECG (65 year old male)

There can be some disadvantages of using this module. Some of these are the impossibility to process data in real time, or to detect if the electrode is detached and there are no algorithms for the QRS detection [3].

III. Description of the Proposed Device

Because of the usefulness of the ADS1298EGG-FE platform, we have decided to design a reduced dimension ADS1298 based ECG signal sampling system.

This module was realized in order to test the integrated circuit ADS1298 (Fig. 4) and to obtain similar results with those from the ADS1298ECG-FE platform.

The communication between the ADS1298 circuit and the microcontroller can be done with the help of the Serial Peripheral Interface (SPI).

The ADS1298 converter ensures the input of the normal electrode, measurements for power supplies, RLD input, differential auxiliary inputs, lead-off signals or single-ended auxiliary inputs.

The settings of each channel can be changed through the CHnSET register and by writing the RLD MEAS bit in a separate configuration [3].

Three integrated amplifiers generate the Wilson Central Terminal (WCT) and Goldberger Central Terminal (GCT), which are necessary for a 12 LEAD ECG.

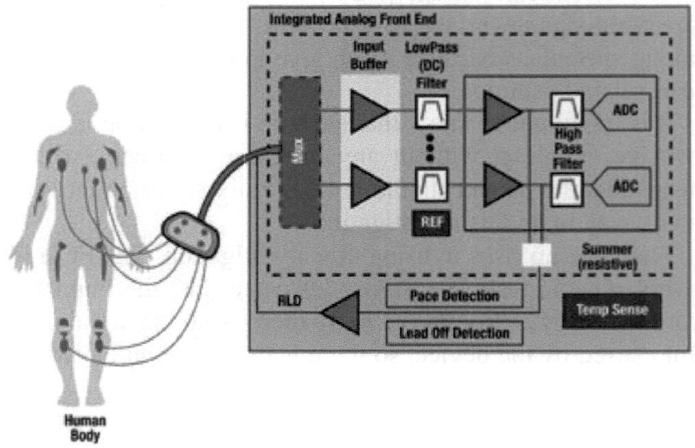

Fig. 4 Bloc diagram of the ADS1298 converter [1]

Common mode interference generated by the power source of an ECG system is reduced by the RLD circuit. [5]

The PACE circuit detection (Fig. 5) can be ensured in two ways: software or hardware.

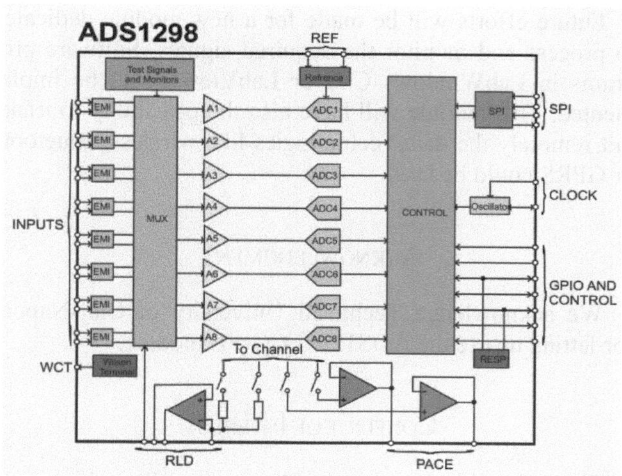

Fig. 5 Detailed structure of ADS1298 [1]

The device has to be supplied by sequential impulses. All digital and analog inputs have to be set at 0. After connecting the power supply, the Clock signal has to be supplied from the CLK pin.

The Analog-Digital Converters from the device offer data rate from 250SPS to 32 kSPS.

The proposed circuit of the ECG acquisition system using ADS1298 was designed in a CAD environment (Fig. 6, Fig. 7).

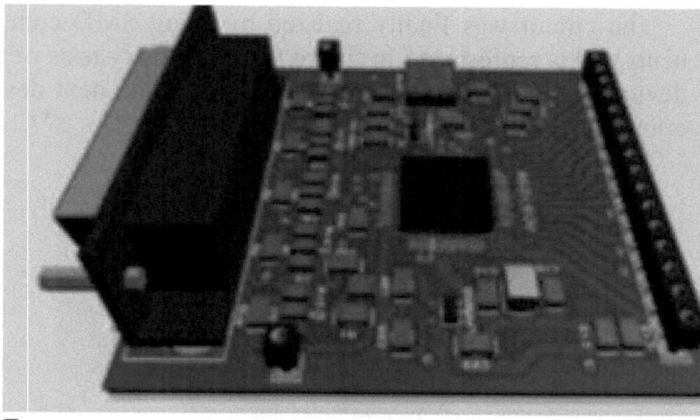

Fig. 7 3D visualization of the printed circuit that contains the ADS1298 circuit [2]

Figure 6 presents the electrical diagram of the acquisition system. The left side of the figure shows the electrodes interface connector and the low-pass signal filtering stage. The ADS1298 uses a 50MHz external oscillator (HC736) represented in figure 6 as OSC1. The lower-right part of the schematic shows the two voltage regulator circuits for the 3.3V analog side (U3) and 1.8V digital side (U2). The PCB design includes both an analog ground and digital ground.

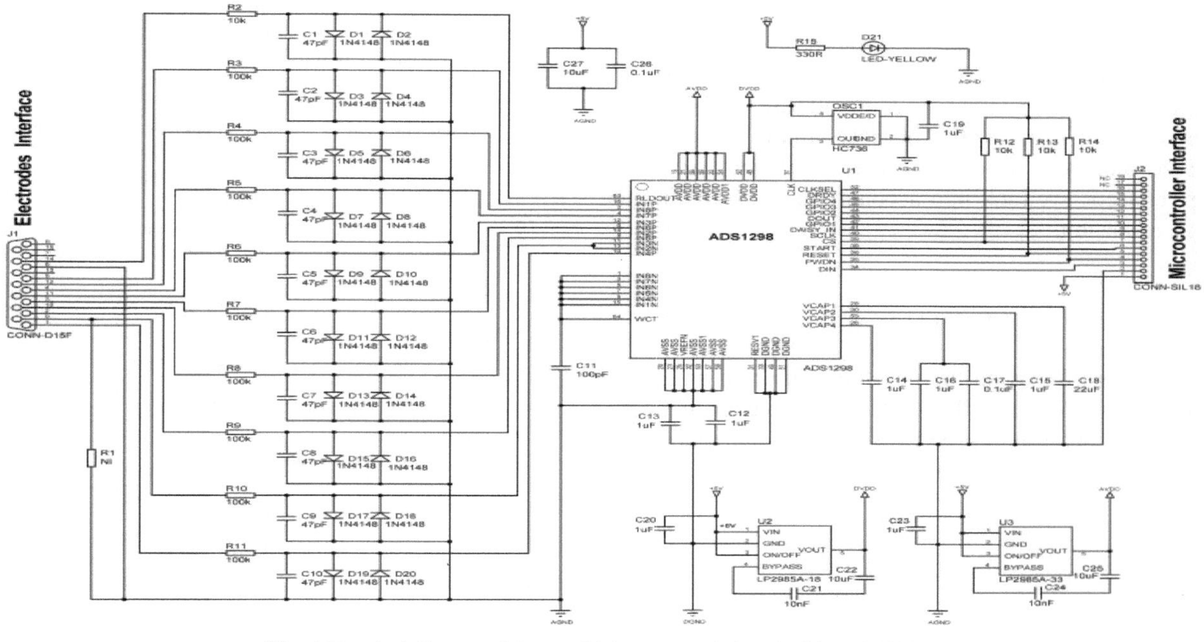

Fig. 6 Electrical diagram of the acquisition system designed with ADS1298

The circuit was finally realized by using SMD components and is represented in figure 8. The primary tests of the device indicated that it works properly and the next developing step can be done.

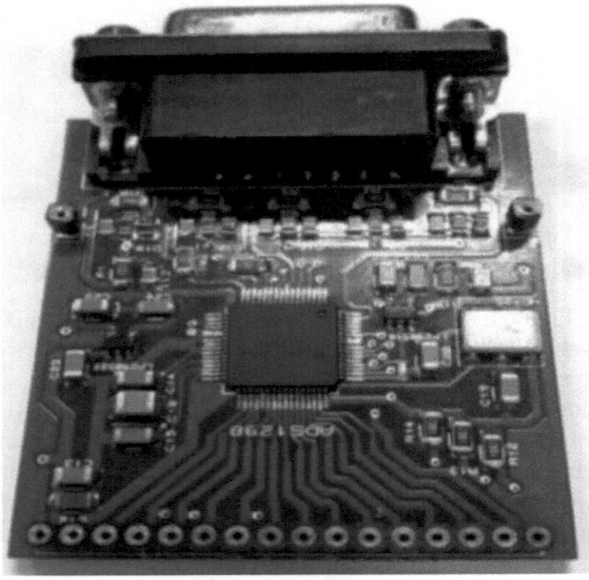

Fig. 8 Practical implementation of the proposed ECH front-end device

The ADS1298ECG-FE device was designed to graphically display the ECG signal on 12 channels. The monitor provided by Texas Instruments can display a virtual oscilloscope, histograms, Fast Fourier Transform (FFT) and a monitor for the ECG display. After post-processing, the ECG data can be printed [3]. Starting from this model, for the proposed device, areal-time monitoring user-interface can be implemented. For this purpose, a new microcontroller-based module can be attached to the main one. In the design concept, we took into account the pin configuration for this extension.

IV. CONCLUSIONS

This paper focuses on the development of an embedded medical device based on the ADS1298 converter that communicates on serial buses, SPI/USB. A miniaturized device (52.9 x 45.8 mm) was designed and realized.

Future efforts will be made for a new module dedicated to process and monitor the acquired signals. Software programs in LabWindows CVI or LabView could be implemented. This module will have also the possibility to transmit remotely the data.Technologies like wireless, Bluetooth or GPRS could be used.

ACKNOWLEDGMENT

We acknowledge Technical University of Cluj-Napoca for letting us use the ADS1298ECG-FE module.

CONFLICT OF INTEREST

The authors declare that they have no conflict of interest.

REFERENCES

1. Ciupe A.M., Roman N.M., " ECG DEVICE BASED ON ADS1298", Annals of the Academy of Romanian Scientists Series on Science and Technology of Information, Volume 8 Number 2, 2015, pp 29-36
2. Ciupe A., "Contribuţii privind realizarea unui sistem de monitorizare şi prelucrare virtuală a semnalului ECG", PhD Thesis, Technical University of Cluj-Napoca, 2016
3. Texas Instruments, „ADS1298ECG-EF – ECG Front-End Performance Demonstration Kit. User's Guide", Literature Number: SBAU171A, May 2010 - Revised January 2011, at www.ti.com
4. Texas Instruments "ADS129x Low-Power, 8-Channel, 24-Bit Analog Front-End for Biopotential Measurements" (datasheet) SBAS459K January 2010 Revised August 2015 at www.ti.com
5. V. Acharya, Improving Common-Mode Rejection Using the Right-Leg Drive Amplifier", Application Report, SBAA188 July2011, Texas Instruments
6. E. P. Vesa and B. Ilie "Equipment for SEMG Signal Acquisition and Processing", International Conference on Advancement of Medicine and Health Care through Technology Volume 44 5-7 June 2014, Cluj-Napoca, Romania
7. Matthew Hann, "Analog Fundamentals of the ECG Signal Chain", a Texas Instruments technical presentation, 2010

Author: Fort Ciprian Mugurel
Institute: Technical University of Cluj-Napoca
Street: 26-28 Baritiu street
City: Cluj-Napoca
Country: Romania
Email: fortciprian@yahoo.com

New Approach for the Electrochemical Detection of Dopamine

M. Tertiş[1], A. Florea[1], A. Adumitrachioaie[1], D. Bogdan[2], C. Cristea[1*] and R. Săndulescu[1]

[1]Analytical Chemistry Department, Faculty of Pharmacy, Iuliu Haţieganu University of Medicine and Pharmacy, 4 Louis Pasteur St., 400349 Cluj-Napoca, Romania
[2]National Institute for Research and Development of Isotopic and Molecular Technologies, 67-103 Donat St., 400293 Cluj-Napoca, Romania

Abstract **An innovative biomimetic electrochemical sensor was elaborated for the dopamine detection using a glassy carbon electrode modified with gold nanoparticles. The molecularly imprinted polymers and nonimprinted polymers were electrochemically generated on the electrode surface after the obtaining of the self-assembled monolayer of the functional monomer - *p*-aminothiophenol through sulfur-gold bonds with dopamine as template molecule (in the case of molecularly imprinted polymer). Cyclic voltammetry and electrochemical impedance spectroscopy were used for the characterization of the sensor considering its response in the presence of hexacy- anoferrate as redox probe, while the morphostructural characterization of the elaborated platform was realized by using atomic force microscopy. Differential pulse voltammetry ex- periments in saline phosphate buffer (0.02M; pH 7.4) were performed after the preconcentration of dopamine in order to test the biomimetic sensor performance.**

Keywords **dopamine, electrochemical sensors, molecularly imprinted polymers, gold nanoparticles**

I. Introduction

Dopamine (DA) is a neurotransmitter that belongs to the catecholamine family with crucial role in humans. It is also a precursor for other neurotransmitters - adrenaline and noradrenaline. Highly abundant in the central nervous system, DA plays an important role in brain circuitry, neuronal plasticity, memory and learning. DA deficiency in the central nervous system can be the cause of serious diseases such as Parkinson, Alzheimer, schizophrenia, epilepsy and ADHD [1].

Due to the physiopathological implications of DA, increasing attention has been recently focused on the determination of DA levels in biological fluids for biochemical and clinical diagnosis. The most commonly used methods are chemiluminescence [2], Rayleigh resonance scattering [3], capillary electrophoresis [4] and fluorimetry [5]. Due to its electroactivity, DA can be readily detected by electrochemical techniques. Several electrochemical sensors for the detection of DA have been recently reported, employing pencil-on-paper-based electrodes [6], calyx[4]arenes [7], polymer/gold nanoparticles (AuNPs) hybrid materials [8] and MIPs modified with graphene and carbon nanotube foam [9].

Molecular imprinting of polymers is a strikethrough technique used to incorporate specific recognition sites into the polymer and therefore to design different biomimetic receptors. The advantages of molecularly imprinted polymers (MIPs) made them an interesting tool for the development of chemical sensors and biosensors. Molecular recognition characteristics of these polymers are attributed to complementary size, shape, and binding sites imparted to the polymers by the template molecules. The fabrication technique is simple and cheap, consisting of polymerization of functional monomers and cross-linkers in the presence of the analyte of interest which serves as template molecule, followed by the removal of the template from the polymer matrix. The resulted cavities possess the ability to recognize and bind the target analyte with high selectivity.

The integration of nanomaterials with unique chemical and physical properties in MIPs can further improve their performance. Metal oxide nanoparticles such as AuNPs, quantum dots or graphene provide better accessibility of the analyte to the recognition sites, enhance sensitivity and improve the limits of detection [10].

The first step in the fabrication of the novel MIP/AuNPs sensor for the detection of DA consisted in the electrochemical deposition of AuNPs on glassy carbon electrodes (GCEs), followed by the functionalization of the gold surface with the monomer, *p*-aminothiophenol. A polymeric film was then electrochemically generated both in the presence (MIP) and absence (non-imprinted polymer, NIP) of the DA. All the modifications of the electrode surface were electrochemically characterized through cyclic voltammetry (CV), differential pulse voltammetry (DPV) and electrochemical impedance spectroscopy (EIS). The morphostructural description of the platform was achieved with atomic force microscopy (AFM).

The results serve as a starting point for the design of point-of-care devices for DA detection, which could significantly improve the quality of life for patients, suffering from neurodegenerative disorders caused by DA deficiency.

S. Vlad and N.M. Roman (eds.), *International Conference on Advancements of Medicine and Health Care through Technology; 12th - 15th October 2016, Cluj-Napoca, Romania*,
IFMBE Proceedings 59,
DOI: 10.1007/978-3-319-52875-5_23

II. Experimental Part

A. Reagents, apparatus and methods

All reagents and chemicals were of analytical grade and were used as received without further purification. Na_2HPO_4, NaH_2PO_4 and *p*-aminothiophenol were purchased from Merck, while H_2SO_4, $K_4[Fe(CN)_6]$), $K_3[Fe(CN)_6]$, NaCl, dopamine hydrochloride and $HAuCl_4$ were purchased from Sigma-Aldrich. All the solutions were prepared using Milli-Q grade water. The supporting electrolyte was 0.02 M phosphate buffer saline (PBS) prepared with Na_2HPO_4, NaH_2PO_4 and NaCl at pH 7.4. The electrochemical studies were performed with a conventional three-electrode system using Ag/AgCl(KCl 3M) reference electrode, a Pt/Ir counter electrode and a glassy carbon electrode from BASi (3 mm diameter). An Autolab PGSTAT 302N equipped with an electrochemical impedance spectroscopy module and controlled by Nova 1.10.4 software was used for electrochemical measurements. CV and EIS measurements were carried out in the presence of 10 mM $[Fe(CN)_6]^{3-/4-}$ in PBS (0.02 M, pH 7.4) as redox probe, while DPV tests were performed in PBS (0.02 M, pH 7.4) at room temperature. CV was employed for the electrochemical generation of AuNPs and for electrochemical polymerization. The EIS measurements were made by the open circuit potential mode, in a frequency range from 100 kHz to 0.100 Hz, in order to characterize the properties of the electrode surface by comparing the values of charge transfer resistance (R_{ct}) during all modification stages.

Open-circuit accumulation experiments were performed using DA solution followed by voltammetric detection after changing the medium to an analyte-free electrolyte solution (PBS 0.02 M; pH 7.4) by DPV, at a scan rate of 10 mV s^{-1}, a modulation amplitude of 50 mV and a modulation time of 0.04 s. The AFM experiments were performed by using a Multimode 8 platform from Bruker (USA), with ScanAsyst and controlled by Nanoscope 9 software in Peak Force Tapping mode, in air. Experiments were conducted by using a ScanAsyst-Air probe (Bruker) with a tip radius of < 12 nm in a silicon nitride cantilever of triangular geometry with a nominal resonance frequency of about 70 kHz and a nominal spring constant of 0.4 N/m.

B. Elaboration of molecularly imprinted sensor

For the elaboration of MIP sensor, the electrode surface was firstly cleaned by polishing with alumina of different particle size, washed with ethanol and distilled water and then cycled ten times between -0.5 and + 1.5 V in 0.5 M H_2SO_4 with a scan rate of 100 mV s^{-1}. After this, the electrode was rinsed with water and was modified with AuNPs electrochemically deposed from a 0.6 mM $HAuCl_4$ solution in 0.5 M H_2SO_4 cycling the potential between -0.2 and 1.2 V vs. Ag/AgCl(KCl 3M) for ten cycles (Figure 1A) [11].

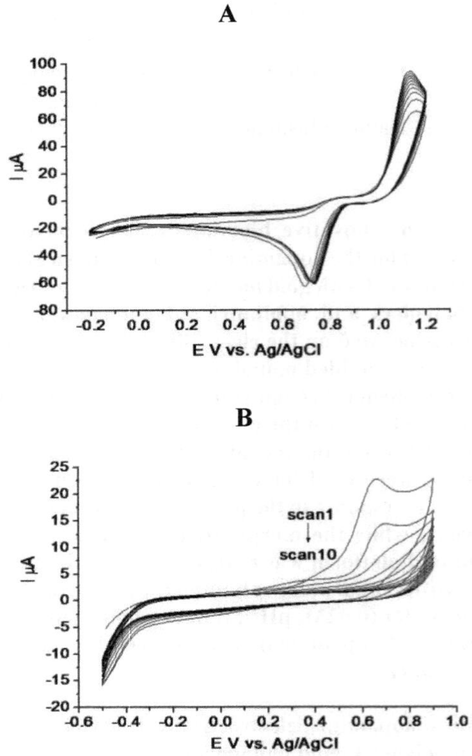

Fig. 1 CVs of the: (**A**) electrochemical deposition of AuNPs on GCE surface; (**B**) *p*-aminothiophenol based film electrochemical generation in the presence of DA

The electrode was soaked overnight in a 50 mM *p*-aminothiophenol solution in ethanol and left overnight at 4°C for the formation of S-Au bonds between the Au from the electrode surface and the -SH groups of the monomer. The electrochemical polymerization of *p*-aminothiophenol was then performed in the presence of DA (0.1 mg mL^{-1}) by cycling the potential between -0.5 and + 0.9 V vs. Ag/AgCl(KCl 3M) for ten cycles. CVs of the *p*-aminothiophenol polymerization in the presence of DA on AuNPs are presented in Figure 1B. DA molecules were removed by washing with PBS for 30 minutes under stirring (800 rpm). Similarly, a non-imprinted sensor was elaborated and tested, in the absence of template molecule.

III. Results and Disscusions

The electrochemical biomimetic sensor for DA detection was elaborated in several steps that are schematically depicted in Figure 2. After the rigorous cleaning of the electrode surface the first step consisted in the generation of AuNPs in order to ensure binding centers for polymer through S-Au bonding. The monomer molecules are then self-assembled and electrochemically polymerized in the presence of dopamine in hydro-alcoholic medium (ethanol:PBS, 1:1).

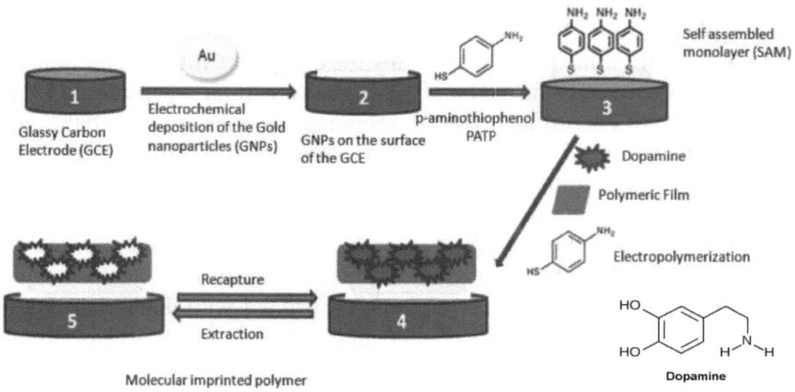

Fig. 2 Development steps of the electrochemical sensor

An irreversible oxidation peak can be observed in the first cycle at about 0.7 V and its intensity decreases during the next scans and completely disappears after four scans (Figure 1B), proving the formation of polymeric film. The intensity of the peak current continuously decreased with the number of cycles until it reached a steady state. The polymerization tests performed in the absence of DA did not revealed any difference regarding the presence or absence of peaks indicating that the co-polymerization of template molecules does not take place in the potential domain used for polymerization. Figure 3 presents the AFM topographic images obtained for GCEs modified with AuNPs before and after polymerization. The features on GCE surface indicate the presence of AuNPs with an average size of 50 nm (line profile not shown here). After polymerization, striking changes in surface morphology and features size are readily apparent. AFM height images clearly indicate that electrode surface is uniformly covered by polymer. Nanomechanical properties, including elastic modulus of the polymeric film and adhesion data, have been evaluated (data not shown here) and indicate a softer and more adhesive region between features (dark areas in topography image). The electrochemical characterization of the novel biomimetic sensor was carried out by using EIS and voltammetric techniques such as CV and DPV. EIS measurements were recorded in the presence of 5 mM $[Fe(CN)_6]^{3-/4-}$ in 0.1 M KCl solution. The electron transfer properties of the modified electrode were evaluated based on the Nyquist representation of EIS. This representation includes a semicircle and a straight line corresponding to the electron transfer and the diffusion limited processes, respectively (Figure 4).

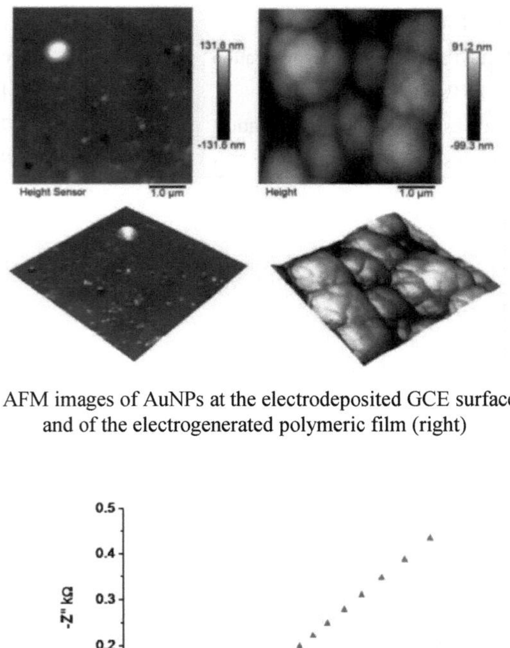

Fig. 3 AFM images of AuNPs at the electrodeposited GCE surface (left) and of the electrogenerated polymeric film (right)

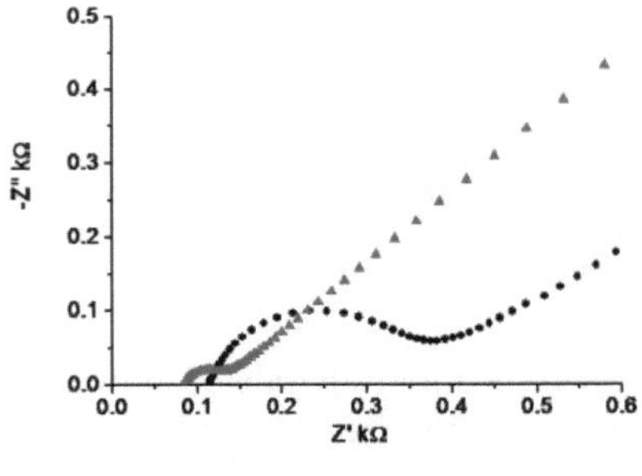

Fig. 4 Nyquist plots for bare GCE (black) and AuNPs modified GCE (red)

The variations in charge transfer resistance after each modification step is presented in Table 1 for both MIP and NIP sensors and compared with the values obtained for bare

GCE and AuNPs modified GCE. It can be seen that the R_{ct} is decreasing from 472.67 Ω to 11.79 Ω after the electrochemical generation of AuNPs onto GCE surface. The R_{ct} values increase after the polymerization process at 870.68 Ω in the case of NIP and at 1067.18 Ω for MIP film, due to the coating of the electrode surface with an isolating film. After the removal of the DA template from the MIP film the R_{ct} increased at 1249.06 Ω, probably due to the cavities formed in the polymeric film, while in the case of NIP a significant variation of this parameter was not observed (Table 1). The electrodes were also tested through DPV in PBS solution (0.02 M; pH 7.4). In the case of MIPs, after polymerization, the DA specific signal is detected through DPV tests at about +0.2 V, signal which disappears after extraction and reappears after immersion of the MIP in 0.1 mM DA solution for 30 minutes.

Table 1 The variation of R_{ct} for different electrode configurations

Electrode configuration	R_{ct} (Ω)
GCE	472.67
AuNPs/GCE	11.79
MIP/AuNPs/GCE after polymerization	1067.18
MIP/AuNPs/GCE after extraction	1249.06
NIP/AuNPs/GCE after polymerization	870.68
NIP/AuNPs/GCE after extraction	880.51

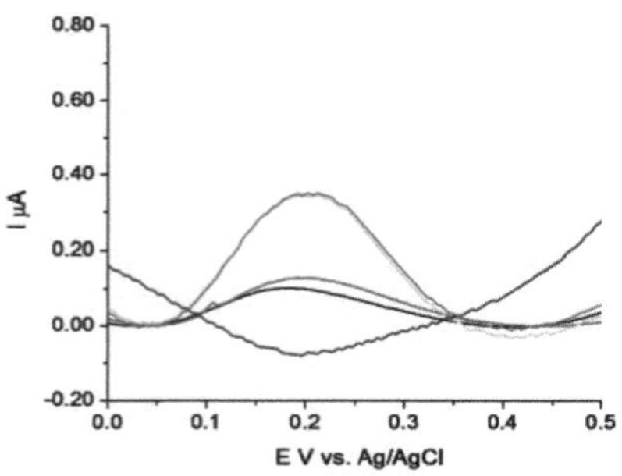

Fig. 5 DPVs for: NIP after polymerization (black); NIP after DA capture for 30 min in 0.1 mM solution (red); MIP after polymerization (green); MIP after dopamine extraction in PBS for 30 min (blue); MIP after DA capture for 30 min in 0.1 mM solution (brown)

The tests performed for NIP did not show a significant difference before and after the accumulation in DA solution (Figure 5), demonstrating that the DA signal obtained for MIP is the result of the template molecule inclusion into the polymeric film and not of the adsorption on the surface of the sensor.

IV. Conclusions

A novel biomimetic sensor based on AuNPs decorated MIP for the dopamine detection was elaborated. The protocol implies one-step polymerization of *p*-aminothiophenol in the presence of dopamine in a hydro-alcoholic solution, preceded by the electrochemical generation of gold nanoparticles onto the glassy carbon electrode and the self-assembling of the monomer monolayer through the S-Au bond. This strategy is very simple and versatile and can be adapted for a wide range of target molecules, from small ones to peptides, proteins and even cells. The polymeric films were successfully obtained both in the presence and absence of the template molecule, higher sensitivity and selectivity being obtained for the polymer imprinted with dopamine. Future prospects include the evaluation of the analytical performance of the sensor (limit of detection, reproducibility, the possibility of multiple use), and the dopamine detection from serum samples.

Acknowledgment

The authors are grateful for the financial support from the Romanian National Authority for Scientific Research UEFISCDI for project no. PN-II-RU-TE-2014-4-0460.

Conflict of Interest

The authors declare that they have no conflict of interest.

References

1. Jackowska K, Krysinski P. (2013) Anal Bioanal Chem. 405(11): 3753–3771.
2. Zhu Q, Chen Y, et al (2015) Sens Actuat B: Chem. 210: 500-50.
3. Dong JX, Wen W, Li NB, et al (2012) Spectrochim Acta A. 86:527-532.
4. Zhao Y, Zhao S, Huang J, et al (2011) Talanta. 99 : 897-903.
5. Wang HY, Sun Y, Tang B. (2002) Talanta. 57(5) :899-907.
6. Li W, Qian D, Li Y, et al (2016) J Electroanal Chem. 769:72-79.
7. Kurzatkowska K, Sayin S, Yilmaz M, et al (2015) Sens Actuat B: Chem. 218:111-121.
8. Khudaish EA, Al-Nofli F, Rather JA, et al (2016) J Electroanal Chem. 761:80-88
9. Li Y, Liu J, Liu M, et al (2016) Electrochem Comm. 64 :42-45
10. Justino CIL, Freitas AC, Duarte AC et al (2015) Trends Environ Anal Chem. 6 :21-30.
11. Florea A, Taleat Z, Cristea C et al (2013) Electrochem Commun. 33: 127-130.

Author: C. Cristea
Institute: Analytical Chemistry Department, Faculty of Pharmacy, Iuliu Haţieganu University of Medicine and Pharmacy
Street: 4 Louis Pasteur
City: Cluj-Napoca
Country: Romania
Email: ccristea@umfcluj.ro

Aptamer-based Electrochemical Sensor for the Detection of Ampicillin

B. Feier, I. Băjan, C. Cristea and R. Săndulescu

Department of Analytical Chemistry, Faculty of Pharmacy, Iuliu Hatieganu University of Medicine and Pharmacy, Cluj-Napoca, Romania

Abstract— **Antibiotics represent an important therapeutic class, but their overuse and erroneous use for humans, animals and agriculture have resulted in increased levels of exposure to sub-therapeutic concentrations of antibiotics, with an increased number of allergies and in the development and spread of antibiotic resistance, a major health problem for the modern world. For these reasons, World Health Organization recommends an urgent improvement in the surveillance of the use of antibiotics, hence the need for developing new analytical sensors, capable to detect selectively low concentrations of antibiotics from different matrices. This study focused on the detection of ampicillin, a β-lactam antibiotic, widely used, both for humans and as veterinary drug, due to its large spectrum of action.**

The purpose of this study was to develop an electrochemical sensor based on the use of an ampicillin-selective aptamer for the detection of ampicillin from environmental and pharmaceuticals samples. Two different strategies for the immobilization of the ampicillin-selective aptamer have been employed: by the grafting of a carboxyl containing diazonium salt by cathodic reduction on a glassy carbon electrode, followed by the chemical reaction with the aptamer containing an amino group and by incubating the aptamer containing a thiol group on a gold electrode, leading to a self-assembling layer of the aptamer. The modified electrodes have been characterized by electrochemical impedance spectroscopy.

The detection of ampicillin using the modified electrodes is a label-free method, using the variation in the impedance signals to quantify the ampicillin concentration.

Keywords — **ampicillin – aptamer – modified electrode – electrochemical impedance spectroscopy**

I. Introduction

Antibacterial drugs have revolutionized the treatment of infectious diseases, but their use and misuse have resulted in the development and spread of antibiotic resistance, a major health problem for the modern world, each year in the European Union alone, over 25 000 people dying from infections caused by antibiotic-resistant bacteria [1]. Another problem associated with the misuse of antibiotics is the spread of allergy reactions related to antibiotics intake, impairing the use of certain antibiotics for certain patients and threatening their health.

The WHO report from 2014 clearly states that resistance to common bacteria has reached alarming levels in many parts of the world. Thus, WHO strongly recommends an intensification of the prevention, including strengthening hygiene, infection prevention and control measures, improving sanitation and access to clean water [2].

Our environment becomes polluted with antibiotics and the runoff from farms and from our own sewers exposes more and more of the world bacteria to low concentrations of antibiotics, increasing the antibiotic resistance, which is a societal problem, deriving from the way we use antibiotics, involving different problems: antibiotic overuse, infection control, surveillance for resistance, antibiotic use in animals and crops, environmental contamination with antibiotics. The statistics show a significant increase in resistant staph, enterococci and *Pseudomonas aeruginosa* over the last 30 years in US hospital intensive care units [3].

The 2015 report of the European medicines agency (EMA) about the consumption of antibiotics for veterinary use showed that penicillins are one of the most employed classes of antibiotics [4].

The most used conventional methods for the detection of antibiotics are instrumental ones [5], such as capillary electrophoresis [6,7], gas chromatography [8,9] and liquid chromatography [10,11] coupled with mass spectrometry [12]. However, these methods are expensive and present limitations, like the need for expensive laboratory instruments, which require skilled technicians, time consuming separation/clean-up methodologies, long analysis time, extensive sample handling with multiple washing steps, use of expensive and pollutant solvents and the impossibility to perform field analyses, making necessary the development of new sensors to overcome these limitations [13]. Electrochemistry based methods appear as an interesting and low-cost alternative for antibiotics detection. Electrochemical sensors are fast and could be easily miniaturized to achieve portable sensors.

Aptamers consist of single stranded-DNA and RNA short chains and they are capable to bind specifically different types of molecules. These properties make them a suitable option for assuring a good selectivity and sensitivity to electrochemical analyses of antibiotics.

Among the sensors developed for the detection of antibiotics the most used are the electrochemical sensors, together with the optical ones. Thus, electrochemical [14] and colorimetric [15] sensors based on the use of aptamers were used for the highly selective detection of antibiotics.

S. Vlad and N.M. Roman (eds.), *International Conference on Advancements of Medicine and Health Care through Technology; 12th - 15th October 2016, Cluj-Napoca, Romania,*
IFMBE Proceedings 59,
DOI: 10.1007/978-3-319-52875-5_24

The purpose of this study was to develop an electrochemical aptasensor for the detection of ampicillin (Figure 1), a β-lactam antibiotic, widely used both for humans and as veterinary drug, due to its large spectrum of action. For this purpose, two different strategies for the immobilization of the ampicillin-selective aptamer have been employed: by the grafting of a carboxyl containing diazonium salt by cathodic reduction on a glassy carbon electrode, followed by the chemical reaction with the aptamer containing an amino group (ss-DNA 5'-CACGGCATGGTGGGCGTCGTGTTTTTTTTTTTTTT-3'-$(CH2)_6$-NH_2) and by incubating the aptamer containing a thiol group (ss-DNA 5'- CACGGCATGGTGGGCGTCGTG TTTTTTTTTTTTTT-3'-$(CH_2)_6$-SH) on a gold electrode, leading to a self-assembling layer of the aptamer. The modified electrodes have been characterized by electrochemical impedance spectroscopy. The detection of ampicillin using the modified electrodes is a label-free method, using the variation in the impedance signals to quantify the ampicillin concentration.

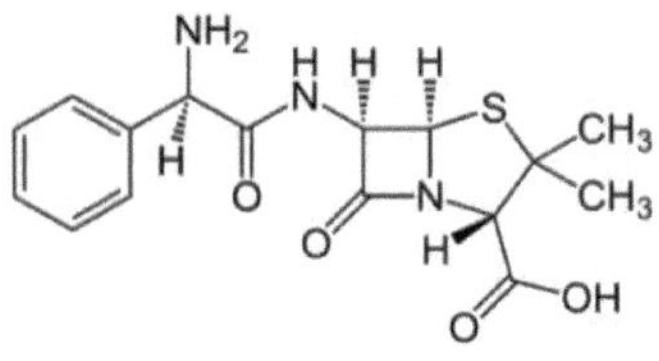

Fig. 1 Chemical structure of ampicillin

II. Materials and Method

All chemicals were of analytical grade and were used as received without further purification. HCl, Na_2HPO_4 and NaH_2PO_4 were purchased from Merck; H_2SO_4, $K_4[Fe(CN)_6]$), $K_3[Fe(CN)_6]$, NaCl, $HAuCl_4$ and ampicillin were purchased from Sigma-Aldrich; N-hydroxysuccinimide (NHS) was purchased from Alfa Aesar and 1-Ethyl-3-(3-dimethylaminopropyl)-carbodiimide (EDC) was purchased from Calbiochem.

All solutions were prepared with ultrapure water (18.2 MΩ, Millipore Simplicity). The supporting electrolyte was 0.02 M phosphate buffer saline (PBS) prepared with Na_2HPO_4, NaH_2PO_4 and NaCl at pH 7.4. The aptamer was diluted in a Tris buffer containing 10 mM tris(hydroxymethyl)aminomethane and 1mM EDTA, with pH=8.

The electrochemical experiments were performed using an AUTOLAB PGSTAT 302N (Ecochemie, The Netherlands) equipped with the associated NOVA 1.10 software. The glassy carbon electrode (GCE), used as working electrodes in the conventional three-electrode cell, along with Ag/AgCl (KCl 3 M) as reference electrode and a Pt wire as counter electrode, were purchased from BAS Inc. (West Lafayette, USA). Before each analysis, the GCE was polished using an alumina suspension and polishing cloth. The screen-printed electrodes (C-SPE) with a carbon-based working and counter electrodes and a silver pseudo-reference were purchased from Dropsens (Spain).

The cyclic voltammetry (CV) experiments were performed in the conventional three-electrode cell of 5 mL, in static mode, at scan rate of 0.1 V s^{-1}.

The electrochemical impedance spectroscopy (EIS) measurements were carried out in the presence of 10 mM $[Fe(CN)_6]^{3-/4-}$ in PBS (0.02 M, pH 7.4) as redox probe. The impedance was measured in a frequency range of 100000 to 0.0100 Hz using the open circuit potential. The EIS measurements were used both for the characterization of the electrode after different steps of modification and for the determination of the ampicillin concentration, the ampicillin trapped by the aptamer leading to a change in the EIS signal.

Prior to its immobilization, the aptamer was brought in its active form, the unfolded one, by heating the aptamer solution at 93° C for 3 min.

The modification with the aptamer of the GCE involved several steps: a stirred solution of 0.5M HCl containing 4-aminophenyl acetic acid and $NaNO_2$ was used for the grafting of the linker molecules by applying a potential of -0.2 V vs. Ag/AgCl(KCl 3M) for 30 s under nitrogen atmosphere; the carboxylated linker was activated by incubation for 15 min with a solution containing 100 μM NHS and 400 μM EDC; then, the electrode was incubated for 30 min with 5 μM solution of the aptamer containing an amino group, resulting an immobilization of the aptamer through an amide bond. In order to prevent the non-specific preconcentration, by adsorption of the ampicillin molecules at the surface of the electrode, the electrode was incubated for 30 min with 1 mM ethanolamine. Between each step the electrode was rinsed with 1 mL with a Tris buffer solution.

The modification with the aptamer of the C-SPE was performed in two steps: first, gold nanoparticles (AuNPs) were electrochemically deposited at the surface of the working electrode by applying 60 μL solution of 0.6 mM $HAuCl_4$ prepared in 0.5 M H_2SO_4 and performing ten cycles of CV, sweeping the potential between -0.2 and 1.2 V vs. Ag/AgCl(KCl 3M) [16] (Figure 2); then, the electrode was incubated with 20 μM solution of the aptamer containing a thiol group, obtaining a self-assembling layer of the aptamer.

The determination of the ampicillin concentration involved two steps: the preconcentration of ampicillin at the surface of the modified electrodes by applying a drop of the solution containing 1 μM ampicillin and incubating for a certain time in a stable atmosphere, followed by an EIS analysis of the electrode with the ampicillin trapped at its surface.

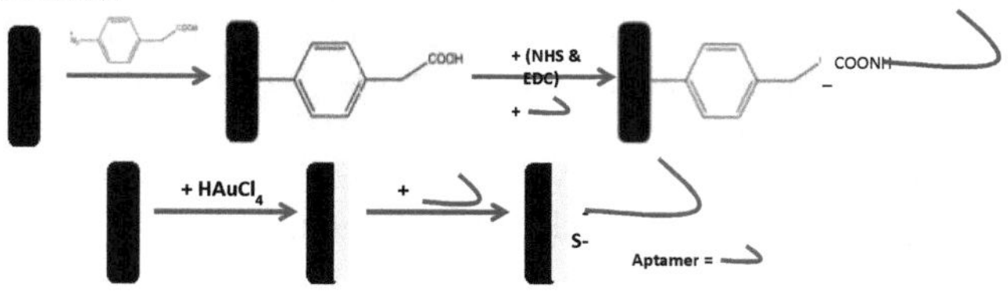

Fig. 2 The two strategies for the modification of electrodes

III. Results and Discussions

A. Modification of the GCE

The electrochemical reduction of the arildiazonium salt formed *in situ* leads to a covalent attachment of the linker molecules and to the formation of multi-layers that impair the electronic transfer. To diminish the number of layers at the surface of the electrode the electrochemical reduction was limited to 30 s. The cycling voltammetry analyses, using $[Fe(CN)_6]^{3-/4-}$ as redox probe, show the passivation of the electrode after the immobilization of the phenyl acetic acid (Figure 3).

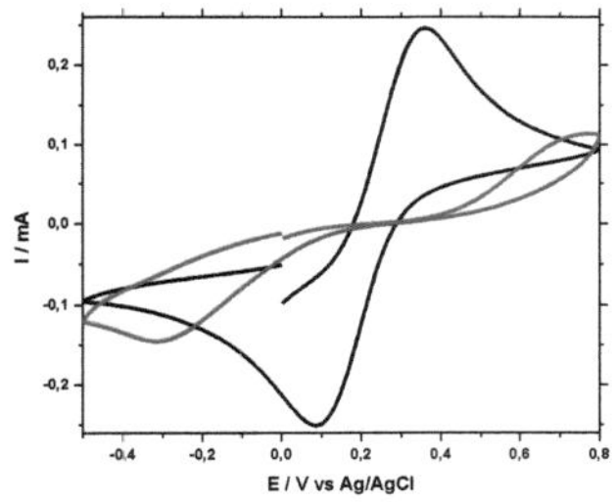

Fig. 3. CVs of 10 mM [Fe(CN)6]3-/4- in PBS on bare GCE (black) and modified with phenyl acetic acid (red). Scan rate 0.1 V s-1.

The EIS measurements were used to characterise the modification of the electrode and as ampicillin detection method. The Nyquist spectrum registered at the electrode modified with the diazonium salt shows a large charge transfer resistance (R_{ct}) (Figure 4), due to the linker layer at the surface of the electrode.

The electrochemical reduction of the arildiazonium salt formed *in situ* leads to a covalent attachment of the linker molecules and to the formation of multi-layers that impair the electronic transfer.

After activation of the carboxylated linker with NHS and EDC, the immobilization of the aptamer at the surface of the electrode seems to facilitate the electron transfer, with a decrease of the R_{ct}. After incubation with an ampicillin solution, the capture of the ampicillin molecules by the aptamer makes it to adopt a conformation that facilitates even more the electron transfer. The variation of the R_{ct} by comparison to the aptamer-modified electrode depends on the concentration of ampicillin, allowing its quantitative determination.

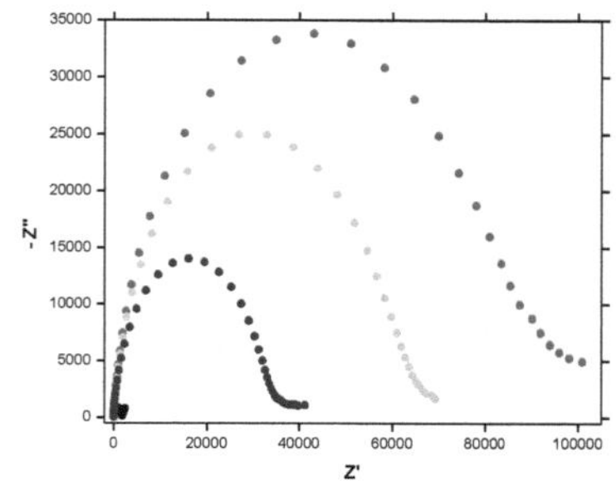

Fig. 4. Nyquist spectra of 10 mM $[Fe(CN)_6]^{3-/4-}$ in PBS registered at bare GCE (**black**), modified with phenyl acetic acid (red), modified with the aptamer (green), modified with the aptamer and incubated with ampicillin (**blue**)

B. Modification of the C-SPE

The modification of the C-SPE was performed using a $HAuCl_4$ solution. The deposition of gold nanoparticles at the surface of the electrode was done by performing 10 cycles of CV between -0.2 V and 1.2 V, allowing the formation of a homogenous layer of gold, hence the stabilisation of the electrochemical signal after the 7th cycle (Figure 5).

The electrochemical reduction of $HAuCl_4$ leads to the formation of Au nanoparticles at the surface of the electrode, which enable the electron transfer, leading to a pronounced decrease of charge transfer resistance (Figure 6). The presence of the Au layer at the electrode surface allows a simple way of immobilization of the ampicillin-selective aptamer that contains a thiol group: an incubation with a solution of the aptamer leads to a strong attachment of the aptamer at the surface, with the formation of a self-assembled monolayer.

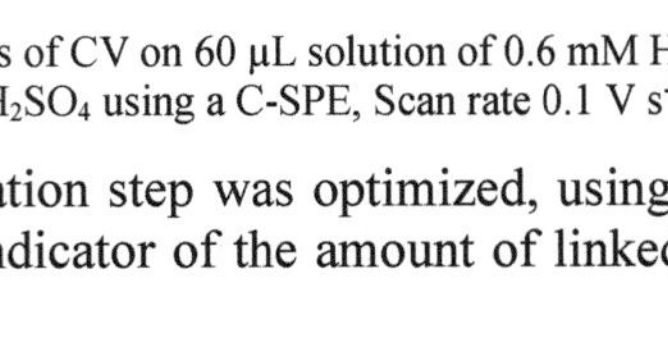

Fig. 5. 10 cycles of CV on 60 µL solution of 0.6 mM $HAuCl_4$ in 0.5 M H_2SO_4 using a C-SPE, Scan rate 0.1 V s^{-1}.

This incubation step was optimized, using EIS measurements as an indicator of the amount of linked aptamer (Table 1).

Table 1. Aptamer incubation time optimization

Aptamer incubation time (min)	Rct (Ω)
30	77.3
80	105.45
1200	132.15

The R_{ct} increases with the incubation time, showing that more aptamer was immobilized, but the small difference between 30 min and 20 h, combined with the need for short procedure, suggests that 30 min are enough for this step.

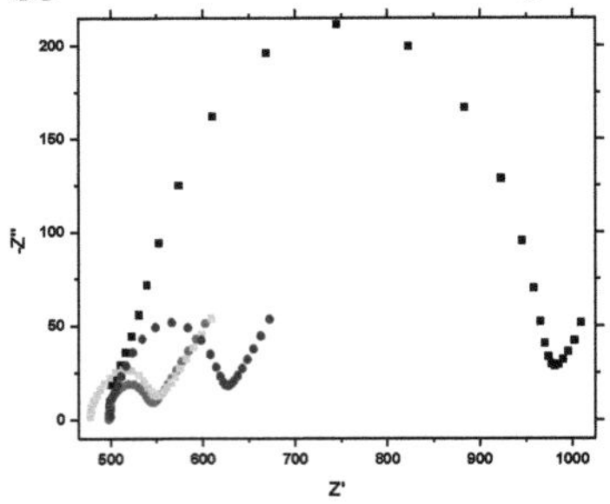

Fig. 6. Nyquist spectra of 10 mM $[Fe(CN)_6]^{3-/4-}$ in PBS registered at C-SPE (**black**), modified with Au-NPs (red), modified with the aptamer (green), modified with the aptamer and incubated with ampicillin (**blue**)

After the incubation with the ampicillin solution, the R_{ct} increases, this increase being used for the quantification of ampicillin. The EIS experiments after different incubation times (Table 2) show that the interaction aptamer-ampicillin occurs quickly, 30 min incubation being enough.

Table 2. Optimization of the incubation time with ampicillin

Ampicillin incubation time (min)	Rct (Ω)
30	130
1440	215.5

For both types of the aptasensor, a change in the EIS signal occurs after ampicillin incubation, which could be used for ampicillin detection. In the case of the sensor obtained by linking the aptamer containing an amino group a greater difference in the EIS signal was obtained after ampicillin incubation compared to the difference in the EIS signal in the case of the immobilization of the thiol-containing aptamer. This suggests a better sensitivity for the first modification method, but the second method presents the advantage of fewer steps in the modification process.

IV. Conclusions

An electrochemical, label-free aptasensor for the detection of ampicillin was developed.

Two different strategies for the immobilization of the ampicillin-selective aptamer have been employed and characterized by EIS: by linking the aptamer containing an amino group through an amide bond and by incubating the aptamer containing a thiol group on a gold electrode, leading to a self-assembling layer of the aptamer. The developed aptasensors presented good affinity for ampicillin.

Acknowledgment

The authors are grateful for the financial support from the Romanian National Authority for Scientific Research UEFISCDI for project no. PN-II-RU-TE-2014-4-0460.

Conflict of Interest

The authors declare that they have no conflict of interest.

References

1. WHO (2011) Tackling antibiotic resistance from a food safety perspective in Europe http://www.euro.who.int
WHO (2014) Antimicrobial resistance: global report on surveillance,http://apps.who.int
2. Shlaes DM (2010) Antibiotics. The Perfect Storm, Springer Science+Business Media B.V., New York
3. European medicines agency-Veterinary Medicines Division (2015) Sales of veterinary antimicrobial agents in 26 EU/EEA countries in 2013. http://www.ema.europa.eu/docs/en_GB/document_library/Report/2015/10/WC500195687.pdf
4. Seifrtova M, Novakova L, Lino C et al. (2009) Anal Chim Acta 649:158–179
5. Herrera-Herrera AV, Ravelo-Pérez LM, Hernández-Borges J et al. (2011) J Chromatogr A 1218:5352– 5361
6. Ge S, Tang W, Han R et al. (2013) J Chromatogr A 1295: 128–135
7. Lacina P, Mravcova L, Vavrova M (2013) J Environ Sci 25: 204–212
8. Migowska N, Caban M, Stepnowski P et al. (2012) Sci Total Environ 441:77–88
9. Lara FJ, del Olmo-Iruela M, Cruces-Blanco C et al. (2012) TrAC 38:52-66
10. Paseiro-Cerrato R, Otero-Pazos P, de Quirós AR-B et al. (2013) Food Control, 33: 262-267
11. Le Bizec B, Pinel G, Antignac J-P et al. (2009) J Chromatogr A 1216: 8016–8034
12. Sanvicens N, Mannelli I, Salvador JP et al. (2011)TrAC 30: 541-553
13. Danesh NM, Ramezani M, Emrani AS et al. (2016) Biosens Bioelectron 75: 123-128
14. Xu Y, Han T, Li X et al. (2015) Anal Chim Acta 891: 298-303
15. Florea A, Taleat Z, Cristea C et al. (2013) Electrochem Commun 33: 127-130.

Author: Cecilia Cristea
Institute: Iuliu Haţieganu University of Medicine and Pharmacy
Street: 4 Pasteur Street, 400349; Cluj-Napoca; Romania
Email: ccristea@umfcluj.ro

Determination of the Electrical Parameters of Some ECG Electrodes

A.R. Iusan [1], N.M. Bîrlea [2], M. Paunescu [1] and A. M. Ciupe[1]

[1] Faculty of Electrical Engineering, Tehnical University of Cluj-Napoca, Cluj-Napoca, Romania
[2] Physics Department, Tehnical University of Cluj-Napoca, Cluj-Napoca, Romania

Abstract— **In this paper we verify if ECG electrodes are adequate for the bioimpedance measurement. A square wave signal (U=1V, *f*=5, 500, 5000 Hz) is applied to a calibrated resistance R=10 kΩ, in series with two identical ECG electrodes glued together by their adhesive part. Using an appropiate model, we find from the data a series resistance with one or more groups of a parallel resistance R_i with a capacitor C_i (i=1, 2, 3).**

Keywords— **electrode, square wave, model, bioimpedance, ECG.**

I. Introduction

Surface biomedical electrodes are used in various forms in a wide range of biomedical applications: detection of bioelectric events such as the electrocardiogram (ECG), application of therapeutic impulses to the body transcutaneous electrical nerve stimulation (TENS), application of electrical potentials for transdermal delivery of ionized molecules and systemic therapeutic effect (iontophoresis), and electrical bioimpedance characterization of body tissues [1].

In applications such as human body's electrical impedance monitoring we inject small currents or voltages into the body and record the resultant voltages or currents. The electrical properties of the body segment can then be calculated. In many of these applications, the magnitude and mismatch of contact impedances can give rise to significant errors or artifacts [2]. As relatively high frequencies are often involved in these techniques, even the series resistance of the gel pad (which is generally ignored) may become significant [2]. Because we are interested in the measurement of the skin impedance, we verify in this paper if the commercially available ECG electrodes are adequate for this purpose.

II. Experimental method

The electrical measurements for impedance spectroscopy are commonly performed using sinusoidal currents over a large frequency range (e.g. 1Hz to 1MHz) [1]. The experimental data are fitted using electrical models or empirical formulas. The electrical models are combinations of electrical resistances and capacitances. Behind these electrical components are physical mechanisms that generate the interesting electrical behavior of the sample versus frequency.

An alternative approach for doing impedance spectroscopy uses square-wave electrical pulses to measure the electrical properties of the material [3]. This time-domain analysis has the advantage of being able to measure in a single shot the frequency characteristics of the sample impedance. This method is well suited for observing impedances which change rapidly in time, and it allows for a more direct and explicit link between the measured quantities (voltages and currents) and the attributed electrical quantities (electrical components, resistances and capacitances).

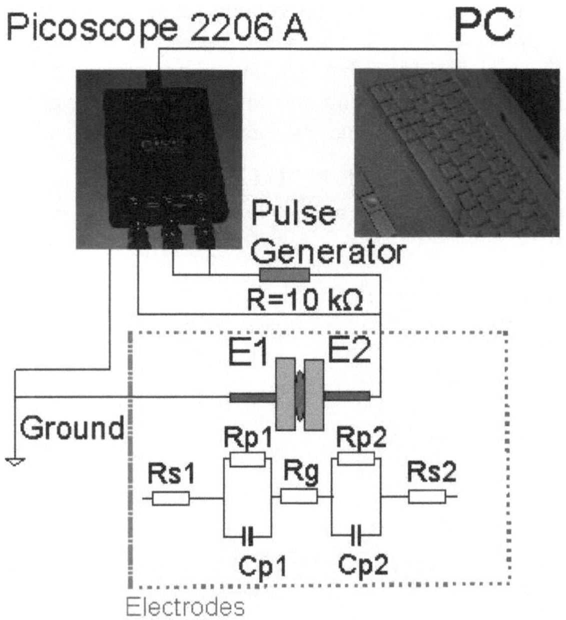

Fig. 1 The experimental arrangement for measuring the two identical ECG electrodes $E_{1,2}$ glued together (equivalent circuit: series resistances, $R_{s1,s2}$, parallel resistances, $R_{p1,p2}$, gel resistance R_g and capacities, $C_{p1,p2}$), in series with a calibrated resistance R=10 kΩ.

Figure 1 presents the experimental arrangement used to measure two identical ECG electrodes glued together by their adhesive part. A digital oscilloscope (Picoscope 2206 A) generates the square wave signal (U=1V, *f*=5, 500, 5000

S. Vlad and N.M. Roman (eds.), *International Conference on Advancements of Medicine and Health Care through Technology; 12th - 15th October 2016, Cluj-Napoca, Romania*,
IFMBE Proceedings 59,
DOI: 10.1007/978-3-319-52875-5_25

Hz) and measures the voltage on the electrodes and on a calibrated resistance R_c=10 kΩ, in series with them for determining the electrical current through circuit. The digital oscilloscope is controlled through a USB link with a computer that displays the waveforms.

Before each measurement, the electrodes were short-circuited to avoid parasite charges on electrodes capacitances. The ECG electrodes tested were: Clinical S55, 3M 2228, and Medi-Trace 210.

III. MODEL AND DATA ANALYSIS

Due to the fact that the calibrated resistance R_c=10 kΩ is much greater than the electrodes impedance, the electrical current through circuit is practically constant. The equivalent circuit model for electrodes [2] has a resistance R_s in series with one or more groups of a parallel resistance R_i with a capacitor C_i (i=1, 2, 3). When the square wave signal change polarity, the current through circuit changes practically instantaneous with $\Delta I=2I$ and so arises a voltage jump (vertical variation of voltage): $\Delta U=U_{up}-U_{down}=\Delta I\ R_s$, where U_{up} is the upper limit of the voltage jump and U_{down} is the lower limit (see Fig.2). This voltage jump is sustained only by the series resistance because the other voltages belong to the capacities in the circuit and cannot change so fast. Thus, the series resistance R_s may be easily computed as:

$$R_s = \Delta U/(2I) \quad (1)$$

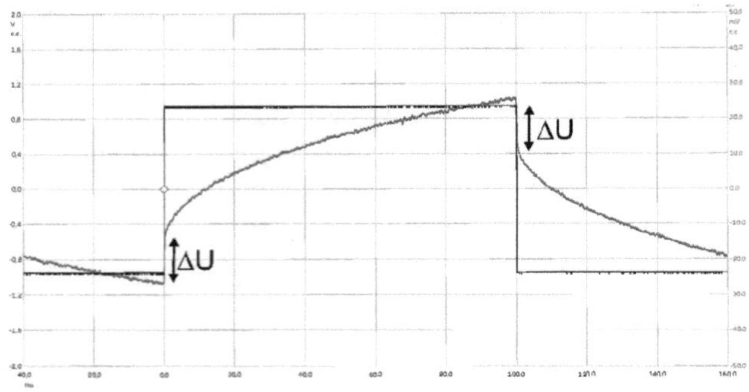

Fig. 2 The oscilloscope's signal (20ms/div.) from Clinical electrodes glued together (red line with voltage jump marked, 10mV/div.) and from calibrated resistance (blue line, 0.4V/div.) at 5 Hz excitation signal.

The solutions for the system of Kirchhoff equations for this circuit are those from [4]. The important difference from [4] is that the applied signal is a biphasic square wave and the "initial" condition is now a condition for periodicity (i.e. the voltages across capacities are identical in absolute value at the beginning and at the end of a semiperiod, but with a different sign):

$$I_i(t=0) = -I_i(t=T/2) \quad (2)$$

where I_i is the current through parallel resistance R_i, and T is the period of the applied signal. As a consequence, the voltage across electrodes is modeled by:

$$U(t) = IR_s + I\sum_i R_i + \sum_i A_i \cdot \exp(-t/\tau_i) \quad (3)$$

where:

$$A_i = -2IR_i / [1+\exp(-T/(2\cdot\tau_i))] \quad (4)$$

$$\tau_i = R_i \cdot C_i. \quad (5)$$

The amplitudes, A_i, and time constants, τ_i, are found by fitting the measured voltage across the electrodes with the function: y0 + $\sum A_i e^{\wedge}(-x/t_i)$ with 1, 2 or 3 time constants. Taking into account that the current through circuit is known: $I= U_{app}/R_c = 1V/10k\Omega = 0.1mA$, the electrical components of the model can be computed from the above equations as:

$$R_i = -A_i \cdot [1+\exp(-T/(2\cdot\tau_i))] / (2I) \quad (6)$$

$$C_i = \tau_i / R_i. \quad (7)$$

$$R_s = y0/I - \sum R_i. \quad (8)$$

IV. RESULTS

The series resistance from the equivalent circuit for 2 electrodes glued together by their adhesive part was calculated with relation (1) for the three types of electrodes at the proposed frequencies. The found values were very stable, with differences between series resistance values at different frequencies < 1 Ω, usually, with the exception of only one case in which a difference of 7.8 Ω have been seen, see Table 1, for average value between 34 and 76 Ω.

Table 1 The series resistances for two identical ECG electrodes glued together by their adhesive part at 3 test frequencies.

Electrode	Test condition	Series resistance R_s(Ω)
Clinical S55	5 Hz (T=200 ms)	58.2
	500 Hz (T=2 ms)	59.8
	5000 Hz (T=0.2 ms)	59.7
	average value	59.2
3M 2228	5 Hz (T=200 ms)	77
	500 Hz (T=2 ms)	76.5
	5000 Hz (T=0.2 ms)	75.4
	average value	76.3
Medi-Trace 210	5 Hz (T=200 ms)	31.5
	500 Hz (T=2 ms)	31.5
	5000 Hz (T=0.2 ms)	39.3
	average value	34.1

Between two consecutive jumps of the voltage across the electrodes, the data were fitted by a generic function: $y0 + \sum A_i e^{\wedge}(-x/t_i)$ with 1, 2 or 3 time constants, using Origin Pro software and monitoring the coefficient of determination R^2. For 3 time constants the fitting procedure has instabilities for some data, a phenomenon known in the literature [5].

In spite of a large coefficient of determination (usually $R^2>0.99$), especially for 5 Hz measurements, plotting the fit in a logarithmic time scale reveals large and systematic deviations between experimental data and calculated values at small values of time (<5ms) for a 1 time constant procedure, but not for 2 time constants procedure, see Fig. 3.

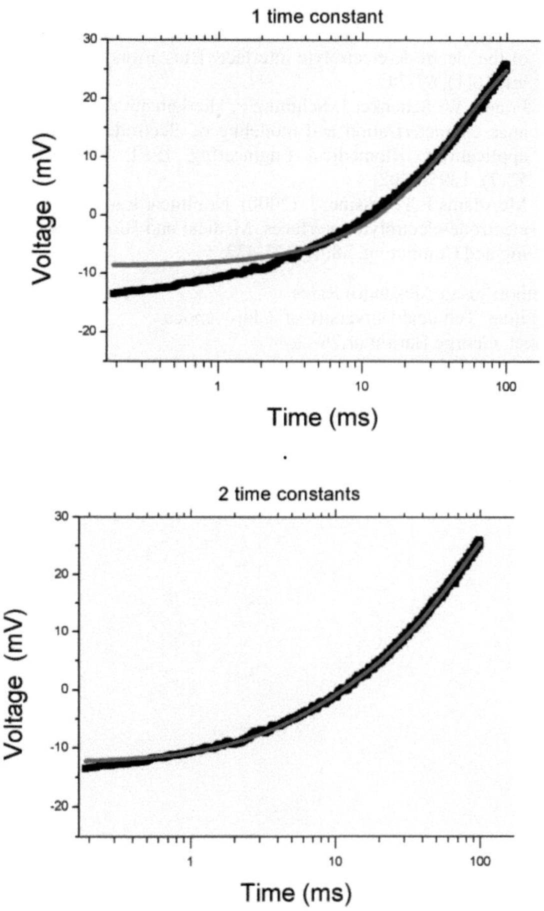

Fig. 3 The results for data analysis with Origin software for 1 time constant (up) and 2 time constants (bottom) for Clinical electrodes at 5 Hz (black-experimental data, red-calculated).

Hence, we concluded that a model with 2 time constants can be enough for describing the electrical behavior of the electrodes. The amplitudes and time constants obtained by fitting procedure using Origin software for data from 5 Hz measurements are displayed in Table 2.

Table 2 The amplitudes, A, and the time constants, T, for two identical ECG electrodes glued together by their adhesive part obtained from fitting procedure for 3 types of electrodes measured with 5 Hz square wave.

Electrode	Clinical S55	3M 2228	Medi-Trace 210
R^2 1 time constant	0.995	0.992	0.986
y0(mV)	30.3	35.8	16.9
−A(mV)	39.1	42.9	23.6
T (ms)	50.6	37.2	60.6
R^2 2 time constants	0.999	0.998	0.989
y0(mV)	36.3	41.3	32.0
$-A_1$(mV)	41.0	40.7	34.4
T_1(ms)	74.5	58.3	168
$-A_2$(mV)	7.90	13.1	5.47
T_2(ms)	5.53	6.36	11.8

The lumped electrical components of the model were computed with equations (6) and (7), and displayed in Table 3, for 5 Hz measurements. The total resistance $R_{tot}= R_s+R_p$ was calculated as $R_{tot}(\Omega)=y0(mV)/I(mA)$.

Table 3 The parallel resistances and capacitances of two identical ECG electrodes glued together by their adhesive part for 3 types of electrodes measured with 5 Hz square wave.

Electrode	Clinical S55	3M 2228	Medi-Trace 210
R^2 1 time constant	0.995	0.992	0.986
$R_{tot}(\Omega)$)	303	358	169
$R_p(\Omega)$	223	229	141
$C_p(\mu F)$	227	162	431
R^2 2 time constants	0.999	0.998	0.989
$R_{tot}(\Omega)$	363	413	320
$R_1(\Omega)$	259	240	267
$C_1(\mu F)$	288	243	629
$R_2(\Omega)$	39.5	65.5	27.4
$C_2(\mu F)$	140	97.1	432

It is important to say that the characteristic values (resistances and capacitances) for a single electrode can be obtained from the tabulated data dividing by 2 the tabulated resistances and multiplying by 2 the tabulated capacities, because of the series arrangement of the electrodes, see Fig. 1.

V. Conclusions

The choice of electrodes for electrical measurements influences to a great extent the signals that are measured and because of that it is important to find the best-suited electrode for the intended use [6]. We have tested ECG electrodes because the silver-silver chloride electrodes tend to have very low interface impedances [7] and have been shown to be particularly stable and resistant to noise [2], useful properties for bioimpedance measurements.

The electrical behavior of the electrodes is usually described by a model with a series resistance and a resistance in parallel with a capacitance or a constant phase element [2, 6-9]. We have chosen a capacitance, instead of a constant phase element because it describes well enough our experimental data.

Our results have shown that a square wave test signal can be used to quickly determine the electrical behavior of the electrodes. This method provides fast and stable results for the series resistance, R_s, over a large spectrum of frequencies. Worth mentioning that the main factor affecting the bioimpedance measurements is the series resistance.

We showed here that the ECG electrodes, usually used to detect bioelectric events (electrocardiogram) can be used to measure the impedance of body tissues.

Conflict of Interest

The authors declare that they have no conflict of interest.

References

1. Grimnes S, Martinsen Ø G, (2015) Bioimpedance and bioelectricity basics. 3rd ed., London: Academic Press. [p405 Ch 10 Selected Applications]
2. McAdams E (2011). Biomedical electrodes for biopotential monitoring and electrostimulation. In Bio-Medical CMOS ICs (pp. 31-124). Springer US.
3. Birlea N M, Birlea S I, Culea E. (2011) The skin's electrical time constants, International Conference on Advancements of Medicine and Health Care through Technology, *IFMBE Proceedings*, **Vol. 36**, Part 2, pp. 160-163, DOI: 10.1007/978-3-642-22586-4_34
4. Bîrlea N M, Bîrlea S I, Toşa V. (2009). The skin's electrical asymmetry. In Journal of Physics: Conference Series (Vol. 182, No. 1, p. 012020). IOP Publishing.
5. Istratov A A, Vyvenko O F. (1999). Exponential analysis in physical phenomena. Rev. Sci. Instrum., **70**(2), 1233-1257.
6. Tronstad C, Johnsen G K, Grimnes S, Martinsen Ø G. (2010). A study on electrode gels for skin conductance measurements. Physiological measurement, 31(10), 1395.
7. McAdams E T, Lackermeier A, McLaughlin J A, Macken D, Jossinet J. (1995). The linear and non-linear electrical properties of the electrode-electrolyte interface. Biosensors and Bioelectronics, 10(1), 67-74.
8. Franks W, Schenker I, Schmutz P, Hierlemann A. (2005). Impedance characterization and modeling of electrodes for biomedical applications. Biomedical Engineering, IEEE Transactions on, 52(7), 1295-1302.
9. McAdams E T, Jossinet J. (2000). Nonlinear transient response of electrode-electrolyte interfaces. Medical and Biological Engineering and Computing, 38(4), 427-432.

Author: Iusan Alexandru Rares
Institute: Tehnical University of Cluj-Napoca
Street: George Baritiu nr.26-28
City: Cluj-Napoca
Country: Romania
Email: iusan_rares@yahoo.com

How to Describe the Skin's Electrical Nonlinear Response

N.M. Bîrlea[1], S.I. Bîrlea[2] and E. Culea[1]

[1] Physics Department, Technical University of Cluj-Napoca, Cluj-Napoca, Romania
[2] Technical University of Cluj-Napoca, Cluj-Napoca, Romania

Abstract—**The skin's electrical nonlinearities found experimentally are related to stratum corneum and modeled by the parallel resistance (R_P) as a linear current dependence in conductance ($1/R_P$). We show that such dependence could occur because the skin's current-voltage characteristic has a non-ohmic linear portion at large voltage, due to pores' conduction, that can be detected as a constant dynamic resistance (dU/dI).**

Keywords—**skin, nonlinearity, dynamic resistance, current-voltage, model**

I. Introduction

The electrical stimulation of the human body is a medical tool for investigation, diagnosis and treatment [1], especially transcutaneous electrical stimulation – with electrodes applied on the skin. The skin-electrode impedance has a direct influence on the investigated parameters values or on the treatment outcome.

The models of the skin-electrode interface are mainly *descriptive models* based on electrical resistive-capacitive circuits or on constant phase elements (Cole's empirical formula) [1]. These models are used on experimental data obtained with sinusoidal low amplitudes currents (or voltages) of various frequencies (usually spread over several decades). An alternative measurement uses square wave stimuli, with the advantage that it is closer to the real stimuli used on applications and it is a faster measurement [2-4]. This type of measurement is better adapted to study nonlinearities associated with larger signals (currents or voltages) applied to the skin [5-6].

In spite of a large palette of applications that use voltages greater than 1V and consequently are in the nonlinear regime of the skin [2, 7], there are few studies on the nonlinear regime of the skin, with the exception of the very large voltages where the electroporation phenomenon arises [8].

In this paper we focus on *lumped parameter models* for the nonlinear electrical properties of the skin, with an *explanatory* flavor, since a better understanding of the physical processes acting within the skin-electrode system is a key factor for development of new devices. We begin with a review of what we consider to be the main landmarks in the field of skin's electrical nonlinearity, then discuss the pores conduction as an explanation for nonlinearity below few tens of volts and the role of current-voltage characteristic in detecting main mechanisms that shape it.

II. Landmarks for nonlinear skin response

In 1963 Stephens [9] describes an *in vivo* experiment with a 7 cm² active liquid electrode and a 20 cm² pad counter (reference) electrode, on the front and back of the forearm, respectively, and a d.c. or square-wave stimulus (10-600 Hz). The voltage across the skin was measured between a probe electrode in the electrolyte and a 3 cm diameter pad electrode placed near the liquid electrode on the skin. He found 2 components in the nonlinearity of the skin resistance: a slow fall in skin resistance dependent on electrical charge passed and a fast resistance fall (without time-lag) modeled as a fixed capacity shunted by a nonlinear resistance.

In 1970 Lykken [2] made an *in vivo* square-wave analysis of skin impedance using active electrodes (0.7 to 10 cm² area) with or without a drilled reference electrode. He applied a square-wave voltage to electrodes in series with a 100 Ω resistance. An oscilloscope monitored the voltage drop on 100 Ω resistance, hence the current through the circuit. Watching the influence of electrode area on model's parameters of the skin-electrode interface (R_s– series resistance, R_p– parallel resistace and C– capacitance) Lykken showed that the series resistance of the model contains 2 area dependent resistances (one for each electrode) and an area independent resistance (common resistance of the body core from electrode-to-electrode, ~500 Ω). Removal of the stratum corneum eliminates the parallel resistive and capacitative elements, and slightly reduces the series resistance (~30%), indicating that R_p and C belong to the stratum corneum, but the area dependent part of R_s has at least 2 anatomically distinct components: one in stratum corneum and other beneath it but yet close enough to the surface so that its conductivity varies directly with electrode area. The nonlinearity of the skin manifests into the parallel resistance, R_p, that held reasonably constant for pulses of 0.2 to 2 V, but decreased sharply above 2 V for all subjects.

In 1981 Yamamoto and Yamamoto studied skin's electrical nonlinearity [7] at low frequencies (0.01 Hz to several kHz) with a 3-electrode technique. Experiments were performed *in vivo* with a constant-current source and Ag-AgCl

S. Vlad and N.M. Roman (eds.), *International Conference on Advancements of Medicine and Health Care through Technology; 12th - 15th October 2016, Cluj-Napoca, Romania,*
IFMBE Proceedings 59,
DOI: 10.1007/978-3-319-52875-5_26

electrodes (1 cm^2 discs) with Beckman paste (NaCl 18%) or PEG solution (polyethylene glycol 91.6%, NaCl 0.9%, H_2O 7.5%,). They obtained lower impedance and more linearity with Beckman paste than PEG solution. They concluded that a linear range exists (where the current dependency disappears) when the current is extremely small, but a point boundary value can not be unconditionally determined. Worth mentioning the asymmetry of their Lissajous figures for positive-negative currents and the electrical breakdown of the skin for very low frequencies (0.01 Hz) and negative currents.

In 1989 Kaczmarek and Webster [10] describe an *in vivo* experiment with a conductive rubber belt which encircles the abdomen (moistened with tap water before the experiment) as reference electrode and 5.5 mm gold-plated active electrode, powered by current pulses (0.4 ms, 1-25 mA). They found that the static resistance (R = steady-state electrode voltage near the end of the current pulse / current i) can be modeled by a series ohmic resistance (R_o) and two parallel resistances, an ohmic one (R_p) and a nonlinear one ($R_v = R_p I_o/i$) depending on current i ($R=R_o+(R_p||R_v)$).

In 1990 Kasting and Bowman [11, 12] describe *ex vivo* measurements for human allograft skin (0.7 cm^2 both sides immersed in a saline buffer) with short bursts (~20s) of direct current of alternating polarity (0 to ±10 μA in 2μA steps, 0 to ±50 μA in 10μA steps, and 0 to ±250 μA in 50μA steps). Their U-j curves (j-current density) were "satisfactorily described" by the relationship $U = (4aRT/F) \sinh^{-1}(bj)$, where *a* and *b* are adjustable parameters; *a* is equal to the number of barriers within the membrane which each ion must cross and *b* is the sum of the rate constants for traversing the barrier (the authors consider the equation "as a phenomenological means of characterizing the data" [11]). They report that the measured voltage was quite stable after 5-10 s for the ±10 μA current range, but for larger currents rather than waiting to achieve stable potential readings (tens of minutes per reading), they chose to record the potential after 15-20 s. Their graphical tool of voltage versus logarithm of the current density is a very cogent argument for the correctness of their formula. For long time effects and mathematical models describing iontophoretic transport through skin barrier see Gratieri and Kalia review [13].

In 1997 Craane-van Hinsberg et al. experimented *in vitro* on *stratum corneum* (SC) samples (0.79 cm^2 area for current transport), exposed to current densities from 0.013 to 13 mA/cm^2, applied as square-wave pulse (5ms positive, 5ms current off, 5ms negative, 5ms current off and repeat) [14, 15]. The *falling parts of the voltage waves* were "satisfactorily modeled" ($R^2 \geq 0.99$) by a series connection of two R||C-circuits. For 0.013 mA/cm^2 the values of R and C remain constant for long times (up to 1h), but for larger current densities the resistances decrease and the capacitances increase. For shorter times (10 μs between voltage samples) the resistances decrease and the capacities increase with the increase of the current density. They concluded that the *electrical field change the ordering of the intercellular lipid lamellae*. This aspect is sustained by the thermal behavior of skin impedance [14]: a ~10°C lowering of the transition point where a sudden drop in resistance arises with the rising current density, and by the structural changes of the intercellular lipid lamellae detected with X-ray diffractograms and electron microscopy on freeze-fracture replicas [15]. They calculated an activation energy (from an Arrhenius plot of the natural logarithm of the conductance versus the inverse of the absolute temperature) that strongly decreases with current density rise. After chloroform-methanol lipid extraction, stratum corneum was characterized by *a single RC circuit*. The resistance of extracted stratum corneum was <1% of the original pre-extraction value, which indicates that the resistance of stratum corneum is mainly determined by the intercellular lipids.

In 1999 Dorgan and Reilly proposed a mathematical model for the electrical impedance of human skin [16] during surface functional neuromuscular stimulation. It consist of the parallel arrangement of a constant linear capacitor with a nonlinear time-dependent resistor, R_p, in series with a constant linear resistor, i.e. the common model for skin, but R_p is modeled by a modified form of the Hodgkin-Huxley equations to take into account the memory effect (slow variation of skin impedance) and fast variation of skin impedance. The model has 15 simulation parameters, a little too much for the taste of an experimenter, but worth mentioning that the nonlinear conductance, $1/R_p$, contains a term proportional with the injected current.

III. Recent Findings and an Explanation

In 2014, Bîrlea et al. [5] used a typical neuromuscular electrical stimulation signal (square wave constant voltage pulses) to study changes in the electrical properties of the skin-electrode interface during a week-long stimulation program. The skin-electrode system was modeled with a series and parallel resistances and a capacitance. From the acquired data it was found a strong inverse relation between the parallel resistance and minimum current: $R_p=R_1+U_1/I_{min}$ (with a coefficient of determination $R^2 = 0.94$) and between the series resistance and peak current: $R_s=R_2+U_2/I_{max}$ (with a coefficient of determination $R^2 = 0.95$). Here R_1, U_1, R_2, U_2 are parameters found from the experimental data. These statistical correlations arise from all the data of 14 different subjects, on 7 consecutive days, in 30 minutes sessions, i.e. the correlations are not limited to the data of a single subject or session, but works globally.

In 2015, Luna et al. [6] published a thorough paper focused on building a model of the skin-electrode interface for transcutaneous electrical stimulation with current or voltage controlled impulses. They found experimentally a linear increase of the parallel conductance G_p ($1/R_p$) with current amplitude (for voltage-controlled stimulation the current at steady state was used as reference, i.e. I_{min}). Their model contains the series and parallel resistances and a capacitance. The parallel resistance, $R_p=R_e+R_o$, includes the nonlinear effects related to instantaneous variations described by $R_e=1/(aI(t)+b)$, due to electroporation, as a current-dependent phenomenon, and the nonlinear effects related to slow changes (as a charge-dependent phenomenon, presumably electro-osmotic) described by $R_o=R_{oi}$ below the threshold q_{th}, and $R_o=R_{oi}\cdot Aa'/(Aa'+q-q_{th})$ for charges above the threshold. Here A is electrode area and a, b, a' are parameters to be determined from the data. The coefficient of determination, R^2, was around 0.99 in a simulation using the proposed dynamic model for both stimulation types.

Birlea and Birlea [17] provide a simple explanation for the nonlinearity and the asymmetry of the current-voltage characteristic of a pore in a membrane, using a Nernst-Planck model and usual approximations from electroporation theory [18, 19]. They found a quasi-ohmic, slow rising linear current at low voltages, a nonlinear region at intermediate voltages, and a non-ohmic, fast rising linear current at large voltages. The asymptotic behavior of the current-voltage relation for a triangular profile of the potential energy inside the pore is:

$$j=u-w/r \quad \text{for } u>>1 \tag{1}$$

$$j=uw/(e^{w}-1) \quad \text{for } u<<1 \tag{2}$$

with $u=qU/(kT)$ as dimensionless transmembrane potential and $j= JL/(cqD)$ as dimensionless current density, where U is the voltage applied to a pore of length L, c, ionic concentration; k, Boltzmann constant, T, absolute temperature, q, elementary charge, $r = d/L$ with d the length of the pore domain where the potential energy varies from 0 to maximum value W, $w=W/(kT)$ dimensionless energy barrier height, and J is the current density (I/S=current /pore section area).

Taking into account Einstein's relation between diffusion coefficient D and electrical mobility of the ions, $\mu= qD/(kT)$ and the electrical conductivity of the electrolyte $\sigma = cq\mu$, the asymptotic relation between U and J for $U>>kT/q$ is:

$$J=\sigma\,[U-W/(qr)]/L=\sigma\,[(U/L)-W/(qd)] \tag{3}$$

$$J=\sigma\,(U/L)\,w/(e^{w}-1) \quad \text{for } U<<kT/q: \tag{4}$$

For small voltages the pore has an ohmic behavior, the equivalent resistence of electrolyte filled pore multiplied by a factor dependent on the energy barrier height $w= W/(kT)$:

$$R=[L/(\sigma S)]\cdot[(e^{w}-1)/w] \tag{5}$$

The maximum energy barrier height W, is related to the pore radius ρ by a simple relation [19]: $W= kT\cdot 5(\text{nm})/\rho(\text{nm})$.

Because the human body temperature is 37°C, the thermal potential, kT/q, is 26.7 mV, hence the pore voltage drop can easily attain the high voltage regime ($U>>kT/q$ or $U\geq 4\,kT/q \approx 0.1$V) and the asymptotic relation seems more useful than the complete formula of the current-voltage for pore's electrical behavior. The relation (3) for large voltages shows that the current through a pore is determined by the difference between the external applied field (U/L) and an internal electrical field ($W/(qd)$) created by the energy gradient at the pore entrance (W/d). Rewriting equation (3) as a formula for voltage U:

$$U=[I/(S\sigma)+W/(qd)]\cdot L \tag{6}$$

we can calculate the resistance of the pore of length L and section aria S, as a simple ratio between voltage and current:

$$R=\frac{U}{I}=\frac{L}{\sigma S}+\frac{LW}{Iqd} \tag{7}$$

The pore resistance (7) has 2 components, the resistance of the electrolyte inside the pore (ohmic) and a nonlinear resistance inversely proportional with the injected current. Connecting in series N pores lead to summing N voltages as (6) thus total voltage has a current proportional part (ohmic) and a current independent part, $NLW/(qd)$, that generates a nonlinear resistance inversely proportional with the current.

We propose such a model as a first approximation of the stratum corneum electrical behavior. In this context a thick stratum corneum (palms) with many layers of corneocytes (~N) has a larger voltage threshold ($NLW/(qd)$) between low and high voltage regimes, than a thin one, with few layers (eyelids, face, lips). Also computing the *dynamic resistance*, dU/dI, instead of a static resistance, seems more appropriate for the nonlinear U-I characteristic. In our case the dynamic resistance of the pore is constant (resistance of electrolyte filled pore) at larger voltages than threshold:

$$R_{dy}=dU/dI=L/(\sigma S) \tag{8}$$

This fact is consistent with Pliquett et al. findings [20] that no changes were observed in dynamic resistance R_{dy} for voltages below 40 V across stratum corneum, only voltages in the region 40-90 V cause dramatic and usually reversible changes of the dynamic resistance due to electroporation.

IV. Conclusions

The skin's electrical properties can be described by a lumped parameter model with a series resistor (R_s) and a parallel combination of a resistor (R_p) and a capacitor (C). The nonlinearities experimentally found belong to stratum corneum and are modeled by the parallel resistance (R_p) as a linear dependence on current of the conductance ($1/R_p$).

To build a model for the nonlinear parallel resistance, R_p, we propose to begin with the current-voltage response of the skin, because current and voltage are the directly measured quantities. A constant dynamic resistance (dU/dI) at voltages above 1V [2] indicates that nonlinearity is due to ionic conduction through pores [17], and a further decrease in dynamic resistance at voltages above 40V [20] indicates the appearance of electroporation, see Fig.1. The numerical values are for a single skin-electrode interface.

Lumped parameter models for the skin-electrode interface are intuitive and easy to use. To elaborate such nonlinear electrical model for the skin the starting point should be the skin's current-voltage response.

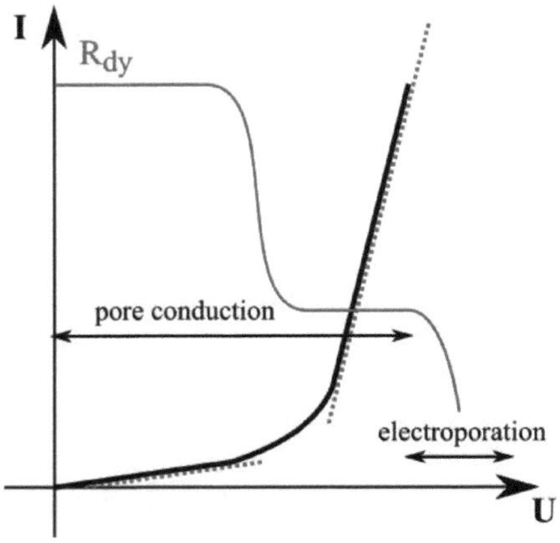

Fig. 1 A schematic current-voltage response of the skin (black line) and the dynamic resistance behavior (dU/dI, red line, with 2 plateaus below and above a threshold voltage), emphasizing the regions for pore conduction and electroporation.

Conflict of Interest

The authors declare that they have no conflict of interest.

References

1. Grimnes S, Martinsen Ø G, (2015) Bioimpedance and bioelectricity basics. 3rd ed., Academic Press. London
2. Lykken DT (1970) Square-wave analysis of skin impedance. Psychophysiology 7(2):262-275.
3. van Boxtel A. (1977) Skin resistance during square-wave electrical pulses of 1 to 10 mA. Med. Biol. Eng. Comput. 15(6) 679-657.
4. Yamamoto Y, Isshiki H, Nakamura T. (1996). Instantaneous measurement of electrical parameters in a palm during electrodermal activity. IEEE Trans. Instrum. Meas. 45(2), 483-487.
5. Bîrlea S I, Breen P P, Corley G J, Bîrlea N M, Quondamatteo F, ÓLaighin G. (2014). Changes in the electrical properties of the electrode–skin–underlying tissue composite during a week-long programme of neuromuscular electrical stimulation. Physiol. Meas. 35(2), 231.
6. Luna JLV, Krenn M, Ramírez JAC, Mayr W (2015) Dynamic impedance model of the skin-electrode interface for transcutaneous electrical stimulation. PLoS One. 10(5), e0125609. doi: 10.1371/journal.pone.0125609.
7. Yamamoto T, Yamamoto Y. (1981) Non-linear electrical properties of skin in the low frequency range, Med. Biol. Eng. Comput. 19(3) 302-310.
8. Chizmadzhev Y A, Zarnitsin V G, Weaver J C, Potts R O. (1995). Mechanism of electroinduced ionic species transport through a multilamellar lipid system. Biophys. J. 68(3), 749-765.
9. Stephens W G S (1963) The current-voltage relationship in human skin. Med. Electron. Biol. Eng. 1(3), 389-399.
10. Kaczmarek K A, Webster J G. (1989). Voltage-current characteristics of the electrotactile skin-electrode interface. In Proc. Annu. Int. Conf. IEEE Eng. Med. Biol. Soc (Vol. 11, pp. 1526-1527). Seattle, WA: IEEE.
11. Kasting G B, Bowman L A. (1990). DC electrical properties of frozen, excised human skin. Pharm. Res. 7(2), 134-143.
12. Kasting G B, Bowman L A. (1990). Electrical analysis of fresh, excised human skin: a comparison with frozen skin. Pharm. Res. 7(11), 1141-1146.
13. Gratieri T, Kalia YN (2013) Mathematical models to describe iontophoretic transport in vitro and in vivo and the effect of current application on the skin barrier. Adv. Drug Delivery Rev., 65(2), 315-329.
14. Craane-van Hinsberg W H M, Verhoef J C, Junginger H E, Bodde H E. (1997). Electroperturbation of the human skin barrier in vitro (I): the influence of current density on the thermal behaviour of skin impedance. Eur. J. Pharm. Biopharm. 43(1), 43-50.
15. Craane-van Hinsberg W H M, et al. (1997) Electroperturbation of the human skin barrier in vitro: II. Effects on stratum corneum lipid ordering and ultrastructure. Microsc. Res. Tech. 37(3) 200-213.
16. Dorgan S J, Reilly R B. (1999). A model for human skin impedance during surface functional neuromuscular stimulation. IEEE Trans. Rehabil. Eng. 7(3), 341-348.
17. Birlea M, Birlea S I (2012) The current-voltage relation of a pore and its asymptotic behavior in a Nernst-Planck model. Journal of Electrical Bioimpedance, 3(1), 36-41.
18. DeBruin KA, Krassowska W. (1999) Modeling electroporation in a single cell. II. Effects of ionic concentrations. Biophys. J. 77(3):1225-33. doi: 10.1016/S0006-3495(99)76974-2
19. Glaser RW, Leikin SL, Chernomordik LV, Pastushenko VF, Sokirko AI. (1988) Reversible electrical breakdown of lipid bilayers: formation and evolution of pores. Biochim. Biophys. Acta, Biomembr. 940(2):275-87.
20. Pliquett U, Langer R, Weaver J C (1995) Changes in the passive electrical properties of human stratum corneum due to electroporation. Biochim. Biophys. Acta, Biomembr. 1239(2), 111-121.

Author: Nicolae-Marius Bîrlea
Institute: Technical University of Cluj-Napoca
Street: Daicoviciu 15
City: Cluj-Napoca
Country: Romania
Email: mbirlea@phys.utcluj.ro

Case Study of Static and Dynamic Postural Balance of an Overweight Pregnant Woman

D. Cotoros, A. Stanciu and I. Serban

Transilvania University of Brasov/Product Design, Mechatronics and Environment Department, Brasov, Romania

Abstract— **Most studies related to the investigation of pregnant women postural balance and stability are statistic analysis performed upon a set of normal weight subjects, with no risk factor regarding their pregnancy. The authors decided to monitor a more complicated case starting from the first weeks of pregnancy until the last ones, by determining the postural stability during stance, and plantar pressure during normal gait. The subject is over 35 and overweight, meaning that she involves more risks than other persons.**

Keywords— **overweight, pregnancy, base of support, postural balance, center of pressure.**

I. Introduction

It is a well-known fact that pregnancy is a normal physiological state for most women; nevertheless it triggers some spectacular changes in the woman's body starting with weight gain, edema, diminished joints mobility, altered posture and balance, also hormonal, cardiovascular and pulmonary changes. [1]

Additionally, when some risk factors are involved even from the beginning of pregnancy, the situation should be carefully studied and monitored. There are several risk factors like: mother's age, pre-pregnancy weight, health problems (diabetes, high blood pressure, HIV, etc.), multiple pregnancy [2] but the ones of interest in our case study concern the age of the mother (over 35) and her overweight since before the pregnancy.

Considering the fact that the weight gain during pregnancy is usually between 9 and 14kg, sometimes even up to 20kg, all located in the abdominal area, it becomes obvious that body posture adaptations are required in order to maintain stability and balance both during stance and during dynamic actions. [3]

The term body posture is used to describe the orientation of a body segment relative to the gravitational force direction while balance refers to body posture dynamics that prevents the person from falling. [4]

In order to maintain equilibrium the neural-muscular control system of the human body works to keep the COP (center of pressure – location of the projection of body center of gravity) within the base of support (BOS – minimum area enclosing the feet's contact with the ground). [4]

Due to the increase of weight in the anterior part of the body during pregnancy, there is a certain risk of altering of COP's position towards outside the BOS, leading to a growing risk of falling, [5] especially in the case of a preexistent overweight in the area.

Even in normal situations it was determined that up to 25% of the pregnant women sustain a fall [6] being thus exposed to complications or even pregnancy loss.

Most studies are generally excluding extreme situations when the investigated subject is overweight already before pregnancy, like shown in [3]. For this reason our team decided to investigate this particular situation, the results being applicable to other persons subjected to similar risk factors.

II. Materials and Methods

The investigation was performed upon a 38 years old woman, height 167cm, mass at the beginning of pregnancy 87kg (BMI = 31,2kg/m^2 – obese class I) and mass towards the end of pregnancy 99kg (BMI = 35,5kg/m^2 – obese class II). She was pregnant the second time and had an increased weight following the first pregnancy and due to an unhealthy nutrition and lack of physical activity.

The subject was tested two times: first time when she was 6 weeks pregnant and second time, 36 weeks pregnant, that is during the first trimester and during the third trimester, wearing different shoes that were comfortable for her at that time (heels between 2cm and 3cm high).

The subject was investigated in the morning, around 10 o'clock each time. She was instructed to assume three types of BOS (small, intermediate and large) and maintain a relaxed standing position with eyes directed straightforward, arms along the body for 30s. For each type of BOS, there were three measurements performed in order to obtain as accurate as possible results.

The experimental setup consisted of a force platform (Kistler) (fig.1) connected to a PC by means of an AC/DC converter. Bioware software was used for data processing.

Each session of measurements started with the force platform calibration, which also provided the exact weight of the subject at the investigation moment, allowing the deter-

S. Vlad and N.M. Roman (eds.), *International Conference on Advancements of Medicine and Health Care through Technology; 12th - 15th October 2016, Cluj-Napoca, Romania,*
IFMBE Proceedings 59,
DOI: 10.1007/978-3-319-52875-5_27

mination of body mass and BMI in order to be able to establish the obesity class of the subject.

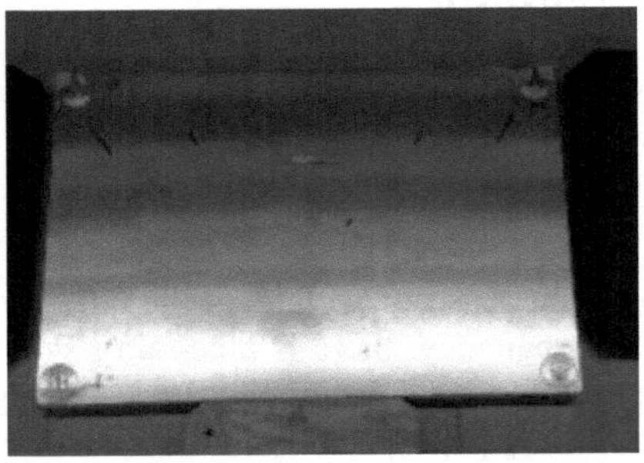

Fig.1 Kistler force platform

The subject is presented while assuming small BOS after six weeks of pregnancy (fig.2) and intermediate BOS after 36 weeks of pregnancy (fig.3).

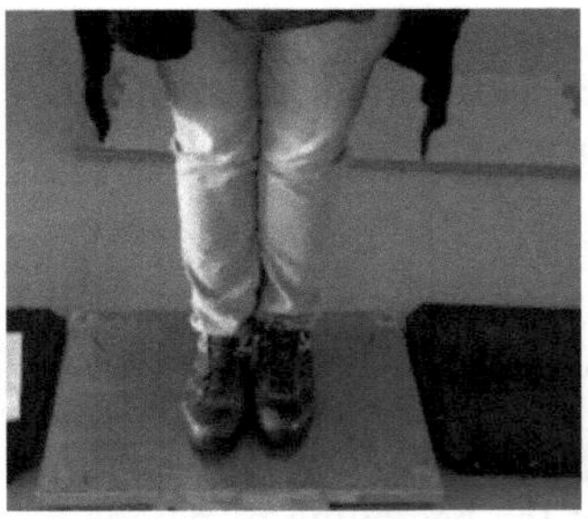

Fig.2 Small BOS 6 weeks

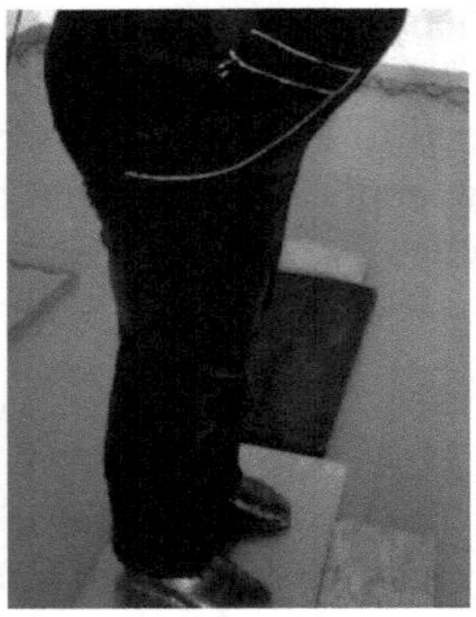

Fig.3 Intermediate BOS 36 weeks

In order to perform the dynamic testing, Kistler platform was used in dynamical conditions. The assembly used for measurement involves besides the Kistler platform, two covered wooden platforms having the role of damping the difference of level between the plate and the floor and also a buffer material. So the subject will step naturally on the plate from the wooden platform without being influenced of the gap.

The subject was instructed to step across the platform three times with the right foot and three times with the left in normal gait.(fig.4 and 5).

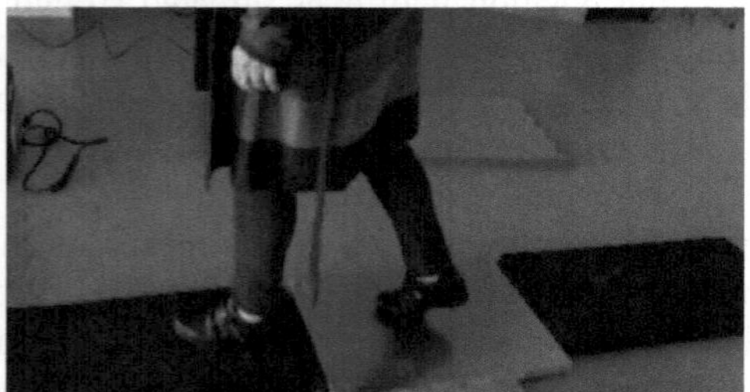

Fig.4 Normal gait at 6 weeks

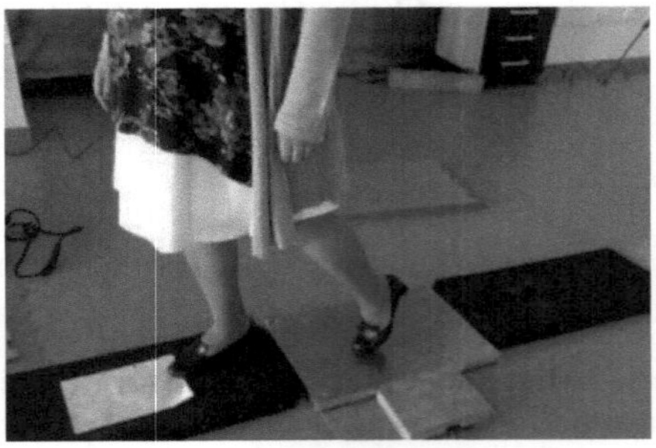

Fig.5 Normal gait at 36 weeks

She was instructed to start walking a few steps before coming in contact with the force platform in order to capture the regular allure of the gait and was tested at 6 weeks and 36 weeks pregnancy.

III. Results and Discussions

Using the dedicated Bioware software, several diagrams can be created based upon the experiments results. The most expressive results are given by the representations of the stability area, showing the positions of the vertical projections of the body center of gravity during stance for a 30s period of time, with different BOS.

In fig.6 and 7, the stability area is shown for a small BOS determined at 6 weeks and respectively 36 weeks of pregnancy.

By analyzing the diagrams it becomes obvious that there is an increased instability at 36 weeks, especially in the sagittal plane, due to the fact that a considerable weight developed in the anterior part of the trunk.

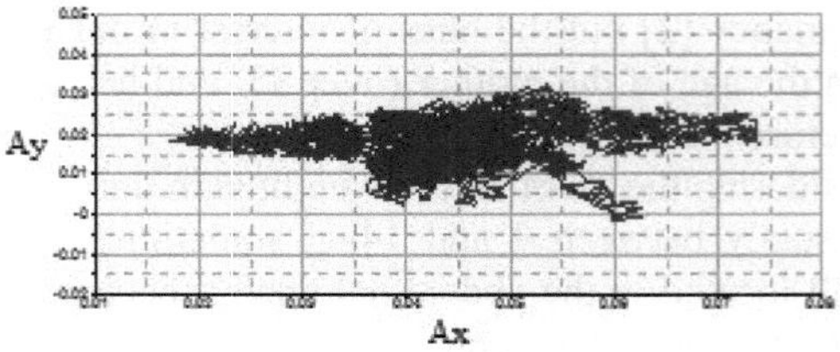

Fig.6 Stability area at 6 weeks, small BOS

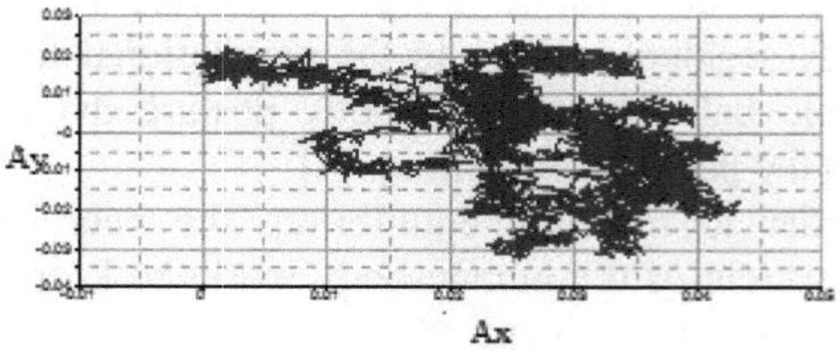

Fig.7.Stability area at 36 weeks, small BOS

At 6 weeks, the stability was almost normal, as the body structure was already adapted to the existing overweight and managed to compensate the unbalance. The posture however is affecting the spinal cord normal position.

For comparison, the stability area for both time periods is presented, this time in large BOS, which allows the subject a more secure and comfortable support area. The diagrams are shown in fig.8 and 9.

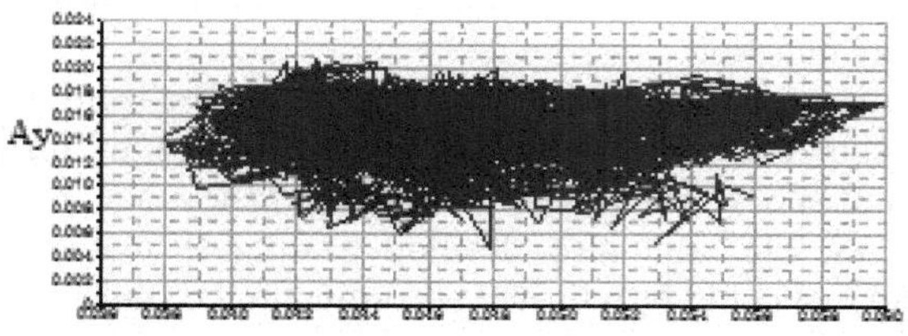

Fig.8 Stability area at 6 weeks, large BOS

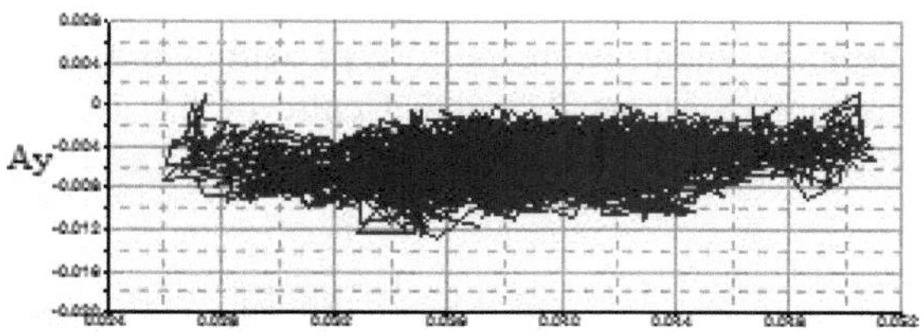

Fig.9 Stability area at 36 weeks, large BOS

The representations are showing the fact that stability is similar in large BOS, at 6 weeks and at 36 weeks, as a larger base of support offers more safety by enlarging the area where the projection of the center of gravity could fall without jeopardizing too much the subject's balance.

Viewing the statistics offered by the software, we found that the range of the projection of COG displacement on the axis Ox, that is anterior-posterior starts at 0,023m at 6 weeks and increases to 0,047 at 36 weeks in small BOS, while the values for large BOS start at 0,013m at 6 weeks to 0,015m at 36 weeks. The values on the axis Oy, expressing lateral balance are within a range of 0,027m at 6 weeks to 0,056m at 36 weeks for small BOS, while for the large BOS the range values remain the same at 0,013m both for 6 and for 36 weeks.

Another interesting parameter to present is the reaction force (Fz) in direct connection to the weight distribution on the support. The diagrams obtained for the force Fz are shown in fig.10-13, following the same conditions as for the stability area (small and large BOS, 6 weeks and 36 weeks pregnancy).

It becomes obvious by analyzing fig. 10-11 that the values of the reaction force Fz are increased at 36 weeks, from an average of 864,5 kgf at 6 weeks to an average of 976,8 kgf at 36 weeks. The values of the reaction force are not significantly different in small BOS or large BOS. However, the force Fx on anterior-posterior direction shows increased values in small BOS.

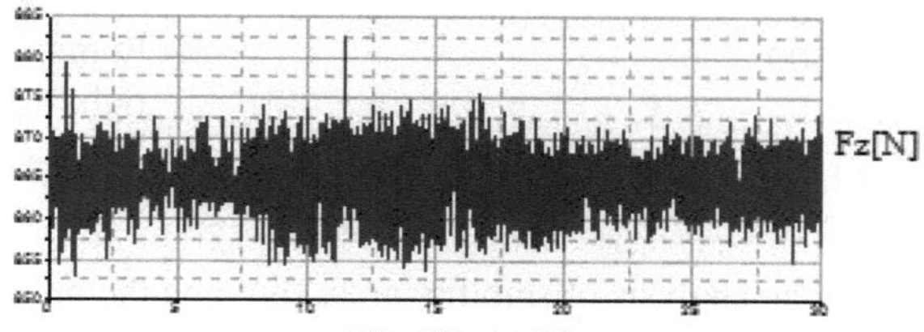

Fig.10 Fz at 6 weeks small BOS

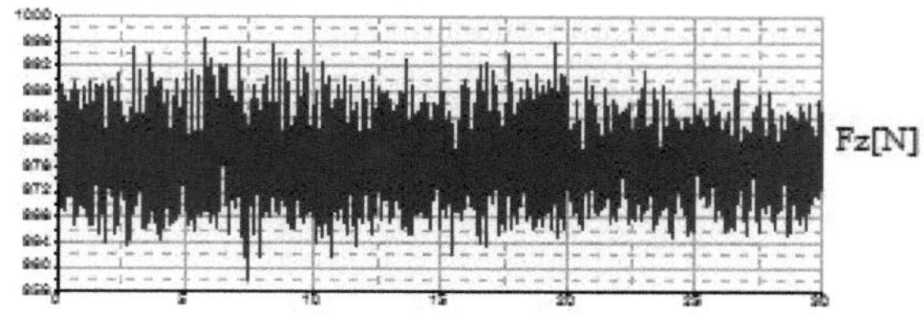

Fig.11 Fz 36 weeks small BOS

In dynamic stance, the representations of the forces on the axes Ox, Oy and Oz are shown in fig. 12 for 6 weeks and in fig.13 for 36 weeks of pregnancy.

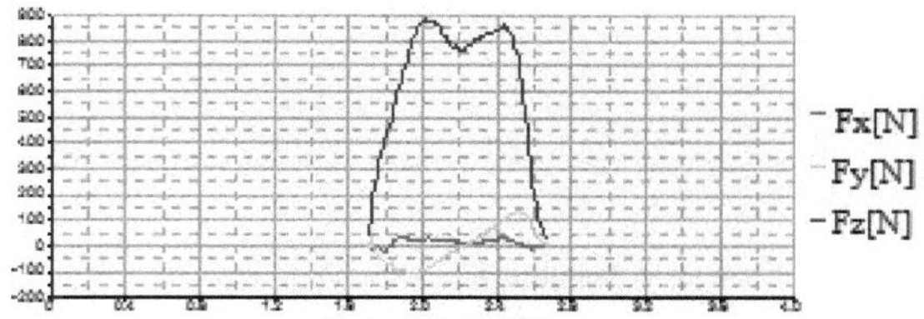

Fig. 12 Stepping with the right foot (6w)

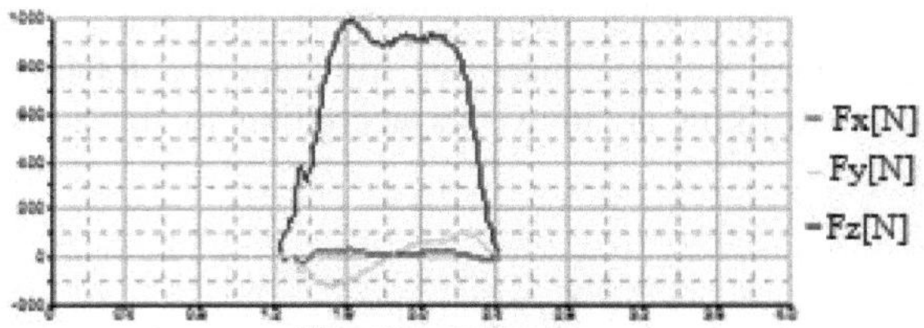

Fig. 13 Stepping with the right foot (36w)

By analyzing the dynamic diagrams of the forces variations during the contact with the platform, the first thing that can be observed is the increase of the reaction force Fz, due to the fact that the subject gained weight. The duration of the contact is longer at 36 weeks as the subject becomes a little more cautious and walks with a little difficulty. The variation of the maximum value of the reaction force for the right foot is shown for comparison in fig.14.

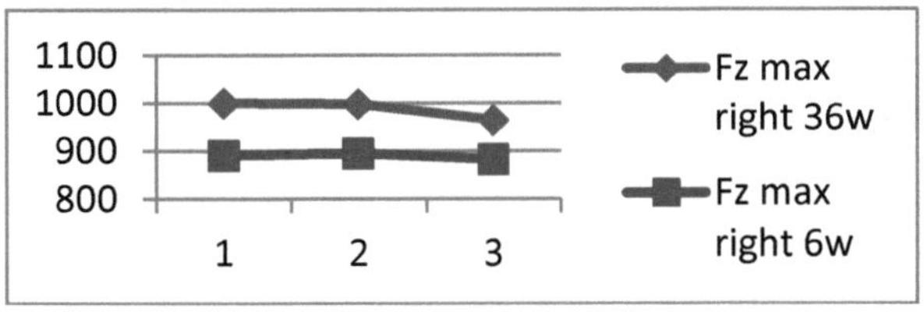

Fig.14 Variation of Fz max

Also the analysis of stability area, showing the projection of the COG on the ground during walking exhibits obvious changes in 36 weeks, the instability is pronounced due to the occurrence of some "wobbling" when the full contact of the foot with the ground takes place.

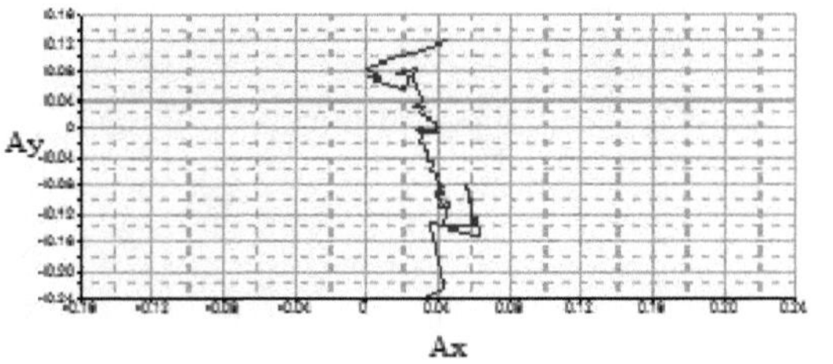

Fig. 15 Stability area at 6w, right foot

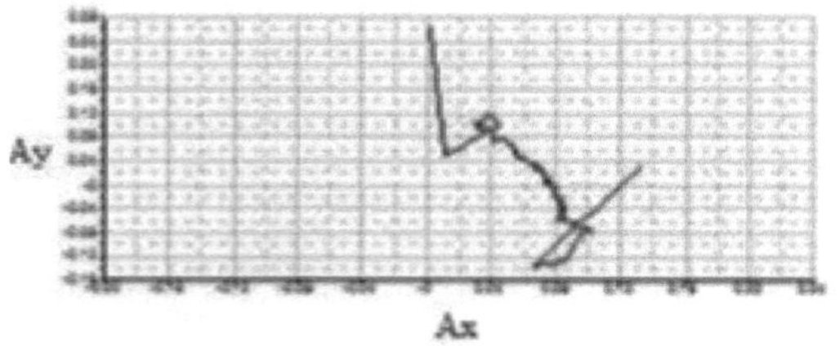

Fig.16 Stability area 36 w, right foot

In order to be able to perform the comparison, in fig.15 and 16, the stability areas are presented for 6 weeks and 36 weeks pregnancy when stepping with the right foot.

The lateral balance increases from approx. 0,04m at 6 weeks to 0,135m at 36 weeks according to the software statistics.

IV. Conclusions

Though generally pregnancy is a normal physiological state that involves some changes of the woman's body, there are situations when higher risk occurs due to several factors. Some of them are related to pre-pregnancy overweight and age over 35 years. These factors together with the postural changes, weight gain and balance difficulties might produce accidental falls leading to miscarriage or other problems.

The methodology proposed by the paper shows in an objective and non-invasive manner, the way in which stability is affected in both static and dynamic conditions, raising awareness of the balance issues and increased demands upon the human body posture, in order to help future mothers and the specialized medical staff to avoid accidents and even miscarriages due to falls during pregnancy.

Our research shows that pre-pregnancy overweight is a risk factor in accidental loss of balance and even falls, thus supporting the recommendation that future mothers should carefully monitor their weight by adequate motion and healthy nutrition.

Future researches will be carried out by the team on several subjects, considering also the influence of different types of shoes, weight gain during pregnancy, age, previous illnesses, etc. and also develop a suitable mathematical model that could be adjusted according to the subject.

Acknowledgment

The experiments were performed within the Advanced Mechatronic Systems Research Centre of the Transilvania University Research Institute.

Conflict of Interest

The authors declare that they have no conflict of interest.

References

1. Ribas SI, Guirro ECO, (2007) Analysis of plantar pressure and postural balance during different phases of pregnancy. Brasilian Journal of Physical Therapy vol.11, no.5, DOI 10.1590/S141335552007000500010
2. The Healthy Woman – A Complete Guide for all Ages, Pregnancy, at https://www.womenshealth.gov/publications/our-publications/the-healthy-woman/pregnancy.pdf
3. Opala-Berdzik A. et al., (2010) The Influence of Pregnancy on the Location of the Center of Gravity in Standing Position, Journal of Human Kinetics 26: 5-11
4. Cotoros D., Baritz M., (2010) Biomechanical Analyzes of Human Body Stability and Equilibrium, World Congress on Engineering, London, UK, pp 1145-1149
5. Cakmak B., Ribeiro A.P., Inanir A., (2016) Postural balance and the risk of falling during pregnancy, The Journal of Maternal-Fetal & Neonatal Medicine 29:1623-1625 DOI 10.3109/14767058.2015.1057490
6. Butler E., Colon I. et.al. (2006) An investigation of gait and postural balance during pregnancy, Gait&Posture 24:128-129

Author: Cotoros Diana
Institute: Transilvania University of Brasov
Street: 29 Eroilor
City: Brasov
Country: Romania
Email: dcotoros@unitbv.ro

Multipoint Wireless Network for Complex Patient Monitoring based on Embedded Processors

T. Sumalan[1], E. Lupu[1], R. Arsinte[1] and E. Onaca[2]

[1] Communications Department, Technical University, Cluj-Napoca, Romania
[2] Family Medicine Dept., "Iuliu Hatieganu" U.M.Ph., Cluj-Napoca, Romania

Abstract— **The present paper presents an approach to the patients or elderly persons monitoring able to oversee some vital signs for more persons in a delimited area. The system is able to collect also the images of patients. Wireless sensors networks (WSNs) became a successful alternative to cabled systems used for surveillance or monitoring. The system is based on the ZigBee wireless technology and using a low-cost Beagle Board, designed with the DM3730 embedded processors. Even if the data rates provided by the ZigBee technology are not very high the application proposed can be successfully achieved using this low-cost approach.**

Keywords— **WSN, ZigBee, embedded processor, vital sign monitoring.**

I. Introduction

In our days the technology reaches a new level of improvement. Medicine is one of the largest areas who are dependent by evolution of technology. One of the biggest problems in hospitals is to monitoring persons, patients with chronic diseases, independent living seniors and the in-patients who have to be cared for in assisted living facilities. WSN technology could be used for monitoring vital signs of some patients on ambulatory, emergency rooms and post-operative care.

Healthcare monitoring: the medical applications might be of two sorts: wearable and implanted. Wearable devices are applied to the body surface of the human or maybe at close proximity from the user. The implantable medical devices are the ones that are inserted inside your body. There are numerous other applications too e.g. body position measurement of the person, overall monitoring of ill patients in hospitals and also at homes. [1]

Researchers from different areas are working towards "smart healthcare" [2]. For instance, some applications are focused on continuous medical monitoring for degenerative diseases (Parkinson's, Alzheimer's) or other cognitive disorders. The "Code Blue" project at Harvard employs WSNs for medical applications in disasters, while other projects focus on high-bandwidth, sensor-rich environments. Another example of application in the Romanian area is presented in [3].

Using WSN technologies for smart healthcare provide some important features, like:

- portability and unobtrusiveness. Very small devices gather data and communicate by wireless connection, network setups can be carried out without fixed infrastructure;
- ease of deployment and scalability. Devices can be used in large numbers with less complexity and cost compared to wired networks;
- real-time and always-on. The continuously monitored data, (physiological and environmental) allow real-time response by workers in healthcare or emergency scenario (it can be accessed by using a centralized monitor);
- reconfiguration and self-organization. The miss of wired connections allow removing or adding sensors which leads to instant reconfiguration of the network. [1]

The wireless technologies [4] differ in a number of dimensions, most notably in just how much bandwidth they provide and how far apart communicating nodes can be. Other important differences include the electromagnetic spectrums they choose and consumed power. The wireless technologies of interest for this type of application are: Bluetooth (802.15.1), ZigBee (802.15.4), Wi-Fi (802.11g), Wi-MAX (802.16), and 3G cellular wireless. Some details of the main features for these technologies can be found in [3] [4].

Our purpose was to implement a wireless system able to monitor some vital signs parameters of patients with chronic diseases or elderly persons and also make a real surveillance. The system was implemented based on the ZigBee technology which provides some suitable features like: simplicity, flexibility and low cost. For a better hard-ware component simplification, we focused on system functionality therefore the values of the parameters are emulated by lookup tables in the acquisition node side.

II. The System Architecture Presentation

The system contains a PC dispatcher and a series of acquisition modules, in a multipoint architecture. The acquisition system is based on two types of modules: the acquisition module based on the BeagleBoard-xM platform (this module is used to gather images and data from patients) and the visualization module employed in data collection from

S. Vlad and N.M. Roman (eds.), *International Conference on Advancements of Medicine and Health Care through Technology; 12th - 15th October 2016, Cluj-Napoca, Romania,*
IFMBE Proceedings 59,
DOI: 10.1007/978-3-319-52875-5_28

acquisition modules (see fig 1). The physiological parameters are scanned from a lookup table for each vital parameter. The range of values for the selected parameters (pulse, blood pressure and body temperature) covers the normal and abnormal values to verify the correct functionality of the system.

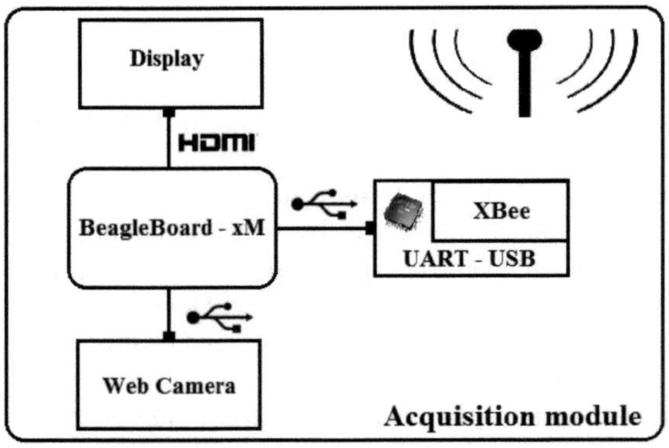

Fig.1 The main architecture of acquisition system (one node)

An XBee-Pro module is also connected to the acquisition platform through an USB-serial adapter. The patient images and parameters are transmitted using XBee-Pro radio modules implementing the Zigbee communication protocol, when an abnormally monitored parameter value occurs. For the collector module, in order to gather data from the acquisition nodes we employ a laptop/PC, where the images and data arrive from multiple acquisition systems (patients). The computer is also connected to an XBee-Pro module in order to be part of the radio communication network with the acquisitions nodes.

A. Hardware module

a) Dual-core DM3730 based Embedded System

BeagleBoard-xM is a single board computer built for the Open Source community and is suitable for health monitoring applications and other embedded applications as previous experiments proved. DM3730 (Texas Instr.), a processor used also in some generations of smart-phones, is based on a dual-core hybrid architecture (ARM + DSP) Digital Media Processor compatible with OMAP™3 architecture and has the following significant properties [6].

The Beagle-Board XM is a DM3730 based development board and contains all the needed components in order to access peripherals such as mouse, keyboard, monitor, memory cards/sticks, internet, USB, WLAN adaptor speakers, microphone [7]. The BeagleBoard has a local disk (MicroSD card) that is loaded with a Linux OS. Angstrom is the most used Linux distribution on BeagleBoard and it is also the recommended option for an operating system [8].

b) ZigBee-Pro module

XBee-Pro PRO RF Module (Radio frequency) meets the IEEE 802.15.4 specifications and supports the basic needs of a low-cost and low-power wireless network. The module operates in the ISM band (Industrial, Scientific and Medical) of 2.4 GHz, and has a fixed RF data rate (250 Kbps). Various network topologies are supported: point-to-point, point-to-multipoint and peer-to-peer [9].

c) ZigBee-ProUSB Explorer

XBee-Pro USB Explorer is an adapter board from USB to UART line for the Xbee modules. Xbee modules must be connected to Xbee Explorer and it will get direct access to serial communication terminals and programming pins of the Xbee unit. [10].

B. Key Tools for Software support

a) X-CTU application

X-CTU is a free multi-platform application designed to enable developers to interact with Digi [11] RF modules through a simple-to-use graphical user interface. X-CTU 6.3.2 a new version of X-CTU tool includes unique features like graphical network view, witch graphically represents the XBee network along with the signal strength of each connection, and the XBee API frame builder, which builds and interprets API frames being used in API mode, combine to make development on the XBee platform easier.

The Frame generator (generate any kind of frame), Frame interpreter (decode a specific frame and see its value), Recovery (recovers radio modules with damaged firmware), Range test (performing a range test between two end points from the same network);

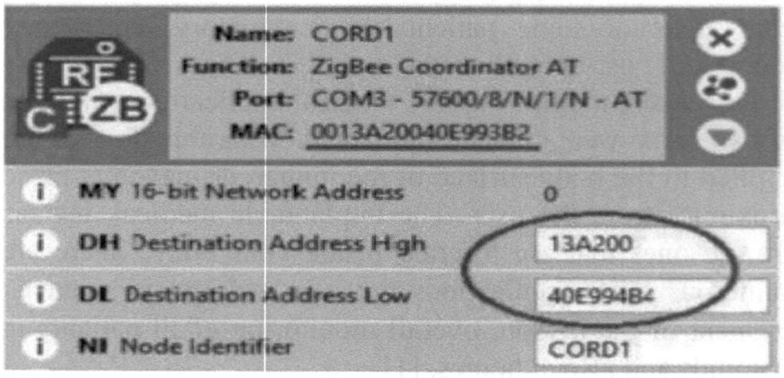

Fig.2 X-CTU tool interface used for modules configuration [11]

b) Open-Source Computer Vision Library

OpenCV [12] is an open source computer vision and machine learning software library. This library was built to provide a common infrastructure for computer vision application and to accelerate the use of machine vision in the commercial products. Being a BSD licensed product, OpenCV makes it easy for user to utilize and modify the code. The library has a lot of optimized algorithms, which includes a comprehensive set of both classic and state of the art computer vision and machine learning algorithms. It has C, Python, Java and MATLAB interfaces and supports Windows, Linux, Android and Mac OS. OpenCV targets real-time vision applications and takes advantage of MMX and SSE instructions when available. OpenCV is written natively in C++ and has a templated interface that works with STL containers [12].

III. The Implementation Of The System. Experiments.

The system is composed from two acquisition parts based on BeagleBoard-xM platform and a data collector part represented by a computer. Communication between devices is performed by ZigBee protocol using the XBee modules. First of all the modules were initialized using X-CTU software tool with the desired rates in order to allow communication.

For experimental purposes, some real strings of values for the physiological parameters (pulse, blood pressure and body temperature) were stored in the acquisition systems like lookup tables. Fig.3. is illustrating the values of abnormal systolic and diastolic blood pressure for a labile arterial hypertension patient.

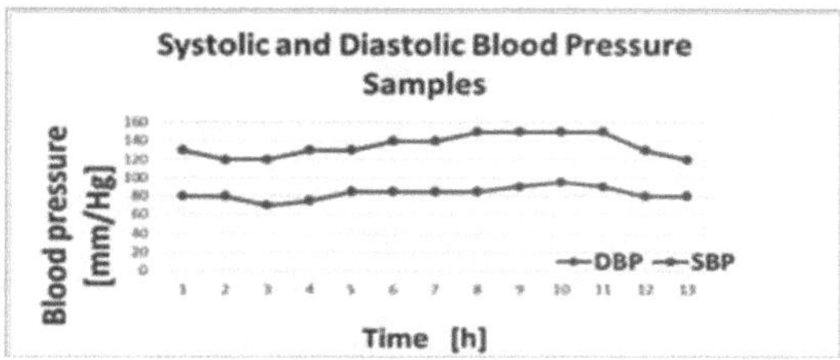

Fig.3 Abnormal blood pressure from experiments

Fig. 4 presents a simplified flowchart of the application with the main steps performed by the acquisition node software.

In this kind of configuration the application running on the collector side allows to display the patient's received image on the computer screen. If the number of acquisition nodes (number of patients) is more than one it will create new frames instances for each patient. In this case the XBee modules can exchange information without any monitoring. The ZigBee network was composed from one XBee module used like router and the other modules, one for each patient, was configured as end points (coordinators). The system works by following algorithm: all images of the patient are captured and the values of vital parameters are scanned at an adequate rate, which may be selected. The sample rate will be set one hour for temperature and blood pressure and for the pulse we choose to sample at every five minutes. Then the values of the vital parameters are compared with the alarm threshold and if an out of range value is detected the subsystem begins to send images with the superimposed parameters value toward the collector system. Because we have two or more acquisition modules we first of all will send an ID, unique for each module. This ID is write as a header in each data packet before begin sent.

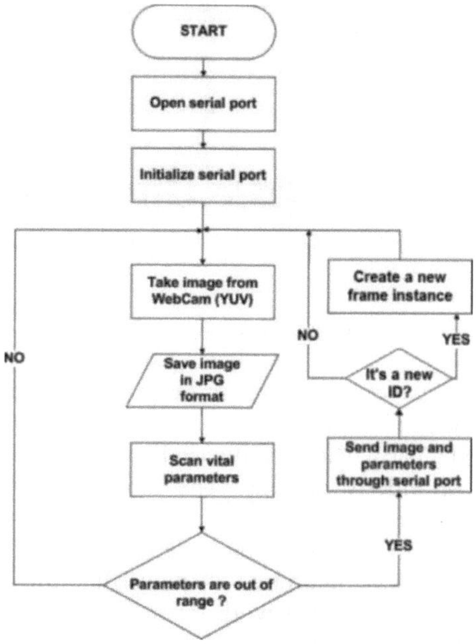

Fig.4 The application flowchart running on BeagleBoard-XM

At the receiver a dynamic matrix is automatically declared for each newly ID that was found. If the number of acquisition modules is more than one, a prioritization algorithm will manage the package prioritization. The alarm threshold may be set by the user depending of patient age and disease. In our experiments we choose the normal range for the temperature (36.5-37°C), for the pulse (60-100 beats/min) and for blood pressure: 90< SBP<140 mm Hg, 70<DBP<90 mm Hg. For retrieving an image from the video camera we used Gst-launch, a tool that builds and runs streams. It is based on integrating different plug-ins for reading and writing in certain file formats and also for converting between different formats. In this case a JPEG encoder is used for converting from video format to JPEG format. For the VGA resolution of (640x480) of the video camera, we transmit a file of 60kB average size. An image processing is necessary for interpolating the values of vital parameters and the date and time stamps on the image. For the interpolation of text on the image the OpenCV library was employed. Fig. 5 presents two instances of patient images with the physiological parameters, received by the collector. The delay introduced in the image transmission, for a detection of out of range value, for one or more vital parameters to the acquisition node, and the image reception to the collector is about 8 seconds for a 57.6 Kbps rate [13].

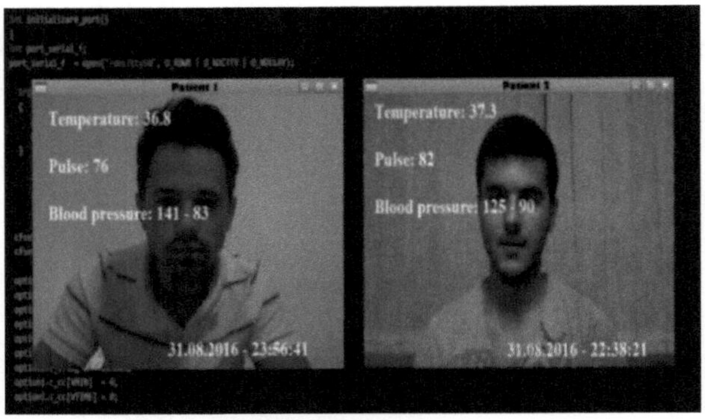

Fig.5 Two patient images received from two acquisitions nodes

IV. Conclusions And Outlook

In this paper we have presented a low-cost, multi-operational and experimental system for monitoring people who need a particular surveillance like patients with chronic disease or elderly persons. The monitoring system was designed to work on a WSN network using the ZigBee technology. The acquisition node is developed around the BeagleBoard-xM platform, a powerful low-cost single board computer. Similar work for long term ECG monitoring using this platform is presented in [14]. To prove the functionality of monitoring system we decide to emulate the selected physiological parameters (pulse, blood pressure and body temperature) by strings of real values and sampled at an adequate rate, set by the user. Additionally, the trend to increase nominal read rate, allows flexible monitoring for a better safety, but it also modify the protocol. For this situation we will realize a TCP/IP communication protocol between the modules. The number of nodes actually implemented is three, and is limited by the number of BeagleBoard modules available in the lab. Increasing the number will be a challenge for the applications and communication capabilities of the system. There are several future directions and open problems. One open problem is the fact that critical systems that rely on computing devices already have a high complexity. If these systems include wireless computing devices, additional precautions are necessary to ensure that the computing devices balance safety with convenience and do not introduce unacceptable risks. Medical device design is one such situation. We will make a serious risk analysis in the next phases of the project.

There are few obvious minor next steps and our research will require innovative actions. This work emphasizes the need for a principled and deeper investigation into prevention mechanisms, detection mechanisms and vital signs determination methods. The application of the system outside hospitals will increase the functionality. Such innovations will become crucial, as the technologies and capabilities for the new monitoring devices continue to evolve.

Conflict of Interest

The authors declare that they have no conflict of interest.

References

1. T. Prashnt, V. Prakas, G. Raj "Wireless Sensor Networks: Introduc-tion, Advantages, Application and Research Challenges" HCTL Open IJTIR, Vol.14,Apr. 2015
2. T. Sumalan, E. Lupu, R. Arsinte, E. Onaca – "Low-Cost Wireless System for Patient Monitoring", The 5-th edition of the International Conference on e-Health and Bioengineering, EHB 2015, 19-21 November 2015, Iasi, Romania
3. O. Morancea, H Costin et al. "Telemon – Romanian Experience for Real Time Telemonitoring of Chronic Patients and Elderly People" Health 2008 - Int. Workshop on Wearable, Micro and Nano Technologies for the Personalised Health, Valencia, Spain, May 2008
4. Crossley GH, Boyle A, Vitense H, et al, CONNECT Investigators. The CONNECT (Clinical evaluation of remote notification to reduce time to clinical decision) trial. J.Am.Coll.Cardio.2011,vol 57: 1181–9.
5. Bowman D. mHealth Summit2013: Remote Monitoring helps CHRISTUS Health slash patient costs. http://www.fiercemobilehealthcare.com/story/mhealth-summit-2013-remote-monitoring-helps-christus-health-slash-patient-c/2013-12-11.
6. ZigBee Alliance Document 053474r17, ZigBee Specification, v. 1.0 r17, Z. Alliance, Editor. 2007.
7. DM3730 datasheet: Texas Instruments. Digital Media Processors. July, 2011. Literature Nr: SPRS685D.
8. BeagleBoard XM System Reference Manual, Rev. C3.0, May 2009.
9. XBee®/XBee-PRO® RF Modules, Product Manual
10. XBee Explorer Serial documentation http://www.sparkfun.com
11. X-CTU, http://www.digi.com/products/xbee-rf-solutions/xctu-software/xctu
12. Open Source Computer Vision, http://docs.opencv.org/
13. E. Lupu et al. "Evaluation of ZigBee Technology for a Low-cost Video Surveillance System", Vol. 44 of IFMBE Proc 2014, pp 233-236
14. Kane JM, Perlis RH et al. First experience with a wire-less system incorporating physiologic assessments and direct confirmation of digital tablet ingestions in ambulatory patients with schizophrenia or bipolar disorder. J Clin Psychiatry. Jun 2013; 74(6): pp. 533-534

Author: Eugen Lupu
Institute: Technical University of Cluj-Napoca
Street: 26-28 Baritiu Str.
City: Cluj-Napoca
Country: Romania
Email Eugen.Lupu@com.utcluj.ro

Automated Titration of Oxygen Fraction in Inspiratory Mixture in Mechanical Ventilation of Life-size Mannequin

M. Rožánek[1], P. Kudrna[1] and V. Králová[1]

[1] Department of Biomedical Technology, Czech Technical University in Prague, Kladno, Czech Republic

Abstract— **Mechanical ventilation is often used in patients suffering inadequate oxygenation. Many ventilator regimens have been already introduced, however mechanical ventilation still causes significant adverse effects. Practicing an intubation and guidance of mechanical ventilation can be crucial for a successful use of mechanical ventilation in the clinical practice. Use of simulators with life-size mannequins represents a unique opportunity to realize simulations with a high fidelity. Aim of this paper is to introduce a scenario prepared for a demonstration of automated ventilatory regimen with automatically controlled fraction of oxygen in a ventilatory mixture with a possibility of studying the effect of ventilatory parameters upon vital signs of the mannequin. The simulator with life-size mannequin and real medical devices used in the simulation increase its fidelity and are used in education of biomedical technicians, biomedical engineers and medical rescuers.**

Keywords—**fraction of oxygen, mechanical ventilation, simulation, close loop system, life-size simulator, mannequin.**

I. INTRODUCTION

Mechanical ventilation (MV) is an important technique that can replace a spontaneous breathing for some time. It is used to deliver oxygen and remove carbon dioxide in patients with inadequate spontaneous breathing or with intentionally inhibited spontaneous breathing. One of the important aims of MV is a maintenance of blood gases inside physiological limits [1, 2].

Preterm born babies require MV very often because of lung immaturity. It is necessary to use a ventilatory mixture with increased fraction of oxygen (FiO_2) in many cases to maintain a proper oxygenation, on the other hand it is advisable to minimize FiO_2 considering adverse effects of higher partial pressure of oxygen upon the lung tissue and the patient's organism [3].

Oxygen saturation of the blood is commonly monitored to evaluate the oxygenation of the organism. It is routinely measured by a monitor of vital signs and too low level of the saturation turns on an alarm. There are cases when the premature infants requiring MV are supported by ventilation with the ventilatory mixture with useless high FiO_2. It can result in a few diseases, e.g. bronchopulmonary dysplasia and retinopathy [4, 5, 6].

There are a few automated systems to control FiO_2 in a close loop system according to the monitored vital signs. One of them is a CLiO2 system that is commercially available in Avea (Carefusion, Yorba Linda, CA) ventilators. CLiO2 represents the close loop system that automatically adjusts the FiO_2 in the ventilatory mixture according to the level of oxygen saturation in the arterial blood. It helps maintain a safe blood oxygen level in a long term MV with an adequate fraction of oxygen in the ventilatory mixture. It can contribute to better care for neonates.

Wilinska et al. describe effects observed during a titration of FiO_2 in the ventilatory mixture in newborns. They compared two manual approaches called attentive and observing with automated system CLiO2 in two ventilated newborns with stable and unstable blood oxygenation. The target range of oxygen saturation was specified at 87-93 %. The results shown that there was less time that newborns spend outside the target SpO_2 range with CLiO2 compared to the manual settings. There was a slight difference for the stable patient while higher differences were seen at the unstable patient. There were also lower nursing times required for CLiO2 period [7].

Education and training is crucial for a proper administration and guidance of many medical devices and approaches. Therefore, simulations have unique importance in the biomedical engineering and simulators and models are very important for the education of the students and the further training and education of a medical staff. They are used also for a calibration of the medical devices or a check of their function. The simulations are also very important for neonatology which is quite specific in many domains [8].

There is a special group of the simulators called patient simulators. These simulators contain life-size mannequin to emphasize the reality of the simulation of taking care about a real patient. Mannequins support a lot of basic procedures required when examine the patient. The mannequins support a connection of a ventilator and support MV of the lungs. Human patient simulator (CAE Healthcare, Sarasota, FL) is one of the commercially available systems equipped with the mannequins.

The Human Patient Simulator (HPS) is intended for the training of practical skills and solution of crisis and severe situations. HPS consists of three components; HPS lab rack,

S. Vlad and N.M. Roman (eds.), *International Conference on Advancements of Medicine and Health Care through Technology; 12th - 15th October 2016, Cluj-Napoca, Romania,*
IFMBE Proceedings 59,
DOI: 10.1007/978-3-319-52875-5_29

instructor workstation with software Müse and life-size mannequin based on the human anatomy. Software Müse is used for a control of the model including parameters of the mannequin.

HPS is equipped with anatomically accurate upper airways that support a practice of difficult airway management techniques. An endotracheal tube can be placed and use of MV is supported. Lungs are formed by two bellows that are placed in Lab Rack and the ventilatory mixture used for the ventilation of the mannequin is moved to the Lab Rack from the mannequin and its composition is analyzed with each breath. It allows to use different FiO_2 in the ventilatory mixture and one can see its effect upon the blood gases of the mannequin. HPS simulates a consumption of oxygen and a production of carbon dioxide. Therefore, HPS allows simulation of end tidal carbon dioxide concentration that can be analyzed by the monitor of the vital signs. One part of HPS is a module OxSim simulating SpO_2 signal that can be also measured by the standard monitor of the vital signs. Mannequin of HPS represents an adult human with its size, weight and other basic parameters of the vital signs, e.g. tidal volume about 8 mL/kg. A lot of parameters can be adjusted in the control software Müse that allows to change the individual parameters of the mannequin, e.g. the consumption of oxygen or the production of carbon dioxide in breathing.

The aim of the paper is to introduce a scenario designed to demonstrate the close loop ventilatory regimen CLiO2. Ventilator Avea and simulator HPS are connected to design a close loop system with controlled FiO_2 according to the oxygen saturation of the arterial blood. The effects of middle and severe desaturation are studied.

II. METHODS

We have used mechanical ventilator Avea to ventilate the life-size mannequin HPS. Automated system CLiO2 can be activated only in the neonatal ventilator mode where tidal volume is limited to 300 mL. Initial ventilatory parameters used in the demonstration are summarized in Table 1.

Table 1 Ventilatory parameters set on Avea ventilator in the neonatal ventilatory regimen.

Ventilatory parameter	Value
Tidal volume	300 mL
Ventilatory frequency	30 bpm
PEEP	4 cmH_2O
Initial fraction of oxygen	25 %

Demonstration of a desaturation was started with a volume-controlled ventilation and normoventilation was achieved by a change of the parameters of HPS that are related to the breathing or ventilation. Because HPS mannequin represents an adult human it was necessary to adjust its parameters corresponding to the lower tidal volume used in the neonatal ventilatory regimen CLiO2. Following parameters of HPS were changed (see Table 2) and held constant in the demonstration of automated ventilatory regimen CLiO2.

Table 2 Parameters set on HPS.

HPS parameter	Value
O_2 consumption	20 mL/min
CO_2 production factor	0.6
$PetCO_2$-$PaCO_2$ factor	1.3
$PaCO_2$ Set-Point	60 mmHg

The consumption of oxygen was decreased to 20 mL/min to simulate a small oxygen consumption of a neonatal patient. The production of carbon dioxide was also decreased corresponding to a smaller amount produced by a neonate. A $PetCO_2$-$PaCO_2$ factor was set to 1.3 increasing partial pressure of carbon dioxide in exhaled gas in contrast to partial pressure of carbon dioxide in the arterial blood. Value of $PaCO_2$ set-point changes the sensitivity of the HPS to level of the partial pressure of carbon dioxide in the arterial blood.

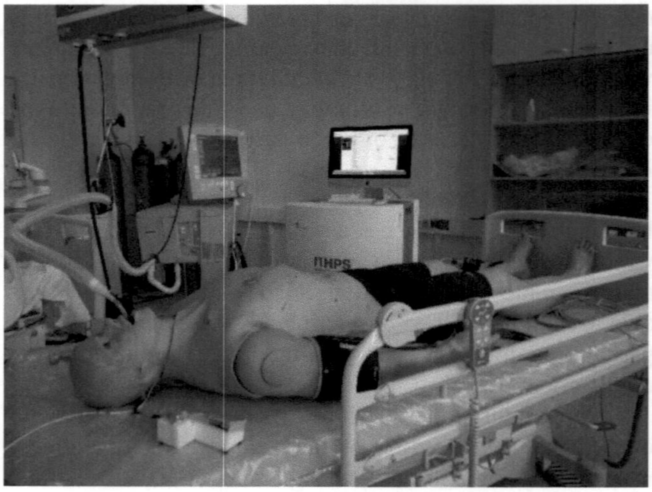

Fig. 1. Experimental settings with HPS and Avea.

A scenario in Müse software was prepared for the experimental demonstration. The scenario starts with a stabilization period where the vital signs become stabilized close to common physiological values. Neuromuscular blockade (NMB) follows in the second part of the scenario. NMB is set on

99%, followed by a reduction of the spontaneous tidal volume. Subsequently, HPS mannequin was intubated with an endotracheal tube and connected to ventilator Avea.

The automated regimen CLiO2 was set on the ventilator and moderate and severe desaturation was simulated. The automatic change of FiO_2 in the inspired ventilatory mixture was observed according to the level of desaturation. The scenario was prepared for each experimental phase including the change of the selected parameters in a specified time. It assures synchronous change of more parameters in one moment.

The values of oxygen saturation and partial pressure of oxygen in the arterial blood were downloaded from the software Müse and the values of corresponding FiO_2 were written down from the ventilator.

III. Results

The results of conducted simulations are depicted in the following figures. A five minute time course of the oxygen saturation of the mannequin and FiO_2 in the ventilatory mixture are depicted in Fig. 2.

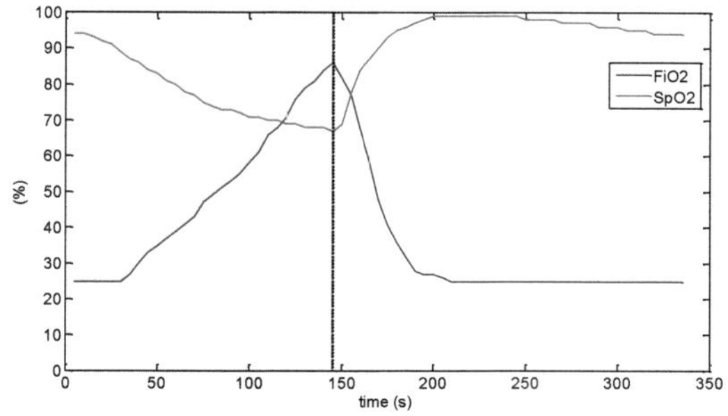

Fig. 2. Time courses of fraction of oxygen in the ventilatory mixture and oxygen saturation.

Corresponding time course of simulated partial pressure of oxygen in the arterial blood is depicted in Fig. 3.

Increased heart rate in the period of desaturation is depicted in Fig. 4.

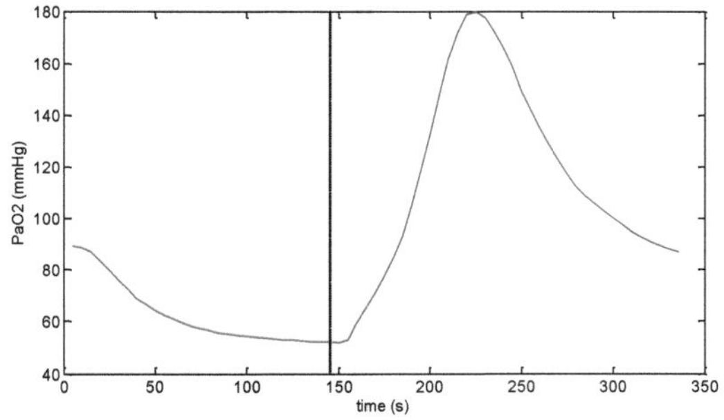

Fig. 3. Time course of partial pressure of oxygen in the arterial blood in severe desaturation.

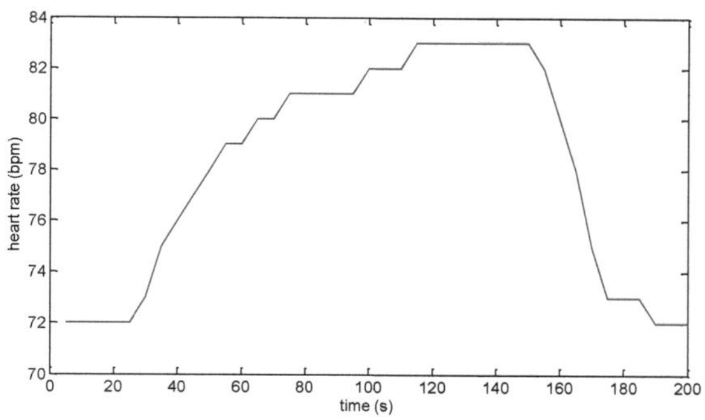

Fig. 4. Time course of the heart rate in severe desaturation.

IV. Discussion

The target range for the oxygen saturation for the purposes of the demonstration was set in 88-95 %. When the oxygen saturation falls under 88 % the ventilator in automated regimen should increase FiO_2 in the ventilatory mixture to compensate a desaturation. This dependence can be seen in Fig. 2 where the time course of the oxygen saturation in the arterial blood is depicted for the simulated scenario of severe desaturation at the patient.

The initial value of FiO_2 in the ventilatory mixture, which was set at 25 % is automatically increasing after a fall of the oxygen saturation in the arterial blood below 88 %. There is a delay approximately 20 seconds in the reaction of the ventilator. The algorithm of the control of FiO_2 takes into account also a time response of the changes in the oxygen saturation. FiO_2 changes quickly (less than 5 seconds) if there is a quick change of the oxygen saturation. It can be seen in 145th second of the time courses of the signals in Fig. 2.

One can see a significant delay in the time course of partial pressure of oxygen in the arterial blood (Fig. 3) in simulated severe desaturation. The value of PaO_2 reached 180 mmHg in maximum.

Rapid changes of the heart rate are depicted in Fig. 4. One can see the increase of the heart rate with decreasing oxygen saturation with a maximum heart rate 83 beats per minute. The heart rate is even quickly decreasing after 150 s of the experiment in finishing desaturation.

Developed scenarios allow a demonstration of the desaturation of an organism and studying of the vital signs of the mannequin and its dependence on the parameters of MV.

V. Conclusions

Connection of the mannequin with the mechanical ventilator and developed scenario of the severe desaturation of the organism represents a perfect tool for the education of medical and technical staff. Medical devices are placed together with HPS in the special laboratory of the simulated intensive care unit and together with the realized scenario will be used for the education of biomedical technicians, biomedical engineers and medical rescuers. Introduced experimental settings gives a unique opportunity to train and practice intubation, setting the ventilator and study the interaction of the ventilator and the patient.

Acknowledgment

This study was supported by grant of Czech Technical University in Prague SGS15/228/OHK4/3T/17.

Conflict of Interest

The authors declare that they have no conflict of interest.

References

1. Jonson B (1999) Mechanical Ventilation and lung mechanics. Anaesthesia, Pain, Intensive care and emergency medicine, Springer, Milan
2. Ch. L. Weber (2002) Pulmonary function, Volume and Ventilation, Loyola University, Chicago
3. Rimensberger P (2015) Pediatric and Neonatal Mechanical Ventilation: From Basics to Clinical Practice, Springer
4. Dort J, Dortová E, Jehlička P (2013) Neonatologie. Karolinum, Prague. ISBN 978-80-246-2253-8
5. Leifer G. (2004) Úvod do porodnického a pediatrického ošetřovatelství. Grada, Prague. ISBN 80-247-0668-7
6. Fendrychová J, Janková M, Ryšavá M, Rybníček O. (2001) Dlouhodobá péče o dítě s bronchopulmonální dysplázií. Pediatrie pro praxi. ISSN 1803-5264
7. Wilinska M, Bachman T, Swietlinski J (2012) Time Required for Effective FiO2-Titration in Preterm Infants: a Comparison. Respiratory Therapy 7:71-73
8. Shukla A, Kline D, Cherian A, et al. (2007) A Simulation Course on Lifesaving Techniques for Third-Year Medical Students. Simulation in Healthcare 2:11-15

A Study of the Effects of Geometry on the Efficiency of Single Slot Microwave Ablation Antennas used in Hepatic Tumor Hyperthermia

V. Neagu

Technical University of Cluj Napoca/Faculty of Electrical Engineering, Cluj Napoca, Romania

Abstract— **Microwave ablation (MWA) has gained appreciation as an alternative to radio frequency ablation in the treatment of tumors. In this paper, COMSOL Multiphysics software is used to perform an analysis of single slot, end-capped MWA antenna with a variable geometry fed at a frequency range between 900MHz and 2500MHz, with the purpose of finding configurations that reduce reflections, increase the power transfer to the hepatic tissue and produce faster heating, giving a more efficient antenna design.**

Keywords— **microwave, ablation, tumor, simulation, optimization**

I. INTRODUCTION

Thermal ablation is the process of destroying unwanted tissue by changing its temperature, either by raising (above ~50-60°C) or lowering it (typically freezing) to cytotoxic levels. This can be performed through a number of techniques, including laser, radio frequency currents (RF), cryoablation and microwave ablation (MWA), the latter gaining more attention in recent years as an alternative to RF [1, 2]. These techniques offer an alternative treatment for patients suffering from malignancies that are not eligible for surgical resection either due to positioning of the tumor close to blood vessels and other structures, insufficient healthy tissue, number of tumor spots or comorbidities. There is absolute evidence of the damaging effects of cancer on the body and studies have found that, if left untreated, hepatocellular carcinoma has a mortality rate of 100% after 5 years, claiming more than 1 million lives per year [3].

MWA operates on the principle of exciting polar molecules (typically water or protein) through the use of varying electromagnetic fields. During MWA, an antenna is inserted into the target tumor laparoscopically, percutaneously or under open surgery with imaging techniques such as ultrasound or CT guidance. The antenna radiates microwave energy resulting in tissue molecules rapidly changing orientation to match that of the EM field, creating heat through friction. As a direct consequence of this, the method is dependent on the tissue's properties, most importantly its water content which is directly linked to the tissue's relative permittivity. Studies have found that MWA gives better results in low conductivity tissues like bone or lung compared to RF ablation in terms of penetration depth and frequency dependent scattering patterns [4]. This paper focuses on an interval of frequencies which includes the industry standard 2.45GHz, shown to offer good results in terms of energy transfer, size of ablation zone and temperature gradients [5, 6].

II. MATERIALS AND METHODS

A. Reflection coefficient and heat transfer

A good measure of an antenna's efficiency is the ratio between feed power and reflected power described by its reflection coefficient, Γ given by:

$$\Gamma = 10 \cdot log_{10}\left(\frac{P_r}{P_{in}}\right)[\text{dB}] \qquad (1)$$

It is desired that this coefficient be as small as possible which denotes a good transfer of power from the generator to the site of the tumor. Antennas operating at high reflection coefficients can cause overheating of the waveguide which cause damage not only to healthy tissue surrounding the antenna but also to the microwave generator [7].

The most commonly used equation for describing heat transfer in biological tissue is the Pennes equation, below:

$$\rho C\,\frac{\partial T}{\partial t} = \nabla \cdot (k_{th}\nabla T) + Q_{met} - Q_p + Q_{ext} \qquad (2)$$

where the first, second, third and fourth right terms denote heat conduction, metabolic heat generation, heat loss due to blood perfusion due to the "heat sink" effect and absorbed heat due to exterior sources [8]. When normalized by tissue density, Q_{ext} is referred to as specific absorption rate (SAR).

B. Mathematical model

The geometry of the problem allows for a 2D axisymmetric rotation model to be built in COMSOL Multiphysics. The coaxial antenna is one of the most preferred applicators in MWA due to its small dimensions which allow for easier use in interstitial spaces, as well as its ease of manufacturing. Dimensions for the antenna were selected to allow for the variation in geometry required for the study. The anten-

S. Vlad and N.M. Roman (eds.), *International Conference on Advancements of Medicine and Health Care through Technology; 12th - 15th October 2016, Cluj-Napoca, Romania,*
IFMBE Proceedings 59,
DOI: 10.1007/978-3-319-52875-5_30

na was modeled with a polytetrafluoroethylene (PTFE) coating to simulate the catheter it would be placed in. Studies have shown the impact this coating has on antenna efficiency [9]. Power is supplied through a Port condition on the top boundary of the antenna using 10W. For the purpose of this paper, the frequency will be variable. A slot with position from antenna tip and height parametrically controlled was then modeled. A sufficiently large cylindrical sample of homogenous hepatic tissue was then modeled around the antenna. As such, Q_p in eq. (2) is constant in the modeled volume. It is important to note then that the response will depend on vascularization, with proximity to major blood vessels greatly increasing this factor. The tissue radius is selected several times larger than the maximum penetration depth of microwaves in hepatic tissue to minimize changes of leftover energy reaching the edges of the model and causing unwanted reflections. The initial geometry and temperature field is illustrated in fig. 1. The 50°C isotherm is the one closest to the antenna tip. Antenna and liver dimensional and material properties can be found in Table 1.

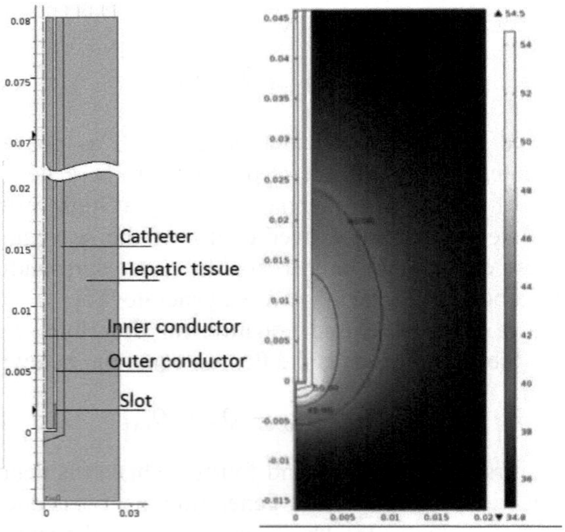

Fig. 1 Base geometry (left) and temperature distribution contours (50°C,45°C,40°C) at 600s (right)

In order to simplify the problem, perfect electric conductor boundary conditions are attributed to the waveguide walls and a scattering boundary condition was applied to the outer boundaries of the hepatic tissue to avoid additional reflections of microwave energy, which would not happen in continuous tissue. For the thermal problem, only the liver tissue was taken into consideration and a thermal insulation boundary was attributed to the PTFE catheter. Antenna heating can be inferred from the reflection coefficient and minimizing this is included in the scope of this paper.

Table 1 Dimensions and properties of antenna and tissue

Parameter	Value
Inner conductor radius	0.255[mm]
Outer conductor radius	1.095[mm]
Antenna length	80[mm]
Slot width	0.25-5[mm]
Slot distance from antenna tip	0-30[mm]
Catheter radius	1.72[mm]
Catheter relative permittivity	2.6
Coax dielectric relative permittivity	2.03
Blood density	1000[kg/m3]
Blood specific heat	3639[J/(kg*K)]
Blood perfusion rate	3.6 e-3[1/s]
Blood temperature	37°C
Hepatic tissue radius	3[cm]
Hepatic tissue relative permittivity	43.03
Frequency	900-2500[MHz]
Feed power	10[W]
Time	0-600[s]

C. Studies

Three studies have been performed within COMSOL focused on determining the effects slot height, slot position from antenna tip and microwave frequency have on antenna efficiency. While the primary focus is the ablation itself since the antenna can be fed through an external impedance matching generator to improve efficiency as well as be equipped with internal cooling to reduce damage to surrounding healthy tissue through unwanted heating of the waveguide, the target of this study was trifold: to observe the geometric configurations that would minimize reflected power, maximize deposited power in the hepatic tissue and provide adequate temperatures in the ablation area. The latter was checked by measuring temperature 5mm away from the antenna in a point centered on the slot.

III. Results

A. Slot width and slot position variations at 2.45GHz

The first study performed centered on the most common frequency used in MWA, namely 2.45GHz. Fig.2 and Fig.3 illustrate the reflection coefficient and dissipated power in hepatic tissue obtained from this study. It is desirable for the attenuation and dissipated power to be maximum. As the two figures illustrate, this can be found at a distance of 4mm from antenna tip with a slot size of 4.8mm. The study has also found a region of minimum efficiency for the antenna, namely centered around 20mm distance from antenna tip, for all slot width values. It is advisable that manufacturers avoid this specific configuration as most feed power will not be transmitted into the tissue and instead will heat up and damage the antenna and surrounding healthy tissue.

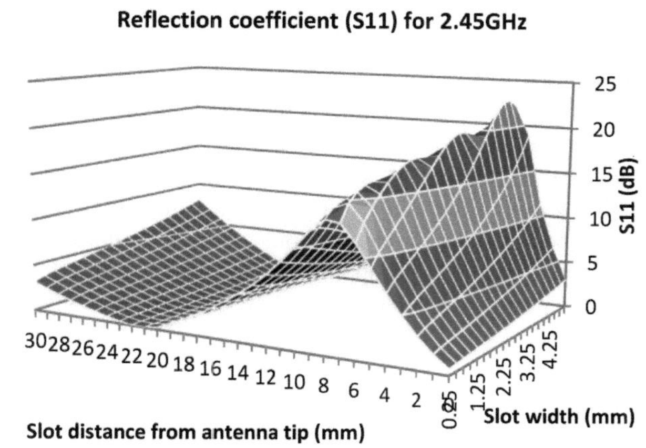

Fig. 1 Attenuation of reflected power (in absolute value) as a function of slot width and slot distance from antenna tip

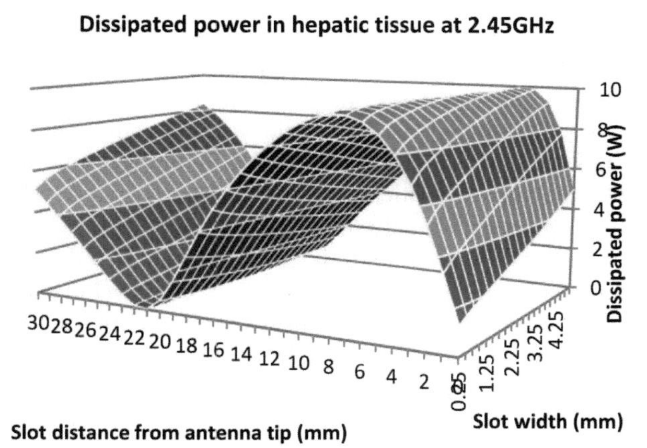

Fig. 2 Dissipated power as a function of slot width and slot distance from antenna tip

During MWA, exposure time is of great importance. Most MWA procedures operate at higher power inputs than this study to reduce this exposure time while still attaining cytotoxic temperatures. Looking at the results, we find that at 300s 35.48% of combinations produce a temperature above 50°C and only 8.11% produce a temperature in hepatic tissue of 60°C or above while at 600s, 52.9% of combinations produce a temperature above 50°C and 39.25% produce one above 60°C, with a maximum reached temperature of 67.97°C.

B. Slot width at 900-2500MHz

Considering the results of the previous test, the distance of the slot from antenna tip was fixed at 4mm. while the slot width was varied from 0 to 5mm. For each of these values, a frequency sweep from 900 to 2500MHz was performed in 25MHz increments. As with the previous study, the reflection coefficient and dissipated power were plotted for each combination of parameters. The study also takes a look at temperature outputs at the measuring point. Figures 4 through 6 illustrate the results.

In terms of power transmission, S11 peaks at -25.39dB at 2.3GHz and a slot width of 5mm while the maximum attenuation obtained for 2.45GHz is -22.78dB which is still considered a good value.

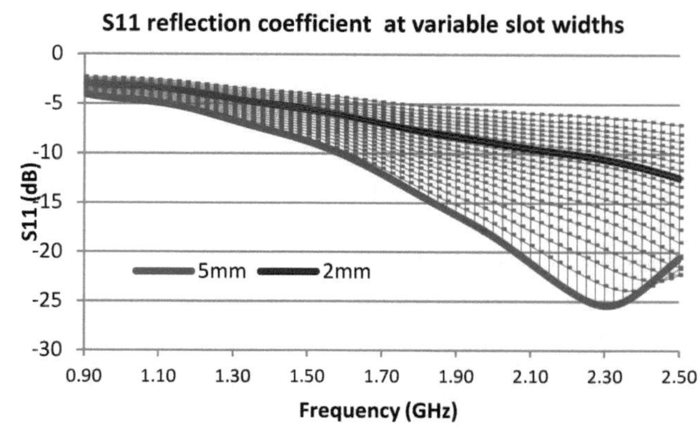

Fig. 3 Attenuation of reflected power as a function of frequency. Each series represents a slot width step

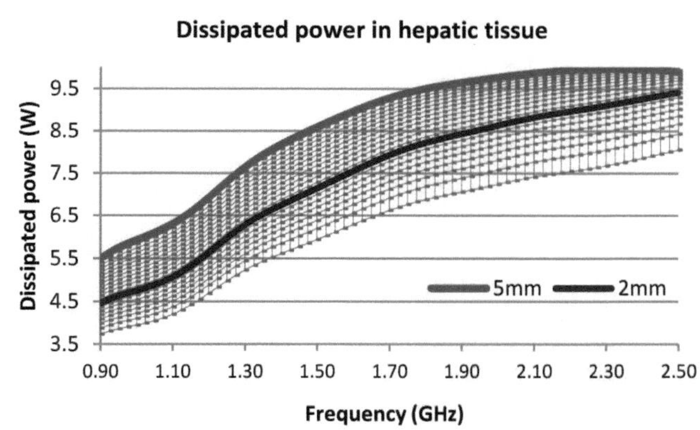

Fig. 4 Attenuation of reflected power as a function of frequency. Each series represents a slot width step

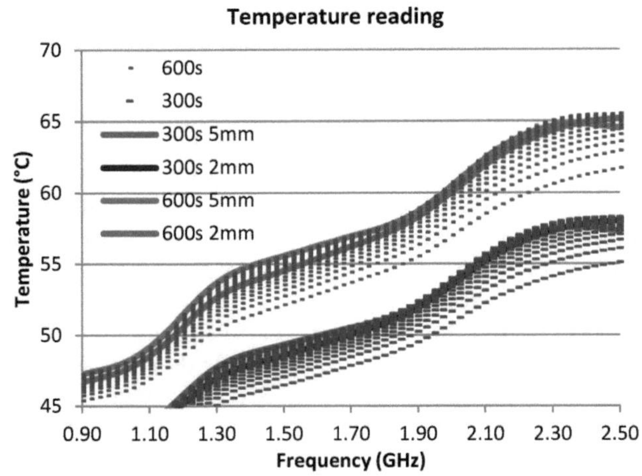

Fig. 5 Temperature at 300s and 600s measured at 5mm from middle of slot as a function of frequency

Dissipated power in tissue (fig. 5) shows a similar situation, with the maximum located at 2.325GHz and 2.3GHz as next maximum, both with over 99.6% of input energy dissipated into the tissue.

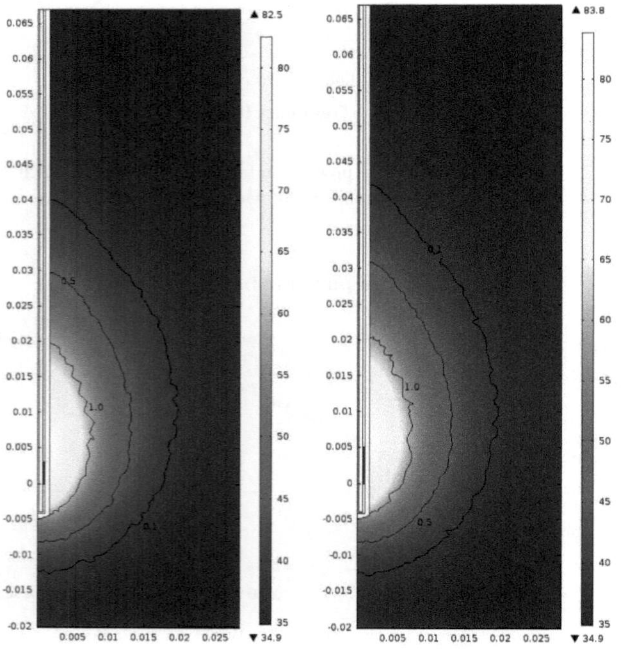

Fig. 6 Temperature and necrosed tissue contours (1.0, 0.5, 0.1) for maximum attenuation (left) and maximum power dissipation (right) at 600s. Slot position is highlighted in blue

Temperature readings were plotted in fig. 6. The maximum temperature attained at 300s was 58.2°C, although only 50.38% of combinations reached temperatures above 50°C and none reached 60°C. At 600s, 82.5% reached 50°C and 30.8% reached 60°C, with a maximum of 65.46°C. The most considerable difference between the previous study and the present one is the absence of any combinations able to reach 60°C in 300s or less, leading to a need for longer procedure times.

An important fact to note is that the temperature maxima are not centered on the slot itself, shown in blue in fig. 7 and, as such, care must be taken during the MWA procedure with regards to the correct positioning of the ablation antenna for best results. A second consequence of this fact is the difference between temperatures maxima obtained at the reading point and overall temperatures maxima visible in fig. 7.

C. Slot position at 900-2500MHz

The slot width was fixed at 2mm while the distance was varied from 0 to 30mm. For each of these values, a frequency sweep from 900 to 2500MHz was performed in 25MHz increments. As with the previous study, the reflection coefficient and dissipated power were plotted for each combination of parameters. The study also takes a look at temperature outputs at the measuring point.

Fig. 8 shows the resulting reflection coefficient for this study. Highlighted are the series corresponding to 4mm distance that was considered as fixed by the previous study, and which gives identical results (-11.886dB at 2.45GHz) in combination with the 2mm slot width, as well as two series which correspond to the first and second maxima, with attenuations of -34.9dB. As with the previous study, transmission efficiency increases with frequency for small distances while larger distances from the antenna tip see an increase in efficiency at lower feed frequencies.

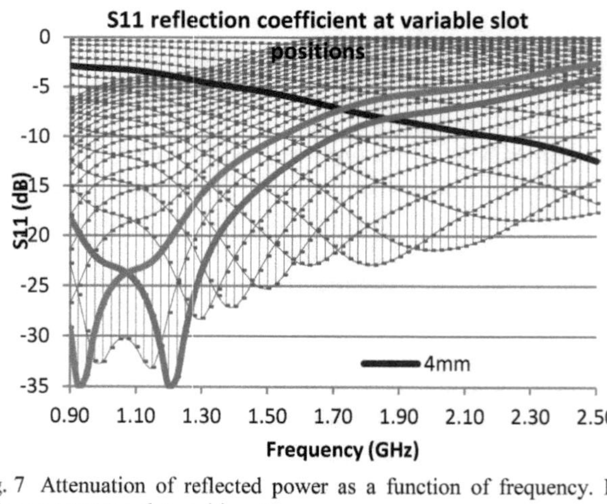

Fig. 7 Attenuation of reflected power as a function of frequency. Each series represents a slot position step

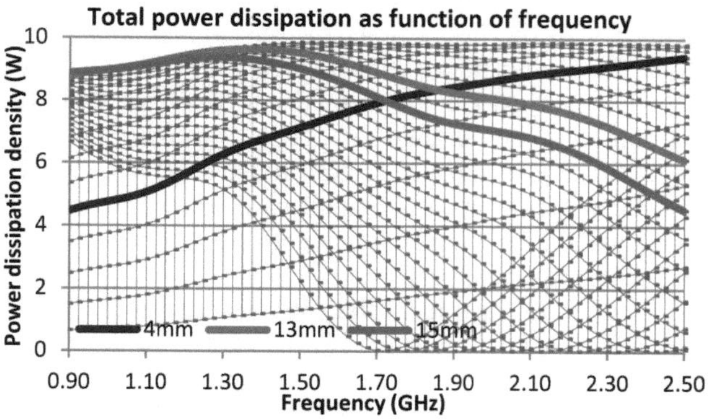

Fig. 8 Attenuation of reflected power as a function of frequency. Each series represents a slot position step

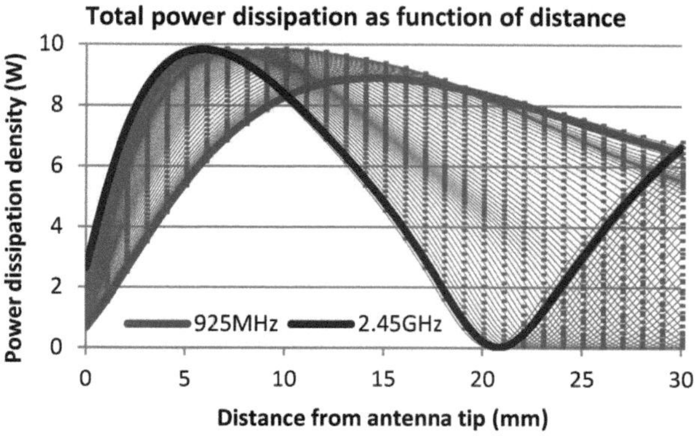

Fig. 9 Attenuation of reflected power as a function of frequency. Each series represents a frequency step

Dissipated power (fig. 9, fig. 10) follows the trend of reflection attenuation, the slope steepness being directly proportional to the feed frequency. The study also shows that higher frequencies provide an overall better power dissipation, with a peak of 98.3% of feed power dissipated for 2.45GHz and only 88.9% for 925MHz. Additionally, it is again found that there is a band of greatly reduced power efficiency at 20mm distance for 2.45GHz.

Temperatures measured at 5mm from the slot are plotted in fig. 11. The 4mm series highlighted in the plot provide a steady increase in temperature over the entire frequency sweep, while the 13mm and 15mm series which were found to give best reflection attenuation present faster rises to cytotoxic levels and a plateau in the middle of the frequency sweep, decreasing to undesirable values at the high end of the sweep. The study has found that 61.04% of combinations have reached a temperature of 50°C at 600s and 32.2% at 300s while 17.56% have gone to 60°C or above at 600s and only 1.14% have reached 60°C at 300s. A maxima of 67.83°C was reached at 600s and 60.48°C at 300s, comparable to the values obtained in the previous study.

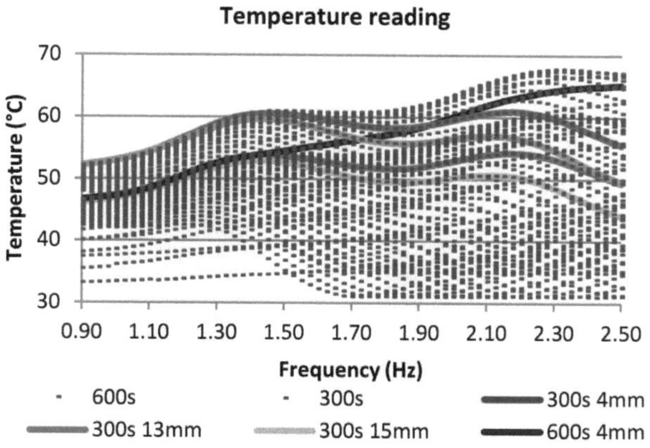

Fig. 10 Temperature at 300s and 600s measured at 5mm from middle of slot as a function of frequency

It must be pointed out that due to how the ablation area is formed, these temperatures are not entirely representative of the overall maxima achieved during the procedure and care must be taken when inserting the antenna to ensure correct positioning in the malignant tissue for optimal coverage. Fig. 12 and fig. 13 show the effective ablation area for 925MHz and 2.45GHz for the 4mm slot position and 15mm slot position.

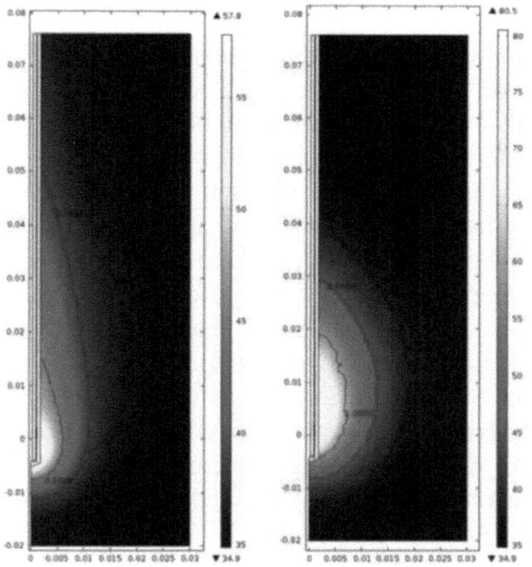

Fig. 11 Temperature and necrosed tissue contours (1.0, 0.5, 0.1) for 925MHz (left) and 2.45GHz (right) at 4mm slot distance. Slot position is highlighted in blue

At the 4mm distance, the higher frequency gives a more spherical volume which helps with better control over the ablated tissue. At the 15mm distance however, the higher frequency antenna fails to heat a large enough volume of tissue although still presenting a small elongation of the heated volume. The higher frequency was also able to produce higher temperatures, reaching 80.5°C for the 4mm distance compared to 57.8°C for 925MHz at the same value.

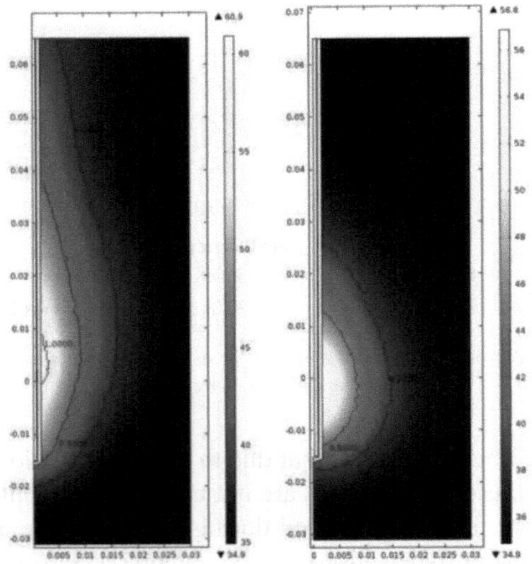

Fig. 12 Temperature and necrosed tissue contours (1.0, 0.5, 0.1) for 925MHz (left) and 2.45GHz (right) at 15mm slot distance. Slot position is highlighted in blue

IV. Conclusions

This paper focused on the effects geometry has on the efficiency of MWA single slot coaxial antennas. Using COMSOL Multiphysics three studies have been performed on a homogenous volume of hepatic tissue to determine how the size of the slot, its position from the antenna tip and frequency impacted the overall characteristics of the antenna, microwave propagation and the ablation zone. While in practice there are limitations to the frequency range used, both physical as generators and antennas cannot operate on the entire spectrum used, and regulatory like the ISM band, this paper wanted to observe antenna behavior over the entire spectrum and compare it to common frequencies used in MWA. As such, during the studies, the 2.45GHz frequency was repeatedly highlighted since this is the most commonly used in MWA therapy. It has been shown that higher frequencies provide a more spherical ablation volume, thus avoiding damaging healthy tissue due to the characteristic "teardrop" shape produced by lower frequencies. The 925MHz frequency has also been highlighted for its proximity 915MHz which previous studies mentioned for its benefits and appears in some manufacturer's medical equipment [10].

This paper has identified several geometric combinations which provide the best results for one of the enumerated factors of overall efficiency however, a single best combination of geometrical elements could not be found. This can be attributed to the fact that the MWA procedure is a complex problem and exterior factors must be taken into account. Such factors include impedance matching feed generators, variable frequency generators, higher feed powers or using multiple antennas.

This paper has also identified an important aspect of the ablation area, namely that it does not center on the slot itself, as shown in fig. 7, 12 and 13 and, as such, temperature readings and antenna positioning must be performed taking this into account. The need for larger slot distances and slot widths must be balanced by the fact that these combinations can lead to increased elongation of the ablation zone which is undesirable.

Conflict of Interest

The author declares that they have no conflict of interest.

References

1. D.M. Lloyd et al. - International multicenter prospective study on microwave ablation of liver tumours: preliminary results, International Microwave Tumour Ablation Group (IMTAG) HPB, Volume 13, Issue 8, p. 579 – 585
2. F. Sterzer (2002) Microwave medical devices. IEEE Microwave Magazine, 3(1), 65-70.
3. J.F. McGahan, G.D. Dodd (2001) Radiofrequency ablation of the liver: current status, American Journal of Roentgenology 176 3–16
4. A.S. Wright et al. (2005) Radiofrequency versus microwave ablation in a hepatic porcine model. Radiology;236(1):132–139
5. A.U. Hines-Peralta (2006) Microwave ablation: results with a 2.45-GHz applicator in ex vivo bovine and in vivo porcine liver, Radiology, 239(1):94-102
6. R.C. Martin (2007) Microwave hepatic ablation: initial experience of safety and efficacy, J Surg Oncol, Nov 1;96(6):481-6
7. M.G. Lubner, MD (2010) Microwave Tumor Ablation: Mechanism of Action, Clinical Results and Devices, J Vasc Interv Radiol. Aug; 21(8 Suppl): S192–S203
8. H.H. Pennes (1948) Analysis of tissue and arterial blood temperatures in the resting human forearm. J Appl Phys, 1: 93–122
9. Bertram et al (2006) Antenna design for microwave hepatic ablation using an axisymmetric electromagnetic model, BioMed Eng Online 5:15. DOI: 10.1186/1475-925X-5-15
10. R. Hoffman, MD et al. (2013) Comparison of four microwave ablation devices: an experimental study in ex vivo bovine liver. Radiology 268:89–97

The Influence of an Orifice Plates as a Flow Sensors on the Removal of Carbon Dioxide in High Frequency Oscillatory and Jet Ventilation

P. Kudrna and M. Rožánek

Department of Biomedical Technology, Czech Technical University in Prague, Kladno, Czech Republic

Abstract— **For the comfortable and safe use of high-frequency ventilation (HFV) it is suitable to use a system for continual monitoring of inspiratory and expiratory gas flow especially for calculating tidal volumes. The orifice plate is one of the usable solutions for experimental practice. But the orifice plate causes an increase in flow resistance in the ventilation circuit, which may affect the elimination of CO_2 from the patient's lungs. Proper compensation for the pressure losses caused by the orifice plate is then necessary.**

Keywords— **High frequency ventilation, orifice plate, CO_2 elimination.**

I. Introduction

High frequency ventilation (HFV) is a technique of mechanical ventilation, which uses a high respiratory rate and low tidal volumes that are comparable to or smaller than the anatomic dead space in the patient's airway. From this perspective, HFV seems to be a safe technique of mechanical ventilation with a minimal risk of volutrauma [1]. HFOV (High Frequency Oscillatory Ventilation) and HFJV (High Frequency Jet Ventilation) are techniques applied especially in therapy of pulmonary disease of extremely preterm infants with typical device representatives: 3100A (SensorMedics, CareFusion, CA) for HFOV and Life Pulse (Bunnell Inc., Salt Lake City, UT) for HFJV.

However, monitoration of tidal volumes or flow, is not a standard use (parameter) in these devices [2]. Suitable sensors for the experimental measurement of flow during HFV are hot-wire anemometers or orifice plates. The commercially available respiratory monitor Florian (Acutronic, Switzerland) which uses a hot-wire for measuring flow and V_T during HFOV is sometimes used in clinical practice but the the monitor is not produced anymore. However, these sensors, especially the orifice plate, can have a negative effect on the course of mechanical ventilation because the measuring elements increase resistance in the ventilation circuit [3].

The aim of this study is to investigate whether the flow sensor (particularly the orifice plate) affect the ability of CO_2 avoided and whether it is possible to compensate the negative effects.

II. Methods

The arrangement of the experiment is presented in figure 1 and figure 2. The experiment was realized in several variations in order to compare HFOV and HFJV with and without the orifice plate and during different frequencies as it is shown in table 1.

Table 1 Variations of the CO_2 elimination experiment.

Type of HFV		Orifice plate	Respiratory Rate [breath/min]
High frequency oscillatory ventilation (HFOV)	High frequency jet ventilation (HFJV)	Without OP	300
			420
			540
			660
		With OP	300
			420
			540
			660
		With OP, compensated	300
			420
			540
			660

A sealed rigid bottle was used as the model of the respiratory system of a newborn patient with a volume 1000 mL, compliance 2.87 mL/cmH_2O, fitted with an endotracheal tube with a diameter of 3 mm. It included ports for monitoring pressure inside the model, for filling the modelled patient's respiratory system by CO_2 and a closed loop for analysing the concentration of CO_2 (an exhaustion gas sample for analysis and return samples of CO_2 gas back to model). Patient monitor S/5 (Datex Ohmeda,Finland) was used as a CO_2 analyzer.

The newborn respiratory system model was continuously infused by 110 mL/min (±1 mL/min) of CO_2 in each configuration. A VT Mobile (FlukeBiomedical, Ohio) electronic flow meter was used to control the dosige rate of CO_2.

S. Vlad and N.M. Roman (eds.), *International Conference on Advancements of Medicine and Health Care through Technology; 12th - 15th October 2016, Cluj-Napoca, Romania*,
IFMBE Proceedings 59,
DOI: 10.1007/978-3-319-52875-5_31

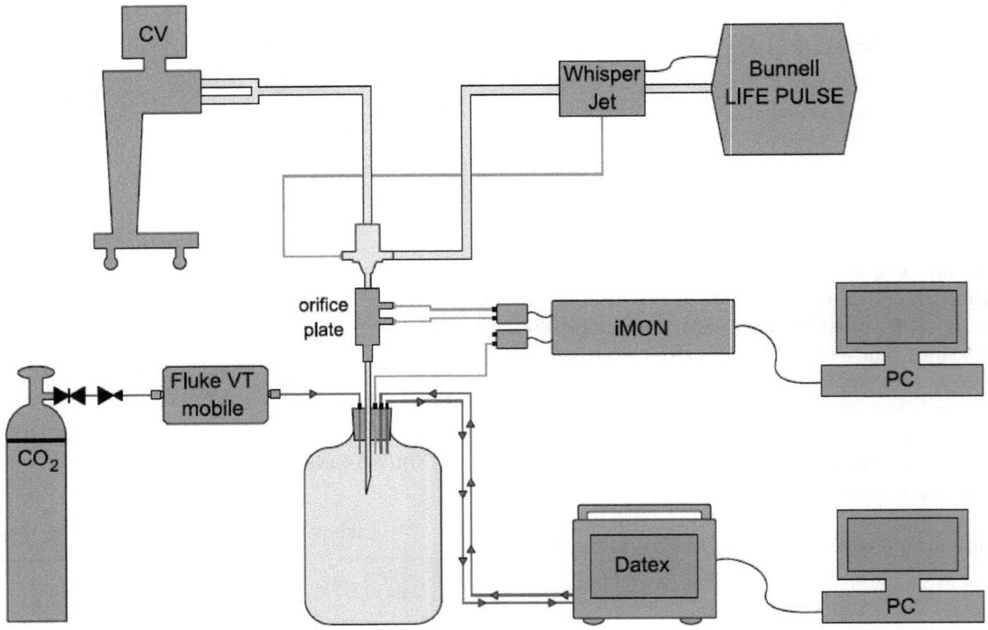

Fig. 1 Setup of the CO_2 elimination experiment using HFJV. We continuously infused 110 ml/min (±10 ml/min) of CO_2 into a rigid bottle using the Fluke VT mobile and in the same time we tried to eliminate it out of the bottle using the Bunnel LIFE PULSE high frequency jet ventilator (PIP = 20 cmH_2O – without compensation). A conventional ventilator was used to produce PEEP (5 cmH_2O) in the system. We measured the concentration of CO_2 in the bottle using the Datex Ohmeda patient monitor and we observed the pressure inside the bottle using the experimental system iMON.

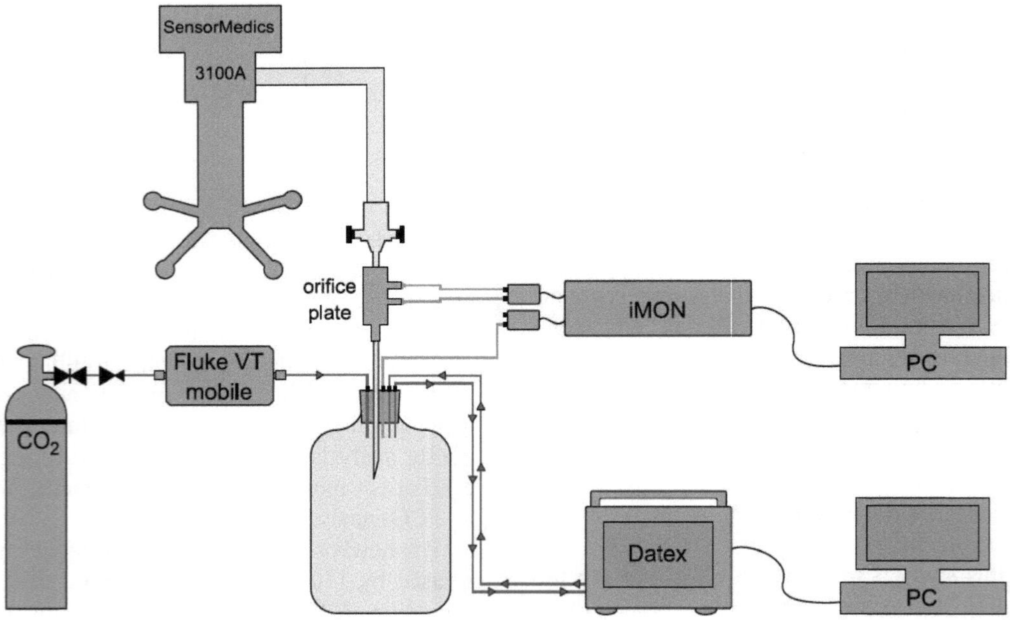

Fig. 2 Setup of the CO_2 elimination experiment using high frequency oscillatory ventilation. We used the SensorMedics 3100A ventilator (Paw = 12,5 cmH_2O, maximal intensity of oscillations).

At the same time we were tried to eliminated CO_2 from the rigid bottle by HF (high-frequency) ventilators according to the Table 1.

The pressure inside of the bottle was measured in order to observe decrease of pressure caused by the orifice plate. Specialized equipment (iMON monitor) with pressure sensors 26PC01(Honeywell, United States) with a pressure range of 1 psi was developed for the simultaneous measurement of up to three pressures at the same time. Signals from the sensors were amplified through instrumental amplifiers INA 128 (Texas Instruments, Dallas, Texas, United States) and recorded by a multifunctional measuring card NIDAQ 6009 (National Instruments, Austin, Texas, United States). The sampling frequency was 1 kHz. LabVIEW Signal Express (National Instruments, Austin, Texas, United States) was used for signal analysis. Pressure losses were compensated by adjusting a higher peak inspiratory pressure on the ventilators (HFJV) or changing the CDP (continual distending pressure) during HFOV.

The actual concentration of CO_2 was recorded by SW and the data were processed using Matlab Curve fitting tool (MathWorks, Natick, Massachusetts, U.S.A.).

A. Sensor – orifice plate

The experimental orifice plate was designed and made of stainless steel. The orifice plate is placed in the ventilation circuit between the jet-adapter and the endotracheal tube. Dimensions of the aperture are shown in Figure 3 and its flow-pressure characteristics are shown in Figure 4. Both connectors located on the orifice plate were attached to the differential pressure sensor but this signal was not further processed.

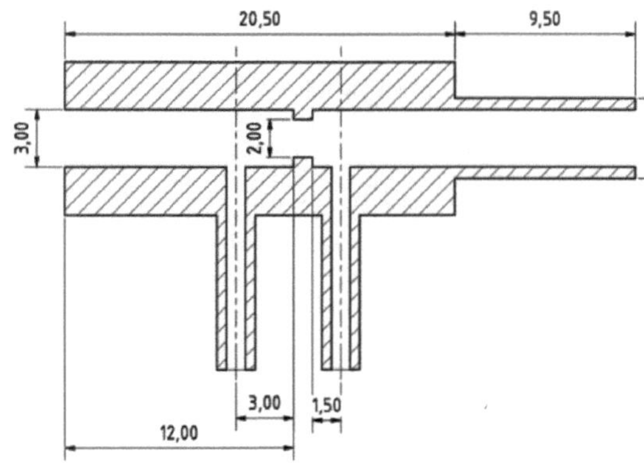

Fig. 3 Orifice plate - cut

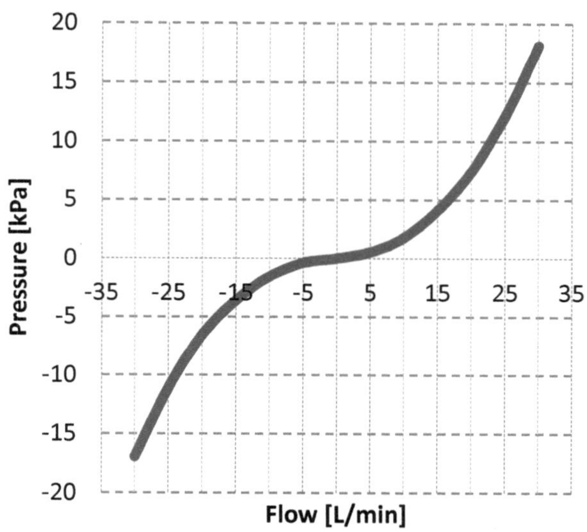

Fig. 4 Pressure-flow characteristics of the experimental flow sensor

III. Results

The increase of CO_2 concentration in the bottle can be described by the following equation:

$$c(CO_2) = c_f \cdot \left(1 - e^{-\frac{t}{\tau}}\right)$$

Values of the final concentration of CO_2 dependent on frequency (Respiratory Rate) and the time constant τ are shown in figure 5.

IV. Discusion

This experiment establishes the effect of an orifice plate on the elimination of carbon dioxide in high frequency ventilation. The orifice plate was used as a flow meter for measuring inspiratory and expiratory flow, respectively volumes, during HFOV and HFJV. Time constants during HFJV were increased when using the orifice plate without compensation. The result of this phenomena was that the final concentration of carbon dioxide in the lung model increased. After the compensation for the pressure loss, deterioration of carbon dioxide was not detected and the system acted as it would without the orifice plate. For clinical use of the orifice plate (as a flow sensor) is compensation of losses inevitable, but difficult for forecast. This plays an important role during practical application in clinics.

The effect of the orifice plate during high frequency ventilation was not as evident as in the previous case with jet ventilation. The embedded sensor caused only small changes in the time constants and did not affect the final concentration of CO_2 in the lung model.

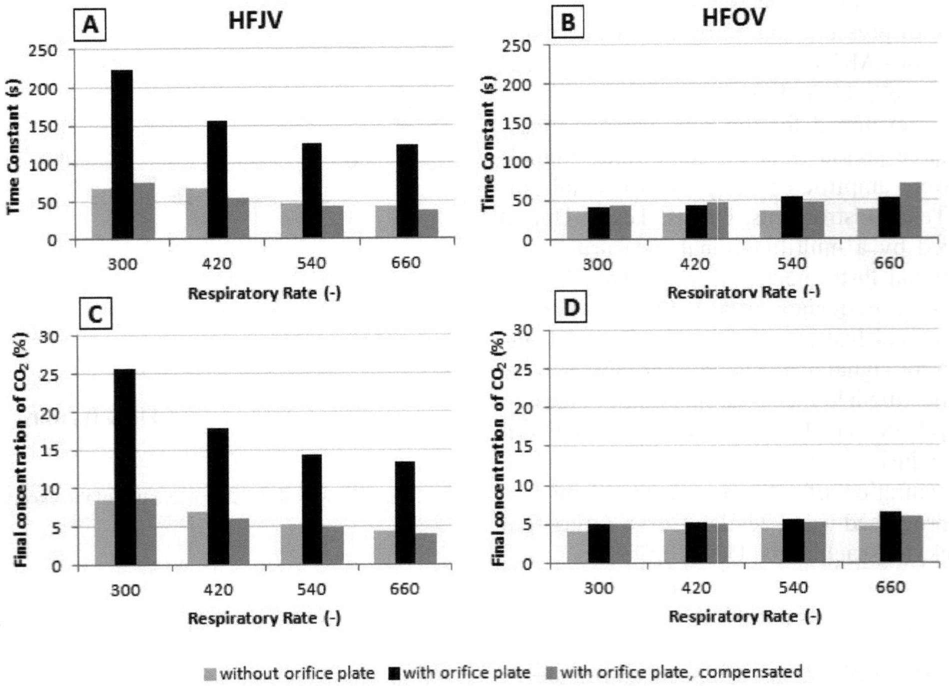

Fig. 5 Values of the time constant (τ) (A, B) and the final concentration of CO_2 (c_f) (C, D) for different variations of the carbon dioxide elimination experiment. These values were found in the Matlab Curve Fitting tool. We smoothed the data using the function (1) $c(CO_2) = c_f \cdot (1\text{-}e^{\frac{t}{\tau}})$. Goodness of fit ($R^2$) intervene between 0,9865 and 0,9994 for different variations of the experiment.

V. Conclusion

We came to the conclusion that ventilation parameters such as flow, resp. tidal volumes, can be monitored by an orifice plate in HFOV, because the orifice plate doesn't affect CO_2 elimination significantly. In HFJV there is a considerable increase in the final concentration of CO_2 when the orifice plate is used. Compensation for the loss in pressure was effective but recognizing how to set up for it in clinical practice could be difficult.

Acknowledgment

This research was supported by project reg. no. CZ.2.16/3.1.00/21564 from OP Prague Competitiveness and grant SGS14/216/OHK4/3T/17.

Conflict of Interest

The authors declare that they have no conflict of interest.

References

1. Gomella T, Cunningham M, Eyal F (2009) Neonatology 7th Edition. Mc Graw-Hill, New York
2. Courtney S E, Asselin J M (2006) High-frequency jet and oscillatory ventilation for neonates: which strategy and when?.*Respiratory care clinics of North America 12*: 453-467.
3. Kudrna P, Rožánek M, Hřibalová B (2014) Flow measuring during neonatal high frequency jet ventilation using orifice plate. *Biomediziniche Technik, 59*: 252-254.

Evaluation of the Electric and Magnetic Field near High Voltage Power Lines

Ş.F. Braicu, L. Czumbil, D. Şteţ and D.D. Micu

Technical University of Cluj-Napoca, Department of Electrotechnics and Measurements, Cluj-Napoca, Romania

Abstract— **The paper studies the magnetic and electric field distribution around a Romanian high voltage overhead power line. Different electrical and geometrical parameters are taken into consideration: power line current load, sky wires, phase wires conductor sag, positioning on electrical towers. Obtained numerical results are related to the appropriate regulations regarding the human exposure to electric and magnetic fields.**

Keywords— **Electromagnetic human exposure, electromagnetic field distribution; power lines; numerical modeling.**

I. Introduction

Developments in technology and industry have simplified human life. However, exposure to electromagnetic fields (EMFs) by using electrical machines, tools, industrial instruments, power lines, and communications devices has occurred as a result of these technological developments and is causing a threat to biological lives [1].

Since the late 1970s, questions have been raised whether exposure to low frequency electric and magnetic fields produces adverse health consequences. As a result, much research has been done, successfully resolving important issues and narrowing the focus of future research. Several interaction mechanisms are well established. These enable extrapolation of scientific results to the entire frequency range and wide-band health risk assessment. They have been used to formulate guidelines limiting exposures to EMF in the entire frequency range from static fields to 300 GHz [1, 2].

There are established biological effects from acute exposure at high levels (above 100 μT) that are explained by recognized biophysical mechanisms. External low frequency magnetic fields induce electric fields and currents in the body which, at very high field strengths, cause nerve and muscle stimulation and changes in nerve cell excitability in the central nervous system. External low frequency (ELF) electric fields similar to static electric fields cause redistribution of electric charges within initially uncharged objects, and consequently charging of the body surface, however, this time oscillating. This leads to periodic electromechanic forces acting upon charged hair and may lead to perception or even annoyance. In addition, alternating electric charging may cause periodic discharges at the body surface or to grounded objects. These repetitive (micro-) electroshocks may also lead to perception or even annoyance. In contrast to static fields periodic recharging induces intracorporeal electric currents and electric fields strengths which, if strong enough may stimulate nerve and muscle cells. ELF magnetic fields induce intracorporeal electric field strengths that according to the induction law increase with frequency and cross sectional area. Consequently, inside the body, the strength of induced electric fields increases from zero at the center to the maximum at the body surface [1, 3].

Most electric power operates at a frequency of 50 Hz or 60 Hz. Close to certain appliances, the magnetic field values can be of the order of a few hundred μT. Underneath power lines, magnetic fields could be about 20 μT and electric fields could be several thousand volts per meter. However, average residential power-frequency magnetic fields in homes are much lower - about 0.07 μT in Europe and 0.11 μT in North America. Mean values of the electric field in the home are up to several tens of volts per meter [2, 4].

The growing public concern about this risk has led several national and international bodies to set prudentially restrictive limitations on permitted exposure levels, even introducing concepts such as "attention levels" and "quality goals" for the magnetic field component [3÷7].

The 1999/519/EC European Council Recommendation (EC, 1999) defines, in its Annex I, the basic restrictions and reference levels for limiting exposure of the general public. This had been added by the directive 2013/35/EU on occupational exposure to EMF. In accordance to EC (1999) and ICNIRP (1998) restrictions on exposure to time-varying electric and magnetic fields that are based directly on established health effects and biological considerations are termed 'basic restrictions'. The main national safety regulation concerning human exposure to low frequency electromagnetic fields is HG 1136 din 30/08/2006, issued by the Romanian government [1, 3, 7].

Therefore, the International Commission on Non-Ionizing Radiation Protection (ICNIRP) [3] and the European Recommendations [5] set the public exposure limit, for electric fields to 5 kV/m, and to 10 μT in case of magnetic fields, according to Table 1 (where f is the frequency).

To respect these limitations, it is necessary to quantify realistically the electromagnetic field environment associated with electric systems, in particular electric power lines that have the widest impact on the territory. Therefore, the current paper studies electric and magnetic field distribution around a Romanian high voltage power line, by numerical modeling

S. Vlad and N.M. Roman (eds.), *International Conference on Advancements of Medicine and Health Care through Technology; 12th - 15th October 2016, Cluj-Napoca, Romania,*
IFMBE Proceedings 59,
DOI: 10.1007/978-3-319-52875-5_32

and on site field measurements. Obtained results are related to the appropriate regulations regarding the human exposure to the electromagnetic fields

Table 1 Reference levels for general public exposure to time-varying electric and magnetic fields (according to ICNIRP)

Frequency range (KHz)	Electric field strength, E (V/m)	Magnetic field strength, H (A/m)	Magnetic flux density, B (μT)
0,025 - 0.8	250/*f*	4/*f*	5/*f*

Due the fact that the accuracy of numerically estimated results depends upon the degree of detail used in simulations, several electrical and geometrical parameters were taken into consideration: power line current load, the presence of sky wires, active conductors sag and positioning on electrical towers.

II. Electric and Magnetic Field Analysis

The accurate 3D analysis of any electrical transmission line requires a great amount of memory and computational power. Therefore, usually simplified 2D cross-section analysis is done to determine the magnetic and electric field distribution around power line phase wires.

A. Evaluation of the magnetic field

The magnetic field is produced when an alternating current flows through a conductor. Applying Biot–Savart law, the magnetic field intensity *H* at point *P* produced by an infinite straight conductor is expressed by [8]:

$$\overline{H} = \frac{I}{2 \cdot \pi \cdot d} \cdot \overline{u}_{\varphi} \quad [A/m] \tag{1}$$

where:

- I is the mean square value of the current flowing through conductor;
- d is the distance from the conductor to observation point P;
- $\overline{u}_{\varphi}$ is a unit vector in the φ-direction.

Since the power line consists of more than one single active conductor, the summation of the magnetic fields by each phase wire current must be repeatedly calculated at the point *P*. Fig. 1 shows the magnetic-field intensity produced by a system of *n* carrying currents conductors ($I_1, I_2, ..., I_n$) in the *z*-direction (perpendicular on the transversal cross-section plan).

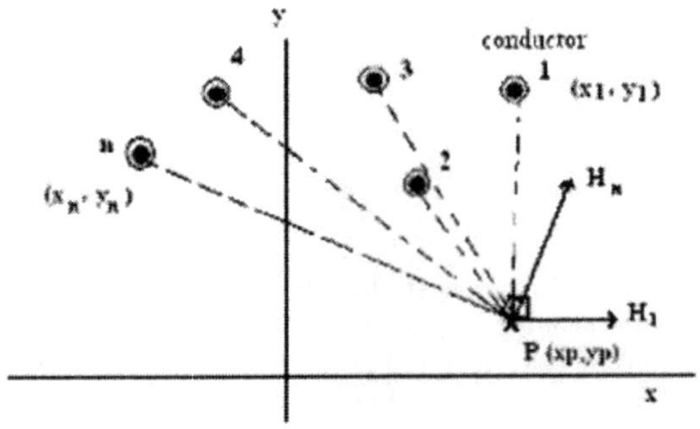

Fig. 1 Magnetic-field intensity for a *n* active conductors system

For A.C. transmission lines, the line currents have sinusoidal variation with time at power frequency. Consequently, the produced magnetic field in the vicinity of the power lines also varies at the power frequency and phasor algebra can be used to combine several components in order to yield the amplitude of the required field (horizontal and vertical vectors). For a three-phase system with one conductor per phase (as in our case), *I* current can be written as follows:

$$[I] = I_m \cdot \begin{bmatrix} \sin(\omega t + \varphi) \\ \sin(\omega t + \varphi - 120°) \\ \sin(\omega t + \varphi - 240°) \end{bmatrix} \tag{2}$$

The magnetic-field intensity at any point (x, y) produced by current I_i can be computed using equation (3) [9]:

$$\overline{H}_i = \frac{I_i}{2\pi} \cdot \frac{(x_P - x_i) \cdot \overline{u}_x - (y_P - y_i) \cdot \overline{u}_y}{(x_P - x_i)^2 + (y_P - y_i)^2} \tag{3}$$

where:

- x_P and x_i are the *x*-coordinates of the observation point *P* and conductor *i* respectively;
- y_P and y_i are the *y*-coordinates of the observation point *P* and conductor *i* respectively;
- $\overline{u}_x$ and $\overline{u}_y$ are unit vector on the *x* and *y*-direction.

The *x*-and-*y* components of the magnetic field intensity in (3) are described in (4) and (5), while equation (6) computes the total magnetic field intensity in the *x* and *y*-directions [10]:

$$H_{xi} = \frac{I_i}{2\pi} \cdot \frac{(x_P - x_i)}{(x_P - x_i)^2 + (y_P - y_i)^2} \tag{4}$$

$$H_{yi} = \frac{-I_i}{2\pi} \cdot \frac{(y_P - y_i)}{(x_P - x_i)^2 + (y_P - y_i)^2} \tag{5}$$

$$H_{xt} = \sum_{i=1}^{n} H_{xi} \qquad H_{yt} = \sum_{i=1}^{n} H_{yi} \tag{6}$$

where n is total number of current-carrying conductors.

Therefore, the magnitude of the total magnetic flux density B_t (rms value) is:

$$B_t = \mu \cdot \sqrt{H_{xt}^2 + H_{yt}^2} \tag{7}$$

where μ is the magnetic permeability of the medium in which the flux density is evaluated.

B. Evaluation of the electric field

To calculate the electric field under the power line, phase conductors are considered as infinite line charges [11]. The line charge densities of the phase conductors are calculated using equation (8):

$$[Q] = [P]^{-1} \cdot [V] \tag{8}$$

where:

- $[Q]$ is a vector representing the line charge densities of each power line conductor (phase wires and sky wires);
- $[V]$ is a vector representing each power line conductor potential regarding remote earth;
- $[P]$ represents Maxwell's potential coefficients matrix, which can be computed using image charge method, equations (9) and (10) [12]:

$$P_{i,i} = \frac{1}{2 \cdot \pi \cdot \varepsilon_r \cdot \varepsilon_0} \cdot ln\left(\frac{2h_i}{r_i}\right) \tag{9}$$

$$P_{i,j} = \frac{1}{2 \cdot \pi \cdot \varepsilon_r \cdot \varepsilon_0} \cdot \ln\left(\frac{d'_{i,j}}{d_{i,j}}\right) \tag{10}$$

with: h_i conductor i height, r_i conductor radius, $d_{i,j}$ and $d'_{i,j}$ the distance between conductor i and conductor j, respectively conductor j image.

After the line charge densities are determined, the horizontal and vertical components of the field, due to the three phase conductors at the desired locations, are calculated separately using equation (11) and (12) [13]:

$$E_{xi} = \frac{q_i}{2 \cdot \pi \cdot \varepsilon_r \cdot \varepsilon_0} \cdot (x_P - x_i) \cdot \left[\frac{1}{D_i^2} - \frac{1}{D_i'^2}\right] \tag{11}$$

$$E_{yi} = \frac{q_i}{2 \cdot \pi \cdot \varepsilon_r \cdot \varepsilon_0} \cdot \left[\frac{(y_P - y_i)}{D_i^2} - \frac{(y_P + y_i)}{D_i'^2}\right] \tag{12}$$

where: D_i and D_i' are the distances from conductor *i*, respectively conductor *i* image to observation point *P*.

Fig. 4 shows the components of the electric field at the observation point *P(x,y)* due to one phase conductor and its image.

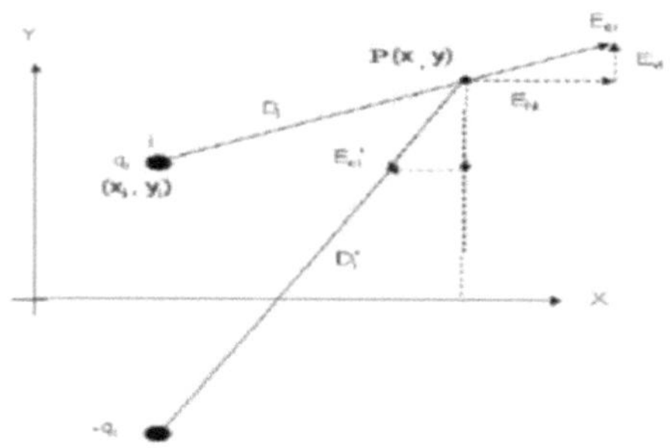

Fig. 2 Electric field produced by conductor i at observation point P

Resultant of horizontal and vertical components of the field gives the total electric field at the desired locations as shown in equation (13) [11]:

$$E_t = \sqrt{E_{tx}^2 + E_{ty}^2} \tag{13}$$

$$E_{tx} = \sum_{i=1}^{n} E_{xi} \quad \text{and} \quad E_{ty} = \sum_{i=1}^{n} E_{yi} \tag{14}$$

III. Numerical Evaluation of the Magnetic and Electric Field Exposure

The investigated power line is a Romanian single circuit 110 kV overhead line. It is one of the main power lines that connect Cluj county to Bistrita-Nasaud county, explicitly the 110/20 kV Dej substation to the 110/20 kV Nasaud substation (see Fig. 3).

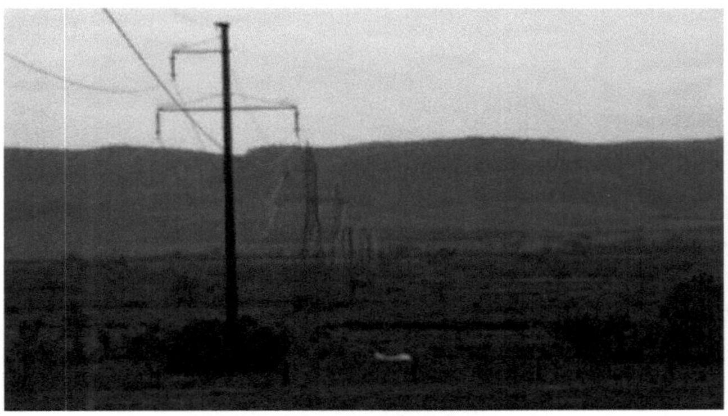

Fig. 3 Dej-Nasaud 110 kV power line

To determine the magnetic and electric field distribution by the above presented relationships, the chosen power line has been implemented in the Maxwell 14, dedicated field analysis software, considering an R-S-T phase distribution, as in Fig. 4:

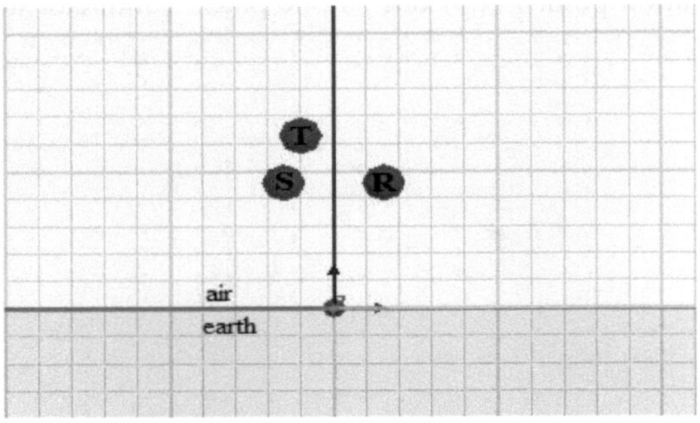

Fig. 4 Numerical model of the studied geometry

Fig. 5 and 6 presents the electric and magnetic field distribution around the power line, considering a maximum 105 A symmetrical current load on each phase wire (20 MW), and a 5.5m conductor sag:

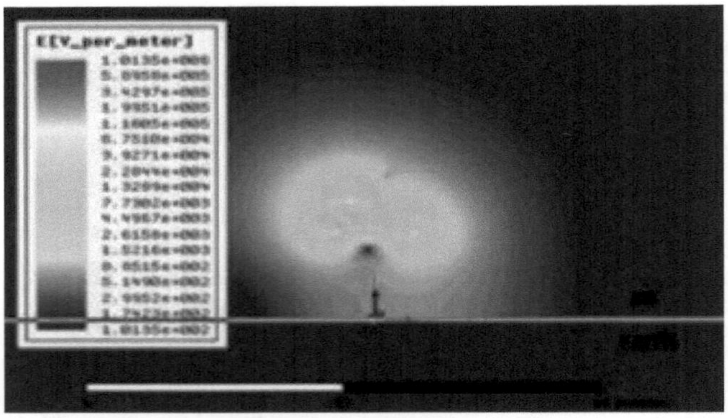

Fig. 5 Electric field distribution around power line (cross-section)

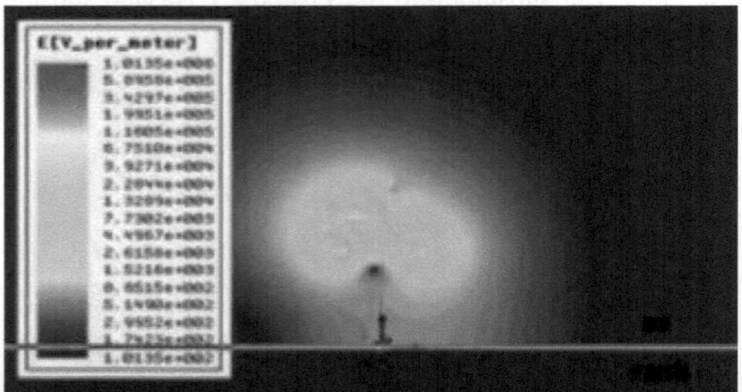

Fig. 6. Magnetic field distribution around power line (cross-section)

For a more detailed analysis, the electric field values had been extracted at 1.7 m and 0.7 m above ground (human medium height and respectively sheep height) for different separation distances on both sides of power line axis (see Fig. 7).

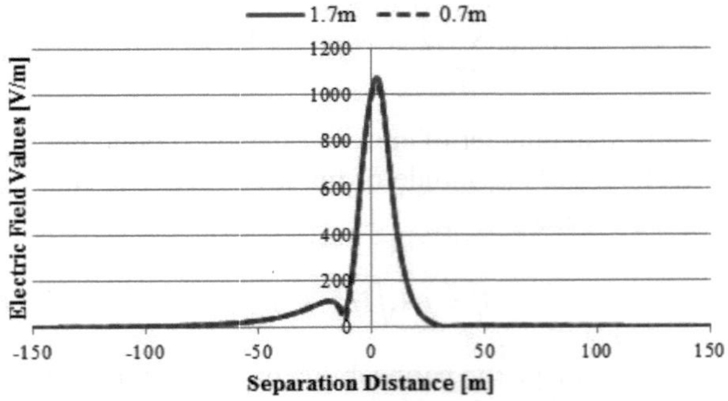

Fig. 7. Electric field values at 1.7 and 0.7 m on both sides of the power line

According to Fig. 7 even under power line phase wires the imposed 5 kV/m electric field limitation for human health are respected [3-7]. The asymmetry one side and another of power line axis is as a result of the phase wires triangle positioning on pylons.

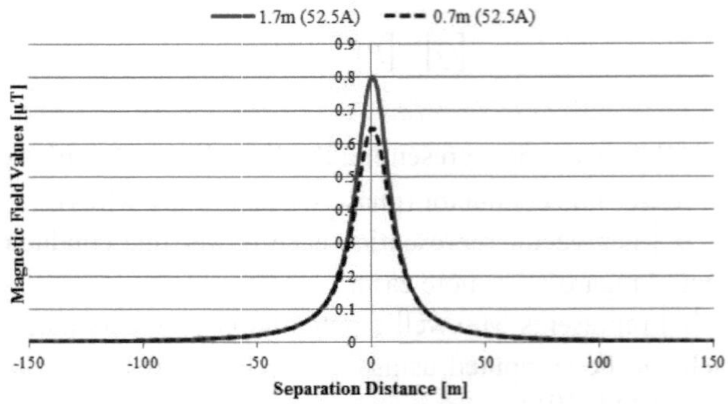

Fig. 8. Magnetic field values at 1.7 and 0.7m for 52.2A current load

Fig. 8 highlights the magnetic field values at 1.7 m and 0.7 m on both sides of the power line axis for the minimum recorded current load on phase wires, 52.5 A (10 MW).

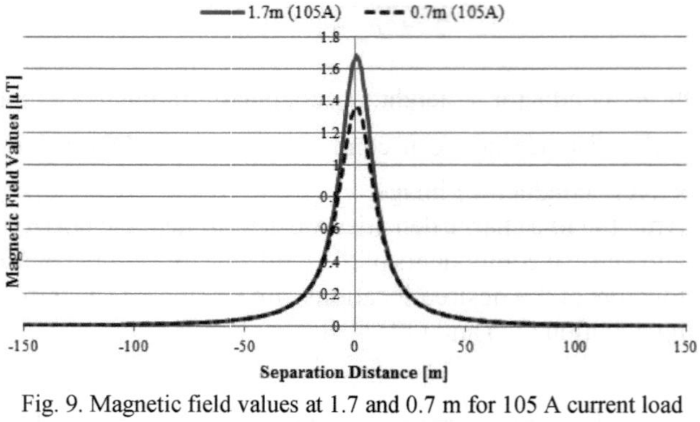

Fig. 9. Magnetic field values at 1.7 and 0.7 m for 105 A current load

Fig. 9 presents the magnetic field values at 1.7 m and 0.7 m on both sides of the power line axis for the maximum recorded current load on phase wires, 105 A (20 MW). As it can be seen, even for maximum current load on phase wires, the imposed 10 μT limitation is not exceeded.

IV. Field Measurements

To test and validate the results obtained by numerical modeling and simulations, magnetic an electric field measurements have been made in open field between Floresti and Mogosesti villages, (Bistrita-Nasaud county), more precisely between pylon No.142 and No.143. The separation distance between the two *SCS1_161* type concrete pylons is 236 m, and conductors sag varies with temperature according to table 2 data:

Table 2 Conductors Sag Variation with Temperature

Opening								
Pylons	Distance	-5°C and frost	0°C	+10°C	+20°C	+25°C	+30°C	+35°C
142-143	263m	638cm	513cm	530cm	547cm	555cm	563cm	571cm

The chosen measurement location is approximately at 600 m from a national road which connects the two villages and it is intersected by the power line.

To determine the magnetic and electric field distribution by the above presented relationships, the chosen power line has been implemented in the Maxwell 14, dedicated field analysis software, considering an R-S-T phase distribution, as in Fig. 5:

The measurements were made on 10th of June 2013, from 10:00 am to 03:00 pm. The average temperature was around +25°C. Therefore, a 555 cm conductor sag could be considered for phase wires. The electrical parameters of the power line, provided by the system operator (*SC Electrica SA*) were the following, during measurements:

- Power line voltage level: 112 kV;
- Power load: 11.2 MW;
- Current load on phase wires: 58 A;

This time, both magnetic and electric fields were measured at 1.7 m above ground, corresponding to human height, using a more precise *ESM–100 3D H/E* field meter.

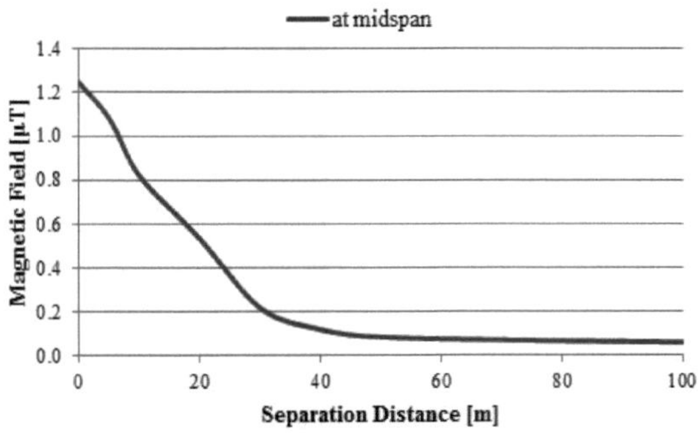

Fig. 10. Magnetic field measurements with respect to separation distance.

Fig. 11 presents the measured magnetic field along a straight perpendicular line placed at midspan and respectively in line with pylon 142, on the right side of the power line axis. As it can be observed, due to the less current load on phase wires, lower magnetic field intensity has been recorded around the power line.

Also due to the presence of iron reinforcement, which concentrates the magnetic flux line inside the pylon, and due to the bigger height of the phase wires, the magnetic field around the pylon is much lower than at midspan.

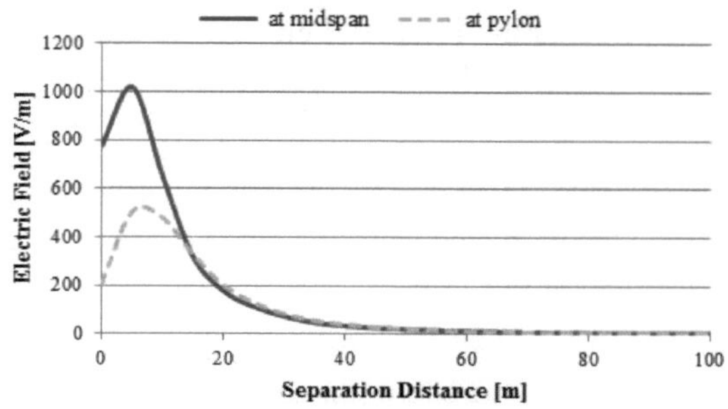

Fig. 11. Electric field measurements with respect to separation distance.

Fig. 11 presents the electric field values measured along a straight perpendicular line placed at midspan and respectively in line with pylon 142. The peak of the electric field values for both cases it was recorded under phase R conductor, where the electric field produced by this conductor is stronger and is not compensated by the electric fields created by the two other phase conductors.

In order to examine the influence of conductor sag on the electromagnetic field distribution, magnetic and electric field measurements had been done along power line axis between pylon 142 and 143 at 1.7 m above ground.

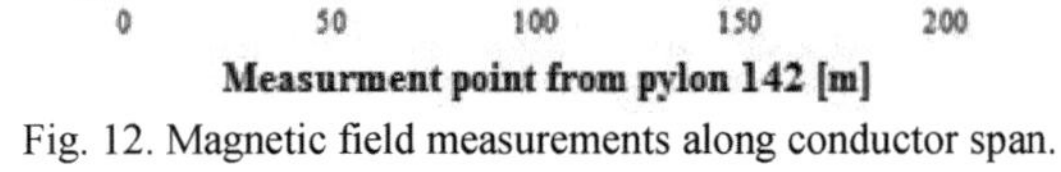

Fig. 12. Magnetic field measurements along conductor span.

Fig. 12 shows the measured magnetic field values along power line axis. The maximum field value was not recorded at midspan point as an effect of the height difference between the two pylons.

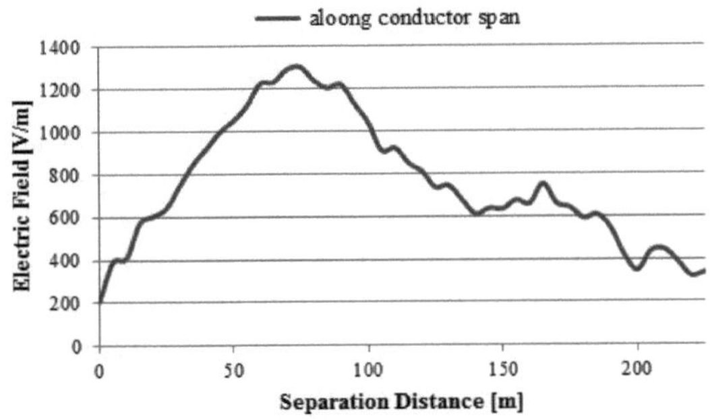

Fig. 13. Electric field measurements along conductor span.

Fig. 13 presents the measured electric field along power line axis. The irregularities on the measurements are as a result of existing bushes and soil bumps under the power line.

Analyzing the measured magnetic and electric field values, form Fig. 10÷13, it can be observed that the measured values are in the predicted variation range determined by numerical evaluation Fig 7÷9.

Conclusions

Overhead high voltage lines are sources of the electric and magnetic fields of low frequency. Near the ground surface, these fields cannot exceed values determined by ecological and health regulations or EMC standards. According to the above regulations, the considered fields should be estimated during the power line designing.

In this paper, an analysis of the electromagnetic field around a Romanian high voltage overhead line has been done, taking into consideration the presence of sky wires, different current loads on phase wires and conductor sag. Electric and magnetic field values obtained by numerical simulations has been compared to on-site field measurements along power line axis, and along a perpendicular straight line placed at midspan position and in line with a lifting pylon.

Both numerical simulation and on-site measurement have confirmed that the produced electrical and magnetic field values are in the imposed limitation values and no risks are present for biological life.

Conflict of Interest

The authors declare that they have no conflict of interest.

References

1. Scientific Committee on Emerging and Newly Identified Health Risks - SCENIHR, "Opinion on Potential health effects of exposure to electromagnetic fields (EMF) ", Health effects of EMF, 20.01.2016
2. World Health Organization – WHO, Electromagnetic fields and public health. Exposure to extremely low frequency fields, 2007 at http://www.who.int/peh-emf/publications/facts/fs322/en/
3. ***ICNIRP guidelines report; "Guidelines for limiting exposure to time-varying electric, magnetic, and electromagnetic fields (up to 300 GHz)", Health Physics Society, vol. 74, pp. 494-522, 1998
4. Matthes, R, Bernhardt, JH, McKinlay, ICNIRP (1999) Guidelines on Limiting Exposure to Non-Ionizing Radiation, International Comission on Non-Ionizing Radiation Prptection, Munchen, 1999, ICNIRP 7/99
5. ***Standard – Electromagnetic Compatibility (EMC). Journal officiel des Communautes europeennes, (EC 89-336) reference no. 1000-4-3, 1995.
6. ***European Council Recommendation of 12 July 1999 on the limitation of exposure of the public to electromagnetic fields 0 Hz to 300 GHz, the Official Journal of the European Communities, 30 July 1999.
7. ***ORDIN nr. 1.193 din 29 septembrie 2006 pentru aprobarea Normelor privind limitarea expunerii populației generale la câmpuri electromagnetice de la 0 Hz la 300 GHz.
8. Kostoff, R.N. M., Lau, C.G.Y. Combined biological and health effects of electromagnetic fields and other agents in the published literature, Technological Forecasting and Social Change, vol. 80, no. 7, pp. 1331-1349, 2013
9. Doni, A, Moro, F. Turri, R, A simplified procedure for computing the environmental magnetic field generated by power lines with complex geometric configurations, 41st Universities Power Engineering Conference, UPEC2006, Newcastle, UK, sept. 2006
10. Dahab, A.A., Amoura, F.K., Abu-Elhaija, W.S. Comparison of Magnetic-Field Distribution of Noncompact and Compact Parrallel Transmission-Line Configurations, IEEE Trans. On Power Delivery, vol. 20, no.3, July 2005
11. Filippopoulos, G, Tsanakas, D, Analytical Calculation of the Magnetic Field Produced by Electric Power Lines, IEEE Trans. On Power Delivery, vol. 20, no. 2, April 2005
12. El Dein, A.Z., The Effects of the Span Configurations and Conductor Sag on the Magnetic-Field Distribution under Overhead Transmission Lines, Journal of Physics, vol. 1, pp. 11-23, 2012
13. D. Şteţ, D.D. Micu, A. Ceclan, L. Dărăbant, "Study of Electromagnetic Interferences Between AC Systems and Metallic Structures", European Electromagnetics, Lausane, Switzerland, July 21-25, 2008.

Author: Levente Czumbil
Institute: Technical University of Cluj-Napoca
Street: George Baritiu
City: Cluj-Napoca
Country: Romania
Email: levente.czumbil@ethm.utcluj.ro

Analysis of Pulse Wave during Magneto-Therapy Session

C.Luca, D.Andrițoi, C. Corciovă and R. Ciorap

University of Medicine and Pharmacy "Grigore T. Popa" Iasi, Faculty of Medical Bioengineering, Iasi, Romania

Abstract— **The aim of this study is to highlight the influence of the therapy with magnetic fields of low-frequency on the human body through the evaluation of the hemodynamic parameters during this type of physiotherapy sessions. Theraphy using low-frequency magnetic fields is one of the procedures of physiotherapy which brings a lot of benefits to the patients and in this paper work we have demonstrated that there is a considerable influence on the circulatory system. In a low-frequency magnetic field, blood circulation to the patient improves, the elasticity of the vessel walls is increasing, and the concentration of oxygen in bloodcells increase with 200%.**

Keywords— **monitoring biomedical parameters, magnetic theraphy, hemodynamic circulatory**

I. Introduction

The energy from magnetic fields used for therapeutic took a tremendous impetus nowadays, which is felt worldwide. Magneto-therapy is a form of physical therapy that uses low frequency magnetic fields energy, noninvasive, being an effective remedy for treating a wide range of rheumatology and beyond.[1]

The principle behind this therapy is that some cells and tissues in the body presents electromagnetic pulses, which in the case of diseases or disorders degrades. Magneto-therapy works by producing different levels of magnetic fields that can penetrate the human body, having healing powers on him.[2]

Monitoring of cardiovascular parameters during magneto-theraphy session can provide information particularly helpful to personalize medical treatment.[3]

II. Study objectives

The evaluation of patients during magneto theraphy session by monitoring biomedical parameters aims to detect changes in functional status of the subject, and the activity of the human body in the electrical, mechanical and magnetic fields.

By measuring hemodynamic parameters we can obtain useful clinical information about cardiovascular function of the body.

Currently, this method of improvement and healing of diseases attracted the attention of specialists, and the studies in this area has intensified proving real qualities of magnets theraphy. However, research towards healing effects of magnetic therapy is still in the early stage. The reason behind the choice of the theme was the desire to bring more studies dedicated to magneto theraphy and its effects on the body.

The monitoring parameters during magneto theraphy session aims to highlight the influence of low frequency magnetic fields on human body by evaluating hemodynamic parameters during this physiotherapy procedure.

Hemodynamic studies referes to the factors that maintain, modify and regulate the movement of blood through the circulatory sistem.

Blood flow (Q) is a fundamental hemodynamic parameter, which is the volume flowing (Δ V) through the unit time (t) in section (D) [3]:

$$Q = \Delta V / D{*}t \quad (1)$$

The flow rate is a derived parameter, represented by the cross-sectional area relative to the volume flow [3]:

$$v = D / S \quad (2)$$

The structural and functional large arteries are vessels to be conductive, while arteries and arterioles are resistance terminal vessels. In turn, the veins are vessels through which blood circulates capacitive under low pressure. Regardless of the vascular territory, the movement of blood through the blood vessels is determined by two main factors.

The difference pressure between the two ends of the vessel (P1 and P2) as the biasing force and displacement of the blood by the pressure within the high to the low pressure;

Many staff who resists blood flow, called vascular resistance.

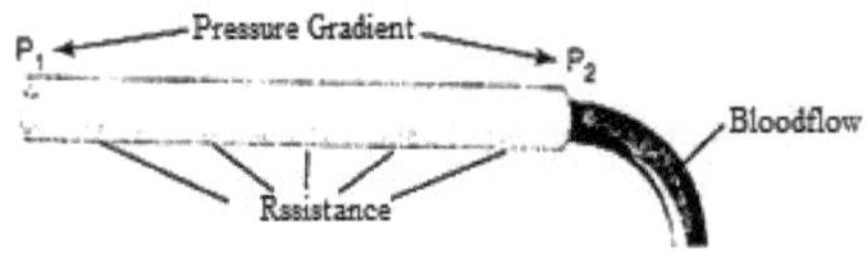

Fig.1 The expression of vascular resistance [3]

P1 is the pressure of blood vessel origin; at the opposite end, the pressure is P2. Resistance occurs due to the friction between the bloodstream and the intravascular endothelium over the entire inner surface of the vessel. The flow through the vessel can be calculated using the formula [3]:

S. Vlad and N.M. Roman (eds.), *International Conference on Advancements of Medicine and Health Care through Technology; 12th - 15th October 2016, Cluj-Napoca, Romania,*
IFMBE Proceedings 59,
DOI: 10.1007/978-3-319-52875-5_33

$$F = Ap / R \text{ (Ohm's law)} \quad (3)$$

F is the blood flow, Ap is the pressure difference (P1-P2) between the two ends of the vessel, and R is resistance. This formula is in effect saying that blood flow is directly proportional to the pressure difference, but inversely proportional to resistance.

It is very important to remember, that the pressure difference between the ends of the vessel, is not absolute pressure in the vessel, which determines the flow rate. For example, if the press-united at both ends of the vessel is 100 mm Hg, and there is no difference in pressure between the two ends of vascular, there will be no flow though a pressure of 100 mmHg. [4]

When the body is under the influence of a magnetic field, blood flow increases and the oxygen is absorbed into the tissues. This is probably one of the mechanisms that helps in healing and one of the reasons why it is helpful in so many different diseases.

III. Results

Magnet has a great influence on our organism, this being discussed and analyzed in numerous documents and publications. The research made so far to make a statement that there is a series of variations in the human body signals during magneto-theraphy session are highlighted by various records during this procedure, and photoplethysmography is one of the body signals who helps as to get information from the circulatory sistem. For a more accurate assessment of biosignals obtained from the pacient in this study we have decided to record the photopletysmography before, during and after magneto-theraphy session.

Venue of research is the Department of Medical Rehabilitation from the Hospital CF, Iaşi, department specialized in all new methods of recovery and physical medicine,.

Magneto theraphy is the physiotherapy procedure chosen for research. During this procedure we monitored the blood flow parameters in patients that received therapy with low-frequency magnetic fields due to their diagnosis of diseases including the treatment procedure.

The device for magneto theraphy used in our study is a product of Romanian origin, and consisting of two solenoids and two inductors coil that blur associated with the following parameters:

Commonly 50Hz;

Intensity fixed: - 4 mT for cervical coil;
- 2 mT for lumbar coil;
- 20 to 23 mT for locating coils.

The effects of therapy with low-frequency magnetic fields device are:

-to continues unmodulated form: sedative, sympathicolitic, trophotrope;

-to interrupted form: excitatory, sympathicotonia, ergotrop.

The patient is placed in a comfortable position (supine) on parallelipipedal component and placed in the magnetic field by placing the coil with diametrically di largest in the lower limbs. Jewelry and the metal objects are removed from the patient.

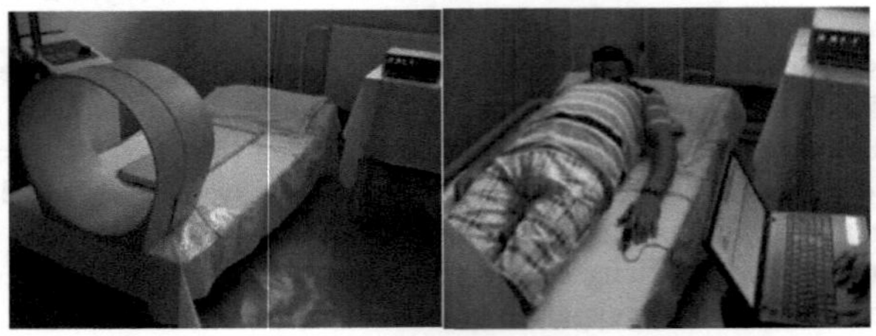

Fig. 2 The position of the pacient in the magneto-theraphy device

Duration and stages of research

For research we monitored during the magnet therapy procedure 37 patients with different diagnoses, in several days (the monitoring was in at least one day and up to six days).

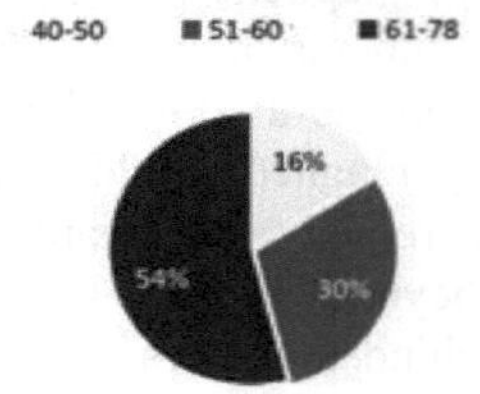

Fig. 3 Age repartition of the patients

For each pacient we recorded the biomedical signals using photoplethysmography before, in time and after the magnto-theraphy session, obtaining a PPG (photoplethysmogram) and a APG (Acceleration PlethysmoGram) wave form.

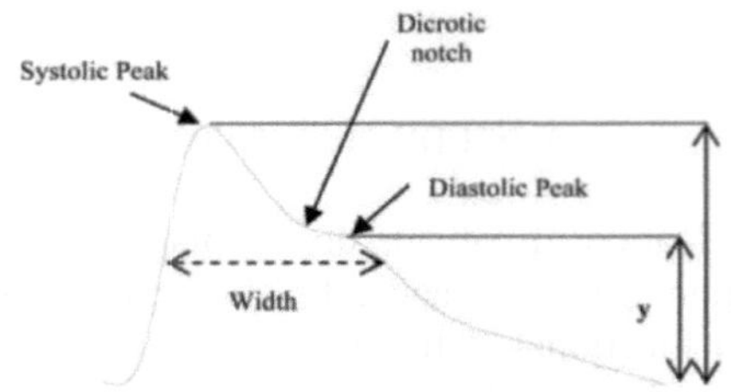

Fig. 4 A typical waveform of the PPG and its characteristic parameters, whereas the amplitude of the systolic peaks is x while y is the amplitude of the diastolic peak [5].

There are different types of APG waveforms. The first APG waveform A (far left) refers to good circulation, whereas the amplitude of B wave is lower than C wave. The last APG waveform G (far right) refers to distinctively bad circulation, whereas the amplitude of C wave is lower than B wave [5].

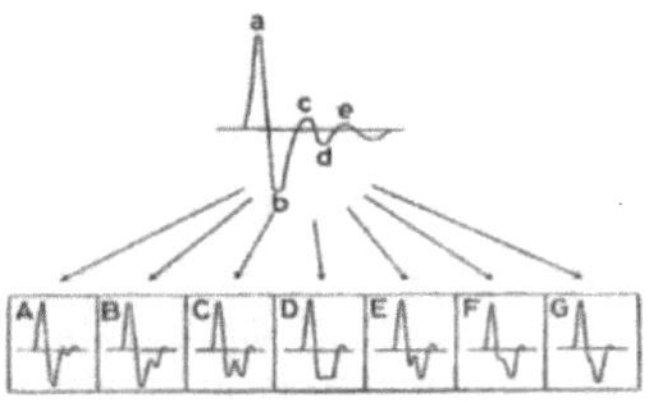

Fig. 5 APG waveforms and types of photoplethysmogram [5]

After collecting all necessary data we have made an analysis of results and graphical method was used to highlight more clearly the level of every patient and its future evolution.

Most indices are based on the second derivative of the finger photoplethysmogram (APG) which seems to provide more information than the first derivative of PPG. The indices calculated from the APG waveforms can be correlated with the distensibility of the carotid artery, age, the blood pressure, the estimated risk of coronary heart disease, and the presence of atherosclerotic disorders

By interpreting the APG form we could decide in which category of hemodynamic risk we can include our pacient. For example in figure 5 we can observe that from the interpretation of APG obtained during theraphy session, the pacient is in a risk category and the blood circulation is getting worse, because the blood pressure is increasing due to the fact that the blood vessels wall narrows.

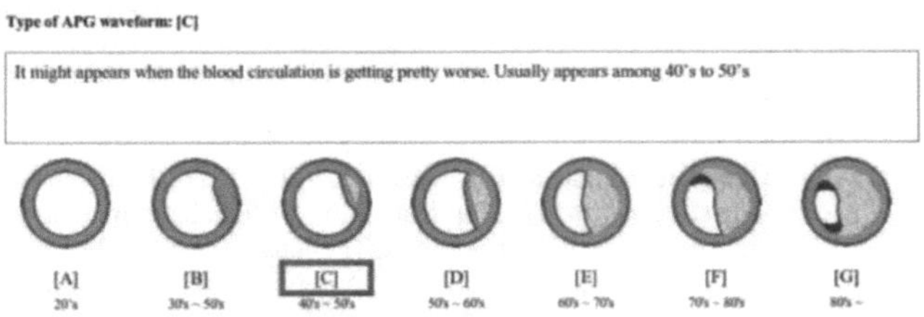

Fig.6 The APG obtained during theraphy session to pacinet A.M.

For each age category we did records, as illustrated in fig.6, fig.7 and fig.8 for wave APG:

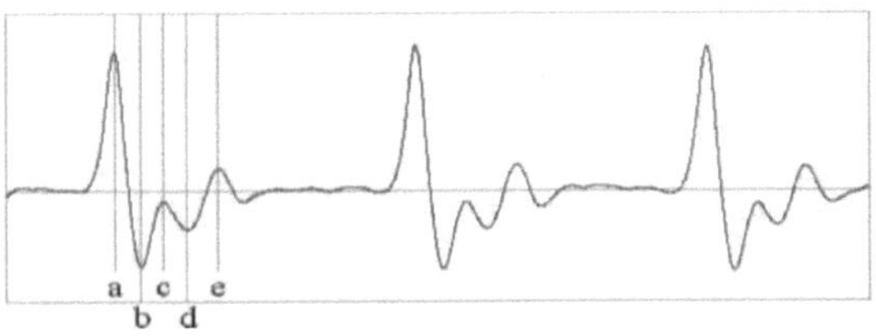

Fig. 7 APG wave for pacients between 40-50 years

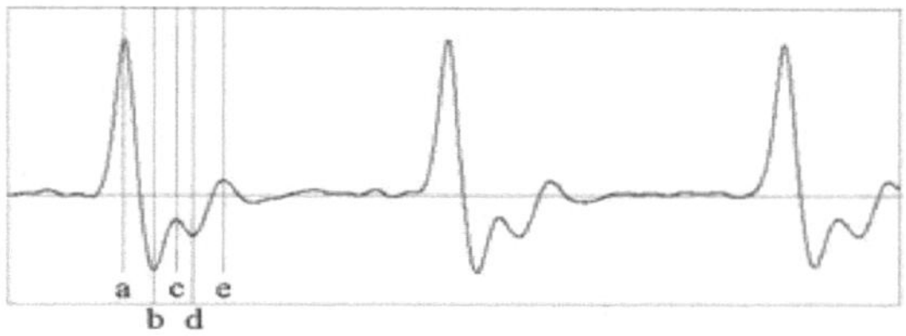

Fig. 8 APG wave for pacients between 51-60 years

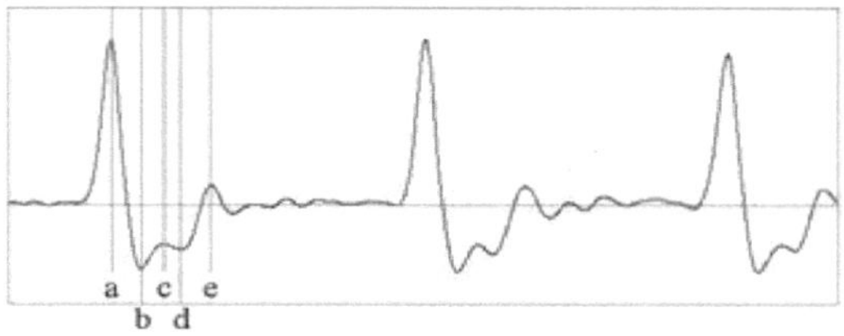

Fig. 9 APG wave for pacients between 61-78years

As we can see from these three graphs, the age of the pacient influences the APG wave form, because the elasticity of the blood vessels is decreasing with age.

For all 37 subjects included in the research, were recorded four individual sheets with daily monitoring of their biomedical parameters that enable better analysis and interpretation of the evolution of each patient during magnetotheraphy and at end of treatment.

The graphical representation of the variation in mean heart rate (HR avg) of the entire group of patients undergoing research:

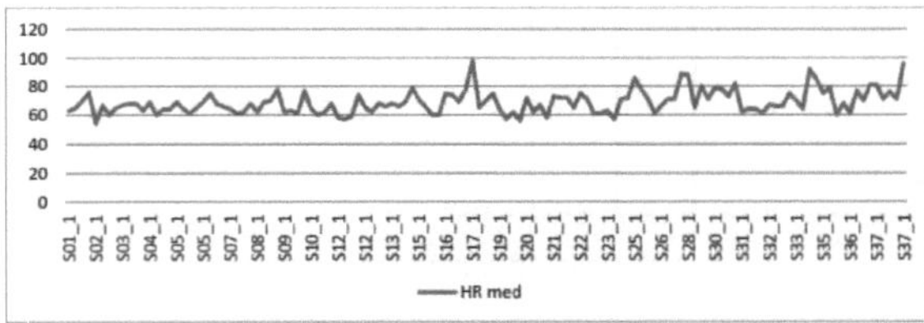

Fig. 10 Change in HR prior magneto therapy session

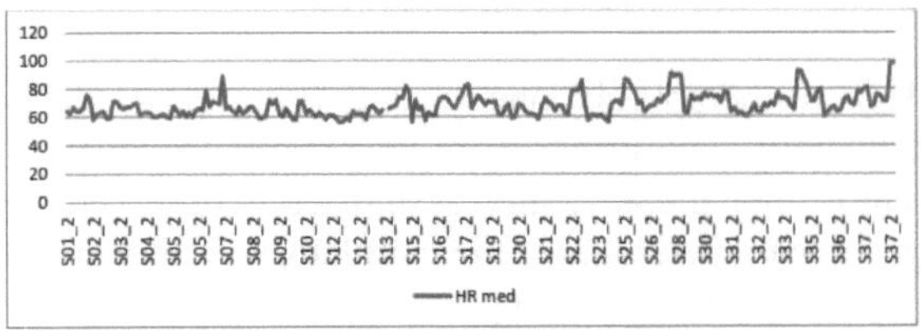

Fig. 11 Change in HR in time of magneto- therapy session

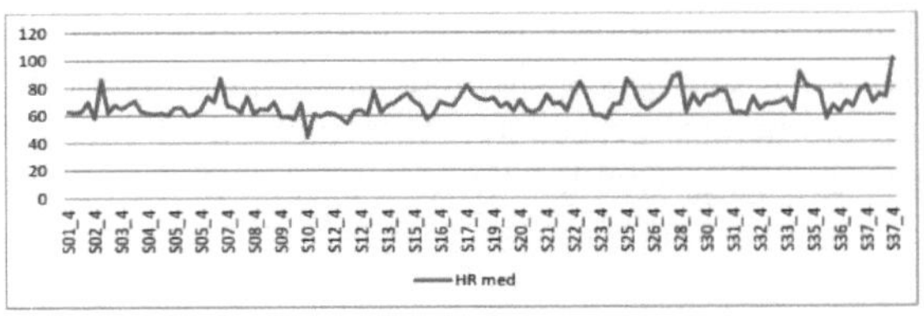

Fig. 12 Change in HR after magneto- therapy session

As we can see from the statistical interpretation of the obtained data, the blood circulation improved, evidenced by regulating heart beat (HR).

Statistics

HR med

N	Valid	125
	Missing	0
Mean		68,85
Median		68,00
Std. Deviation		8,199
Variance		67,227
Skewness		1,072
Std. Error of Skewness		,217
Kurtosis		1,514
Std. Error of Kurtosis		,430
Minimum		54
Maximum		98

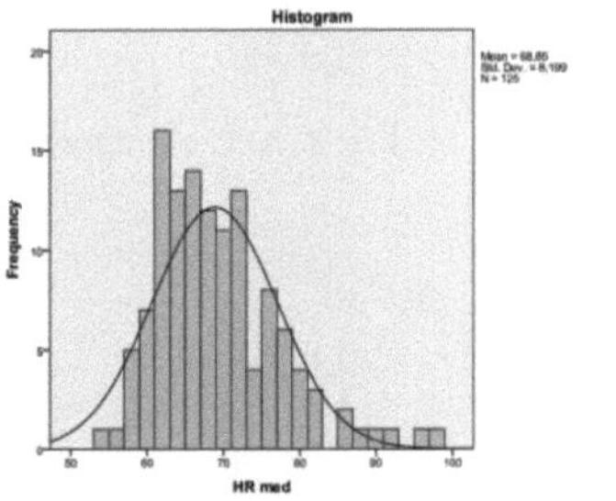

Fig. 13 HR mean before magnetoteraphy session

Statistics

		HR med	HR min	HR max
N	Valid	249	249	249
	Missing	0	0	0
Mean		68,20	55,1478	84,7473
Median		67,00	57,9700	77,4200
Std. Deviation		7,979	14,89950	29,73272
Variance		63,664	221,995	884,035
Skewness		1,165	-,265	3,164
Std. Error of Skewness		,154	,154	,154
Kurtosis		1,612	-,789	10,800
Std. Error of Kurtosis		,307	,307	,307
Minimum		56	30,08	59,70
Maximum		98	90,23	240,00

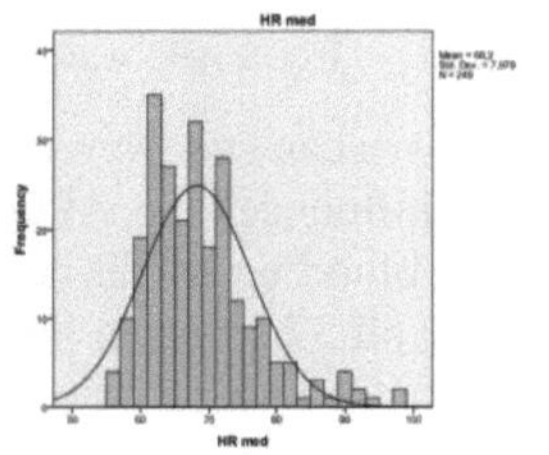

Fig. 14 HR mean in time of magnetoteraphy session

Statistics

		HR med	HR min	HR max
N	Valid	125	125	125
	Missing	0	0	0
Mean		68,38	53,2470	86,7114
Median		67,00	56,8700	76,9200
Std. Deviation		8,510	15,04563	34,16111
Variance		72,416	226,371	1166,982
Skewness		,846	-,041	2,924
Std. Error of Skewness		,217	,217	,217
Kurtosis		1,612	-,580	8,609
Std. Error of Kurtosis		,430	,430	,430
Minimum		44	30,06	47,43
Maximum		101	99,17	240,00

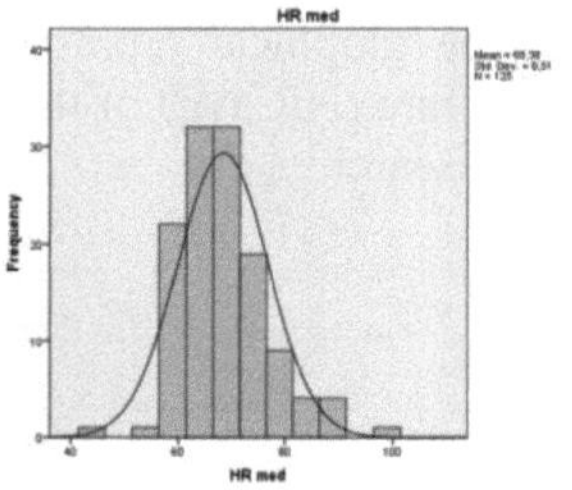

Fig. 15 HR mean after magnetoteraphy session

IV. Conclusions

Magneto-therapy, is one of the basic pro-cedures on physiotherapy, and brings a lot of benefits to patients who can enjoy this therapy, and as has been observed in our study, the parameters from the circulatory system are modified, and helps on the healing of the pacient.

Photoplethysmography used as an objective method for registration of biomedical parameters has failed to identify magneto-theraphy impact on the human body. APG wave illustrates the changes in hemodynamic parameters during this physiotherapy procedure. This method of biomedical signals recording, enabled better analysis of the impact of this therapy on the human body. Thus we have observed an improvement in blood circulation, evidenced especially by regulating heart rate.

In conclusion, we can say that the therapy with low frequency magnetic fields is a safe, tackle low and surprising benefits for treating various diseases. It is undeniable the influence of magneto-theraphy to human body. Because of the many indications in a wide variety of diseases and the few contraindications, magnet should be one of the most popular and most used methods of treatment both prophylactically and therapeutically.

Conflict of Interest

The authors declare that they have no conflict of interest.

References

1. Smith David V., Sălceanu A., Ciorap R. – "Acquisition and Analysis of Biomedical Signals in Case of Peoples Exposed to Electromagnetic Fields", in Mukhopadhyay Subhas Chandra, Postolache Octavian A. (Eds.) – "Pervasive and Mobile Sensing and Computing for Healthcare", Series: Smart Sensors, Measurement and Instrumentation, Vol. 2, Springer-Verlag Berlin Heidelberg 2013, p.269-297
2. Ciorap R., Andriţoi D., Corciovă C., David V.- Recording of biomedical parameters during magnetotherapy, 4th International Conference on Advancements of Medicine and Health Care through Technology, Cluj-Napoca, Romania, 5th – 7th June 2014, IFMBE Proceedings 44, Springer International Publishing Switerland 2014, p. 163-166, DOI:10.1007/978-3-319-07653-9_33
3. Andritoi Doru, Matei Dana, Luca Catalina, Corciova Calin, Ciorap Radu, Preliminary study of HR analysis on patients recovering after stroke, 9th International Symposium on Advanced Topics in Electrical Engineering (ATEE), 7-9 mai 2015 Bucureşti, p. 23-26
4. Munteanu M., Bechet P., Rusu C., Micu D.D., Munteanu R.A., Moga R., Amza C.- Application of Virtual Instrumentation for Transmitting and Processing ECG Signals, în IFMBE Proceedings of the 4 th International Conference on Advancements of Medicine and Health Care through Technology, Springer, 5th – 7th June 2014, Cluj-Napoca, Romania, p. 215-219
5. Mohamed Elgendi, "On the Analysis of Fingertip Photoplethysmogram Signals", Curr Cardiol Rev. 2012 Feb; 8(1): 14–25, doi: 10.2174/157340312801215782

Author: Luca Catalina
Institute: University of Medicine and Pharmacy "Grigore T. Popa" Iasi, Faculty of Medical Bioengineering
Street: Kogalniceanu Street, nr. 9-13
City: Iasi
Country: Romania
Email: luca.katalina@yahoo.com; catalina.luca@bioinginerie.ro

Three Element Windkessel Model to Non-invasively Assess PAH Patients: One Year Follow-up

A. Lungu[1,2,3], D.R. Hose[2,3], D.G.Kiely[4], D. Capener[2], J.M Wild[2,3] and A.J Swift[2,3]

[1]Faculty of Electrical Engineering, Technical University of Cluj-Napoca, Cluj-Napoca, RO
[2]Immunity, Infection and Cardiovascular Diseases Department, University of Sheffield, Sheffield, UK
[3]Institute for in-silico medicine, INSIGNEO, Sheffield, UK
[4]Pulmonary Vascular Disease Unit, Sheffield Teaching Hospital, Sheffield, UK

Abstract-**Pulmonary arterial hypertension (PAH) is a severe, low survival and rapidly progressive disease, characterised by an increase in the distal pulmonary vascular resistance and decrease in pulmonary compliance. The current standard procedure for PAH diagnosis and therapy response assessment is right heart catheterisation (RHC). Although if performed in a specialist centre, the severe complications associated with RHC are reduced, non-invasive alternatives are desirable. Windkessel models have been previously proposed[1], [2] to estimate the overall pulmonary system resistance and compliance.**

The aim of this study was to evaluate whether the pulmonary resistance and total vascular compliance computed using a Windkessel model can be used to assess the therapy response in PAH patients using MRI input data.

56 treatment naïve patients, diagnosed with PAH at RHC, underwent MRI of the main pulmonary artery (MPA) at baseline and one year follow-up. A plug-in implemented in MATLAB was used to segment the MPA images at baseline and follow-up, extract the area and flow waveforms and compute the values of the Windkessel model.

At follow-up, the computational results showed statistically significant increase of the compliance, C_{Wk}($p<0.05$), and decrease in resistance, R_{Wk} ($p<0.01$). Separated according to the patient's sex, the femalesub-group showed a statistically significant increase of the compliance ($p<0.01$) and decrease of the resistance ($p<0.01$). However, the male sub-group showed statistically significant reduction of the resistance ($p<0.05$) but no significant increase of the model's compliance ($p=0.19$). When separated upon patient's age, younger patients (age≤50 years) showed statistically significant decrease of the Windkessel resistance ($p<0.01$) and increase of the compliance ($p<0.05$), while older patients (age>50 years) showed statistically significant reduction of the resistance ($p<0.01$) but no significant increase of the Windkessel compliance ($p=0.21$).

The non-invasive proposed metrics have the potential to assess the response to PAH therapy, reducing the RHC interventions at follow-up.

Keywords— **PAH, Windkessel, non-invasive, follow-up, MRI**

I. Introduction

Pulmonary hypertension (PH) is a condition defined by an increased mean pulmonary arterial pressure (mPAP≥25 mmHg), measured at rest, by right heart catheterisation (RHC).

According to pathophysiology, clinical presentation, and therapeutic approaches, PH wasdivided at the Dana Point congress into 5 groups [6] as follows: Group 1: Pulmonary arterial hypertension (PAH), Group 2: Pulmonary hypertension due to left heart disease (PH-LHD), Group 3: Pulmonary hypertension owing to lung disease and/or hypoxia (PH-Lung), Group 4: Chronic thromboembolic pulmonary hypertension (CTEPH), Group 5: Pulmonary hypertension with unclear or multifactorial etiologies. Only group 1 (PAH) and group 4 (CTEPH) have a defined clinical treatment, whereas for the other three groups, the optimal treatment is not clear, being determined mainly by the treatment of the underlying cause.

Pulmonary arterial hypertension (PAH) is a severe, low survival and rapidly progressive disease [7], characterised by an increase in the pulmonary vascular resistance (PVR) and decrease in the compliance (C). Both are contributing to an increase in the heart afterlod, leading to heart failure, which is one of the most common death causes in PH[8].

According to the guidelines, once the PAH diagnosis is established at baseline, a 6 to 12 months RHC follow-up is recommended. RHC presents risks to the patient, including bleeding, hematoma formation, vessel puncture, reaction to the contrast dye, abnormal heart rate and, in extreme cases, heart attack, stroke and death [9],[10]. Although the severe complications are reduced when the procedure is performed in a specialist centre[11], non-invasive methods for PH diagnosis and assessment are highly desirable to reduce the risks and improve patient's life quality.

A three element (R_c-C-R_d) electrical analogue Windkessel model was previously proposed by the authors [2] to estimate the overall pulmonary system resistance and compliance based on MRI flow and anatomy data and showed promising results for differentiating between healthy volunteers, patients without PH and clinical patients with stratified PH.

The aim of this study was to evaluate whether the pulmonary resistance and total vascular compliance computed using the Windkessel model (Fig. 1) can assess the therapy response in PAH patients using MRI.

S. Vlad and N.M. Roman (eds.), *International Conference on Advancements of Medicine and Health Care through Technology; 12th - 15th October 2016, Cluj-Napoca, Romania,*
IFMBE Proceedings 59,
DOI: 10.1007/978-3-319-52875-5_34

II. Methods

A. Patients

56 treatment naïve patients, 32 women and24 men, diagnosed with PAH at RHC, underwent magnetic resonance imaging (MRI) of the main pulmonary artery (MPA) at baseline and one year follow-up.

B. Right heart catheterization

RHC was performed via the internal jugular vein using a Swan-Ganz catheter. PH was defined as mPAP $\geq$ 25 mmHg at rest with PAH being diagnosed when the pulmonary capillary wedge pressure (PCWP) $\leq$ 15 mmHg[12].

C. Magnetic Resonance Imaging

MRI images of the main pulmonary artery (MPA) were acquired for all the subjects, under breath hold, using phase contrast (PC) and balanced steady state free precession (bSSFP) sequences. The two sets of acquired images were co-registered in time (same number of temporal phases) and space (same matrix dimensions) and were used to obtain simultaneous time varying flow and pressure (from the measured radius as previously proposed [2]).The PC and bSSFP images were spatially and temporarily synchronised, using the same pixel size (256x 128 matrix dimensions, 480x288 mm FOV) and same number of cardiac images (40). For the PC sequence a value of V_{enc}= 150cm/s, 5.85 ms repetition time (TR) 2.87 ms echo time (TE) and 10% arrythmia rejection. For the bSSFP acquisition, a 3.73ms TR and 1.62 ms TE were used.

D. Image processing

Using a semi-automatic registration based segmentation method[13] implemented under ShIRT (Sheffield University Registration Toolkit), the images were post-processed in MATLAB(R2014a, The MathWorks Inc.) in order to extract the MPA cross-sectional area and quantify the flow variation during the cardiac cycle. The applied method is using an average image as a fixed image, as previously described in [14].

E. Windkessel model

The total vascular compliance and distal resistance were estimated by optimising the electrical parameters of a three element Windkessel model (R_c-C-R_d), using as input MRI derived flow and area waveforms. The Windkessel model offers a global representation of the entire pulmonary circulation through the means of electrical analogy. The components of the proposed electrical circuit are: the proximal resistance, R_c, representing the characteristic resistance of the main pulmonary artery (MPA), the total pulmonary vascular compliance, C and the distal resistance, R_d, representing the pulmonary resistance of the distal vasculature. The sum of the two resistors is equal to the total vascular resistance and it is referred in this article as the Windkessel resistance, R_{Wk} (R_{Wk}=R_c+R_d). The computation method, proposed in [2], returns the best set of electrical parameters that minimizes the cost function between the measured and model computed pressure (radius used as surrogate) waveforms.

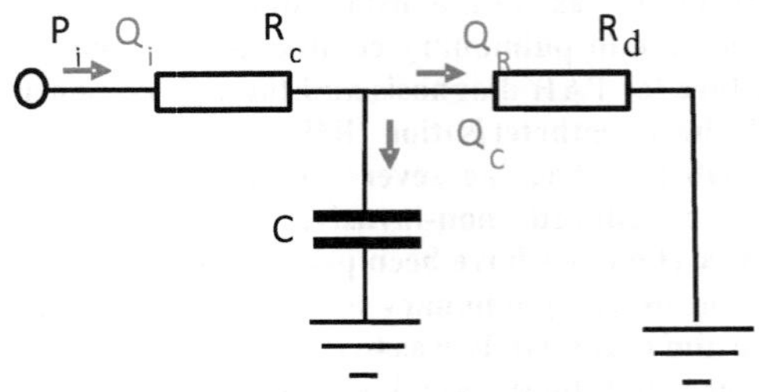

Fig. 1 The three element Windkessel model (R_cCR_d) used for the analysis of the pulmonary circulation in PAH at baseline and follow-up

A graphical user interface (GUI) was implemented in MATLAB to integrate the segmentation of the MRI images, computation of the area and flow waveform and the optimization of the Windkessel parameters. The plug-in allows the user to upload the MRI images, perform and correct the segmentations and compute the Windkessel parameters.

F. Statistics

IBM SPSS 20 (SPSS, Chicago,IL) was used for statistical analysis and GraphPad Prism 6.0 (San Diego California USA)was used for data presentation.

The normality condition was tested by visual inspection of histograms and confirmed by the Shapiro-Wilk normality test. Since the normality condition was violated, the non-parametric Wilcoxon statistical test for 2 related samples was applied. A *p-value*<0.05 was considered significant for all statistical tests.

III. Results and Discussion

The RHC baseline hemodynamic data according to patient's sex is displayed in Table 1. No statistically significant differences were found between any of the measured metrics, evaluated using independent group Mann-Whitney U non-parametric test.

Table 1 RHC hemodynamic data for the analysed cohort, according to patient sex

	F, n=32	M, n=24
age, y	52	59
mPAP, mmHg	52 ±13	50 ±11
CO , l/min	4.6 ±1.3	4.5 ±1.1
PVR, WU	10.2 ±4.5	8.2 ± 3.1

The Wilcoxon signed-rank test was used to evaluate the baseline to follow-up differences between the Windkessel resistance (R_{Wk}) and compliance (C_{Wk}). The results for the entire cohort (n=56), showed statistically significant increase of the compliance, C_{Wk}($p<0.05$), and decrease of the resistance, R_{Wk} ($p<0.01$).

Separated according to the patient's sex, the female subgroup showed a statistically significant increase in pulmonary compliance ($p<0.01$) and decrease of the resistance ($p<0.001$). However, the male sub-group showed statistically significant reduction of the resistance ($p<0.05$) but no significant decrease of the model's compliance ($p=0.19$).
The mean values for the Windkessel resistance and compliance at baseline and follow-up, together with the *p*-value returned by the statistical signed-rank test are displayed in Table 2. The C_{Wk} metric increased at follow-up for 75% of women (24/32) and for 63% of men (15/24). The R_{Wk}metric decreased at follow-up for 81% of (26/32) women and 67% (16/24) of men. In one female patient, the R_{Wk} metric remained constant, while for other two women, the increase was only of 1%.

Table 2 Changes in the non-invasive computational pulmonary resistance and compliance at follow-up in PAH naïve patients, separated based on sex

parameter	**F, n=32**			**M, n=24**		
	base-line	**follow up**	**p value**	**base-line**	**follow up**	**p value**
R_{Wk}, mmHg s/ml	0.88	0.57	<0.001	1.21	0.74	0.04
C_{Wk}, ml/mmHg	0.69	1.06	<0.001	1	0.92	0.19

Separated upon patient's age, younger patients (age≤50 years, n=19) showed statistically significant decrease of the Windkessel resistance ($p<0.01$) and increase of the compliance ($p<0.05$), while older patients (age>50 years, n=37) showed statistically significant reduction of the resistance ($p<0.01$) but no significant decrease of the Windkessel compliance ($p=0.21$).

The scatter plot from Fig. 2 shows the distribution of the changes in the Windkessel resistance and compliance between baseline (R_{Wk1} and C_{Wk1}) and follow-up ($R_{Wk2}$and C_{Wk2}) in PAH patients separated according to their age and sex. The figure was divided in four, by two dotted vertical and horizontal lines, marking no change in the Windkessel compliance and resistance at follow-up.

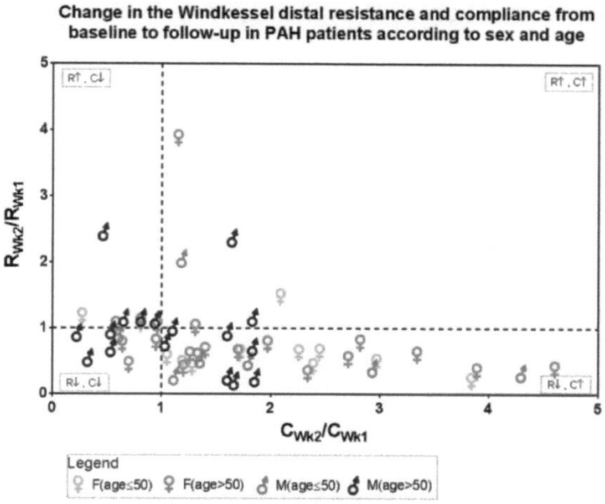

Fig.2 The distribution of the changes in the Windkessel resistance and compliance from baseline to follow-up in PAH patients separated according to their age and sex.

Considering that a lower resistance and a higher compliance at follow-up are suggesting an improvement in the heart afterload and of the patient's condition, it can be argued that the patients found on the top-left panel of Fig. 2 are doing the worst, while the patients from the lower-right panel are doing the best at follow-up. It can be noticed from the figure, and confirmed by Table 2than most of the patients have a lower resistance at follow-up, while a smaller number of patients were improving their Windkessel compliance.

Separated according to patients' age and sex, the results indicated that younger patients (light colors) are mainly positioned in the lower-right side of the graph. Additionally, the proportion of female patient found in the area suggesting follow-up improvement is higher than the male patient proportion. A study of Gabler et al. [3] concerning the response to therapy according to patient's race and sex, showed that female patients have better outcome following PAH treatment.Jacobs et al.[15] showed that although male and female patients had similar reduction in PVR at one year follow-up, the female patients had a better improvement of the ventricular functions. Similar findings were also noted by Swift et al. [16] in patients withidiopathic pulmonary arterial hypertension (IPAH). According to these studies, although PAH is prevalent in female patients, male patients have a worse therapy outcome. This idea is often referred clinically as the "estrogen paradox" [17], suggesting that the female hormone might favor the PAH development, but it also might have a positive influence on the response to treatment.Several pulmonary hypertension registry studies [4], [5] have been shown that age isalso an independent marker of poor outcome in patients with PAH. In the study of Benza et al. [5], male patients over 60 years of age were revealed to have a worse outcome than female patients regardless of their age, while the study of Ling et al. [4]showed that patients younger than 50 years old had better survival comparing to older patients.

IV. Conclusions

These results are in agreement with previously reported invasive findings[3],[4], [5], suggesting that the non-invasively computed resistance and compliance could be used for the PAH assessment, in order to reduce the frequency of the RHC interventions at follow-up

V. Compliance with Ethical Requirements

A. Conflict of Interest

The authors declare that they have no conflict of interest.

B. Statement of Informed Consent

Informed consent was waived for this retrospective study.

C. Statement of Human and Animal Rights

This study was undertaken following approval from the local research ethics committee.

Acknowledgment

The authors gratefully acknowledge the support of INSIGNEO- Institute for *in-silico* medicine and Sheffield Hospitals Charity for funding this project.

References

1. Lankhaar, J.W., et al., *Quantification of right ventricular afterload in patients with and without pulmonary hypertension.* Am J Physiol Heart Circ Physiol, 2006. **291**(4): p. H1731-7.
2. Lungu, A., et al., *MRI model-based non-invasive differential diagnosis in pulmonary hypertension.* J Biomech, 2014. **47**(12): p. 2941-7.
3. Gabler, N.B., et al., *Race and Sex Differences in Response to Endothelin Receptor Antagonists for Pulmonary Arterial Hypertension.* Chest, 2012. **141**(1): p. 20-26.
4. Ling, Y., et al., *Changing demographics, epidemiology, and survival of incident pulmonary arterial hypertension: results from the pulmonary hypertension registry of the United Kingdom and Ireland.* Am J Respir Crit Care Med, 2012. **186**(8): p. 790-6.
5. Benza, R.L., et al., *Predicting survival in pulmonary arterial hypertension: insights from the Registry to Evaluate Early and Long-Term Pulmonary Arterial Hypertension Disease Management (REVEAL).* Circulation, 2010. **122**(2): p. 164-72.
6. Simonneau, G., et al., *Updated clinical classification of pulmonary hypertension.* J Am Coll Cardiol, 2009. **54**(1 Suppl): p. S43-54.
7. Kiely, D.G., et al., *Pulmonary hypertension: diagnosis and management.* BMJ, 2013. **346**: p. f2028.
8. Voelkel, N.F., et al., *Right Ventricular Function and Failure: Report of a National Heart, Lung, and Blood Institute Working Group on Cellular and Molecular Mechanisms of Right Heart Failure.* Circulation, 2006. **114**(17): p. 1883-1891.
9. 9.Ranu, H., et al., *A retrospective review to evaluate the safety of right heart catheterization via the internal jugular vein in the assessment of pulmonary hypertension.* Clin Cardiol, 2010. **33**(5): p. 303-6.
10. Glowny, M.G. and F.S. Resnic, *What to Expect During Cardiac Catheterization.* Circulation, 2012. **125**(7): p. e363-e364.
11. Hoeper, M.M., et al., *Complications of right heart catheterization procedures in patients with pulmonary hypertension in experienced centers.* J Am Coll Cardiol, 2006. **48**(12): p. 2546-52.
12. Galie, N., et al., *Guidelines for the diagnosis and treatment of pulmonary hypertension: the Task Force for the Diagnosis and Treatment of Pulmonary Hypertension of the European Society of Cardiology (ESC) and the European Respiratory Society (ERS), endorsed by the International Society of Heart and Lung Transplantation (ISHLT).* Eur Heart J, 2009. **30**(20): p. 2493-537.
13. Barber, D.C. and D.R. Hose, *Automatic segmentation of medical images using image registration: diagnostic and simulation applications.* J Med Eng Technol, 2005. **29**(2): p. 53-63.
14. Lungu, A., et al., *Automatic, Simultaneous, Non-invasive Measurements of Flow and Area in the Human Pulmonary Arteries from MRI Images,* in *International Conference on Advancements of Medicine and Health Care through Technology; 5th – 7th June 2014, Cluj-Napoca, Romania*, S. Vlad and R.V. Ciupa, Editors. 2014, Springer International Publishing. p. 259-264.
15. Jacobs, W., et al., *The right ventricle explains sex differences in survival in idiopathic pulmonary arterial hypertension.* Chest, 2014. **145**(6): p. 1230-6.
16. Swift, A.J., et al., *Right ventricular sex differences in patients with idiopathic pulmonary arterial hypertension characterised by magnetic resonance imaging: pair-matched case controlled study.* PLoS One, 2015. **10**(5): p. e0127415.
17. Manes, A., et al., *[Female gender and pulmonary arterial hypertension: a complex relationship].* G Ital Cardiol (Rome), 2012. **13**(6): p. 448-60.

Author: Angela Lungu
Institute:Technical University of Cluj-Napoca
Street: G. Baritiu, 26-28
City: Cluj-Napoca
Country:Romania
Email: Angela.Lungu@ethm..utcluj.ro

Thermal Rehabilitation Influence upon the Comfort in Hospitals

A. Abrudan, T. Rus and R. Mare

Technical University of Cluj-Napoca/Building Services Department, Cluj-Napoca, Romania

Abstract— **In Romania, most of the hospitals still have a relatively low level of thermal insulation, thus inside of building the microclimate conditions are continuously deteriorating, due to vapors condensation producing also an increase in heat losses, energy consumption and operational costs.**

The rehabilitation and modernizing can be applied successfully using energy efficient methods together with latest materials and technologies.

The rehabilitation solutions are strictly binding to the required level of comfort required by a certain area, its occupancy pattern, its geographical location (urban or rural areas, etc.), etc.

The thermal rehabilitation of hospitals buildings is a must in order to achieve the required interior microclimate conditions, increase the degree of environmental protection and reducing operational costs, regarding as well the investment costs involved.

A special attention has to be given to the interior microclimate conditions required by the hospital specific activities conditions which are different compared to other buildings.

This paper intends to present some of the possibilities to improve the thermal protection, the measurements being performed on a wall structure used for the construction of most hospitals in Romania, and for the thermal insulation two of the most used materials have been considered. The results of measurements have been processed through a mathematical modelling software, and the conclusion are demonstrating the need to reduce or eliminate the thermal bridges of any kind, especially in the intersection zone of building elements and around the openings for windows and doors in order to ensure optimal thermal comfort.

Keywords—**Hospitals, thermal comfort, thermal rehabilitation, condensing, numeric modeling.**

I. Introduction

Thermal Comfort as explained by the BS EN ISO 7730 [6] is "Thermal comfort is that condition of mind which expresses satisfaction with the thermal environment". Due to considerable individual differences, it is impossible to define a thermal comfort (not only air temperature) that will satisfy everybody, those individual parameters will help ultimately to define the "human thermal environment". The effort made by the human body to maintain the functional equilibrium may be severely influenced by excessive conditions, having negative influence upon human health.

As it establishes a dual link between external thermal parameters and the human body capacity of self-regulation (heat gain or loss) the thermal comfort comprises two components: one is physiologic and the other is economic (increases work productivity).

II. Considerations Regarding the Main Parameters Influencing Thermal Comfort

Those parameters can be divided in two categories:

1. Environmental parameters:

-radiant temperature,

- air temperature,

-air humidity,

-air velocity.

2. Personal parameters:

-clothing insulation,

-metabolic heat (the metabolic rate allows the thermal risk evaluation in relation with the activity level, age, sex, gender, body weight)

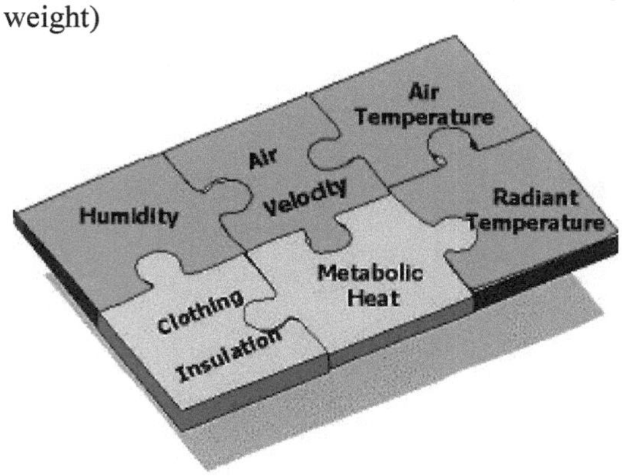

Fig.1 The main parameters influencing the thermal comfort

The human being is homoeothermic, having a complex thermal-regulation capacity, maintaining a relatively constant temperature (< 37 °C), independent of the variation of the surrounding climate conditions, provided that the variation is not an excessive one.

Where the variations are important, the human body capacity of self-regulation is exceeded, therefore it is necessary to use additional measures to restore the thermal equilibrium, like adequate clothing and climate control using heating, ventilation and air-conditioning systems.

The human body maintains its thermal balance through:

S. Vlad and N.M. Roman (eds.), *International Conference on Advancements of Medicine and Health Care through Technology; 12th - 15th October 2016, Cluj-Napoca, Romania*,
IFMBE Proceedings 59,
DOI: 10.1007/978-3-319-52875-5_35

• Modifying the metabolic rate, namely the heat production → ***chemical regulation***;

• Regulation of heat loss through physical mechanism like radiation, convection, conduction and vaporization → ***physical regulation.***

When exposed to cold environment the heat loss regulation is being made mainly through chemical regulation, whereas when exposed to heat the regulation is being made physically.

Obviously those processes are not exclusive but compensate each other.

A remarkable progress related to the global evaluation of the hygro-thermal comfort is achieved through usage of the Fanger equation [8] (rectified by Olesen) which is based on the thermal balance of human body, starting from the equality between the heat produced by the body and the heat exchanged with the environment.:

$$S = M \pm W \pm R \pm C \pm K - E - RES \quad (1)$$

where:

S represents the heat accumulated by the body;
M - Metabolic heat production;
W - External mechanical power;
R, C, K – heat exchange through radiation, convection, conduction;
E, RES – heat loss through sweat and respiration.

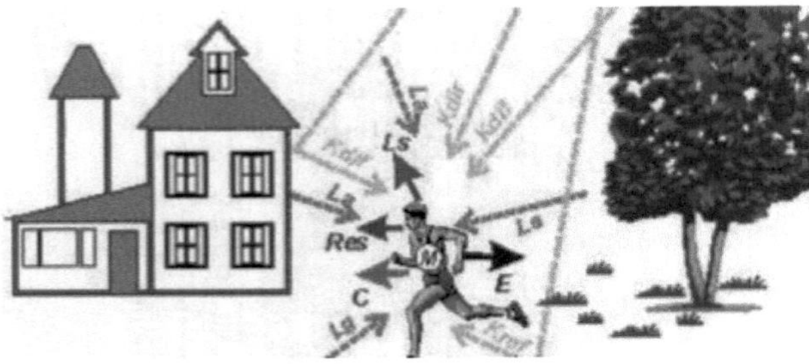

Fig.2 Thermal balance of human body

Considering the case of dressed people, the thermal balance becomes a double equation:

$$M \pm W - E - RES = \pm K_{imb} = \pm R \pm C \quad (2)$$

where K_{imb} is the heat passing through clothing.

This double equation is based on the equality between the metabolic heat produced added or subtracted by the heat lost through mechanical power, sweating and breathing and the heat received or given to the clothing respectively to environment through radiation and convection. The conduction component has a negligible value therefore it will not be taking into consideration.

The variables of Fanger's equation will be briefly explained below:

• **M** is the energy released into the body through oxidation processes, which is partially converted into mechanical power (W) but mainly into internal body heat. The value of **M** may suffer variation between 45W/m^2 skin surface, in resting state, and 500 W/m^2 for running man. Metabolism is being expressed in "met"; 1met =58.15W/m^2 being defined as the metabolism of a person during resting. The literature is specifying the values of **M** for different activities.

• External mechanical power **W** may be positive or negative. If the energy is used by the human being for a certain activity then **W** >0, and if the energy used is transformed into heat (muscles for example) then **W** <0.

• The heat lost through evaporation (sweat) **E** may be expressed as :

$$E = E_d + E_{tr} \quad [W/m^2] \quad (3)$$

where:

$\mathbf{E_d}$ - heat lost through water vapor diffusion through skin [W/m^2] or insensible perspiration:

$$E_d = 3.05 * 10^{-3} (p_s - p_v) = 3.05 * 10^{-3} (256T_p - 3373 - p_v) \quad (4)$$

p_s – saturated water vapor pressure at the skin temperature (T_p) [Pa];
p_v - water vapor pressure in the environment [Pa].

This component (E_d) is being permanently produced and it is not controlled by the human body thermo-regulation system.

$\mathbf{E_{tr}}$ – is the heat lost through evaporation of sweat on the skin surface [W/m^2].

Component (E_{tr}) is has large variations conditioned by the physical activity from 0 W/m^2 during rest, to a maximum of 400W/m^2, during high physical activities, in a warm and dry environment; it is mainly influenced by the environmental temperature and its relative humidity.

• The heat lost through respiration **RES** is due to the fact that the temperature of exhaled air (cca. 34°C) is generally higher than the one inhaled and more humid as well.

$$RES = 0.0014M(34 - T_a) + 1.72 * 10^{-5} M(5867 - p_v) \, [W/m^2] \quad (5)$$

where:

M – metabolism rate [W/m^2];
T_a = environmental temperature [°C];
p_v = inspired water vapor pressure [Pa].

Generally for normal activities, at $T_a \cong 20$°C , RES =2÷5 W/m^2 therefore negligible.

• The heat lost through conduction through clothing $\mathbf{K_{imb}}$ [W/m^2] is:

$$K_{imb} = \frac{T_p - T_{imb}}{0.155 R_{cl}} = \frac{T_p - T_{imb}}{R_{imb}} \quad [W/m^2] \quad (6)$$

where:

T_p – skin temperature [°C];
T_{imb} – clothing surface temperature [°C];
R_{cl} – clothing thermal resistance in "clo", 1clo = 0.155 m^2K/W;
R_{imb} – clothing thermal resistance in [m^2K/W].

Heat exchanged by the body through radiation "**R**" [W/m^2] between the body surface and environment is being calculated using Lambert, Stefan-Boltzman and Kirchhoff laws.

• Heat exchanged by the body through convection "**C**" due to the surrounding air flowing on the body surface. It is being calculated using Newton law where the thermal transfer coefficient through surface α_{cv} results from using the phenomenon analysis and using criteria formulas obtained from the theory of similitude related to the fluid flow.

III. Experimental tests and discussions

To ensure the optimal thermal comfort conditions in hospitals is necessary to solve problems one set of environmental factors and specific humidity.

The measurements and their interpretation have been made for a hospital building with the structure mono-layer from bricks BCA-GBN 35, 40 cm thickness bound with mortar M 25, and plastered internally and externally with M 50 mortar having a thickness of 1 cm respectively 2 cm (A) and two alternatives for externally mounted thermal insulation, respectively expanded polystyrene with 15 cm thickness(solution1) (B) and mineral wool G.100 in rigid plates protected with polyethylene foil with 0.15 mm thickness (final thickness15 cm)(solution 2)(C).

The comparison criterion is the overall behaviour related to hygro-thermal parameters. Also, it is obvious that achieving higher efficiency levels, it is required to make a correlation between the thermo-physical features, their dimensions and their construction, but also the disturbing elements (thermal bridges, air infiltration, etc.)

Because the marginal influence on the occurrence of condensation is minimized, a 60x60 cm perimeter was defined for each of the three segments of the analyzed panel, centered on the transverse axis of each segment. Table 1 shows the risk of condensation expressed through maximum allowable relative humidity of the interior air, for prevention of the interior surfaces' condensation.

The risk of condensation is less as the value of maximum allowable relative humidity is higher.

An optimal solution for building thermal protection has to be established, prior to rehabilitation in order to ensure optimal thermal comfort. Therefore, the measurements of 3 panel segments have been numerically modelled [7]. The numeric modelling allows both the influence analysis of the various external factors and optimizing the technical solutions for closing elements.

Table 1 Maximum allowable relative humidity of interior air, adjacent to internal surfaces

Panel segment	Average temperature of the interior surface [^{0}C]	Average temperature of air adjacent to the area [^{0}C]	Maximum allowable relative humidity [%]
(A)	15.3	17.6	86.4
(B)	18.1	19.1	94.0
(C)	18.4	19.0	96.4

Modelling involves the input of several material types, their dimensions and heat loads. The software [7] allows inputs for punctual or surface heat loads and tempe-ratures and convection loads (temperatures and conductive transfer coefficients). The software used for numerical modelling is a meshing and automatic data input, writing programs of elementary equations, their assembly into the overall system and solving the obtained data. Thus, on the existing and studied structural frame, the simulation was done with the use of two types of externally mounted thermal insulation where the indoor temperature is T_i=20 ^{0}C and the outdoor temperature is T_e= -15 ^{0}C.

The results achieved for the base structure and solution 1 are shown in figure 3.

The results for base structure and solution 2 are shown in the figures 4, 5 and 6.

Comparing the two alternatives where the structure is identical, but the thermal insulation is composed of expanded polystyrene and the second one in mineral wool plates, having the same thickness, it can be noticed that for the same building and same temperature conditions, the density of thermal flux is almost identical, with a difference of 0.2 %.

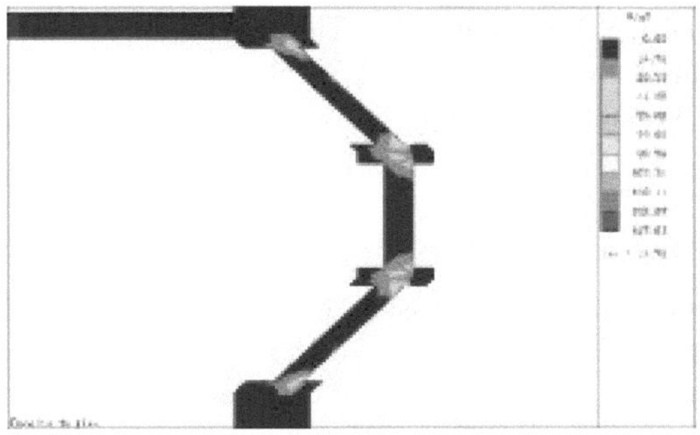

Fig.3 Detail with areas with maximum flux density

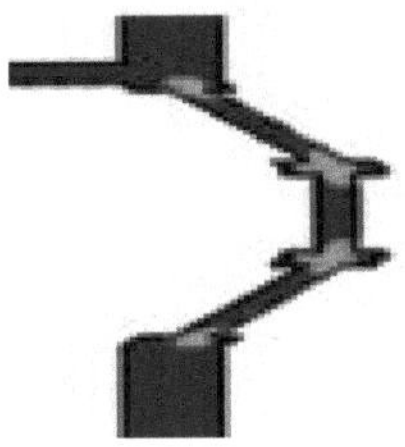

Fig.4 Equal thermal flux for the considered section

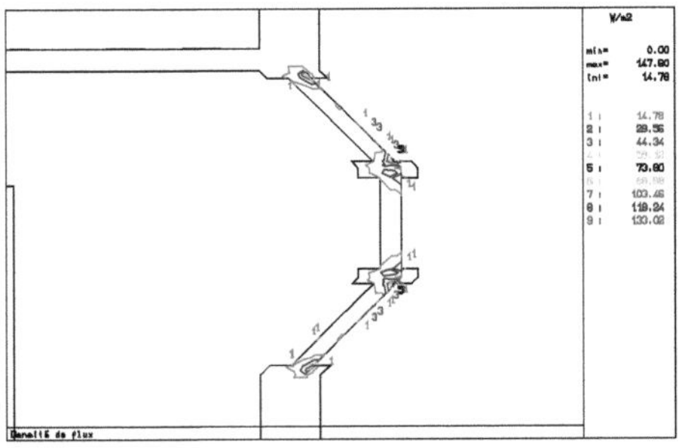

Fig.5 Equal density thermal flux lines for the considered section

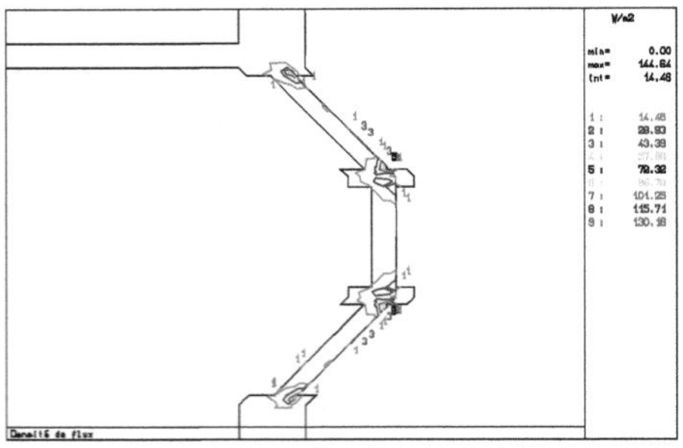

Fig.6 Equal density thermal flux lines for the most unfavorable area at the junction between the window and wall

The maximum value for the thermal flux is in both cases in the same sections (at the joining between wall and window frame). Variation of the lines of equal thermal flux density is obvious in the jointing areas between the building structure (external wall) and windows. The maximum values, for the solutions 1 and 2 are 147.80 W/m^2 and 144.64 W/m^2 respectively, with a 3% difference.

IV. Conclusions

1. It is absolutely necessary to improve the thermal behavior of the building elements which are composing the building envelope in order to reduce the heat losses and avoiding to the extent possible the condensation.

2. The maximum allowable relative humidity is higher, the lower is the risk of condensation. For the studied materials, the highest value of allowable maximum relative humidity is for the mineral wool (2.1 % higher than the expanded polystyrene). Considering this criterion only, it has been concluded that the optimal solution is the one with mono layer brick masonry and thermal insulation with mineral wool.

3. The lines of equal thermal flux density are showing its variation for the studied structure. This change in the lines shapes is obvious in the intersection areas between the construction elements, around the windows and doors openings, and where the material properties are different. In those areas the thermal flux density is the highest, with a 3% difference between the two insulation solutions.

As a conclusion, it is obvious that from the thermal point of view, there is a major need to eliminate or reduce at its most the presence of thermal bridges, especially in the intersection areas and around the windows and doors in order to ensure the thermal comfort in the buildings with a structure and insulation similar to the studied ones.

Conflict of Interest

The authors declare that they have no conflict of interest.

References

1. Abrudan A, (2003) , PhD Thesis "Reduction of the heat losses in the building envelope", Cluj-Napoca
2. Abrudan A, Domnita F (2009) " Heating installation, elements of building thermal engineering", U.T. Press, Cluj-Napoca, 2009 ISBN 978-973-662-512-1
3. Domnita F, Abrudan A (2009) "Ventilation and air conditioning in hospitals", U.T. Press, Cluj-Napoca, 2009 ISBN 978-973-662-511-4
4. Mârza C, Abrudan A, (2012), "Thermotechnics construction elements ",UT Press Cluj-Napoca, ISBN 978-973-662-745-3
5. Enache L, Bunescu I, (2011), "Thermal comfort important environmental factor in the treatment centers" A IX a Conferinţă Naţională de Balneologie 12 - 14 mai 2011
6. British Standard BS EN ISO 7730:2005
7. Software RDM 6
8. Poul O. Fanger (1982), "Thermal Comfort. Analysis and Applications in Environmental Engineering". Krieger, Malabar, ISBN 0-89874-446-6

Author:Ancuta ABRUDAN
Institute:Technical University of Cluj-Napoca
Street:28 Memorandumului,
City: Cluj-Napoca,
Coutry:ROMANIA,
Email:ancuta.abrudan@insta.utcluj.ro

Modelling the Passive Behavior of the Nervous Cell. Influence of Electric Parameters Variation

M. Crețu, L.Darabant and A. Răcășan

Technical University of Cluj-Napoca/Electrotechnics and Measurements Department, Cluj-Napoca, Romania

Abstract — **The main role of nerve and muscle cells is to contribute to the electrical impulses conduction, known as action potentials. In conditions of very weak excitation, under the sensory threshold (subliminal), passive waves are propagated along the cells. In the case of nerve cells, the time and space variations of the membrane potential occur at the axon level, subjected to the action of stimulus with the low intensity, below the neuronal excitability threshold, or in the dendrites, which receive synaptic signals from other neurons.**

The paper will analyze the propagation mechanism of passive wave (of the transmembrane potential) along nerve fibers with known geometry and electrical properties.

Keywords — **Transmembrane potential, Passive waves, Subthreshold response of the nerve fiber, Electric parameters variation.**

I. Introduction

The cell remains in polarized (passive) state, as long as there is no action exercised by any external factor, in order to disturb the balance of the membrane (the so-called rest state) [1], [2]. These external factors that can cause depolarization of the membrane cell are called stimuli or stimulus factors. Their action is called stimulation. Artificial stimulation of excitable tissues is an important tool in restoring muscle and nerve functions lost due to different accidents [3], [4]. The stimulation is also important in cardiac defibrillation [5].

The membrane cell depolarization is initiated locally, on a small area, by an electrical process (the value of the transmembrane potential changes). The increase of the transmembrane potential value above a certain threshold to the rest level, triggers depolarization of the cell membrane in the form of an impulse, called action potential. The response of the membrane is characterized by a sudden initial increase of the transmembrane potential; it reaches a maximum followed by a slow return to its resting value [1], [2].

In this paper, the propagation mechanism of the passive waves (the transmembrane potential) along the nerve fibers will be analyzed. The geometrical and electrical properties of the fiber are known. We also consider possible inhomogeneity's of the membrane cell; these will be modeled by varying its electrical parameters along the nerve fiber. This variation has a significant influence on the membrane response during stimulation of the nerve fiber, which can lead to changes in transmembrane potential, e.g. modification of the nervous excitability threshold.

II. Theoretical Background

From the electrical point of view, the cell behaves similarly to a coaxial cable: the core conductor of the cable is the cytoplasm, with good electrical conductivity; the membrane is an insulator coaxial layer and the external environment (interstitial fluid) is a coaxial conductor new layer, with a higher electrical conductivity than the cytoplasm, but with the same order of size [6], [7]. In order to model the electrical properties of the nerve fiber we will use the well kwon cable equation that modeled the electrical properties of the nerve fiber [1], [6], [8], [9]. The solution of the passive cable equation provides a direct determination of membrane voltage, so the passive cable model specifies the behavior of the membrane in subliminal state [1], [6], [8], [9].

The nerve fiber is considered infinitely long, and it can be approximated by an electrical network made up of resistive and capacitive elements each compartment of the cable having the same length – Fig. 1 [1], [6], [8], [9]. The output of a section is the input for the next section. Electrical network modeling the axon is similar to a two-conductor transmission line [6].

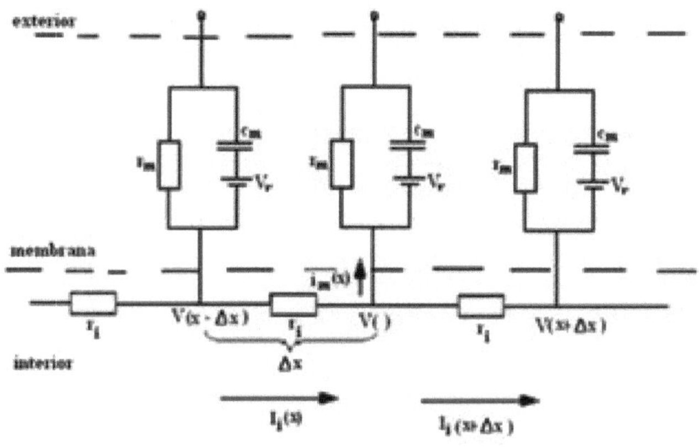

Fig. 1 The electrical circuit of the passive cable for the nerve fiber [6]

S. Vlad and N.M. Roman (eds.), *International Conference on Advancements of Medicine and Health Care through Technology; 12th - 15th October 2016, Cluj-Napoca, Romania*,
IFMBE Proceedings 59,
DOI: 10.1007/978-3-319-52875-5_36

The quantities from the model are:
- I_i the longitudinal current from the intracellular medium [μA];
- i_m the total transmembrane current per unit length of the fiber [μA/cm];
- V_r = -65 [mV] the resting potential of the membrane.

Knowing the values for the resting potential, the membrane capacitance per unit area - C_m=1.0 [μF/cm^2], the axoplasma resistivity - ρ_i=0.0354 [kΩ·cm], the specific resistance of the membrane - R_m=0.0354[kΩ·cm^2] and the fiber radius - a=0.005[cm], we will compute the following parameters of the membrane per unit lenght:

$$\begin{cases} c_m = 2\pi a C_m = 0.0314\ [\mu F/cm] \\ r_m = \dfrac{R_m}{2\pi a} = 106.0926 [k\Omega \cdot cm] \\ r_i = \dfrac{R_i}{\pi a^2} = 2202.704\ [k\Omega / cm] \end{cases} \tag{1}$$

The transmembrane voltage of an excitable cell is defined as the difference between the electric potential of the inner surface of the cell membrane, V_i, and of the outer surface, V_e. The outer surface of the membrane potential is considered as a reference potential (V_e = 0). Therefore, instead of the concept of the transmembrane voltage, we will use the term of transmembrane potential or membrane potential.

The equation that describes the variation of the membrane voltage (transmembrane potential) in time and space is [1], [6], [8], [9]:

$$\lambda^2 \frac{\partial^2 V_m}{\partial x^2} - \tau \frac{\partial V_m}{\partial t} - V_m = 0 \tag{1}$$

, where $\lambda^2 = \dfrac{r_m}{r_i}$, λ=0.1294[cm] is the spatial constant of the fiber and $\tau = r_m c_m$ = 3[ms] is the time constant. Using the above equation, it can be described the membrane voltage variation along the fiber below the depolarization threshold.

III. Electrical stimulation modeling of the nerve fiber

A. Stimulus represented by an impulse current

In order to study the behavior of passive nerve fiber, the fiber is intracellular stimulated at x=0 (the left extremity), with a current source. At the right extremity of the fiber the transmembrane potential is set to zero. The passive wave propagation from the stimulated electrode (left extremity) to the opposite side, must be characterized through time representation.

Figure 2 shows the train of impulses used to stimulate the nerve fiber. We will consider three excitation pulses and an inhibitory one. The impulses have the same length but different amplitudes. Duration of stimulation is 40 [ms], and the time step is 0.004 [ms].

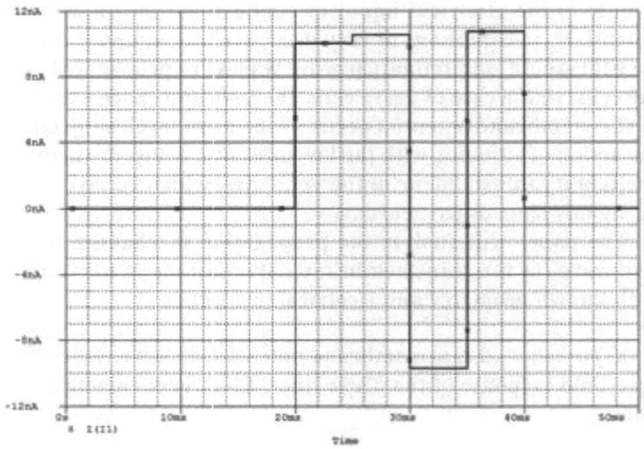

Fig. 2 The train of impulses used to stimulate the nervous fiber

The time variation of the transmembrane potential was studied using an electrical circuit analysis program. The electric circuit of the fiber is illustrated in the Fig. 3. The length of the fiber is L=2[cm] and the electric cable is composed of 10 compartments.

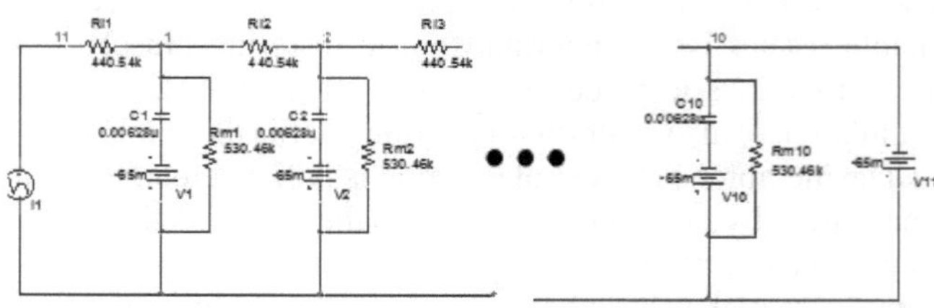

Fig. 3 The equivalent electrical circuit of the fiber

From the simulation analysis – Fig. 4, one can notice that, when an inhibitory impulse is applied, the value of the transmembrane potential becomes negative; this represents the areas where the membrane is hyperpolarized (inhibition of the nervous impulse). Also, the transmembrane potential rapidly decreases along the fiber (V(1)>V(2)>V(3)>V(4)>V(5)).

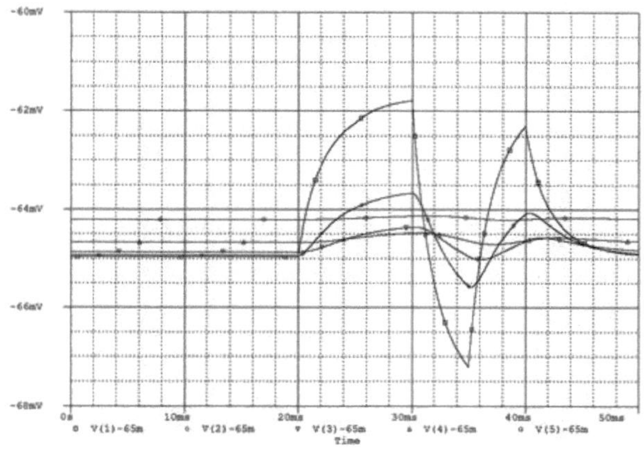

Fig. 4 Time variation of the transmembrane potential. (Representation is made for the first 5 compartments of the cable.)

B. Stimulus represented by the transient current from the RLC series circuit

The stimulation circuit can be modeled through a series RLC circuit, working in transient regime. Considering the coil inductance $L = 0.165$ [mH], the capacitance $C = 200$ [μF] and the resistance $R = 3$ [Ω], knowing that the damping factor is $\omega_1 = \frac{R}{2L} = 9.091[\text{ms}^{-1}]$ and the pulsation $\omega_2 = \sqrt{\left(\frac{R}{2L}\right)^2 - \frac{1}{LC}} = 7.235[\text{ms}^{-1}]$, the circuit works in overdamped regime, because $\left(\frac{R}{2L}\right)^2 > \frac{1}{LC}$. The waveform of the current through the coil is represented in Fig. 5.

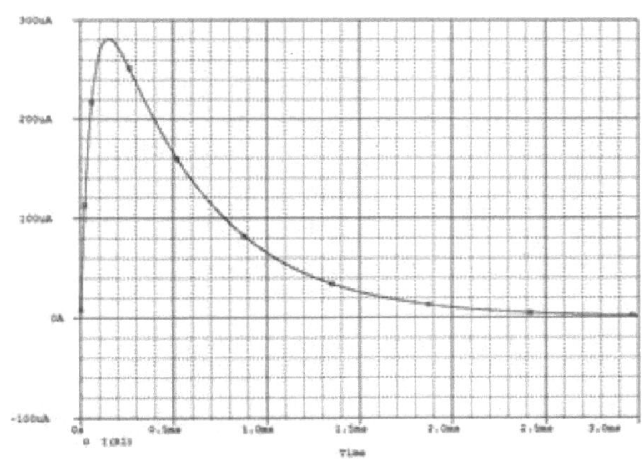

Fig. 5 The current pulse generating the nerve fiber stimulation

The current pulse generated by the RLC series circuit, determines the stimulation of the nerve fiber and the transmembrane potential changes. The stimulation is excitatory or inhibitory, depends on the stimulus applied.

For a lower intensity of the applied stimulus, the transmembrane potential will not reach the threshold value, and the membrane is not activated.

To describe the subliminal behavior of the fiber inside the tissue, we will use the passive cable model. The electrical circuit representing the nerve fiber is shown in Fig. 6, having the same finite length L = 2 [cm], and the cable was still considered to be composed of 10 compartments. One ca see that the stimulus is not apply at one end of the fiber as in the case described in paragraph *A*, but in the middle. The necessary stimulation signal is taken through a current source controlled in current. The amplifying of this source is considered unitary.

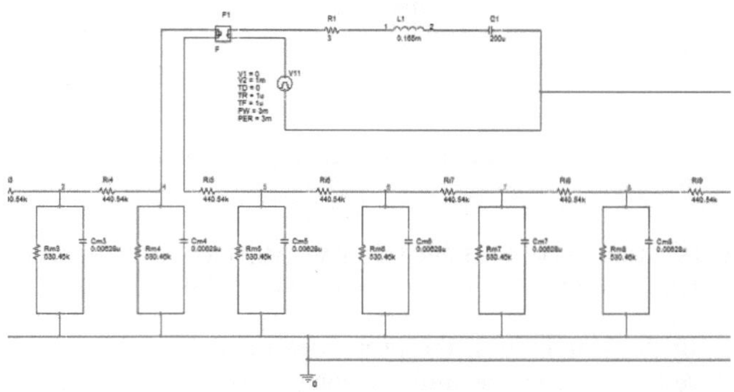

Fig. 6 The equivalent circuit of the nerve fiber; stimulation impulse is generated by a series RLC circuit, working in transient regime

The response of the membrane cell is shown in Fig. 7 and represents the transmembrane potential determined on each section of the cable.

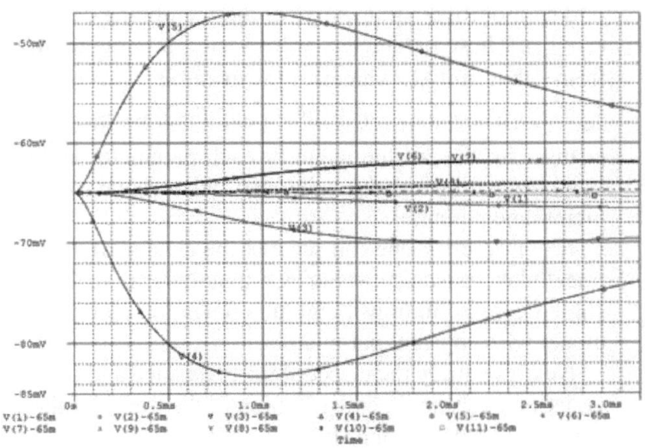

Fig. 7 The subliminal response of the nerve fiber

One can easily notice that at the 5 level, where stimulus is applied, the transmembrane potential has the highest value, decreasing gradually as the intensity of the stimulus decreases.

Three-dimensional representation of the transmembrane potential, V_m, as a function of space and time along the nerve fiber, is illustrated in Fig. 8.

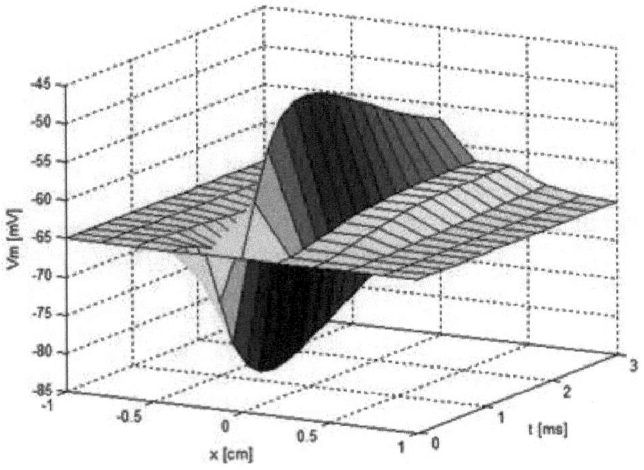

Fig. 8 The transmembrane potential variation

IV. Influence of the Electric Parameters Variation of the Membrane Cell over the Nerve Fiber Response

In the simulations, the properties of the membrane cell were considered to be uniform along the fiber. Further on, we will consider possible inhomogeneities in the membrane cell, shaped by varying its electrical parameters along the nerve fiber [9]. This can have a significant influence over the nerve fiber response during stimulation and will lead to changes in transmembrane potential, with the possibility to modify the nerve excitability threshold [11], [12], [13].

The modified parameters' of the membrane cell were c_m, r_m, şi r_i. These parameters were varied in a range of 2-20% from the initial value: for example $r_{i1} = r_i \pm 2\% \cdot r_i$, $r_{i2} = r_i \pm 6\% \cdot r_i$, $r_{i3} = r_i \pm 10\% \cdot r_i$ etc. First, we began with the change, in turn, of the value of each parameter and studied how this will affect the value and pulse shape of the transmembrane potential.

From figure 9, one can see that the change of the axial intracellular resistance value per unit length, will lead to a slight decrease in transmembrane potential, compared to the model with constant parameters.

Next, we study the effect of the resistance and capacitance variation over the time distribution of the transmembrane potential – Fig. 10 (a) and (b).

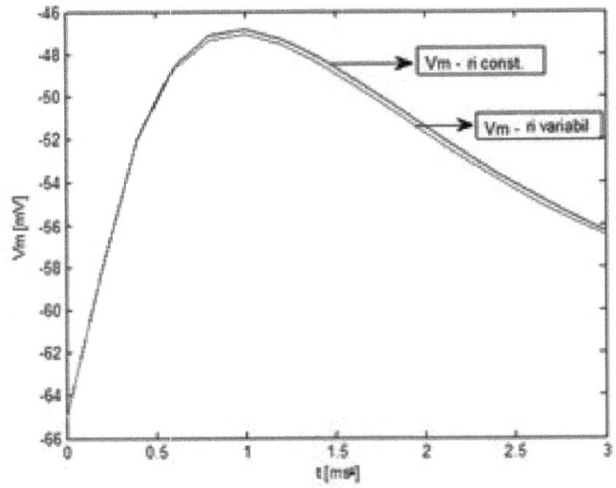

Fig. 9 Time variation of the transmembrane potential for the node 5 of the fiber, when the intracellular resistance changes

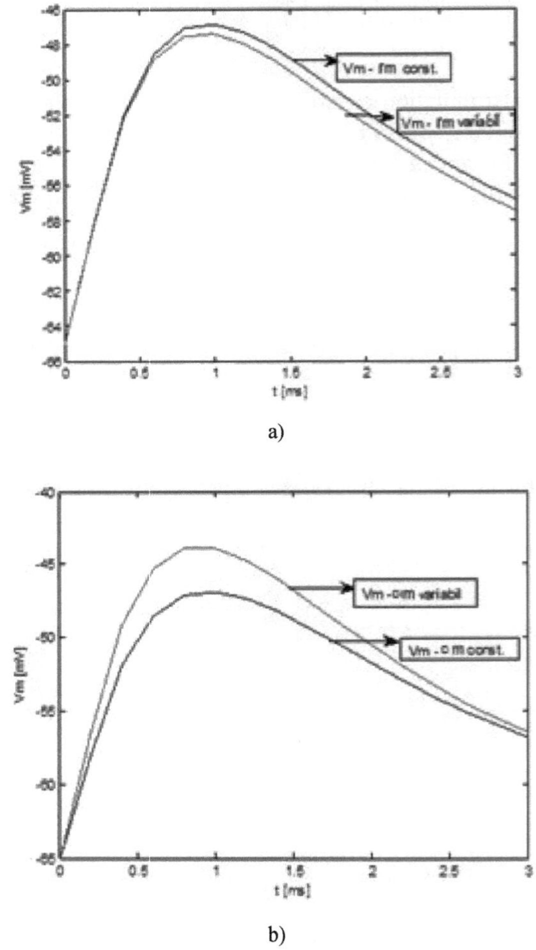

Fig. 10 Transmembrane potential variation. a) the membrane resistance, rm , varies; b) the membrane capacitance, cm, varies.

The variation of the r_m and c_m leads to different effects on the cell membrane behavior, under subliminal conditions.

The membrane resistance variation leads to a decrease of the transmembrane potential value compared with its initial value, when r_m was constant along the nerve fiber.

On the other hand, changing the membrane capacitance along the nerve fiber leads to a potential increase of the V_m amplitude, compared to the case when the parameter was constant.

The most significant variation of V_m can be observed for the variation of c_m, the transmembrane potential increases about 4 [mV] to the case of constant parameters.

Simultaneous modification of these three parameters, determines a higher value of the membrane potential V_m = -44.5 [mV] compared to the case when the cell membrane properties were uniform throughout the fiber V_m = -47 [mV] – Fig. 11.

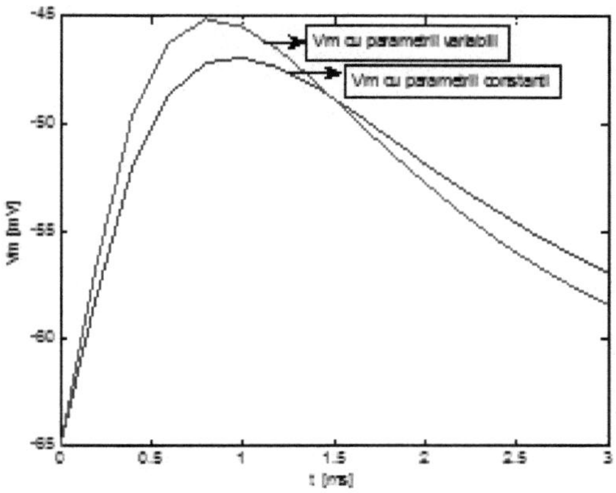

Fig. 11 Transmembrane potential resulting from the simultaneous variation of the three parameters of the cell membrane - compared with the model with constant parameters

Figure 12 shows the time variation of the transmembrane potential V_m, as a function of distance along the nerve fiber, computed using the Matlab software.

When the stimulus intensity is below the threshold, the nerve fiber behaves passive and the membrane voltage local growth, determined by the stimulus, is dissipated very quickly. Comparing the chart below – Fig. 12 - with that of Fig. 8, one can notice an increase in the value of V_m with about 6%.

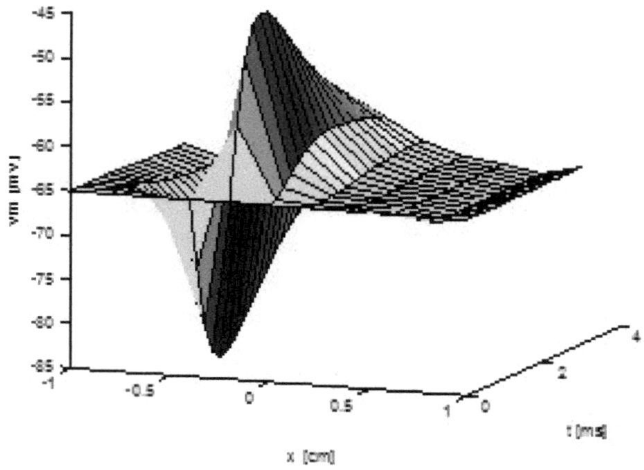

Fig. 11 V_m at the electrical parameters variation of the cell membrane

V. Conclusions

Knowing the effects of the stimulation mechanism on the neural structures provides a better understanding of how to realize the nervous excitability. In this paper we studied the behavior of the nerve fiber in subliminal regime, and we analyzed the propagation mechanism of the action potentials along the nerve cells.

The nerve fiber was electrically stimulated using both a train current pulse and a current impulse generated by a RLC series circuit working in overdamped transient regime.

For the stimulation with the train of impulses, we used both excitation and inhibition impulses, that leads to significant changes in the amplitude of V_m.

By applying an inhibitory pulse, V_m takes values lower than -65 [mV], this being the area where the cell membrane is hyperpolarized or zones of inhibition of nerve impulses.

The areas where the membrane potential has values greater than -65 [mV] represents the depolarization areas, these are stimulation areas.

Also, in this paper, we analyzed the influence of the membrane electric parameters variation on the transmembrane potential (nerve fiber response). There is an increase up to 6% of V_m, when the cell membrane parameters vary, compared to the case where they are kept constant.

Conflict of Interest

The authors declare that they have no conflict of interest".

Acknowledgment

This work was supported by a grant of the Romanian National Authority for Scientific Research and Innovation,

CNCS – UEFISCDI, project number PN-II-RU-TE-2014-4-0199".

REFERENCES

1. Rafiroiu D., Munteanu R. A., Munteanu M. S. (2007), Bioelectromagnetism. Teorie si aplicatii, Ed. Mediamira
2. Roth B. J. (2000), Mechanism of electric stimulation of excitable tissue, Crit Rev Biomed Eng. 22 (3-4): 253-305
3. Gargiulo P. (2011), 3D Modelling and monitoring of denervated muscle under FES, European Journal Translational Myology - Basic Applied Myology, 21: 31-94
4. Langhals N. B., Shoshana L. W., Moon J. D., et all, (2014), Electrically stimulated signals from a long-term Regenerative Peripheral Nerve Interface, Engineering in Medicine and Biology Society, pp. 1989 - 1992
5. Lu J., Toshifumi N., Takashi A., et all. (2006), The Influence of Activation Time on Contraction Force of Myocardial Tissue: a Simulation Study, Engineering in Medicine and Biology Society, pp. 2900 - 2903, DOI: 10.1109/IEMBS.2006.260804
6. Morega M. (1999), Bioelectromagnetism, Editura Matrix ROM
7. Papadopoulos T.A., Christoforidis G.C., Micu D.D. & Czumbil L. (2014), Medium-Voltage Cable Inductive Coupling to Metallic pipelines: A Somprehensive Study, 49th International Universities Power Engineering Conference, (UPEC), ISBN: 978-1-4799-6556-4, Cluj-Napoca, Romania, September 2-5
8. Roth B.J., Basser P.J. (1990) A Model of the Stimulation of a Nerve Fiber by Electromagnetic Induction. IEEE Transactions on Biomedical Engineering, vol. 37, no. 6
9. Nagarajan S., Durand D., Warman E. (1993) Effects of Induced Electric Fields on Finite Neuronal Structures: A Stimulation Study. IEEE Transactions on Biomedical Engineering, vol. 40, no. 11
10. Cretu M, Ciupa R. V. (2014), Influence of the Electrical Parameters Variation of the Membrane Cell over the Nerve Fiber Activation, MediTech, pp. 209-214
11. Cretu M., Darabant L, Ciupa R. V., (2012), Modeling the Activation of a Non-Homogenous Nerve Fiber by Magnetic Stimulation, BIBE, pp. 651-656
12. Corlan A., D., Amuzescu B., Milicin I., et all. (2011), Intercellular conductance variability influences early repolarization potentials in a model of the myocardial tissue with stochastic architecture, ATEE, pp. 1-4
13. Struijk J. J., Schnabel V., (2000) Influence of Parameter Variability on Stimulus Thresholds in Nerve Fiber Models, Proceedings of the 5th conf. of the IFESS, pp. 245-248.

Author's details: Mihaela Cretu
Technical University of Cluj-Napoca, Faculty of Electrical Engineering
Baritiu Street, no. 26-28
Cluj-Napoca
Romania
Mihaela.Cretu@ethm.utcluj.ro

Simulation of Teeth Movement in the Case of Orthodontic Treatment Procedures

T. Coloşi[1], V. Mureşan[1], O. Nemeş[2], M. Olt[3] and N. M. Roman[4]

[1] Technical University of Cluj-Napoca/ Automation Department, Cluj-Napoca, Romania
[2] Iuliu Hatieganu University of Medicine and Pharmacy/ Orthodontics Department, Cluj-Napoca, Romania
[3] Technical University of Cluj-Napoca, Cluj-Napoca, Romania
[4] Technical University of Cluj-Napoca/Electrotechnics and Measurements Department, Cluj-Napoca, Romania

Abstract— **In this paper, the authors propose an original method for the simulation of the teeth movement in the case of orthodontic treatment procedures. In this approach, the orthodontic treatment procedures are considered medical processes being modeled using mathematical functions. The proposed mathematical solution is a general one due to the fact that it remains valid for both the rotation and roto-translation movement. For the implementation of the obtained mathematical model, in order to be simulated, a procedure based on transfer functions is used. The main objective of the present research activity is to open the premise of the apriority approximation through simulation of the orthodontic treatments duration.**

Keywords— **Simulation, orthodontic treatment, transfer function, medical process, distributed parameter process.**

I. INTRODUCTION

The orthodontic treatment [1] consists in the application of external forces to the teeth in order to imply their movement. One of the most challenging research directions in Orthodontics is referring to the precise approximation of the duration of the orthodontic treatment. This problem is a very difficult one, due to the fact that the mathematical model of the teeth movement process (which is a medical process) is hard to be obtained. The main explanation of the previous remark is due to the fact that the structure parameters (time and length constants) of the biological tissues vary from a person to another one. In this contest, we consider that the approach of the modeling-simulation problem of the medical orthodontic process is an appropriate one.

In this paper, the case of using the dental braces with a high level of elasticity is considered. Also, as case study, the movement process associated to a central incisive is considered.

II. THE THEETH MOVEMENT PROCESS

In order to describe the teeth movement process, the example from Fig. 1 is considered. The significance of the notations from Fig. 1 is: u(t) – input signal representing the external force applied to the tooth; y(t,p) – output signal representing the tooth movement and depending both on time (t) and on the position from the tooth longitudinal symmetry axis (p) – resulting that the considered medical process is a distributed parameter one [2,3]; α-β – longitudinal symmetry axis of the tooth; $p_a' = 0$mm – reference position representing the tooth top; p_0 – the position from the α-β axis where the u(t) signal is applied; p_a – the position from the α-β axis representing the gum level; p_{C1} – the position from the α-β axis of the tooth rotation centre in the case of the rotation movement; C_1 – rotation centre of the tooth in the case of the rotation movement; p_f – reference position representing the tooth apex (the distance on the α-β axis between the tooth top and the tooth apex); p_{f1} - the distance on the α-β axis between the point where the input signal is applied and the tooth apex; p_{C2} - the position from the α-β axis of the tooth rotation centre in the case of the roto-translation movement; C_2 – rotation centre of the tooth in the case of the roto-translation movement; $y_\alpha' = y(t,p_a')$ – – tooth movement (the distance passed through of the tooth) in relation to time in the position corresponding to $p = p_a'$; $y(t,p_i)$ (for $i \in \{1; 2\}$ — tooth movement in relation to time in the intermediary positions from the α-β axis corresponding to $p = p_0$ and $p = p_1$; $y_\beta = y(t,p_f)$ - tooth movement in relation to time in the position corresponding to $p = p_f$ ($y_\beta \leq \leq 0$mm in the case of the rotation movement and $y_\beta \geq 0$mm in the case of the roto-translation movement). In Fig. 1, the external force u(t) (which is considered the input signal in the medical process) is applied to the tooth (central incisive) at the distance $p_0 - p_a' = p_0$ from its top. Depending on the treatment type, the imposed movement can be either rotation or roto-translation. In the case of the rotation movement, the rotation centre C_1 belongs to the α-β axis, more exactly to the interval $\{p_0; p_f\}$. In the case of the roto-translation movement the rotation centre C_2 belongs to the continuation of the α-β axis above the p_f point (practically the position of C_2 is outside from the tooth volume). In order to simplify the presentation and due to the fact that p_f has a much bigger value than the y(t,p) signals, only the rectilinear movement of the tooth is considered in the evaluation of the output signal value. In Fig. 2, the input signal u(t) and its components are presented. The significance of the numerical notations from Fig. 2 is: 1 – elastic decreasing force of the resort; 2 – plastic remanent increasing force; 3 – u(t) force which activates the orthodontic treatment (resultant of 1 and 2 components).

S. Vlad and N.M. Roman (eds.), *International Conference on Advancements of Medicine and Health Care through Technology; 12th - 15th October 2016, Cluj-Napoca, Romania,*
IFMBE Proceedings 59,
DOI: 10.1007/978-3-319-52875-5_37

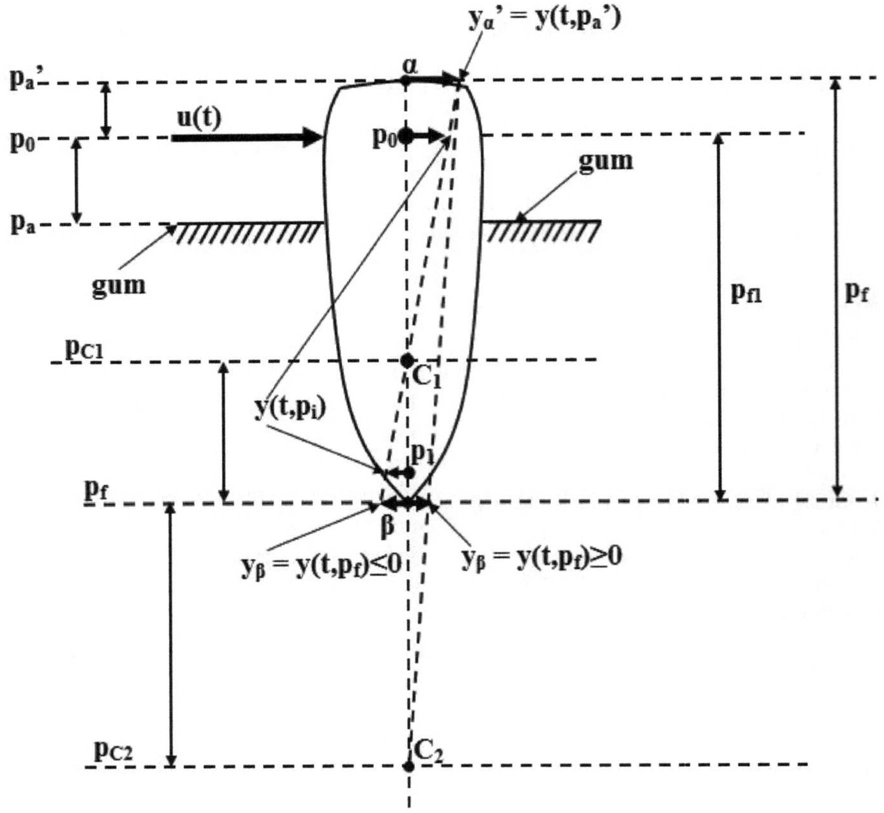

Fig. 1 Case study for the central incisive movement

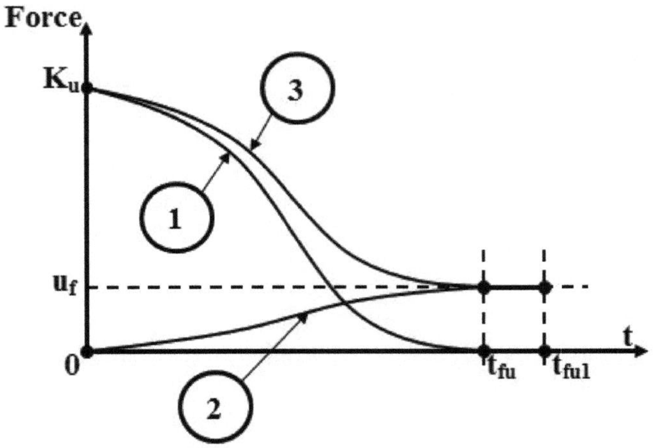

Fig. 2 Components of the u(t) input signal and u(t) signal

The other notations from Fig. 2 are: K_u – initial value of the elastic decreasing force of the resort and implicitly of the input signal u(t) measured in [grf]; u_f – steady state value of the plastic remanent increasing force; t_{fu} – settling time of the component 1; t_{fu1} – settling time of the component 2. From Fig. 2, it can be remarked the fact that we consider the case when the component 2 is slower than the component 1 ($t_{fu1} > t_{fu}$). Also, the value of u_f can be considered as percentage from the initial value K_u of the u(t) signal. The plastic remanent increasing force is due to the disturbed tissue (through compression – depression).

In order to obtain mathematical model of the u(t) signal evolution, the Laplace transformation for null initial conditions is used. The model of the component 2 (notated with u_R) from Fig. 2 is presented in Eq. 1:

$$U_R(s) = \frac{1}{(T_{3u} \cdot s+1)\cdot(T_{4u} \cdot s+1)} \cdot U_f(s) \quad (1)$$

where the transfer function $H_1(s) = \frac{1}{(T_{3u} \cdot s+1)\cdot(T_{4u} \cdot s+1)}$ makes the connection between the signals $U_R(s)$ and $U_f(s)$, T_{3u} and T_{4u} being the corresponding time constants. Practically, the signal $U_f(s)$ can be written as $U_f(s) = u_f \cdot \frac{1}{s}$, where $\frac{1}{s}$ represent the Laplace transformation of the unit step signal. The model of the component 1 (notated with F_E) from Fig. 2 is presented in Eq. 2:

$$F_E(s) = \frac{K_u}{s} \cdot (1 - \frac{1}{(T_{1u} \cdot s+1)\cdot(T_{2u} \cdot s+1)}) \quad (2)$$

where $\frac{K_u}{s}$ represents a step signal with the steady state value equal to K_u, respectively T_{1u} and T_{2u} represent the time constants of the transfer function $H_2(s) = \frac{1}{(T_{1u} \cdot s+1)\cdot(T_{2u} \cdot s+1)}$. Due to the fact that $t_{fu1} > t_{fu}$, T_{1u} and T_{2u} are smaller as value than T_{3u} and T_{4u}.

Considering Eq. 1 and Eq. 2, the input signal U(s) (U(s) is the Laplace transformation for null initial conditions of u(t)) is given by:

$$U(s) = F_E(s) + U_R(s) = \frac{K_u}{s} \cdot (1 - \frac{1}{(T_{1u} \cdot s+1)\cdot(T_{2u} \cdot s+1)} + \frac{u_f / K_u}{(T_{3u} \cdot s+1)\cdot(T_{4u} \cdot s+1)}) \quad (3)$$

where u_f/K_u represents the ratio between the two constant values.

The mathematical model of the orthodontic process, which makes the connection between the applied force U(s) (considered input signal in the orthodontic process) and the distance passed through by the teeth, as effect of the applied force, Y(s) (considered output signal from the orthodontic process) is presented in the following equation:

$$H_3(s) = \frac{Y(s)}{U(s)} = \frac{K_y}{(T_1 \cdot s+1)\cdot(T_2 \cdot s+1)} \quad (4)$$

where K_y is the proportionality constant of the orthodontic process, respectively T_1 and T_2 are the time constants of the orthodontic process. Analyzing the structure of the element from Eq. 4, it results that the orthodontic process is a second order one (modeled using a second order transfer function). Eq. 4 describes only the process dynamic in relation to time. Introducing, also, the dynamic in relation to the independent variable (s), the output signal Y(s,p) is given by:

$$Y(s,p) = F_{OP}(p) \cdot \frac{K_y}{(T_1 \cdot s+1)\cdot(T_2 \cdot s+1)} \cdot U(s) \quad (5)$$

where the linear function $F_{OP}(p)$ introduces in the model the effect of (p) independent variable, being given by:

$$F_{OP}(p) = \gamma_0 + \gamma_1 \cdot p\,. \quad (6)$$

In Eq. 6, the constants can be computed with the formulae: $\gamma_0 = y'_\alpha$ (the imposed movement in steady state regime for the tooth top) and $\gamma_1 = -\frac{y'_\alpha - y_\beta}{p_f}$ (the slope of the $F_{OP}(p)$ function). Applying the inverse Laplace transformation to Eq. 5, we obtain the output signal written in time domain:

$$y(t,p) = F_{OP}(p) \cdot [(K_y \cdot F_{OT}(t)) * u(t)] \quad (7)$$

where "*" represents the convolution product between the signals u(t) and $F_{OT}(t)$. The exponential function $F_{OT}(t)$ is given by:

$$F_{OT}(t) = \frac{1}{T_1 - T_2} \cdot (e^{-\frac{1}{T_1} \cdot t} - e^{-\frac{1}{T_2} \cdot t})\,. \quad (8)$$

In other words, in Eq. 7, the expression of the analytical approximating solution which models the y(t,p) deformation is presented. Also, the analytical solution from Eq. 7, depending on two independent variables (t) and (p) represents practically the solution of a partial differential equation [4,5] which can be determined in order to express the complete model of the process. The evolution of the analytical solution, in relation to both independent variables (t) and (p), is presented in Fig. 3.

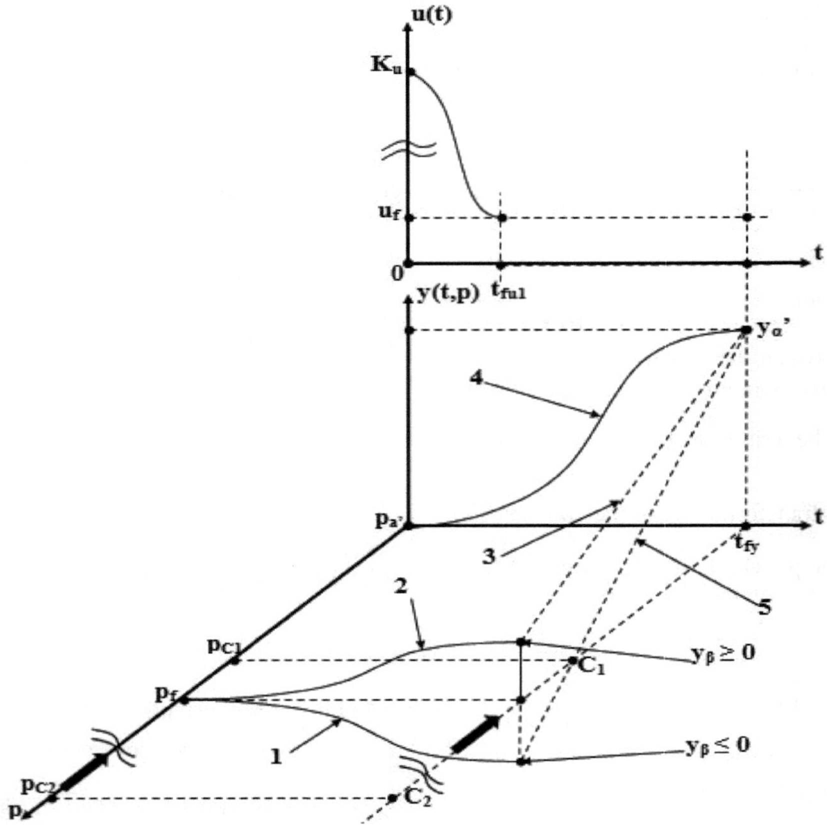

Fig. 3 The evolution of the analytical solution in relation to both independent variables (t) and (p)

In Fig. 3, the sine parallel curves signify the fact that the distances from the corresponding axes are much bigger (the scale of the graph is not respected on the mentioned intervals). Also, in Fig. 3, the increasing evolution of the analytical solution in relation to time (t), respectively its decreasing evolution in relation to (p) independent variable, are highlighted. The significance of the new notations used in Fig. 3 is: 1- the curve y_β in the case when it is ≤ 0mm; 2 – the curve y_β in the case when it is ≥ 0mm; 3 – the linear variation of the analytical solution in relation to (p) independent variable for the case when $y_\beta \geq 0$mm; 4 - the curve $y_{\alpha'}$ in both cases ($y_\beta \geq 0$mm and $y_\beta \leq 0$mm); 5 – the linear variation of the analytical solution in relation to (p) independent variable for the case when $y_\beta \leq 0$mm; t_{fy} – the settling time of the y(t,p) signal.

From Fig. 3, it results that $t_{fu1} << t_{fy}$, implying the fact that the input signal can be assimilated with an impulse type signal. Practically evolution form from Fig. 3 represents the y(t,p) signal response at u(t) signal and the u(t) signal represents the response of the element $\left(1-\frac{1}{(T_{1u}\cdot s+1)\cdot(T_{2u}\cdot s+1)}+\frac{u_f / K_u}{(T_{3u}\cdot s+1)\cdot(T_{4u}\cdot s+1)}\right)$ (from Eq. 3) at the $\frac{K_u}{s}$ step input signal. The wide arrows from Fig. 3 show the position evolution of the rotation centre C_2 (case of the roto-translation movement) with the increase of the ratio between y_α' and y_β. Also, in the case of the rotation movement, the C_1 centre presents the evolution according to the arrows at the increase of the same ratio.

III. Simulations Results

The simulations of the teeth movement process are made in MATLAB/Simulink.

The simulation structure implemented in Simulink is presented in Fig. 4. In the left part of the structure, the step signal with the final value K_u is generated and applied to the medical process.

The time constants and the proportionality constants which occur in the presented model (Eq. 1-8) are initialized according to some measurements practically obtained (through some experiments). These values are not given in the paper in order to simplify the presentation.

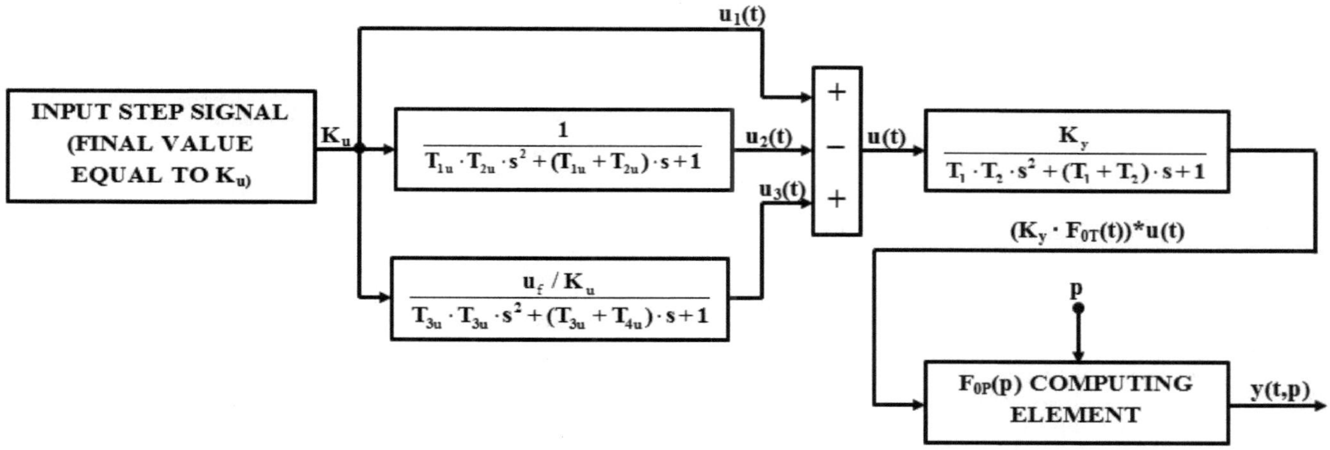

Fig. 4 The simulation structure implemented in Simulink

Between the step signal generator and the adder, the u(t) signal is formed as:

$$u(t) = u_1(t) + u_2(t) + u_3(t) \tag{9}$$

practically implementing Eq. 3. In this context, $u_1(t) = L^{-1}\{\frac{K_u}{s}\}$, $u_2(t) = L^{-1}\{\frac{K_u}{s\cdot(T_{1u}\cdot s+1)\cdot(T_{2u}\cdot s+1)}\}$ (the two components of $F_E(t)$) and $u_3(t) = L^{-1}\{U_R(s)\}$ (from Eq. 1). The notation $L^{-1}\{\}$ represents the inverse Laplace transformation of the function between the {}. It can be remarked the fact that in Fig. 4, all the signals are presented in time domain and the elements models are presented using transfer functions (for a more intuitive understanding of the structure). The element $H_3(s)$ models the orthodontic process (Eq. 4), the output signal from it being $((K_y \cdot F_{OT}(t))*u(t))$. Finally, the signal $((K_y \cdot F_{OT}(t))*u(t)$ is multiplied with the value of $F_{OP}(p)$ function (Eq. 6), value which is computed (in relation to (p) independent variable) using the computing element from the right-down part of the structure. The output signal from the mentioned element is the final form of the y(t,p) output signal from the medical process.

In Fig. 5, the results of the simulations of the medical process are presented, in the case of the teeth rotation movement. In this figure, the variation form of the output signal y(t,p) is presented for 9 different values of the (p) independent variable. In Fig. 5 it is highlighted again the increasing evolution of the y(t,p) in relation to time (t) and its decreasing evolution at the increase of the (p) independent variable value.

From the figure, it can be remarked that the rotation centre is placed at p_{C1} = 18 mm from the teeth top (case figured with yellow color on Fig. 5). Practically, in this case, the value of y(t,p = 18mm) = 0mm the entire period of simulation ($t \in [0,7]$ weeks) due to the fact that the rotation centre remains immovable.

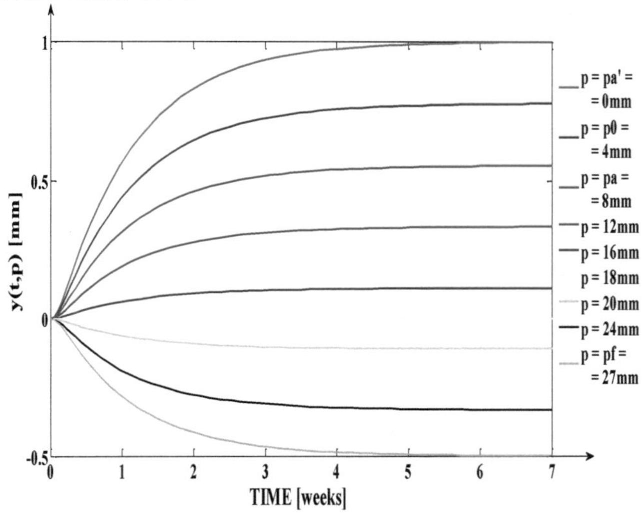

Fig. 5 The evolution of the y(t,p) signal in relation to both independent variables, for the rotation movement case

In Fig. 6, the results of the simulations of the medical process are presented, in the case of the teeth roto-translation movement.

The same remarks as in the case of the rotation movement are valid regarding to the evolution of the y(t,p) signal. In contrast with the previous case, the y(t,p) signal evolution corresponding to the position of C_2 rotation centre is not presented due to the fact that C_2 is placed outside from the tooth volume. For the simulation from Fig. 6, p_{C2} = 54mm. Also, the curves from Fig. 6 present only positive values. The steady state values of the curves presented in Fig. 5 and Fig. 6 are presented in the Table 1.

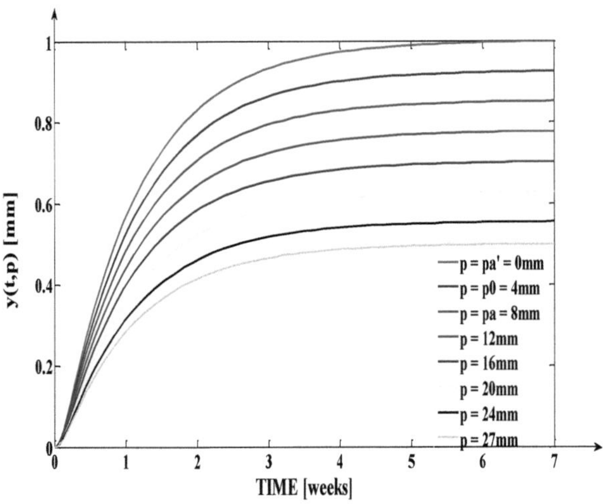

Fig. 6 The evolution of the y(t,p) signal in relation to both independent variables, for the roto-translation movement case

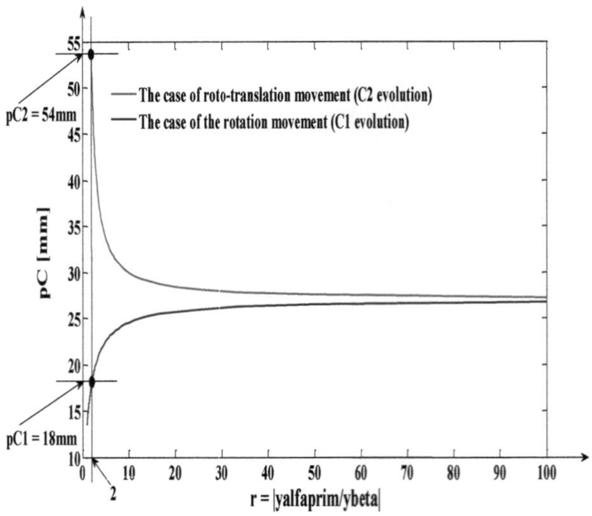

Fig. 7 The evolution form of the p_{C1} and p_{C2} positions in relation to the ratio $r = |y_\alpha'/y_\beta|$

Table 1 The steady state values of the curves from Fig. 5 and Fig. 6

p	$y(t = t_{fy},p)$ (Fig. 5)	$y(t = t_{fy},p)$ (Fig. 6)
p_a' = 0mm	1 mm	1 mm
p_0 = 4mm	0.7773 mm	0.9253 mm
p_a = 8mm	0.5552 mm	0.8513 mm
p =12mm	0.3331 mm	0.7773 mm
p =16mm	0.111 mm	0.7033 mm
p =18mm	0 mm	-
p =20mm	-0.111 mm	0.6292 mm
p =24mm	-0.3331 mm	0.5552 mm
p =27mm	-0.5 mm	0.5 mm

The values of $y(t = t_{fy}, p)$ from Table 1 represent the distance passed through by different points from the symmetry axis α-β after 7 weeks.

In Fig. 7, the evolution of the position of the rotation centres C_1 and C_2 (for the two movement cases: rotation and roto-translation) is presented in relation to the ratio r $= |y_\alpha' / y_\beta|$. In both cases $y_\alpha' = 1$mm value is maintained. In the case of rotation, y_β is initialized at the value -1mm and it is increased progressively with the value of 0.01mm to 0mm. In the case of roto-translation, y_β is initialized at the value 0.5mm and it is decreased progressively with the value 0.005mm to 0mm.

In Fig. 7, the positions of the two rotation centres from Fig. 4 and Fig. 5 is also highlighted (p_{C1} and p_{C2}). For rotation movement (the blue curve from Fig. 7), the value of the rotation centre position increses at the increase of r and in the case of roto-translation movement (the red curve from Fig. 7), the value of the rotation centre position decreases at the increase of r.

IV. Conclusions

The paper proposes an original method for the modeling and the simulation of a medical process (in particular an orthodontic process). In Paragraph III, some interesting simulation results of the proposed mathematical model are presented. The medical process is simulated both for rotation and roto-translation movement. In order to apply the simulation method for predicting the duration of the orthodontic treatment, a study about the resistance of the biological tissue of each subject has to be made. This study is necessary in order to determine the time constants and the proportionality constants of the model presented in Eq. 1-8.

Conflict of Interest

The authors declare that they have no conflict of interest.

References

1. Colosi H., Achimaş A., Roman N. M. (2011) Evaluarea Biomecanicii Ortodontice prin Modelare şi Simulare. Galaxia Gutenberg, Cluj-Napoca
2. Coloşi T., Abrudean M., Ungureşan M.-L., Mureşan V. (2013) Numerical simulation of distributed parameter processes. Springer
3. Li H.-X., Qi C. (2011) Spatio-Temporal Modeling of Nonlinear Distributed Parameter Systems: A Time/Space Separation Based Approach. Springer
4. Krstic M. (2006) Systematization of approaches to adaptive boundary control of PDEs. Int. J. of Robust and Nonlinear Control, 16: 801-818
5. Morris K. A. (2010) The Control Theory Handbook, Control of Systems Governed by Partial Differential Equations. ed. W. S. Levine, CRC Press

Part III
Biomedical Signal and Image Processing

Non-Linear Analysis of Heart Rate Variability

Z. German-Sallo

"Petru Maior" University of Tirgu-Mures/Department of Electrical Engineering and Computers, Tirgu-Mures, Romania

Abstract— **HRV signals can be viewed as discrete time series and treated as well through accepted mathematical procedures in order to find specific properties. These mathematical procedures can be linear or non-linear. Lately, non-linear analysis methods brought new and valuable results in HRV analysis and prediction. This paper deals with approximate entropy and sample entropy calculations in order to find unrevealed properties of these signals. The used signals are obtained from the MIT-BIH Long-term ECG database. The aim of this paper is to measure information theory based parameters as different entropies for different signals to emphasize non-linear dynamics in HRV in order to help cardiology specialists.**

Keywords— **HRV, nonlinear dynamics, approximate entropy, sample entropy.**

I. Introduction

From over hundred years electrocardiogram (ECG) plays an important role in the analysis of human heart activity and the identification of different cardio-diseases. In an attempt to obtain a better understanding of the mechanisms of ECGs, procedures based on different theories such as information theory, chaos and fractal theory have been used to extract linear and nonlinear information from these signals.

Heart rate variability (HRV) analysis is a relatively new method for measuring the effects of interactions with the environment of human body. It is measured as the time difference between heart beats (named R peaks on regular ECGs) and its variations are correlated to health status. High HRV is an indication of healthy autonomic and cardiovascular response. Low HRV may indicate that the sympathetic and parasympathetic nervous systems aren't properly coordinating to provide an appropriate heart rate response [8].

In 1996 a Task Force of the European Society of Cardiology (ESC) and the North American Society of Pacing and Electrophysiology (NASPE) defined and established standards of measurement, physiological interpretation and clinical use of HRV. Time domain indices, geometric measures and frequency domain indices nowadays constitute the standard clinically used parameters [15].

Electrophysiological time series (as HRV) are usually stochastic; lately using different new theories these have been identified as fractal-like and as being generated by scaling phenomena [14], [6].

There are many methods to study and analyze HRV signals; these are usually grouped under linear and non-linear methods. The linear methods are defined in time-domain (based on the beat-to-beat or NN (normal in sinus rhythm) intervals, which are analyzed through parameters as standard deviation of different intervals or differences, root mean square of successive differences, the number or proportion of different pairs of successive NNs that differ by more than a fixed time interval [15]) and frequency-domain (power spectral density computation by several parametric or non-parametric methods in different frequency bands of interest, which are typically high frequency (HF) from 0.15 to 0.4 Hz, low frequency (LF) from 0.04 to 0.15 Hz, and the very low frequency (VLF) from 0.0033 to 0.04 Hz) [1].

The most commonly used non-linear method of analyzing HRV is the Poincaré plot which quantifies by fitting mathematically defined geometric shapes to the data represented as a pair of successive beats. The graphical representation means that on x-axis is represented the current RR interval, while on the y-axis is the previous RR interval [2].

In this paper an information theory approach to supporting the analysis of HRV signal is proposed. Information theory parameters as sample entropy and approximate entropy of R-R intervals extracted from regular ECG signal were calculated and analyzed [9]. These parameters of R-R interval dynamics can exhibit different patterns. This paper presents approximate entropy and sample entropy computation applied to three different long term ECG signals obtained from MIT-BIH database.

II. Nonlinear methods in HRV analysis

A. Heart Rate Variability

The HRV recorded as time duration between two heartbeats or as a distance R-R (R being the peak of QRS complex) on a surface electrocardiogram (ECG) is strongly related to the activity of autonomic nervous system. This is irregular if measured in milliseconds. This variation is significant and is related to physiological (controlled by the autonomous nervous system) conditions. A reduction of HRV has been reported in several diseases.

S. Vlad and N.M. Roman (eds.), *International Conference on Advancements of Medicine and Health Care through Technology; 12th - 15th October 2016, Cluj-Napoca, Romania,*
IFMBE Proceedings 59,
DOI: 10.1007/978-3-319-52875-5_38

Moreover, HRV also may have a prognostic value and is therefore very important in risk stratification [12]. Previous studies demonstrated a fractal-like complexity pattern in the variability of heart rate (HRV) which is possible to be measured, evaluated and quantified [9]. Fast variations (fluctuation) of HRV can reflect changes of sympathetic and parasympathetic activity; in other words, HRV is a noninvasive index of the autonomic nervous system's control on the heart. Many studies suggested that mechanisms involved in the regulation of cardiovascular system interact with each other in a nonlinear way and that it is possible to study these mechanisms with several algorithms for non-linear signals and systems [10], [11]. Recent data suggest that non-linear analysis in comparison to standard HRV measurements seems to detect abnormal patterns of RR fluctuations more efficiently [13].

B. Nonlinear dynamics in time series analysis

a) Approximate Entropy:

The approximate entropy is a statistical parameter inspired on the chaotic systems measures used to quantify the degree of regularity and the unpredictability of fluctuations over time-series data. This entropic measure was first proposed by Pincus [2], and it exhibits a good performance in the characterization of randomness even when the data sequences are not very long. In order to compute the approximate entropy, the embedded dimension m, that is, the length of the vectors to be compared, and a noise filter threshold r are required. Given N data points $u(1), u(2), \dots u(N)$ of an HRV signal, a sequence of vectors $x(1), x(2), \dots x(N-m+1)$ is formed, where

$$x(i) = [u(1), u(2), \dots\, u(i+m-1)] \tag{1}$$

Using the previous defined sequence $x(i)$ for each i satisfying $1 \leq i \leq N-m+1$, on construct

$$C_i^m(r) = \frac{nr\ j<N-m+1\ such\ that\ d[x(j),x(i)]<r}{N-m+1} \tag{2}$$

where $d[x(j), x(i)]$ represents the distance between the vectors $x(j)$ and $x(i)$, given by the maximum difference in their respective scalar components. It's important to observe that j takes on all values, so the match provided when i=j will be counted (the subsequence is matched against itself). This distance is calculated as follows

$$d_{ij} = \max_{k=0,\dots,m-1} (|x(i+k)| - |x(j+k)|) \tag{3}$$

Than the parameter approximate entropy $AE(m, r, N)$ is defined as follows:

$$AE(m,r,N) = \begin{cases} \Phi^m(r) - \Phi^{m+1}(r)\ for\ m > 0 \\ -\Phi^{-1}(r)\ for\ m = 0 \end{cases} \tag{4}$$

where

$$\Phi^m(r) = \frac{1}{N-m+1} \sum_{i=1}^{N-m+1} lnC_i^m(r) \tag{5}$$

Parameter selection as length of data m and noise filter threshold r hardly depends on the chosen application. Approximate Entropy reflects the likelihood that similar shapes of observations will not be followed by additional similar observations [5].

b) Sample Entropy:

The sample entropy is the negative natural logarithm of the conditional probability that two sequences similar for m points remain similar for $m+1$ points, where self-matches are not included in calculating the probability. Thus, a lower value of sample entropy also indicates more self-similarity in the time series. To be defined, sample entropy requires only that two templates similar for m samples remain similar for $m+1$ samples. Distance between every pair of vectors x_i and x_j is computed as before (equation (3)). Then, for given x_i, a probability function is computed as:

$$C_i^m(r) = \frac{1}{N-m} \sum_{j=1,x\neq 1}^{N-m+1} H(r - d_{ij}) \tag{6}$$

Where H is the Heaviside function, defined as

$$H(z) = \begin{cases} 1\ if\ z > 0 \\ 0\ if\ z \leq 0 \end{cases} \tag{7}$$

The probability that two sequences match for m points

$$\Phi^m(r) = \frac{1}{N-m+1} \sum_{i=1}^{N-m+1} C_i^m(r) \tag{8}$$

For $m+1$, $C_i^m(r)$ and $\Phi^m(r)$ are calculated. Finally, sample entropy is:

$$SE(n,r) = -lg \frac{\Phi_{m+1}(r)}{\Phi_m(r)} \tag{9}$$

It is clear from the definition that $\Phi_{m+1}(r)$ will always have a value smaller or equal to $\Phi_m(r)$, Therefore, $SE(n,r)$ will be always either be zero or positive value. A smaller value of $SE(n,r)$ also indicates more self-similarity in data set or less noise.

III. Procedure

The long term ECG signal is first filtered (regular noise, baseline wandering) than R peaks are detected as local maxima in the signal. Both time moments and R peak values are introduced in a bi-dimensional vector, after that the R-R intervals are revealed. These time series are ready to be evaluated through non-linear procedures. The RR intervals are considered as discrete time series (one dimensional vectors) and they are evaluated through computing sample entropy and approximate entropy for different embedded lengths and thresholds. The main idea is to find a relationship between regularity or unpredictability of fluctuations over these HRV data and their computed entropies.

IV. Results

A. Approximate Entropy calculation

In this paper are presented results obtained with signals 14184 (101543 samples, standard deviation 0.1638), 15814 (103354 samples, standard deviation 0.1032) and 14172 (66006 samples, standard deviation 0.2911) from the MIT BIH Long term ECG database. The histograms (graphical representation of the distribution) of these signals (128 equal sized bins) are presented on figure 1.

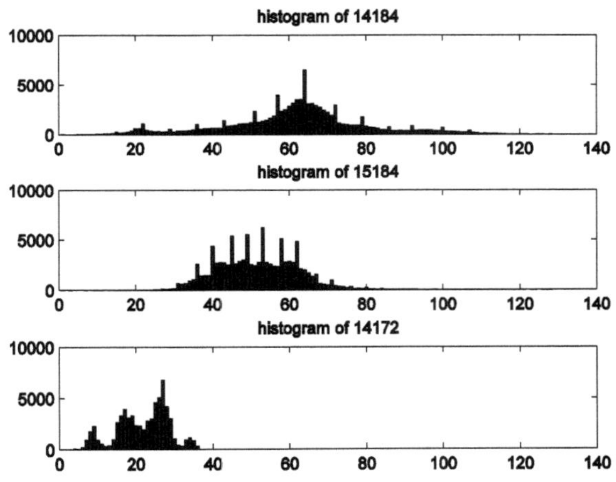

Fig. 1 The histogram of studied signals

Using the already presented mathematical background the approximate and the sample entropies were calculated for various lengths of signal (chosen to be a power of two in order to have better results in signal processing. The computational procedures were performed in Matlab environment using specific toolboxes. The chosen threshold for sample entropy was 0.2 and 0.2 of standard deviation for approximate entropy as recommended in literature [7].

The approximate entropy values were computed for different lengths (embedded dimensions), these lengths were chosen in six steps in order to see how the obtained values are influenced by these lengths. The obtained approximate entropy values are presented on figure 2

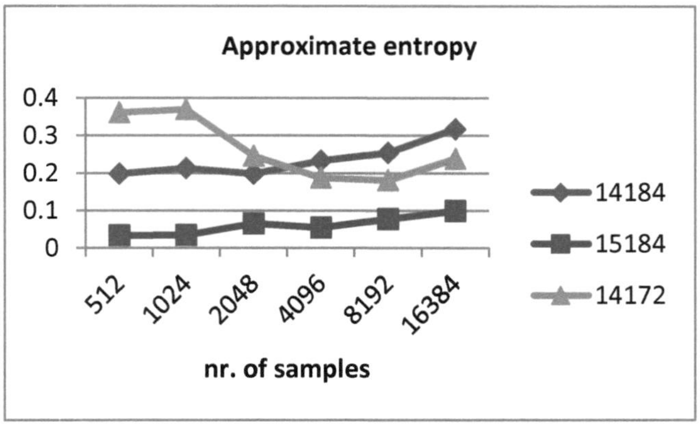

Fig.2 Approximate entropy versus number of samples

A time series containing many repetitive patterns has a relatively small value of approximate entropy; a less predictable process has a higher [4].

B. Sample entropy computation

The sample entropy values were obtained, using the presented computational framework (equations (6) to (9)) for different lengths (embedded dimensions), these lengths were chosen in eight steps as presented on figure 3. Their variations present similarities with the approximate entropy.

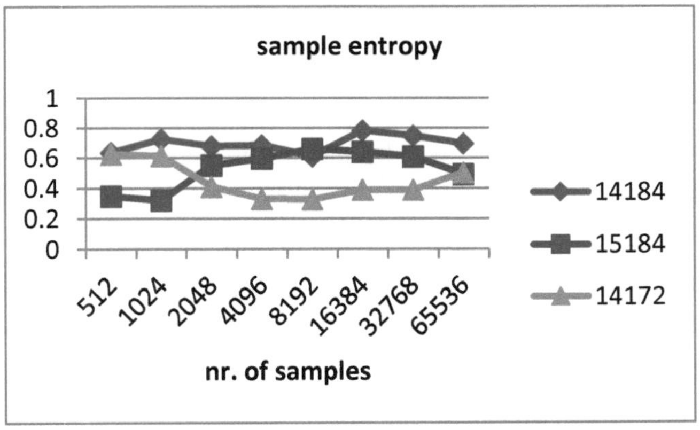

Fig.3 Sample entropy versus number of samples

To avoid a significant effect of noise in entropies calculation, one must choose threshold r larger than most of the noise [3]. The dependence between sample entropy and different values of chosen threshold is presented on figure 4.

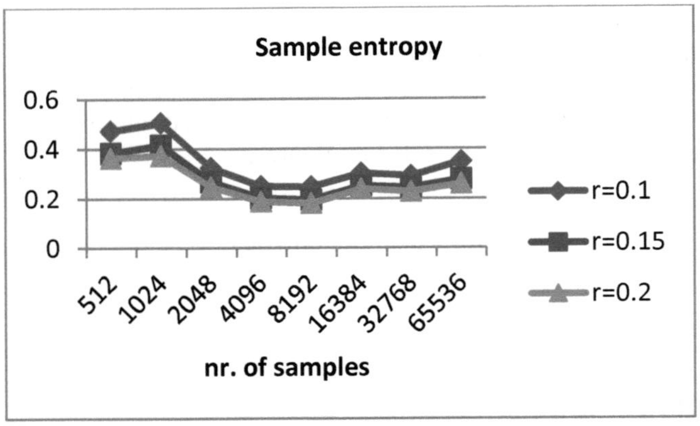

Fig.4 The variation of sample entropy with the threshold *r*

V. Conclusions

Approximate entropy and sample entropy are nonlinear indexes of heart rate dynamics that describes the complexity of R-R interval behavior, meaning regularity, unpredictability of fluctuations and self-similarities and can be helpful when others such as mean or variance cannot distinguish between discrete time series. Accurate entropy calculation of HRV signals usually requires vast amounts of data, and the results can be influenced by the accuracy of R peak detection and system noise. The HRV signals obtained from long term observations are more valuable from a medical point of view to, lower values indicating presence of various diseases. There is an organic relationship between sample values distribution (seen on histograms) and obtained entropies, lower entropy values indicates more regularity, higher values means more unpredictability.

The criteria for selecting threshold *r* can be adapted in different heart rate studies depending on the followed parameters. Usually electing the *r* value which maximizes approximate entropy seems to be a reasonable approach, because this choice would allow quantifying more of the time series irregularity than any other. In any case, whatever will be the criterion for selecting r, it is hardly recommended a preliminary quantification the whole entropy to get a more complete view of the phenomenon

As further work these entropies can be extended in multiscale domain through time-frequency (wavelet) transformation in order to get more accurate information about their non-linear dynamics.

Conflict of Interest

The authors declare that they have no conflict of interest.

References

1. Kitney, R. I., Rompelman, O, Coenen, A. J. R. M.(1977), Measurement of Heart Rate Variability. MBEC, vol. 15, pages 233–239
2. Akay, M.(2000) Nonlinear Biomedical Signal Processing Vol. II: Dynamic Analysis and Modeling. Wiley-IEEE Press, NY, USA
3. Costa, M; Goldberger, AL; Peng, CK (2002). "Multiscale entropy analysis of complex physiologic time series.". Physical Review Letters. 89 (6): 068102.
4. Pincus, S.,M.(1991) Approximate entropy as a measure of system complexity. Proc. Natl. Acad. Sci., vol. 88, pages 2297–2301
5. Pincus, S., M., Viscarello, R. (1992) R. Approximate Entropy: A Regularity Measure for Fetal Heart Rate Analysis. Obstetrics and Ginecology, vol. 79, pages 249–255.
6. Peng CK, Havlin S, Stanley HE, Goldberger AL. Quantification of Scaling Exponents and Crossover Phenomena in Nonstationary Heartbeat Time Series. Chaos, vol. 5, pp. 82-87, Jan. 1995
7. Castiglioni, P. Di Rienzo, M.(2008) How the threshold "r" influences approximate entropy analysis of heart-rate variability Computers in Cardiology, DOI: 10.1109/CIC.2008.4749103
8. Ho, K. K.; Moody, G. B.; Peng, C.K.; Mietus, J. E.; Larson, M. G.; Goldberger, A. L. (1997). "Predicting survival in heart failure case and control subjects by use of fully automated methods for deriving nonlinear and conventional indices of heart rate dynamics". Circulation. 96 (3): 842–848
9. Malik M, Camn AJ. (1993) Components of heart rate variability—what they really mean and what we measure. American Journal of Cardiology;72:821–2
10. Richman, JS; Moorman, JR (2000). "Physiological time-series analysis using approximate entropy and sample entropy". American Journal of Physiology. Heart and Circulatory Physiology. 278 (6): H2039–49
11. Acharya UR, Min LC, Joseph P.(2002) HRV analysis using correlation dimension and DFA, Innov Tech Biol Med (ITBM-RBM) 23:333–339,
12. .Smith J, Jones M Jr, Houghton L et al (1999) Future of health insurance. N Engl J Med 965:325–329 DOI 10.10007/s002149800025
13. Pincus, S., M. Goldberger, A., R. (1994). Physiological time-series analysis: what does regularity quantify? Am. J. Physiol. Heart. Circ. Physiol., vol. 35,pages 1643–1656.
14. Oppenheim A.V.,(1992) Signal processing in the context of chaotic signals, IEEE Int. Conf. ASSP, vol. 4, pp. 117-120.
15. Heart rate variability: standards of measurement, physiological interpretation and clinical use. Task Force of the European Society of Cardiology and the North American Society of Pacing and Electrophysiology. Circulation. 1996; 93:1043-65.

Author: Zoltan German-Sallo
Institute: "Petru Maior" University of Tirgu-Mures
Street: Nicolae Iorga nr.1
City: Tirgu-Mures
Country: Romania
Email: zoltan.german-sallo@ing.upm

Dependency of Tidal Volume on Mean Airway Pressure in High-Frequency Oscillatory Ventilation

J. Matejka and M. Rozanek

Department of Biomedical Technology, Faculty of Biomedical Engineering, Czech Technical University in Prague, Kladno, Czech Republic

Abstract— **Recent studies have shown that there exists a dependence of tidal volume on a mean airway pressure in high-frequency oscillatory ventilation. Objective of the present study was to examine if the dependence is caused by changing the mean airway pressure value itself or if it is caused by a change of the mechanical properties of the respiratory system according to a change of the mean airway pressure. Ventilator 3100B and rigid respiratory system models of volumes 25 L, 35 L, 50 L and 120 L with constant mechanical properties were used in the experimental circuit. Volume flow and tidal volume was measured with custom-made orifice and 2100 Respiration Monitor. Mean airway pressure was increased from baseline value by 4 cmH₂O every 1.5 min. It was shown that there is a statistically significant relationship between tidal volume and the mean airway pressure in constant mechanical properties of the respiratory system.**

Keywords— **Tidal volume, mean airway pressure, high-frequency oscillatory ventilation (HFOV), 3100B, rigid respiratory system model.**

I. Introduction

High-frequency oscillatory ventilation (HFOV) is a mode of unconventional mechanical ventilation intended for pediatric and adult patients with acute respiratory distress syndrome and for neonatal patients with infant respiratory distress syndrome. HFOV function is based on an application of relatively high mean airway pressure (P_{AW}) which keeps ventilated lungs open and on application of high-frequency pressure oscillation superimposed on P_{AW}. These pressure oscillation ensures exchange of ventilator mixture in respiratory system. Ventilators 3100A and 3100B (Carefusion, Yorba Linda, CA) are most commonly used ventilators for HFOV in the clinical practice. Recent studies have shown that tidal volumes (V_T) delivered by the ventilators are affected by set P_{AW} value [1, 2]. Link between these two HFOV variables can be direct or indirect. Direct relationship means that V_T will change its value with P_{AW} regardless of changes in the mechanical properties of the respiratory system induced by P_{AW}. Indirect relationship means that changes in V_T are caused by changes in respiratory mechanics which in turn are induced by change in P_{AW}.

The aim of the present study was to examine dependence between P_{AW} and V_T in HFOV under the constant mechanical properties of the respiratory system.

II. Methods

A. Measurements

Measurements were carried out with 3100B ventilator which was connected to one of used rigid respiratory system models. Models of volumes: 25 L, 35 L and 50 L were used. Measurement was also conducted with one model based on respiratory system anatomy with overall volume of 120 L [3]. Rigid respiratory system models with specified volumes were chosen because of their particular compliance ranges from 24.2 mL/cmH_2O to 116.2 mL/cmH_2O.

Flow sensor based on measurement of pressure difference was placed at joint of ventilatory circuit and connecting tube of the given respiratory system model. Volume flow was measured with a steel custom-made orifice specially designed for HFOV measurements. Data from orifice were digitized (DAQCARD 6009, National Instruments, Austin, TX) at sample rate 1 kHz and collected with custom-built software developed in Signal Express software (National Instruments). Mentioned measurement system including custom-made orifice is described in detail in [4]. Hot-wire anemometer 2100 Respiration Monitor (SLE, Croydon, UK) was placed next to the orifice in order to validate the measured data. Value of P_{AW} was taken over from 3100B ventilator. Scheme of the measurement setup is presented in Fig. 1.

B. Mapping P_{AW}-V_T Relationship

Baseline setting of 3100B ventilator prior to start of an experiment was: P_{AW} value 17 cmH_2O (13 cmH_2O in case of 120 L model), bias flow 25 L/min, inspiration time 50 %, frequency of pressure oscillations 5 Hz and pressure oscillations amplitude (ΔP) varied in range from 67 cmH_2O to 78 cmH_2O in dependence on used respiratory system model.

P_{AW} was changed every 1.5 min by 4 cmH_2O to maximal value 57 cmH_2O (45 cmH_2O in case of 120 L model). P_{AW} was changed by increasing expiratory valve resistance.

S. Vlad and N.M. Roman (eds.), *International Conference on Advancements of Medicine and Health Care through Technology; 12th - 15th October 2016, Cluj-Napoca, Romania,*
IFMBE Proceedings 59,
DOI: 10.1007/978-3-319-52875-5_39

Control voltage of ΔP was held constant throughout experiments. Despite this fact ΔP varied with P_{AW}. List of ΔP values for individual models and P_{AW} values in course of experiments is summarized in Table 1.

The flow was recorded continually throughout the whole course of conducted experiments. Value of tidal volume measured with 2100 Respiration Monitor was recorded before each change in P_{AW} value.

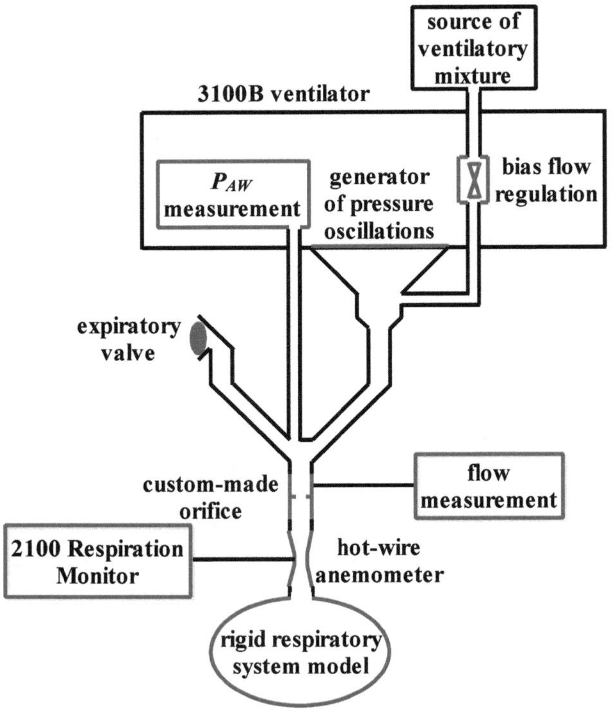

Fig. 1 Scheme of measurement setup, crucial elements are highlighted by red color

Table 1 Values of ΔP (cmH_2O) for different models and P_{AW} values

P_{AW} value (cmH_2O)	Respiratory system model 25 L	35 L	50 L	120 L
13				73
17	77	67	78	80
21	80	81	81	85
25	83	84	84	87
29	85	86	86	89
33	87	88	88	90
37	88	88	89	91
41	89	89	90	92
45	89	89	90	92
49	89	89	90	
53	88	89	89	
57	89	89	89	

C. Data processing

Flow signal measured with custom-made orifice was numerically integrated to compute a volume. Flow signal was not filtered during processing, because it wasn't considered necessary due to negligible amplitude of noise compared to amplitude of desired signal, see Fig. 2. Delivered V_T was calculated by subtracting maximal and minimal volume during the same respiratory cycle. Calculated V_T values were compared with values of V_T measured by 2100 Respiration Monitor.

Set of 200 V_T values was selected for each P_{AW} level in order to carry out statistical testing. Selected data were tested for normality using Chi-Square Goodness of Fit test and statistical significance of differences between V_T values on different P_{AW} was tested using one-way ANOVA. Dunn and Sidaks's post-test was applied to all ANOVA analyses. Value of p less than 0.05 was considered statistically significant. Statistical testing was performed using Statistics and Machine Learning Toolbox of Matlab R2015b (MathWorks, Natick, MA).

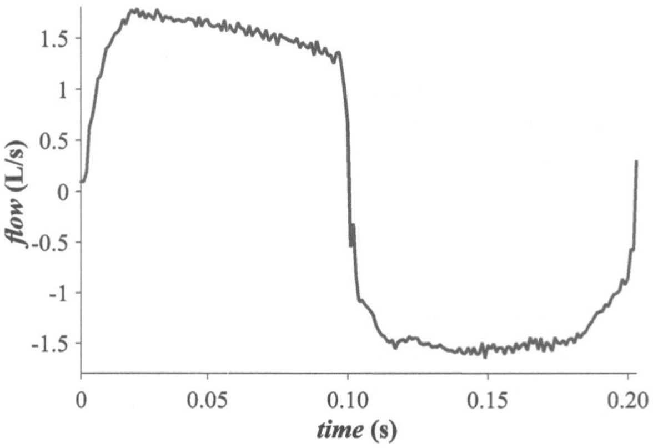

Fig. 2 Example of flow signal with superimposed noise in course of one respiratory cycle

III. Results

Mean values of sets of V_T measured with custom-made orifice (red line) and V_T values measured with 2100 Respiration Monitor (black line) for 25 L respiratory system model are depicted in Fig. 3 as a function of P_{AW}.

Same data are presented for 35 L, 50 L and 120 L model in Fig. 4, Fig. 5 and Fig. 6 respectively.

Standard deviations of sets of V_T measured with custom-made orifice had values of two to four tenths of milliliter. All standard deviation values are summarized in Table 2.

All sets of V_T had normal distribution (p > 0.06). Differences between V_T on each P_{AW} level were statistically significant for all used models ($p < 1.57 \cdot 10^{-9}$).

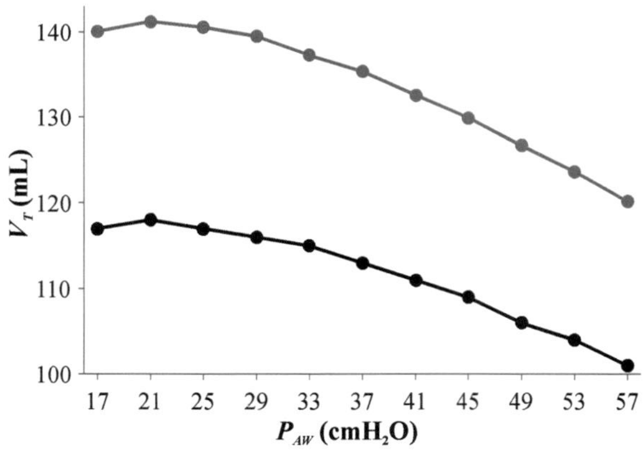

Fig. 3 VT measured with custom-made orifice (red line) and VT from 2100 Respiration Monitor (black line) as functions of PAW for 25 L model

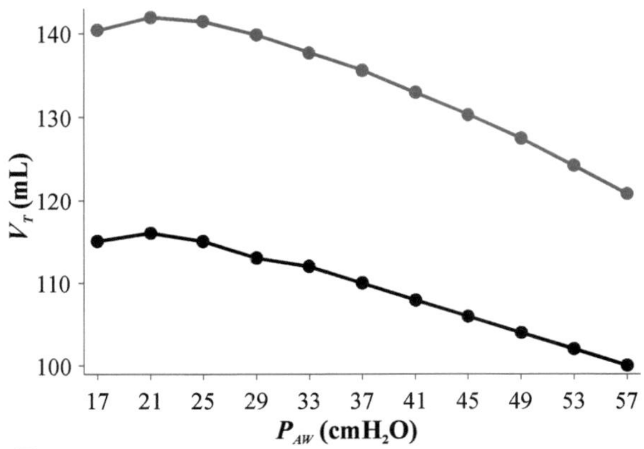

Fig. 4 VT measured with custom-made orifice (red line) and VT from 2100 Respiration Monitor (black line) as functions of PAW for 35 L model

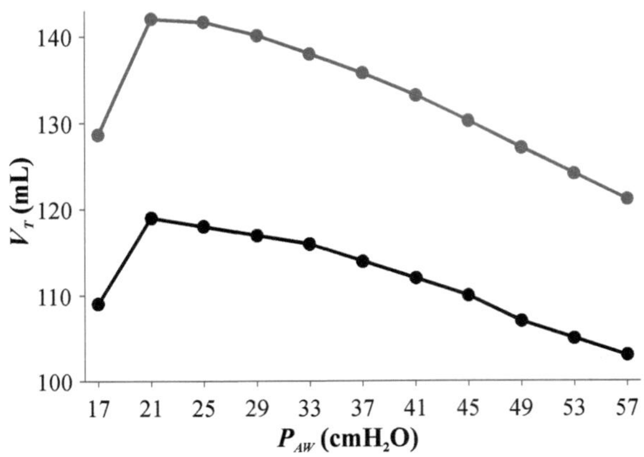

Fig. 5 V_T measured with custom-made orifice (red line) and V_T from 2100 Respiration Monitor (black line) as functions of P_{AW} for 50 L model

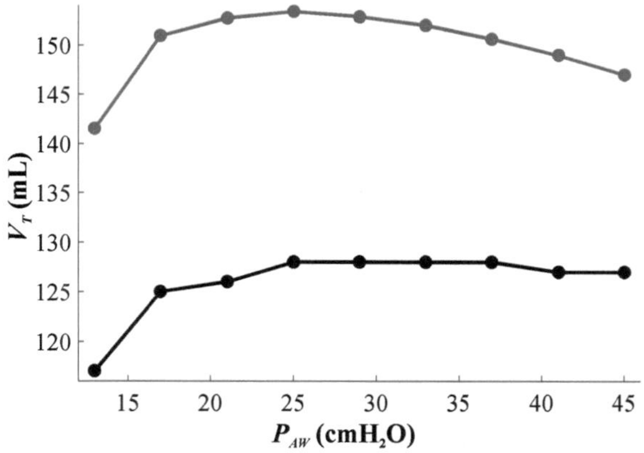

Fig. 6 V_T measured with custom-made orifice (red line) and V_T from 2100 Respiration Monitor (black line) as functions of P_{AW} for 120 L model

Table 2 Standard deviations of V_T (mL) for different models and P_{AW} values

P_{AW} value (cmH$_2$O)	Respiratory system model			
	25 L	35 L	50 L	120 L
13				0.26
17	0.29	0.38	0.28	0.24
21	0.27	0.27	0.30	0.25
25	0.28	0.27	0.27	0.26
29	0.27	0.28	0.28	0.27
33	0.26	0.24	0.27	0.25
37	0.25	0.24	0.26	0.28
41	0.26	0.25	0.26	0.29
45	0.25	0.26	0.26	0.31
49	0.26	0.28	0.33	
53	0.27	0.27	0.25	
57	0.22	0.26	0.28	

IV. Discussion

It was shown that there exists a statistically significant direct dependence of V_T in HFOV on P_{AW} under the constant mechanical properties of the respiratory system.

Figures in section Results show that V_T increased with P_{AW} value to 21 cmH$_2$O, or to 25 cmH$_2$O in case 120 L model. In higher P_{AW} values V_T decreased with P_{AW}. Initial rise in V_T was clearly caused by rise in ΔP, see Table 1. Subsequent decrease in V_T was probably due to ongoing increase in P_{AW} which wasn't sufficiently compensated by rise of ΔP. (Detailed explanation of this phenomenon: P_{AW} was increased by changing expiratory valve resistance. With help of electroacoustic analogy and Ohm's law one can establish relationship between flow, pressure and acoustic impedance. Higher pressure means higher flow and higher acoustic impedance means lower flow. If acoustic impedance (P_{AW}) rises faster than pressure (ΔP) then flow (after numerical integration V_T) will have downward trend.)

It can be also seen from Figures 3 to 6 that V_T measured with custom-made orifice differed from V_T measured with 2100 Respiration Monitor. Mean value of this difference is 22.9 mL. This could be caused by inaccurate calibration function from voltage to volume flow of custom-made orifice, or by filtration of flow signal in 2100 Respiration Monitor. However, data from custom-made orifice and 2100 Respiration Monitor possessed the same trend, except 120 L rigid respiratory system model. In this one particular case measured V_T values differed by less than 1 mL between some of the set P_{AW} values. This difference is under the measurement resolution of 2100 Respiration Monitor, which is 1 mL.

The values of P_{AW} higher than 40 cmH_2O are used only rarely in the clinical practice because of possible barotrauma.

Major limitation of this study is the use of rigid respiratory system models instead of animal models. Rigid models were chosen because of their constant mechanical properties which is the feature that cannot be assured in case of real lungs. However, this choice resulted in almost negligible standard deviation in V_T values on the same P_{AW} level. This in turn led to the fact that even the smallest change in V_T between two P_{AW} levels caused statistical significant difference. Conclusion of this study is that there exists statistical significant direct dependence of V_T on P_{AW}, but authors proved, on the basis of the above, that this dependence is not clinically significant. Almost negligible standard deviation in V_T also resulted in minimal p values.

V. Conclusion

Statistical significant dependence of V_T on set value of P_{AW} under the condition of constant mechanical properties of the respiratory system in HFOV was described in this study. We proved that the dependence has insignificant clinical impact upon the ventilated patients.

It was also proved that used custom-made orifice is suitable for measurement of tidal volumes in HFOV.

Acknowledgment

This study was supported by grant of Czech Technical University in Prague SGS16/258/OHK4/3T/17 and SGS15/228/OHK4/3T/17.

Conflict of Interest

The authors declare that they have no conflict of interest.

References

1. Zannin E, Ventura M L, Dellaca L D et al. (2014) Optimal mean airway pressure during high-frequency oscillatory ventilation determined by measurement of respiratory system reactance. Pediatric Research 75:493–499
2. Tingay D G, Mills J F, Morley C J et al. (2013) Indicators of Optimal Lung Volume During High-Frequency Oscillatory Ventilation in Infants. Critical Care Medicine 41:237–244
3. Rožánek, M., Hajný, O., Čech, M. (2014) Distribution of the ventilatory pressure in high-frequency oscillatory ventilation in the anatomically based model of the respiratory system. 48th DGBMT Annual Conference Proceedings, Walter de Gruyter GmbH & Co. KG, Hannover. 59:S998–S1000
4. Roubik K. (2011) Measuring and evaluating system designed for high-frequency oscillatory ventilation monitoring. Czech Technical University in Prague, Kladno

Author: Jan Matejka
Institute: Department of Biomedical Technology, Faculty of Biomedical Engineering, Czech Technical University in Prague
Street: nam. Sitna 3105
City: Kladno
Country: Czech Republic
Email: jan.matejka@fbmi.cvut.cz

Towards a Trial-based, Time-scale Dynamic Detection of M1 and M2 Components from the EMG Stretch Reflex Response

M. Tarata[1], M.S. Serbanescu[1], D. Georgescu[1], D.O. Alexandru[1], and W. Wolf[2]

[1] University of Medicine and Pharmacy of Craiova/Medical Informatics, Craiova, Romania
[2]Universität der Bundeswehr München, EIT-3-2, Neubiberg, Germany

Abstract— **The paper shows a new approach to the dynamic detection of the M1 & M2 electromyographic stretch reflex evoked activity (SR EMG), based on the detection of abrupt changes within the SR EMG signal on a trial-by-trial basis in the time-domain, using the generalized likelihood ratio test (AGLR). This algorithm was experimented on 16 healthy subjects (8 males and 8 females). The method makes possible the detection of the M1 & M2 responses in single, individual trials, on a trial-by-trial basis. The novelty which the method brings consists in using only the time-domain to provide the real time detection of the M1 & M2 in specific experimental closed loop paradigms, comparing to the complexity and time-consumption while using frequency/scale domains.**

Keywords— **stretch reflex, automated, trial-based, dynamic detection, noninvasive.**

I. Introduction

A. T-reflex and its importance

To develop force, the striate muscle elicits the muscular fibers contraction through the neural command received from motor neurons. The motor behavior is controlled at lower levels by spinal reflexes [1]. A significant reflex is the stretch reflex (SR), representing the contraction of the muscle while being abruptly lengthened by external forces. Mechanically, SR consists of a short-lasting (phasic) contraction determined by the speed of the length change and a longer-lasting (tonic) contraction determined by the actual static length of the muscle. Within the SR EMG response, two distinct components can be seen: M1 (short-latency) and M2 (long-latency) respectively. It was shown [2] in experiments with human subjects that M2 originates in skin and/or subcutaneous nerve terminals and accordingly, only M1 is elicited by the muscle stretch receptors. The reported latencies [2] are 30-35 ms (M1) and 50-60 ms (M2) for the First Dorsal Interosseus muscle (FDI). The assessment of the clinically relevant integrity of the spinal neural paths, can be accomplished through the detection of SR M1 & M2 in single trials. Till now M1 & M2 could be recorded only through coherent averaging of the SR EMG, when the stimulus time location is known. It allows only statistical (averaged) results. In this way, the individual relationship of the events with time is lost. With coherent averaging many trials are needed, which is time-costly. The detection of SR M1 & M2 in single trials is difficult because of (i) background EMG and noise, (ii) their shape and amplitude variability. To overcome the above difficulties and prepare for a dynamic, trial-by-trial detection of SR M1 & M2 from the EMG evoked during SR, we used previously the wavelet transform related techniques due to their ability to locate events in time, to extract time dependent spectral properties of the signals and to detect changes within signals [3, 4, 5, 6, 7] together with using a new experimental paradigm [8].

In a relaxed hand there are trials with no reflex response, therefore the subject was asked [5] to elicit a little voluntary muscular pre-activation, which improved the sensitivity to stretch and reduced the number of passive trials. Such voluntary pre-activation induces background EMG noise superimposed onto the SR EMG, which makes the onset detection even more difficult. This was the main drawback of the wavelet approach [5], because the spectral composition is similar for the M1, M2 and for the pre-activation EMG. The present work shows it is possible to detect the SR M1, M2 in single trials, only with processing the SR EMG in the time domain.

B. Aim of the paper

We aimed to develop a method for a time-scale dynamic, trial-by-trial detection of SR M1 & M2 from the evoked SR EMG, to alleviate the above reported drawbacks. Therefore we considered the signal in the time domain and used the approximated generalized likelihood ratio test (AGLR), to detect the SR M1, M2 as abrupt changes within the signal. Instead of using the cumulative sum decision rule (CUSUM) test, used in [6], we used the AGLR method [7]. With this method it is easier to approximate the statistical parameters for real signals, as the SR EMG.

II. Material and methods

A. Informed Consent and of Human and Animal Rights

The noninvasive experiments were performed with the consent of the subjects and in accordance with the ethical

S. Vlad and N.M. Roman (eds.), *International Conference on Advancements of Medicine and Health Care through Technology; 12th - 15th October 2016, Cluj-Napoca, Romania,*
IFMBE Proceedings 59,
DOI: 10.1007/978-3-319-52875-5_40

standards of the responsible committee on human experimentation (institutional and national) and with the Helsinki Declaration of 1975, as revised in 2000 and 2008.

B. Acquisition setup

A hardware and software acquisition setup was developed in order to trigger the stretch reflex of the FDI of the right hand and to acquire the EMG response of the muscles together with other parameters describing the event (torque, angle, trigger signal), whose description can be found in our pilot study [5] based on our new experimental setup [8].

The subjects (dominant right hand) were 8 females (age 19.6 ± 0.74) and 8 males (age 21.88 ± 5.18), healthy and motivated. The subject was comfortably seated in a chair, with hand and forearm supported by a table and strapped to a heavy plastic plate. The subject's index finger was immobilized within an orthopedic finger splint fixed on a lever. Two surface electrodes were placed on the abrazed, clean skin, longitudinally above the FDI muscle. The lever was attached to a torque motor. At randomized time intervals, unexpected impulse-like load changes (square signal of 350 ms duration) were applied by the torque motor causing full extension of the FDI muscle (Fig. 1). For each subject, 100 trials were performed. Two more parameters were logged: torque and finger angle.

The subjects kept a small muscular pre-activation before the stretch, to improve the sensitivity of the spindle transducers [1] and thus to increase the chance to elicit a SR EMG response.

C. Data acquisition

The signals were acquired during 2 seconds in each trial, at 2000 Hz sampling rate on all the channels (EMG, torque, angle, trigger signal) simultaneously, via NI 6052 board (National Instruments Inc., USA).

The EMG signal was amplified (gain 5000) (BIOPAC SYSTEMS INC, USA), filtered with a built-in 10-500 Hz band-pass filter and normalized against the maximum value.

The first second (2000 samples) of each trial was acquired to appreciate the level of pre-activation (Fig. 1, Pre-activation). The onset of the stretch-trigger was set after the first acquired second and had a duration of 350 ms. This window of 350 ms is also the time-window where the M1 & M2 can be seen (Fig. 1, Stretch-reflex). The rest of the acquired signal (650 ms) was acquired to appreciate the pre-activation within the post stretch reflex (Fig. 1, Post-activation).

The acquired EMG signals were normalized against the maximum value. The acquisition software was developed in Matlab (Mathworks, USA).

Fig. 1 shows an example of the signals.

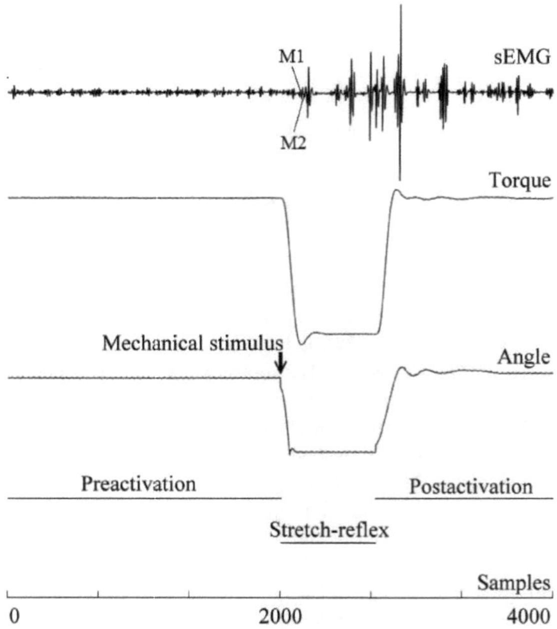

Fig. 1. Timing and acquired signals. Top to bottom: surface electromyography channel, mechanical engine torque and finger angle.

D. Manual onset detection of M1 and M2 components

For each trial, when elected, the onset of M1 and M2 of the stretch reflex were marked by skilled operators in order to be used as reference for the proposed automated method.

E. AGLR – computing the DETECTION signal

The rectified EMG signal was used to detect the onset of the muscular activity, as the moment when a change in the statistical properties, occurred according to the following.

Accepting an approximation of the model parameters as valid, a CUSUM type decision rule can be implemented by comparing the cumulative sum

$$S_j^k = \sum_{i=j}^{k} s_i(j) \qquad (1)$$

of the log-likelihood ratios

$$s_i(j) = \ln \frac{p_{\mu 1}(\varepsilon_i, j)}{p_{\mu 0}(\varepsilon_i)} \qquad (2)$$

with a threshold. In (2), $p_{\mu i}$, $p_{\mu 0}$ are the probability density functions of the i-th random variable before and after a possible change at moment j. Assuming a Gaussian density distribution, they are described by the variance and mean of the process. Since the position of the change is not known, it is replaced by its maximum likelihood estimate, i.e. a maximum operator selects the largest value of the test function with respect to all possible change times $1 \le j \le k$. With the above observations, in the AGLR implementation [5], (1) becomes:

$$\hat{S}_j^k = \frac{1}{\sigma^2}\left[\frac{\left(\sum_{i=j}^{k} u(i,j)\varepsilon_i\right)^2}{2\sum_{i=j}^{k} u^2(i,j)} - \sum_{i=j}^{k}\mu_0(i)(\varepsilon_i - \frac{\mu_0(i)}{2})\right] \quad (3)$$

where:

u – the average profile of the signal (either real or estimated);

ε_i – the rectified EMG signal at moment i;

$\mu_0(i)$ – actual signal value at moment i;

σ – the variance of the signal preceding the moment j.

The input sequence is analyzed by a growing observation window, from the beginning up to the actual observation k. A test window with the bounds j and k respectively, proceeds reversely in time, computing the log-likelihood ratios. The time j, at which the maximum value is obtained, acts as the maximum likelihood estimate of the unknown change time, namely the onset time in our case.

F. Automated onset detection of M1 and M2 components

(i) The AGLR based decision signal (AGLREMG) is computed from the SR EMG.

(ii) Next, from the AGLREMG signal a new signal (DETECTION signal) is computed as a moving standard deviation of 5 samples following each point within the signal (Fig.2, DETECTION).

(iii) Two different elements are revealed from the DETECTION signal: a) the highest peaks from M1 and M2 time windows and, b) the potential silent periods preceding M1, M2, processed within the M1 and M2 time windows:

a) the highest peak is considered as the maximum positive amplitude within M1 and M2 windows and stays for the maxim probability of a coherent change within the signal (Fig. 2, M1 & M2 maximal peak).

b) using the signal standard deviation, within the first second (2000 samples) before the mechanical stimulus, as a variable threshold relative to the highest peak detected in each M1 and M2 time windows of the DETECTION signal, we consider as a potential silent period all samples lower than the threshold. Several potential silent periods are thus detected, having an onset and an offset (Fig. 2, Silent periods).

(iv) The criteria to decide on the M1, M2 onset is the ratio between the current silent period duration and the duration from its offset to the next maximum peak within the DETECTION signal. M1 and M2 onsets are considered when this ratio is maximal (Fig. 2, Detected M1 & M2).

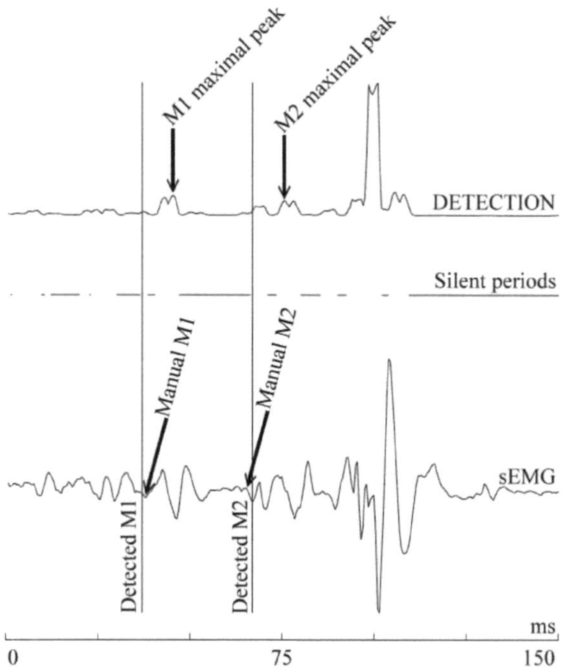

Fig. 2. Automated detection. Top to bottom: DETECTION signal, computed silent periods, and surface electromyography channel.

III. RESULTS

A. Manual onset detection of M1 and M2 components

From all the 1980 trials, both M1 and M2 were detected manually in 1112 trials, from the original SR EMG signal (Table 1).

Table 1 M1, M2 onsets (F- females, M- males)

	SR EMG M1 onset (ms)	SR EMG M2 onset (ms)	AGLR M1 onset (ms)	AGLR M2 onset (ms)
F	30.91 ± 6.93	61.19 ± 9.03	30.79 ± 9.49	59.77 ± 18.81
M	33.71 ± 7.12	65.83 ± 7.69	29.28 ± 12.57	64.50 ± 14.12

The M1 component could be identified in other 216 trials and the M2 component in other 356 trials, individually.

B. Automated onset detection of M1 and M2 components

On the 1112 trials where both components were identified by the human operator, the mean values were 30±11 ms for the M1 component and 62±16 ms for the M2 component (for males and females, together).

The results, separated on gender, are shown in Table 1.

IV. Discusion

Initially we attempted to detect the SR M1, M2 components from within the time-scale domains, as shown in our pilot study [5], based on our new experimental setup [8]. Which is new now, is the detection of M1, M2 from within the time-domain, working directly on the SR EMG signal, to avoid the incapacity of the wavelet-based approach to deal efficiently with the noise-like infestation of the signal, due to the voluntary pre-activation. Because some voluntary pre-activation is necessary to improve the rate of elicited SR responses, this also acts as noise, making more difficult the detection, also because it alters the silent periods within the EMG. The silent periods, occurring before the M1, M2 components, play an important role within the detection process.

Having no control mechanism for the automatic detection accuracy, when taking into consideration only the 544 trials where automated detection was within 10 ms from the manual detection on both M1 & M2,mean values were 32±7 ms for M1 component and 63±8 ms for M2 component. The average error was 3.03 ms for the M1 component and 3.06 ms for the M2 component. To conclude, in 28% from all the trials, the automatic detection was close to the human detection (time deviation less than 10 ms), in another 28.2% the time deviation was greater. In total, from 1980 trials, in 868 trials the human operator could not decide on the onsets, i.e. 43.83 %. The main reason of detection failure is the noise within the EMG signal, i.e. also the pre-activation signal, as discussed. A better detection of the silent periods is one way to further improve the algorithm.

V. Conclusions

The actual implementation improves the refined experimental setup (hardware & software) to be further used in physiological and clinical research and the algorithmic basis to proceed to the dynamic (automatic) detection of the M1 & M2 onsets from the SR EMG, in the time-domain on single trials. The novelty which the method brings consists in using only the time-domain to provide the real time detection of the M1 & M2 in specific experimental closed loop paradigms, comparing to the complexity and time-consumption while using frequency/scale domains.

The advantages of the actual approach:

- the use of the time domain, which improves the speed,
- the use of human-mind logic, based on the specificity of the SR EMG, which adds flexibility.

We shall further consider refining the method, in the sense of introducing exclusion decision on trials that are inappropriate for manual and automated detection, together with improving the detection of the silent periods preceding the SR M1, M2.

Acknowledgment

We are thanking the University of Medicine and Pharmacy of Craiova, Romania for having provided part of the equipment, facilities, subjects and the Universität der Bundeswehr, München, Germany for having provided part of the equipment to perform this research.

Conflict of Interest

The authors declare that they have no conflict of interest.

References

1. Gordon J, Ghez C (1991) Principles of Neural Science, Kandel ER, Schwartz JH, Jessel TM. eds. 3d ed., Appleton & Lange, Norwalk CT, pp 564-580
2. Matthews PB (1991) The human stretch reflex and the motor cortex. Trends Neurosci 14:87–91
3. Kurtzer IL (2015) Long-latency reflexes account for limb bio mechanics through several supraspinal pathways, Frontiers in Integrative Neuroscience 8, article 99, pp 1
4. Corden DM, Lippold OCJ, Buchanan Katie, Norrington Caryll (2000) Long-Latency Component of the Stretch Reflex in Human Muscle Is Not Mediated by Intramuscular Stretch Receptors, J. Neurophysiology 84:184-8
5. Tarata M, Serbanescu M, Georgescu D, Alexandru D, Wolf W, A New Wavelet Based Approach for the Noninvasive Dynamic Detection of M1 & M2 EMG Stretch Reflex Response Components – Preliminary Results, IFMBE Proc. vol. 57, Mediterranean Conference on Medical and Biological Engineering and Computing, Paphos, Cyprus, 2016, pp 46-49
6. Staude G, Wolf W (1999) Objective motor response onset detection in surface myoelectric signals, Medical Engineering & Physics 21: 449-467
7. Basseville M, Nikiforov IV (1993) Detection of Abrupt Changes – Theory and application Prentice-Hall, Inc. Upper Saddle River, NJ, USA
8. Tarata M, Serbanescu M, Georgescu D, Alexandru D, Staude G, Wolf W (2010) A new experimental concept for the quantitative exploration of the stretch reflex electromyographic response, Biomed Tech 2010; 55 (Suppl. 1) Walter de Gruyter • Berlin • New York. DOI 10.1515/BMT.2010.597

Corresponding author:
Author: Mihai Tarata
Institute: University of Medicine and Pharmacy of Craiova
Street: Petru Rares 2-4
City: Craiova, 200499
Country: Romania
Email: mihaitarata@yahoo.com

Discriminate Animal Sounds Using TESPAR Analysis

G.P. Pop

Comm. Dept., Technical University of Cluj-Napoca, Romania

Abstract— **Identification of animal species by their sounds is important for biological research and biodiversity assessment. In this paper we investigate the use of a dedicated TESPAR analysis, which does not use directly the acoustic signal from animals, but cepstral coefficients derived from it (MFCC and T-MFCC), to discriminate between different species. Our experiments shows that TESPAR S-matrices of some cepstral coefficients can be successfully used to discriminate between different animal species.**

Keywords— **animal species identification, acoustic analysis, time domain analysis, TESPAR analysis, cepstral coefficients.**

I. Introduction

In our daily life, we can hear, besides human speech, a variety of animal's sounds, including bird songs, dog barks, frog calls, cricket calls, etc. Many animals generate sounds either for communication or to accompany their living activities such as eating, moving, flying, etc. Identification of animals by their sounds is important for biological research and biodiversity assessment, especially in detecting and locating animals [1]. Some research difficulties when processing animal vocalizations are connected to noisy data, imperfect data labeling and poor knowledge about how animals produce and perceive sound. The incorporation of noise models is important since the recording environment is usually populated with many interfering noise sources. This noise can significantly reduce classification accuracy, especially when the characteristics of the noise vary across the dataset. Detecting state of an animal is a challenging task since humans can only guess as to what an animal is trying to communicate acoustically [2].

One of the important tasks when analyzing animal sounds is the measuring of acoustically relevant features. Majority of bioacoustics signals processing systems use time-frequency techniques such as the short-time Fourier transform, wavelets and energy distributions [3]. Most authors use the Mel frequency cepstral coefficients (MFCC) as acoustic characteristics for training and then testing under different classification systems.

In this paper we investigate the use of certain MFCC coefficients with TESPAR analysis to differentiate the sounds of different animal species. The choice is justified by the fact that only some of the MFCC coefficients contain specific information about the emitter of sound, while the rest containing information about the message. On the other hand, TESPAR analysis allows obtaining a specific fingerprint, of fixed length, for the sound emitter.

II. Cepstral Coefficients

In order to obtain spectral features, usually the acoustic signal is pre-processed before extracting features by [4]:

- preemphazis: the signal samples are filtered by a high pass digital filter;
- frame blocking: the acoustic signal is blocked into frames of samples with an overlap factor of frames;
- windowing: favor the samples towards the center of the window; this fact coupled with the overlapping analysis performs an important function in obtaining smoothly varying parametric estimates.

Mel cepstral analysis [4] use Mel scale and a cepstral smoothing in order to obtain the final smoothed spectrum. First, the short-term spectrum of the vocal segment is evaluated. Then, this spectrum is integrated over gradually widening frequency intervals on the Mel scale using a triangular filter bank. The resulting Mel-warped spectrum is projected on a cosine basis in order to obtain an uncorrelated cepstral coefficients MFCC (Mel Frequency Cepstral Coefficients).

The first cepstral coefficient (C_0) describe the shape of the log spectrum independent of its overall level. The second cepstral coefficient (C_1) measures the balance between the upper and lower halves of the spectrum while higher order coefficients are concerned with increasingly finer features in the spectrum.

Another type of coefficients are obtained if, first, apply the Teager energy operator (TEO) on acoustic signal and then repeat the same operations described before. In this way, we obtain so-called Teager MFCC coefficients (T-MFCC) [5]. The Teager Energy Operator (TEO), is a nonlinear energy-tracking signal operator used to estimate the amplitude envelope of an AM signal and the instantaneous frequency of a FM signal [6]. For discrete signals, TEO is defined as:

$$\Psi[x_n] = x_n^2 - x_{n-1}x_{n+1} \tag{1}$$

S. Vlad and N.M. Roman (eds.), *International Conference on Advancements of Medicine and Health Care through Technology; 12th - 15th October 2016, Cluj-Napoca, Romania*,
IFMBE Proceedings 59,
DOI: 10.1007/978-3-319-52875-5_41

The TEO has important applications in energy and time frequency estimation and has been widely used in speech signals analysis.

III. TESPAR ANALYSIS

TESPAR (Time Encoded Signal Processing and Recognition) is a technique which classifies time domain signals based on some specific signal shape parameters. The TESPAR method is based on the approximations of the locations of the signal zeroes (real and complex). The real zeroes correspond to the zero crossings of the signal while the complex zeroes are associated with local minima, maxima, points of inflexion etc. The real zeroes of a signal and some complex zeroes can be easily detected by visual inspection of signal waveform (Fig. 1), but the detection of all complex zeroes is difficult and time consuming. This drawback can be overcome in this way: the waveform is segmented between successive real zeroes, thereby generating a number of *epochs* with a certain durations (lengths); then, this duration information is combined with simple approximations of the shape between two successive real zeroes.
In this way an important number of complex zeroes may be identified by analyzing the shape of the waveform between its successive real zeroes.

In the simplest implementation of the TESPAR method [7], two descriptors (attributes) are associated with each epoch of the waveform:

- the *duration* (D) between two successive real zeroes expressed as the number of samples;
- the *shape* (S) between two successive real zeroes expressed as number of minima of that epoch.

Most signals can be described by a series of discrete numerical descriptors based on TESPAR symbol alphabets.

The standard alphabet can be used to convert the sequence of epochs into an equivalent TESPAR symbol stream, mapping the duration/shape (D/S) attributes of each epoch to a single descriptor or symbol by a coding process [6] (Fig. 2).

Another approach use an additionally descriptor A, for each epoch, such as epoch maximum amplitude, epoch energy, etc. In this case, the coding is based on a comparison of two successive epochs (for each descriptor D, S, A), as shown in Fig. 3. In this case, we get a fixed number of symbols (27) regardless of the duration or complexity of an epoch. This is TESPAR DZ alphabet [8].

The resulting TESPAR symbols string may be converted into a variety of fixed-dimension matrices [6]. The *S*-matrix is in fact a histogram of TESPAR symbols. Given a stream *s(i)* of symbols *Ti*, the elements of S matrix can be expressed as:

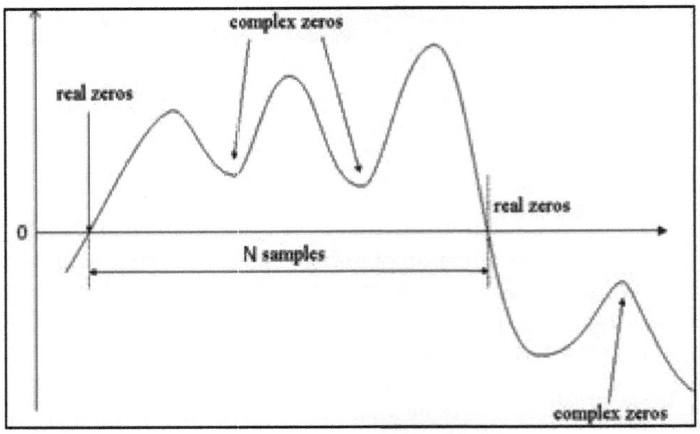

Fig.1. TESPAR waveform analysis

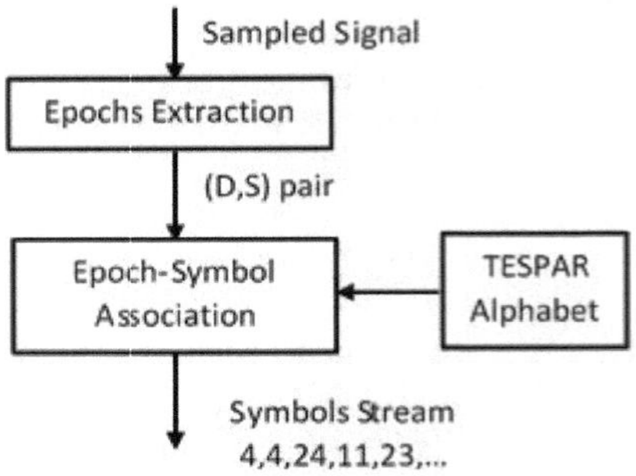

Fig.2. TESPAR coding process

$$S_n = \frac{1}{N}\sum_{i=0}^{M} T_i, \quad 1 \le n \le N \tag{2}$$

where: $$T_i = \begin{cases} 1\, if\, s(i) = n \\ 0, otherwise \end{cases}$$

The contribution of each symbol to the S-matrix values can be weighted by the value of the associated A descriptor.

Another type of matrix is the *A*-matrix, a two dimensional *N x N* matrix that contains the number of times each pair of symbols appears, with a possible lag of *L* symbols between the pair elements:

$$A_{mn} = \frac{1}{N}\sum_{i=l+L}^{M} T_i, \quad 1 \le m,n \le N \tag{3}$$

where: $$T_i = \begin{cases} 1\, if\, s(i) = m \ and \ s(i-L) = n \\ 0, otherwise \end{cases}$$

Again, the contribution of each pair of symbols can be weighted with a value that implies values of *A* descriptor from each epoch associated with that symbols.

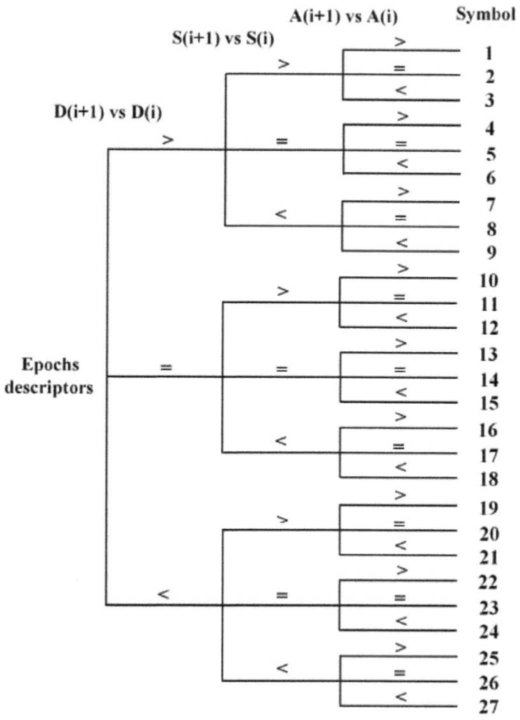

Fig.3. TESPAR DZ alphabet with fixed number of symbols

IV. Experiments And Results

For our experiments, a dedicated application was designed that allows:

- selecting a file with an acoustic signal;
- determine and eliminate silence zones;
- pre-processing the acoustic signal, with a selected frame length (ms);
- selecting a type of features (LPC, LPCC, MFCC, T-MFCC) and computing a specified number of coefficients for each frame;
- TESPAR analysis of a selected feature values, with the possibility to vizualize the epochs;
- generating symbol stream (coding) specifying the alphabet used (standard or DZ) and the type of additional epoch descriptor (maximum amplitude, average energy);
- generate and vizualize TESPAR matrices, *S* and *A* (for different values of the lag parameter *L*), with the possibility of applying a weight to each symbol or pair of symbols.

In our experiments, we used sounds from different animal species (domestic and wild: pig, sheep, bear and hawk) [9], [10]. For all animal sounds, 16-bit mono audio recordings, at 22,050 KHz sampling frequency were used.

We performed several experiments with our application, using 10*ms* signal frames, computing 12 MFCC and T-MFCC coefficients, using DZ TESPAR alphabet with maximum amplitude as additional descriptor for each epoch.

At this stage, we used visual comparison of *S* matrices. In all cases, the use of weighting lead to greater differences between the animal sounds. The best results were obtained using C_3, C_4 and C_8 coefficients. Figures 4-6 shows TESPAR *S*-matrices for T-MFCC coefficients (a-pig, b-sheep, c-bear, d-hawk) while figures 7-9 shows same matrices for MFCC coefficients.

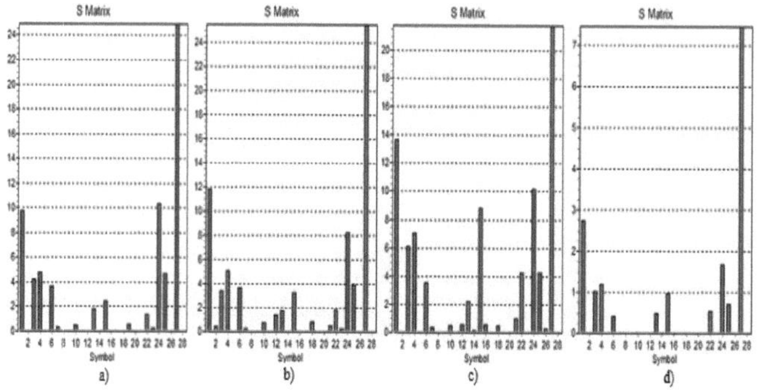

Fig.4. TESPAR DZ S matrix for T-MFCC C3 coefficient

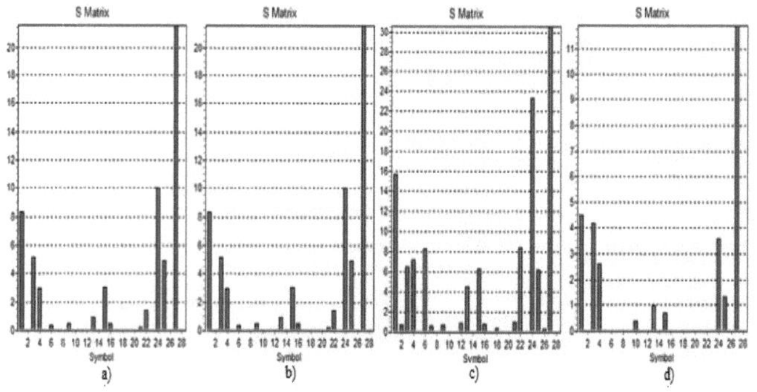

Fig.5. TESPAR DZ S matrix for T-MFCC C4 coefficient

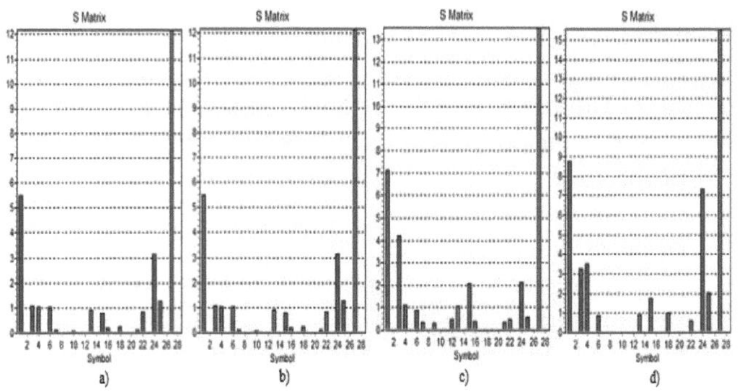

Fig.6. TESPAR DZ S for T-MFCC C8 coefficient

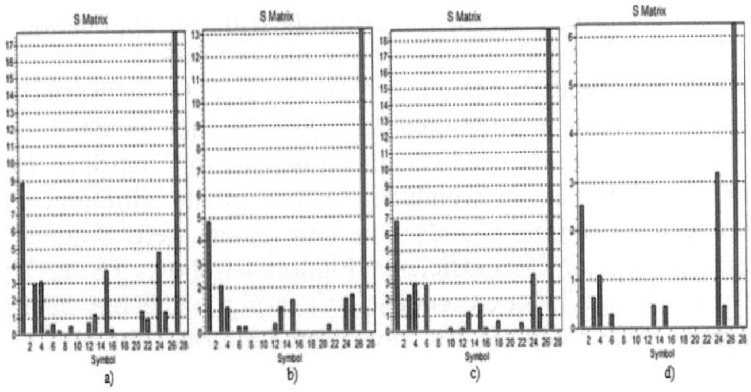

Fig.7. TESPAR DZ S for MFCC C3 coefficient

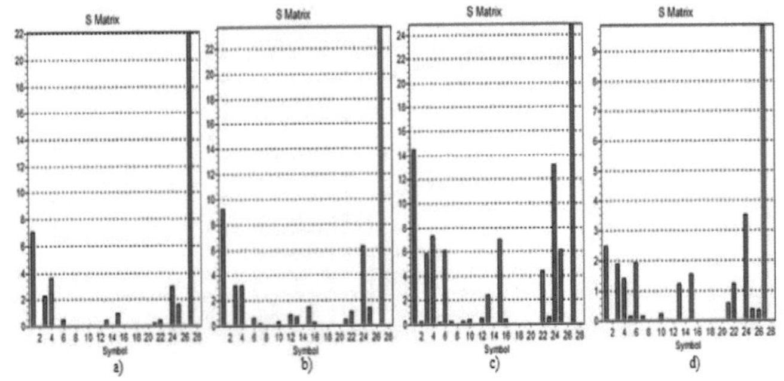

Fig.8. TESPAR DZ S matrix for MFCC C4 coefficient

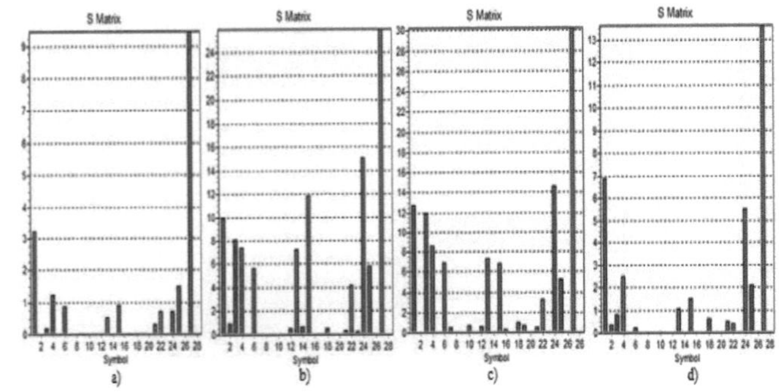

Fig.9. TESPAR DZ S matrix for MFCC C8 coefficient

Visual interpretation of these matrices should consider the following:

- first and last symbol occurring more frequently for this type of alphabet, which emphasizes the normal evolution of the acoustic signal: early vocalization sounds supposed epochs of increased complexity (symbol 1), while the end of sounds vocalization generates epochs of low complexity (symbol 27);
- matrices differ both in terms of their form (symbols appearing and the relative values of the number of symbols) and in terms of absolute values of histograms.

Remarkable obvious differences between mammals and birds, for both coefficients. In mammals, T-MFCC coefficients allow obtaining high complexity matrices (number of symbols and associated values) which allows better differentiate between species.

V. Conclusions

In this work, we investigate the use of TESPAR *S*-matrices to discriminate between animal species based on their sounds, using cepstral coefficients (MFCC, T-MFCC) in TESPAR analysis. First results show that the TESPAR *S*-matrices can be successfully used for this purpose. Some of coefficients allow better discrimination between species. More experiments on a larger database with animal sounds are needed, using a classifier to automate discriminate between different animal species.

Conflict of Interest

The authors declare that they have no conflict of interest.

References

1. Chang-Hsing Lee, Yeuan-Kuen Lee, Ren-Zhuang Huang (2006), Automatic Recognition of Bird Songs Using Cepstral Coefficients, Journal of Information Technology and Applications Vol. 1 No. 1, May, 2006, pp.17-23.
2. Deshmukh O., Rajput N., Singh Y., Lathwal S. (2012), Vocalization patterns of dairy animals to detect animal state. 21st Int. Conf. Pattern Recognition (ICPR 2012) November 11-15, 2012. Tsukuba, Japan.
3. E. D. Chesmore (2004). Automated bioacoustic identification of species. An. Acad. Bras. Ciênc. 76(2): 435 – 440.
4. Huang, X., Acero, A., Hon, H. (2001), Spoken Language Processing. Prentice Hall.
5. H.A. Patil, T. K. Basu (2008), Identifying perceptually similar languages using teager energy based cepstrum. Engineering Letters, 16(1):151–159.
6. P. Maragos, J. F. Kaiser, and T. F. Quatieri (1993), Energy separation in signal modulations with application to speech analysis. IEEE Trans. Signal Processing 41, 3024.
7. R.A. King, T.C. Phipps (1998), Shannon, TESPAR And Approximation Strategies. ICSPAT 98, Vol. 2, pp. 1204-1212, Toronto, Canada, Sept. 1998.
8. E. Lupu, S. Emerich, F. Beaufort (2009), On-line signature recognition using a global features fusion approach, Acta Tehnica Napocensis, Electronics and Telecomunications, *Vol.50,* no..3, pp. 13-20, 2009.
9. http://www.grsites.com/
10. http://soundbible.com/

Author: Petre G. Pop
Institute: Comm.Dept., Technical University of Cluj-Napoca
Street: G.Baritiu, 26-28
City: Cluj-Napoca
Country: Romania
Email: petre.pop@com.utcluj.ro

Robust Analysis of Non-stationary Cortical Responses: tracing Variable Frequency Gamma Oscillations and Separating Multiple Component Input Modulations

A. Dăbâcan[1,2] and R.C. Mureşan[2]

[1] Technical University/ Faculty of Electronics, Telecommunications and Information Technology, Cluj-Napoca, Romania
[2]Romanian Institute of Science and Technology/Theoretical and Experimental Neuroscience Laboratory, Cluj-Napoca, Romania

Abstract— **Natural signals have a complex nature and most often encode information both in the frequency and time domain. Neuronal signals in particular have a very nonlinear behavior, with features of interest appearing sparsely and discontinuously. Therefore, methods that characterize and enable the visualization of these data are of great importance. Here, we present two algorithms that act on different dissociation problems in neuroscience: Firstly, the definition of trajectories in a time-frequency-power three dimensional space and secondly, the dissociation of modulatory effects of different time scales. The methods have the advantage of preserving the transient nature of neuronal features and of providing a practical computational implementation. We apply these methods on cortical response to visual stimuli where multiple parameters are manipulated. Results show that such response characteristics reveal features that are not explained by current theories of underlying mechanisms of oscillatory response.**

Keywords— **neuroscience, feature extraction, spectral pattern, time-domain decomposition.**

I. Introduction

Neuronal activity has complex dynamics, its behavior resembling that of chaotic systems, where small perturbations trigger highly a nonlinear response [**Error! Reference source not found.**]. Electrophysiological signals recorded from cortical structures reflect this by showing a high level of non-stationarity [**Error! Reference source not found.**]. Moreover, coding in the brain is achieved through time-related features, but also through spectral features such as oscillatory activity and coherence [**Error! Reference source not found.**].

The analysis and visualization of this type of data is often difficult due to the multiple relevant dimensions of the extracted information. For example, in order to analyze the neuronal response to a particular stimulus from a spectral point of view, the average power spectrum of the response period will reveal general spectral components of the response, but will hold no information about the temporal localization of the spectral feature. Also, such averaging cannot dissociate between a strong, short burst of oscillatory activity and a weak prolonged oscillation. Moreover, frequency variation within response period will appear as a broad spectrum response in a time-averaged spectrum.

For these reasons, a time-resolved analysis of spectral patterns is of interest. But in this case, the response pattern is a three dimensional component, defined by time, frequency and power. Also, multiple oscillatory modes coexist, each representing either a different underlying cortical process or a harmonic of the main response component. In order to independently isolate these three dimensions and further isolate the main response from multiple oscillatory modes, we introduce a new method to structurally define the trajectory of neuronal activity through this three dimensional space, rendering the independent analysis of each dimension possible. Further, we describe a method of dissociating modulatory effects on these individual parameters via a time-domain spectral decomposition method, without being perturbed by the non-stationary nature of the analyzed signals.

We apply these methods to analyze gamma-band oscillatory response in the visual cortex. Gamma oscillations occur in the range of 30-120 Hz and are associated with multiple processes in the brain, from perception to high level cortical processes such as attention and memory [**Error! Reference source not found.**]. In the visual cortex, this component is known to be modulated by visual input strength, such as contrast, but the nature of this modulation is not yet understood [**Error! Reference source not found.**]. Specifically, frequency and power increase with input strength. The relationship between frequency, power and input strength of gamma oscillations represent hallmarks for underlying mechanisms. For example it is hypothesized that intrinsic membrane properties of neurons within the cortical volume of interest affect the frequency stability and power of gamma [**Error! Reference source not found.**].

We implemented a series of methods that can evaluate the relationship between frequency and power in the local field potential (LFP) spectral response. We apply these methods in the study of transient oscillatory responses. Also, we look at the evolution of these parameters with respect to different stimulus characteristics to test whether they establish a codependent relationship in all circumstances.

S. Vlad and N.M. Roman (eds.), *International Conference on Advancements of Medicine and Health Care through Technology; 12th - 15th October 2016, Cluj-Napoca, Romania,*
IFMBE Proceedings 59,
DOI: 10.1007/978-3-319-52875-5_42

II. Methods

All the experiments were conducted in accordance with the European Communities Council Directive of 24 November 1986 (86/609/EEC), according to the guidelines of the Society for Neuroscience and the Romanian law for the protection of animals, approved by the local ethics committee and overseen by a veterinarian.

We acquired electrical signals using silicon probes from the visual cortex of isoflurane anesthetized mice while they were presented moving orientation gratings. We had two types of stimuli, one where contrast of the gratings was fixed and the spatial and temporal frequencies were low (0.1 cycles/degree, 1.75 cycles/s) and another where contrast was following a triangular modulation and spatial and temporal frequencies were higher (0.28 cycles/degree, 5 cycles/s). The acquired signal was filtered with a low pass filter with a cutoff frequency of 300 Hz.

III. Spectral pattern detection

We defined a method capable of following an oscillatory pattern through a three-dimensional space, based on the assumption that the movement through this space happens smoothly on all axes. For this purpose, we computed a time-resolved Fourier decomposition and computed the spectral power. On this three-dimensional space, we traced the power crest of the response.

Specifically, we split our response period into windows which we multiplied with a Blackman window to minimize border effects. Then, we adjusted the length of the window with zero padding to have enough resolution in frequency. We computed the fast Fourier transform and computed the power for each time and frequency bin.

Our method makes, several assumptions:

- Response is defined by increase in power with respect to baseline conditions. Therefore, we normalized the spectrum to a baseline period, where no stimulation was provided.
- The point of maximum power is part of the response of interest.
- In two successive time bins, the closest maxima in frequency is part of the same oscillatory component.

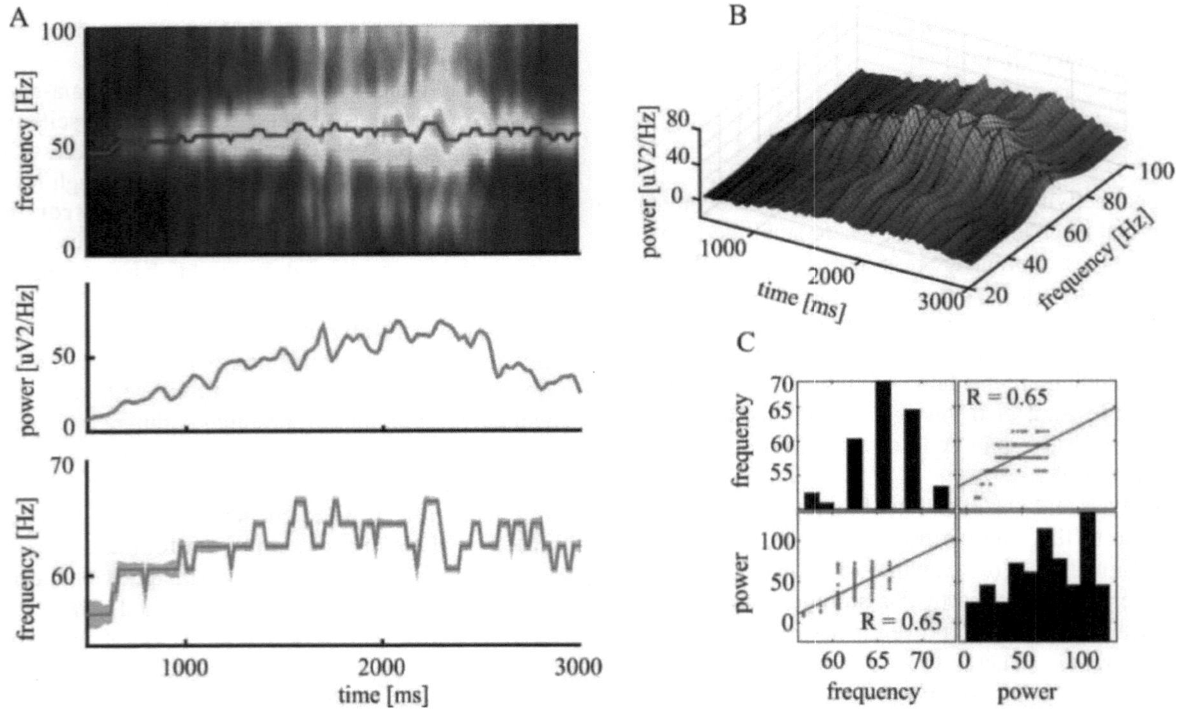

Fig. 1. Pattern analysis of the time-resolved FFT of simulation LFP: A - time-resolved FFT across response period. Red line mark the selected trajectory in peak following; below are the power and frequency of the followed peak across time; B - A three-dimensional view of the response and the crest-detection algorithm. C - Scatter plots of power versus frequency of the followed peak and histograms of each measure; Red line marks the linear correlation and the coefficient value is noted for each plot.

We mention that the time-frequency response could also be defined using other decomposition methods, such as a wavelet transform.

Therefore, the definition of spectral component is determined taking the following steps:

- The time and frequency band of interest are defined. **Note** that the presence of a response within these bands of interest is necessary for the effectiveness of the method. A good way to determine response time is through a power threshold, therefore eliminating periods of time where there is no relevant pattern to detect. Limiting the frequency band can be of interest when dissociating between multiple oscillatory components of different power ranges.
- The coordinates of the point of maximum power is detected. This will be the starting point for tracing the response trajectory.
- Through an iterative process, the closest maxima on the frequency axis is determined for each time bin while moving away from the point of origin towards the beginning and towards the end of the response period respectively.
- For each point, define the time, frequency and power.

Fig. 1shows an application of this algorithm on electrophysiological local field potentials (LFP) recorded in the primary visual cortex of anesthetized mice while they were presented a visual stimulus composed of moving gratings of variable contrast. The response pattern shows that power and frequency vary across time. From here on, the shape of each trajectory parameter can be assessed independently. In this case, the correlation between the two parameters is computed and the histogram of each is displayed.

IV. Empirical mode decomposition

We wanted to analyze the differential effect that stimulus features had on power and frequency of the LFP spectral pattern. We introduced two degrees of variability in our stimulus: one was a moving sinusoidal grating. The passage of the grating through the receptive field of the recorded brain area causes local luminance fluctuations, altering both power and frequency of the response. The second variable was contrast: the difference between the brightest pixel and the darkest one was modulated by a triangular carrier. Contrast varied in a slow timescale (one period = 4.5 s) while local luminance varied rapidly (200 ms). We needed a method to reliably separate the modulations induced by each factor, when we knew the timescale of each modulatory effect. We therefore needed to break down signals which were non-stationary and non-linear, with no assumptions of periodicity or sinusoidal approximation.

For this, we applied an algorithm of empirical mode decomposition, which represents an alternative to spectral decomposition methods [**Error! Reference source not found.**]. It offers the advantage of an easy implementation operating integrally in the time domain.

The basic principle is an iterative filtering and subtraction of independent mode functions (IMFs), also called the sifting process.

An IMF is defined as a function that

- Has one extreme between zero crossings and
- Has a mean value of zero.

The algorithm comprises of the following steps:

- For a signal $X(t)$, the local minima and maxima are detected. The definition of locality determines the effectiveness and calculation time of the EMD.
- The upper and lower envelopes are determined by cubic spline interpolation of the points of local maxim and minima.
- The average of the upper and lower envelopes $M_{11}(t)$ is computed and subtracted from the original signal.

$$H_{11}(t) = X(t) - M_{11}(t)$$

- The residual H_{11} is then treated as the input data in an iterative process of subtraction of mean envelopes until H_{1k} is an IMF, that is:

$$Nr(extremes) = Nr(zeros) \pm 1$$

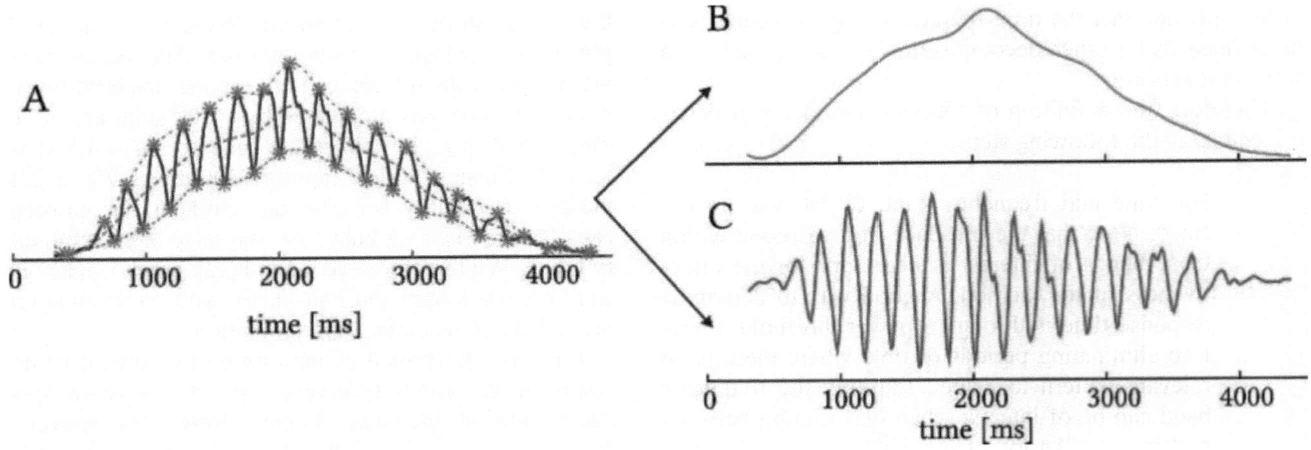

Fig. 2. Adapted variant of Empirical mode decomposition algorithm example: A – a power profile of neuronal response to moving gratings of variable contrast. Blue markers indicate the detected minima and maxima. Red dotted lines are the computed envelopes and the blue dotted line is their mean. B – the slow component of the decomposition resulted by the subtraction of the first mode from the original signal. C – the detected first mode, using a definition of locality restricting maxima and minima that are at least 100 ms apart.

- Therefore H_{1k} is the first intrinsic mode function, containing the shortest period component of the signal.

$$IMF_1 = H_{1k}$$

- This component is subtracted from the original signal:

$$R_1 = X(t) - IMF_1$$

And the same process is performed on the residual until the residual does not contain any fluctuations, that is:

$$Nr(extremes) = 0$$

The components $IMF_1 \dots IMF_n$ are the modes of the signals and create a nearly orthogonal basis of the signal.

In our experimental conditions, we wanted to separate between a fast and a slow component of the data, without making any assumption on the harmonic structure of the oscillation, its stationarity or its stability in frequency. Therefore we adapted the EMD algorithm so that we could achieve this in the fastest, simplest way.

We first limited the range of timescales of the decomposition by limiting the number of local minima and maxima detected. We therefore imposed a minimum distance in time between two maxima and minima respectively so as to ignore components that are above our frequency of interest, but still preserve the features for further analysis.

Second, we only needed to dissociate between two timescales. Therefore, we extracted the first mode as the fast modulatory effect and the first residual as our slow modulatory effect. Fig. 2 shows an example of this decomposition applied on power fluctuations in LFP in response to fast luminance (Fig. 2 C) and slow contrast (Fig. 2 B) variation.

V. Discussion

The structural detection of spectral components is relevant when each element represents a different underlying mechanism. In our case, we were interested in the isolation of an oscillatory component of neuronal responses which has a large range of frequency variation, but represents the same underlying process. To characterize this process without limiting the frequency range of its fluctuation or smearing its properties by averaging across a wide range of frequencies, we chose to structurally follow the pattern of the response within the three dimensional space of time, frequency and power. We found this algorithm useful for independent analysis of the power and frequency dimension of the oscillatory response in particular, eliminating any artefacts caused by the variation of one with respect to the other.

This algorithm was especially useful when oscillatory response was non-stationary. For example, we looked at response properties of gamma oscillations where the spatial and temporal frequency of the stimulus was low enough to elicit transient responses at each grating passage through the receptive field (Fig. 3). In this case, our algorithm successfully traced the power and frequency patterns of the response, revealing a complex trajectory. Frequency and power in this case did not follow the same pattern, as predicted by other studies.

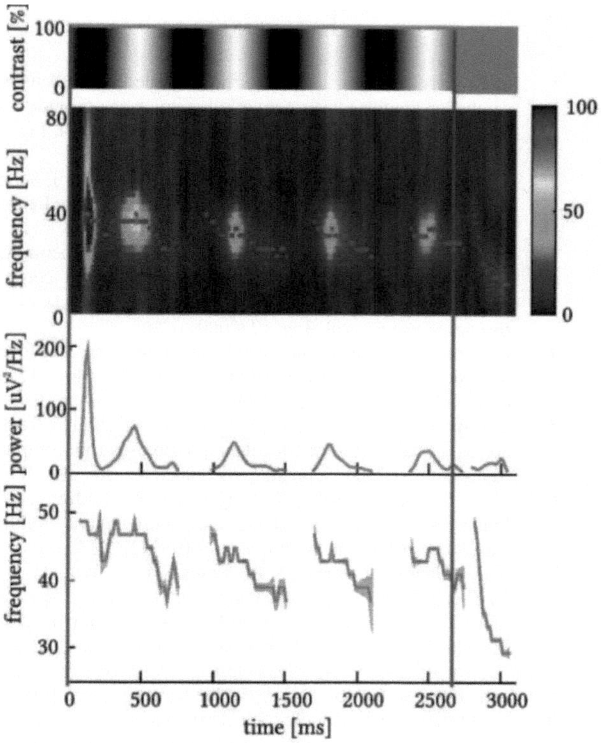

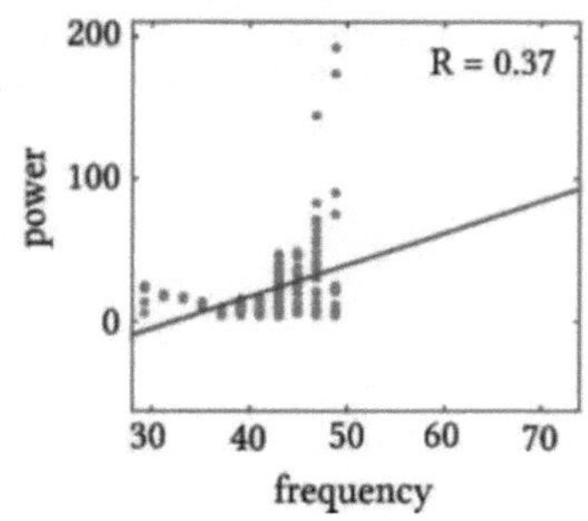

Fig. 3. Pattern analysis of transient oscillatory responses. From top to bottom: visual stimulus profile presented; time-resolved Fourier transform of the response period. Red dots mark the selected points in peak following. Note that a power threshold was selected so as only to look for patterns where there is a response; Power and frequency of the followed response pattern. Red vertical lines show start and end of visual stimulation; Scatter plot of power versus frequency of the followed oscillatory component. Red line represents the linear correlation of the two values whereas the correlation coefficient r is listed.

Further, we looked at the relationship between frequency and power when different stimulus manipulations occurred. By separating the effects induced by luminance and contrast variation using the adapted variant of empirical mode decomposition, we were able to independently test the correlation between frequency and power for each of the varied parameter.

We found that power and frequency are differently correlated as a function of local luminance and contrast level respectively. Specifically, power and frequency were highly correlated with respect to contrast, but luminance of the receptive field induced a lower correlation between the two. This fact corresponds to our observations when looking at the response pattern at lower spatial and temporal frequencies (Fig. 3), where we see a low correlation between power and frequency when only luminance is varied.

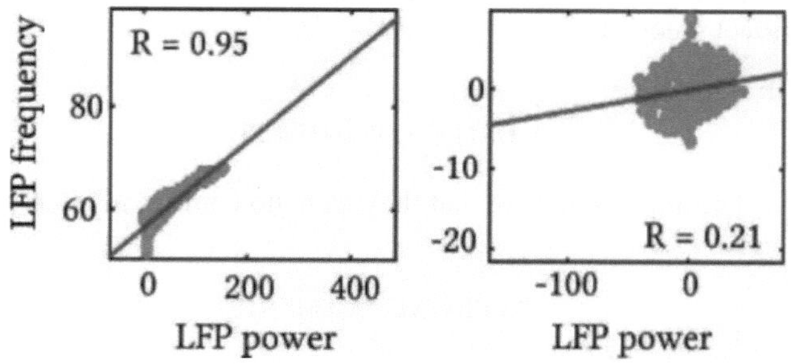

Fig. 4. Power and frequency correlations as a result of modulatory causes of different timescales. Scatter plots of frequency versus power of the response pattern in slow timescales (*Right*), corresponding to contrast modulation, and fast timescales (*Left*) corresponding to the passage of the grating through the receptive field.

These observations have important implications in the study of mechanisms underlying oscillatory behavior in the cortex. They suggest that existing theories about interactions giving rise to synchronization and increase in local field potential power within a specific frequency range fail to explain all features that are observed experimentally. In particular, the Pyramidal-INterneuron Gamma (PING) mechanism [**Error! Reference source not found.**] predicts that a stronger input is associated to a larger gamma power and a higher frequency [**Error! Reference source not found.**] [**Error! Reference source not found.**]. Our results indicate that this seems not to be the case when the activity of the cortical circuit is modulated by the local luminance fluctuation in the receptive fields of underlying cells.

VI. Conclusions

The study of oscillatory components across time and their dependence on input parameters within cortical networks is extremely important, impacting directly on our understanding of the functional role of such oscillations. Here, we proposed two methods which aim to characterize transient oscillatory responses more precisely and to disambiguate between dimensions of these responses and the various causes that lead to modulations of the response. We showed the application of these algorithms in the spectral analysis of local field potentials recorded in the visual cortex of anesthetized mice, while being presented a series of moving stimuli with variable contrast and local luminance. With the aid of these methods, we were able to determine the trajectory of the response through a three-dimensional time-frequency-power space and separate the effects of modulation of different timescales on each of these dimensions. Our results indicate that such analysis methods reveal features which are not explained by current theories about mechanisms of gamma oscillatory responses and are therefore of great relevance in the development and testing of novel theories.

Conflict of Interest

The authors declare that they have no conflict of interest.

Acknowledgements

This work was supported by a grant from Consiliul Național al Cercetării Științifice (CNCS) - Unitatea Executivă pentru Finanțarea Învățământului Superior, a Cercetării Dezvoltării și Inovării (UEFISCDI) project number PNII-RU-TE-2014-4-0406/2015 contract no. 169/2015.

References

1. C. Rössert, P. Dean, and J. Porrill, "At the edge of chaos: How cerebellar granular layer network dynamics can provide the basis for temporal filters," *PLoS Comput Biol*, vol. 11, no. 10, p. e1004515, 2015.
2. M. Lundqvist, J. Rose, P. Herman, S. L. Brincat, T. J. Buschman, and E. K. Miller, "Gamma and beta bursts underlie working memory," *Neuron*, vol. 90, no. 1, pp. 152–164, 2016.
3. P. Uhlhaas, G. Pipa, B. Lima, L. Melloni, S. Neuenschwander, D. Nikolic, and W. Singer, "Neural synchrony in cortical networks: history, concept and current status," *Frontiers in integrative neuroscience*, vol. 3, p. 17, 2009.
4. P. Fries, "Neuronal gamma-band synchronization as a fundamental process in cortical computation," *Annual review of neuroscience*, vol. 32, pp. 209–224, 2009.
5. S. Ray and J. H. Maunsell, "Differences in gamma frequencies across visual cortex restrict their possible use in computation," *Neuron*, vol. 67, no. 5, pp. 885–896, 2010.
6. V. V. Moca, D. Nikolic, W. Singer, and R. C. Muresan, "Membrane resonance enables stable and robust gamma oscillations," *Çerebral Cortex*, vol. 24, no. 1, pp. 119–142, 2014.
7. N. E. Huang, Z. Shen, S. R. Long, M. C. Wu, H. H. Shih, Q. Zheng, N.-C. Yen, C. C. Tung, and H. H. Liu, "The empirical mode decomposition and the hilbert spectrum for nonlinear and non-stationary time series analysis," in *Proceedings of the Royal Society of London A: Mathematical, Physical and Engineering Sciences*, vol. 454, pp. 903–995, The Royal Society, 1998.
8. C. Börgers and N. Kopell, "Synchronization in networks of excitatory and inhibitory neurons with sparse, random connectivity," *Neural computation*, vol. 15, no. 3, pp. 509–538, 2003.
9. B. V. Atallah and M. Scanziani, "Instantaneous modulation of gamma oscillation frequency by balancing excitation with inhibition," *Neuron*, vol. 62, no. 4, pp. 566–577, 2009.

Comparison of Classifiers for Brain Tumor Segmentation

L. Lefkovits[1,3], Sz. Lefkovits[2], M. F. Vaida[3], S. Emerich[3] and R. Măluţan[3]

[1] Department of Electrical Engineering Sapientia University, Tîrgu-Mureş, Romania
[2] Department of Computer Science "Petru-Maior" University, Tîrgu-Mureş, Romania
[3]Faculty of Electronics, Telecommunication and Information Technology, Technical University of Cluj-Napoca

Abstract— **Nowadays numerous efforts and promising results are obtained in medical imaging processing, although reproducible segmentation and classification of tumors is still a challenging task. The difficulty consists of the different shapes, locations and image intensities of these tissues. In this article we present our discriminative segmentation system for brain tumor delimitation from multimodal MR images. The detection of tumor requires a well-defined process-sequence on every analyzed MRI including preprocessing, feature extraction, classification and post-processing. The discriminative models are trained from annotated image databases and build their decision function around a classifier algorithm. In machine learning there are a lot of advanced classifiers that can be used for segmentation task. The choice of the most adequate classifiers is not straightforward. The SVM, the AdaBoost and the Random Forest (RF) are among the most 10 best classifiers and are often used in image segmentation. The goal of this paper is to analyze and compare these three classification techniques and their obtainable performances or the same segmentation framework. First, we present our framework for brain tumor segmentation. In the theoretical part we briefly present each classifier, emphasizing the advantages and disadvantages of them. In practice, we trained all these three classifiers on the same data set and tested them on 10 image sets, which were not used during training phase. The segmentation performance was evaluated with the Dice coefficients, computing them in each test case separately. Finally, we statistically compared the provided results. At the end, we evaluated the dependence of segmentation accuracy on training set size, providing practical information for possible users of the classifiers created.**

Keywords— **brain tumor segmentation, random forest, AdaBoost, SVM.**

I. Introduction

The spread of MRI equipment creates new possibilities in preventive medicine. The early diagnosis of most diseases can change and improve life quality. In this domain the MRI image processing will play always an important role. The brain tumor segmentation from MRI images is focused only on detection and delimitation of cancerous tissues. The tumor segmentation can be very helpful in clinical diagnosis, drug or radiotherapy treatment planning and in tracking tumor evolution. The automat segmentation system can enhance the diagnostic capabilities of physicians and reduce the time required for accurate diagnosis. Manual segmentation methods are time consuming, can take around 3 hours to complete. Furthermore, there are large variations between expert segmentation even though they use an accurate annotation protocol. In lots of cases an efficient computer based system is required that accurately examines the boundaries of brain tissues with little any human interaction or even without it. Despite numerous efforts and promising results obtained in medical imaging processing, reproducible segmentation and classification of tumors still remains a challenging task. It is considerably influenced by different shapes, locations and image intensities of the analyzed tissues. In this article we present our discriminative segmentation system for brain tumor delimitation from multimodal MR images. The main part of this system is the classification function built obtained by a learning algorithm. There are lots of algorithms used for the same segmentation task; the choice of the most adequate classifiers is not straightforward. The top 10 classifiers were analyzed in [1]. The ranking based on classifiers performances is very difficult, because the evaluation of them is task dependent. These classifiers were selected by numerous researchers in the domain without any ranking criteria. A. N. Mizil in [2] compared the relationship between the predictions made by different learning algorithms and true posterior probabilities, on 8 binary classification problems. The empirical results show that boosted trees, random forests, and SVMs predict the best probabilities, of course after calibration. Following this work R. Caruana et. al. [3] extended the empirical evaluation of supervised learning on high dimensional data. They concluded that boosted trees do very well in modest dimensions, but lose ground to random forests, neural nets, and SVMs as dimensionality increases.

The AdaBoost [4, 5] with boosting variants, the SVM [6, 7] and the RF [8, 9] are classifiers intensively used in image segmentation and also in brain tumor segmentation.

The paper is organized as follows: after a short introduction of the similar systems in the state of the art we briefly present our approach (section II) and the three algorithms compared in this papers: random forest (section III), AdaBoost (section IV) and Support Vector Machines (section V). The theoretical sections are followed by our compara-

S. Vlad and N.M. Roman (eds.), *International Conference on Advancements of Medicine and Health Care through Technology; 12th - 15th October 2016, Cluj-Napoca, Romania,*
IFMBE Proceedings 59,
DOI: 10.1007/978-3-319-52875-5_43

tive experiments and results concerning the MR brain tumor segmentation.

II. THE PROPOSED DISCRIMINATIVE MODEL

The proposed discriminative model is similar to previously used model (fig. 1) in [10].

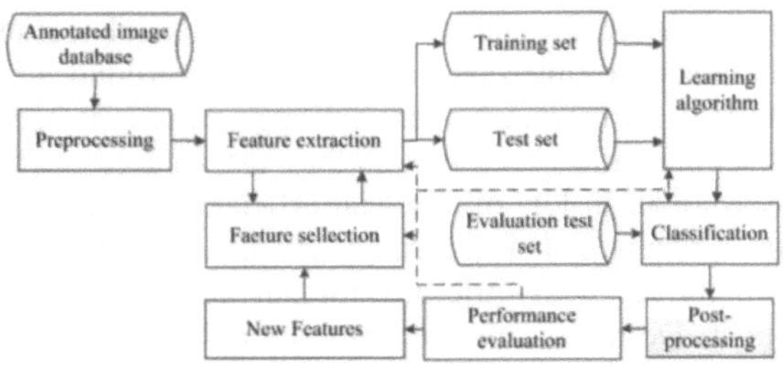

Fig. 1 Components of our system

The performances of our segmentation model, built on a discriminative function, are mainly determined by three important issues: the quality of annotated image-database, the classification algorithm applied and feature set used.

The BRATS 2015 [11] dataset contains 220 high grade (HG) and 54 low grade (LG) brain images with gliomas, assures sufficient diversity, requirement for a performant database. All cases were acquired with similar protocol and contain four types of images: *T1*, *T1c* (with contrast material Gadolinium), *T2* and *FLAIR*. A dataset for one patient contains these four types of 3D images and the annotation image. In our approach we consider three classes for performance evaluation used in BRATS Challenges. These classes are: whole tumor - *WT* (including all four tumor structures), tumor core – *TC* (including all tumor structures except edema) and active tumor - *AT* (only the enhancing core).

In our work we have analyzed three important artifacts: inhomogeneity, noise and intensity nonstandardness. For inhomogeneity reduction in MR images, we have applied the *N4* filter implemented in the ITK package [12]. For noise reduction we used the anisotropic filtering from the same package. Intensity normalization was done by histogram linear transformation in such a way that the first and third quartiles have predefined values.

In our approach we started with defining a large feature set, but this is later reduced. We defined, for each feature, many low-level characteristics that describe the intensities in the neighborhood of the voxels studied. In our application we have used the following features: first order operators (mean, standard deviation, max, min, median, Sobel, gradient); higher order operator (Laplacian, difference of Gaussian, entropy, curvatures, kurtosis, skewness); texture features (Gabor filter); spatial context features.

By extracting all of these features for every voxel in all modalities, we transform the image segmentation task into a statistical pattern recognition problem. The segmentation process obtained with this statistical model also requires the analysis of variable importance. The appropriate selection of the attributes has to be done according to the target objects. First, we extracted 240 image features of each modality and we obtained a feature vector with 960 elements.

Our algorithm [13] was created to manage this big database and to select a set of adequate features for the given segmentation task. We applied our algorithm several times by evaluating the overall *OOB* (out-of-bag) error, in order to determine the optimal number of attributes (*M*) used.

III. RANDOM FOREST ALGORITHM

The random forest is an ensemble classifier built from binary decision trees [14]. The RF classifier is built on two random processes: the random built of bootstrap set and the random feature selection in each node. The creation of RF is based on two sets: the bootstrap set, containing the instances for building a tree and the *OOB* set (out-of-bag set), containing test instances not included in bootstrap set. The maximization of information gain is the splitting criterion applied in every node. Applying this criterion each node splits the incoming in-stances in two sets. In order to evaluate the information gain, the RF uses in each node only a small number of variables (m_{tries}) out of all existing variables (*M*). These m_{tries} variables are chosen randomly and the splitting criterion is maximized only with these variables. The RF algorithm has two main parameters: the number of trees K_{trees} used in forest and the number of randomly chosen variables in each node m_{tries}. In the state of the art there are no indications regarding the choice these parameters. They are dataset dependent. Determining the appropriate values of these variables may be the objective of an optimization framework [10]

IV. ADABOOST ALGORITHM

One of the most used algorithms in images processing in the last decade is the AdaBoost algorithm, proposed by Freund and Shapire [15]. It constructs an ensemble of classifiers and uses a voting mechanism for the final classification. The idea of boosting is to use several weak classifiers to form a highly accurate prediction rule by calling the weak classifier repeatedly on different distributions of the training set. AdaBoost was the first adaptive boosting algorithm, which automatically adjusts its parameters of the algorithm according to the data used in the current iteration. Initially, all the weights are set equally, but each round the weights of incorrectly classified examples are increased so that the images which were incorrectly classified by the previous classifier, will receive greater weight on the next iteration. This forces the learner to concentrate on the hard examples. The weight of the weak learner is computed, in fact, from the classification error of the current weak classifier. The final classifier reduces the statistical dispersion of the decision and at the same time reducing the classification error too.

This algorithm [15] is an iterative method. In each iteration, a weak classifier having the lowest error rate on the training set, is selected. This step is followed by the re-weight of the input instances, putting an accent on hard examples. The restriction of the used weak classifiers is related to their performance which has to be better than the random decision. Thus, weak classifier has to eliminate more than half of the backgrounds. This means that the final classifiers formed of N weak classifiers will have a very small false detection rate.

The most important theoretical propriety of AdaBoost concerns in its ability to reduce the training error. The AdaBoost converts a set of weak classifiers into a strong learning algorithm which can generate an arbitrarily low error rate on the training set. Practically this statement is limited in two ways. First, the number of used classifiers is finite, thus an arbitrary low error rate is not possible to obtain. Second, the computational complexity of training phase increases with each classifier added. By obtaining and equilibrium between the two factors we are able to combine enough weak classifiers in order to create the desired strong classifier [16].

The most important drawback of the algorithm is the overfitting. On the phenomenon of overfitting we understand the fact that the training set is much better approximated. The classification surface lies exactly on the training entities and underperformes for the real data. To avoid overfitting, the task for the algorithm therefore should not be to find the best possible classifier for the underlying training sample, but rather to find the best prediction rule for a set of new observations [17].

V. Support Vector Machines

The Support Vector Machines [18] are supervised learning machines for binary classification problems. They are able to separate the inputs linearly, or if they are not linearly separable they can map them in a higher dimensional feature space, where the linear separation is possible. The learning algorithm finds the best hyperplane, which separates the entities included in the training set. In other words, it finds the hyperplane which maximizes the distance to the nearest entities in each class. The larger the separating margin between the classes the lower is the generalization error of the obtained classifier [19]. The optimization problem consists of maximizing the distance between the closest data points.

Given k inputs in the training data set

$$S = (x_i, y_i) \mid x_i \in \mathbb{R}^n, y_i \in \{+1, -1\}; i = 1, 2, \ldots, k \quad (1)$$

The classification is achieved by a hyperplane of this form:

$$w^T \Phi(x) + b = 0, w \in \mathbb{R}^n, b \in \mathbb{R} \quad (2)$$

where Φ is the transformation of the inputs in a higher-dimensional space, b is the bias, the translation of the hyperplane from origin and the w is the normal vector of the hyperplane [20].

The distance from a point x_i to the hyperplane P is the length of the perpendicular segment from the point x_i. Or it can be computed as the distance of the projection of x_i on the normal vector of the plane and any point on the plane $x \in P$ the distance has the form:

$$dist = \frac{1}{\|w\|}\left|w^T\left(\Phi(x_i) - \Phi(x)\right)\right| = \frac{1}{\|w\|} \quad (3)$$

The optimization problem becomes the maximization of the distance

$$\max\left(\frac{1}{\|w\|}\right) \text{ with the constraint } y_i\left(w^T\Phi(x_i) + b\right) \geq 1 \quad (4)$$

where $\|w\|^2 = w^T w$ The solution is obtained from the *Lagrangian* of the problem with respect to k inequality constraints.

$$\mathrm{L}(w, b, \lambda) = \frac{1}{2}w^T w - \sum_{i=1}^{k} \lambda_i \left[y_i\left(w^T\Phi(x_i) + b\right) - 1\right] \quad (5)$$

The solution will be given by the quadratic programming with Sequential Minimal Optimization SMO [21].

The most important advantages of SVM is its robustness and classification accuracy for the training data set. In case of a sufficiently general training data set it also offers correct classification of the future data instances. It can handle classification in two different classes regardless the dimensionality of the data. If the linear separation is not possible several kernels may be used to transform the original non-separable data into a higher dimensional space where the linear separation is possible. The classification of new instances is very simple; it only verifies the position of them relative to the hyperplane. SVM has also considerable disadvantages. The optimization of the quadratic programming problem is not obvious. It can be solved only with iterative methods. The analytical solution is not possible. The multiclass classification can be done only with pairwise two class decisions. The final classification is a binary decision which can be transformed in a weighted decision if the distance of the analyzed instance to the hyperplane is taken in consideration.

VI. Experiments and results

We have measured the obtained performances of the above presented three classifiers. Each algorithm created its classifier by using the same training set. This training dataset is a random subsample 50:1 of the total information from 20 HG images used in BRATS 2013 Challenge [11]. Thus, the training set size is about 2% of the whole dataset. The test set contains all information of 10 HG images. In order to transpose the image segmentation into a statistical pattern recognition task, we applied a voxelwise classification, in each voxel we evaluated 120 low level image features. These features were obtained from a large set by evaluating their importance for brain tumor segmentation [13]. Our optimized RF classifier is composed of $K_{trees}=100$ trees, each having a size of $T_{size}=2048$ nodes [10]. The splitting criterion is evaluated with $m_{tries}=9$ randomly chosen features from the whole $M = 120$ feature set. The classification performance can be easily converted in Dice coefficient, which is used to compare segmentation performances:

$$Dice = 2 \cdot |S_1 \cap S_2| / (|S_1| + |S_2|) \tag{6}$$

where: | | is the cardinality, S_1 the true region, S_2 the obtained segmentation. The segmentation results obtained on 10 test images are graphically given in fig. 2.

In order to test the AdaBoost classifier we used decision stamps and 12 iterations, the same depth as used for tree size in RF. The SVM used a polynomial kernel with optimized exponent. For these two classifiers we defined two class classification tasks: WT-vs.-all and TC-vs.-all. The segmentation results obtained on the same test set are shown in fig. 3 and fig. 4. Table 1 presents a statistical evaluation of Dice coefficient obtained with each of the three classifiers. Overall, we can conclude, based on these results, that the RF classifier reaches significantly more accurate performances then the other two classifiers.

Table 1. Statistical parameters of the compared algorithms

	RF		SVM		AdaBoost	
	Mean	Std.	Mean	Std.	Mean	Std.
WT	0.905	0.035	0.736	0.050	0.720	0.094
TC	0.887	0.046	0.817	0.072	0.791	0.094

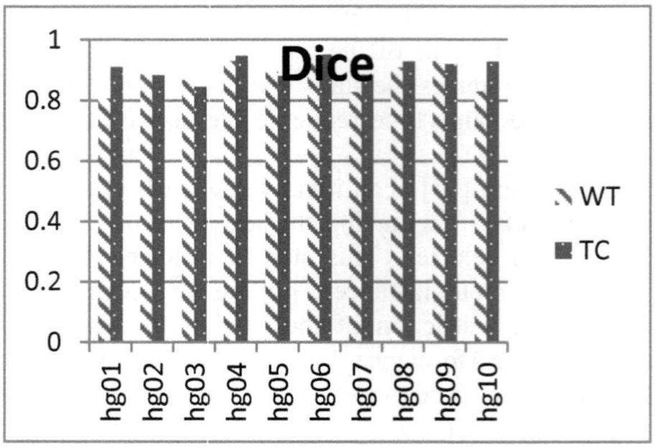

Fig. 2 Dice coefficients of Random Forest

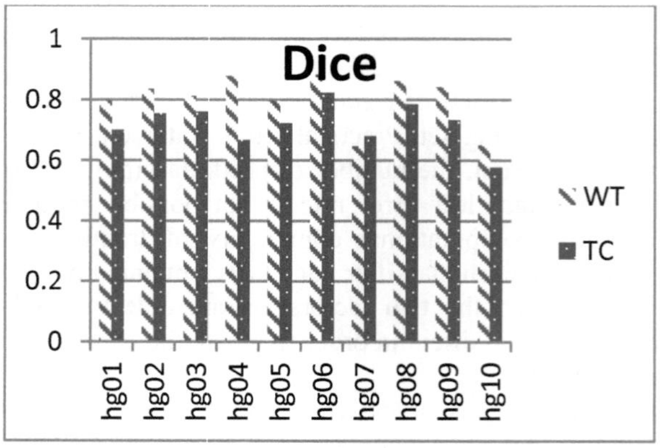

Fig. 3 Dice coefficients of SVM algorithm

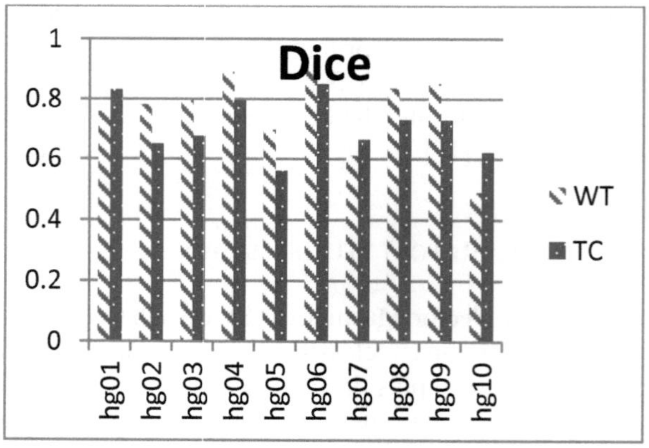

Fig. 4 Dice coefficients of AdaBoost

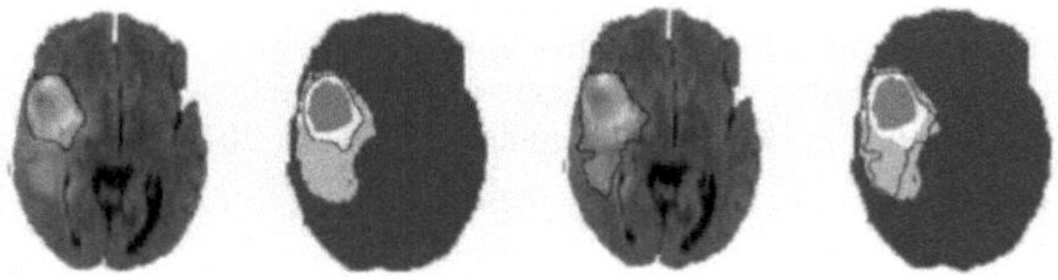

Fig. 5 Segmentation on the test set – usual example

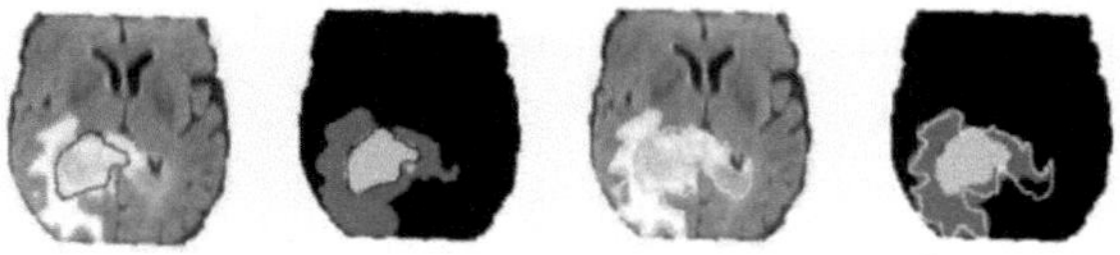

Fig. 6 Segmentation on the test set – hard example

VII. Conclusions

The segmentation performances obtained by our disriminative model built on RF are explainable by the most important characteristics of this classifier:
- efficient run on big data sets;
- easy handling of multi classification task;
- smooth transition between class borders [22].

Following the results obtained, during our research described in this work and also in the previous articles [10, 13] we have built a segmentation system. In fig.5 and fig.6 we graphically presented our segmentation results on a brain slice of the test set. The black line is the contour of the annotation. The light gray region is the detection of the edema (WT); the white region is the result for the tumor core (TC) and dark grey is the necrotic part of tumor. The segmentation obtained by our approach has performances comparable to state-of-the-art systems (table 2) [11].

In the future we intend to adapt and integrate the proposed system for biometric images, more exactly for dorsal hand vein segmentation.

Table 2. Comparison of segmentation results

	Our clas-sif.	**Brats2012** [11]	**Brats 2013** [11]
WT HG	75-86%	63-78%	71-87%
CT HG	71-82%	24-37%	66-78%

Acknowledgment

This work was supported by a grant of the Romanian National Authority for Scientific Research and Innovation, CNCS – UEFISCDI, project number PN-II-RU-TE-2014-4-2080.

Conflict of Interest

The authors declare that they have no conflict of interest.

References

1. Wu X, Kumar V, Quinlan JR, Ghosh J, Yang Q, Motoda H, et al. Top 10 algorithms in data mining. Knowledge and information systems. 2008; 14(1): p. 1-37.
2. Niculescu-Mizil A, Caruana R. Predicting good probabilities with supervised learning. In Proceedings of the 22nd international conference on Machine learning; 2005. p. 625-632.
3. Caruana R, Karampatziakis N, Yessenalina A. An empirical evaluation of supervised learning in high dimensions. In Proceedings of the 25th international conference on Machine learning; 2008. p. 96-103.
4. Nivetha P, Vaijayanthi N. Detection and segmentation of brain tumors based on multifractal features. 2015.
5. Rangini M, Jiji GW. Identification of Alzheimer's Disease Using Adaboost Classifier. In Proceedings of the International Conference on Applied Mathematics and Theoretical Computer Science; 2013. p. 229.
6. Nichat AM, Ladhake SA. Brain Tumor Segmentation and Classification Using Modified FCM and SVM Classifier. Brain. 2016; 5(4).
7. Shahare PD, Giri RN. Comparative Analysis of Artificial Neural Network and Support Vector Machine Classification for Breast Cancer Detection. 2015.
8. Reza S, Iftekharuddin KM. Improved Brain Tumor Tissue Segmentation Using Texture Features. In MICCAI-BRATS Challenge on Multimodal Brain Tumor Segmentation; 2014.
9. Zikic D, Glocker B, Konukoglu E, Shotton J, Criminisi A, Ye D, et al. Context-sensitive classification forests for segmentation of brain tumor tissues. In MICCAI-BRATS Challenge on Multimodal Brain Tumor Segmentation; 2012.
10. Lefkovits L, Lefkovits Sz, Szilágyi L. Brain Tumor Segmentation with Optimized Random Forest. In Medical Image Computing and Computer Assisted Intervention (MICCAI) BrainLes Workshop; 2016, under review.
11. Menze BH, Jakab A, Bauer S, Kalpathy-Cramer J, Farahani K, Kirby J, et al. The Multimodal Brain Tumor Image Segmentation Benchmark (BRATS). IEEE Transactions on Medical Imaging. 2015 Oct; 34(10): p. 1993-2024.
12. The Interactive Learning and Segmentation Toolkit ITK..
13. Lefkovits L, Lefkovits Sz, Emerich S, Vaida MF. Random Forest Feature Selection Approach for Image Segmentation. In Advanced Concepts for Intelligent Vision Systems ACIVS; 2016, under review.
14. Breiman L. Random forests. Machine learning. 2001; 45(1): p. 5-32.
15. Schapire RE. The boosting approach to machine learning: An overview. In Nonlinear estimation and classification.: Springer; 2003. p. 149-171.
16. Lefkovits Sz, Lefkovits L. Distance based k-NN Classification of Gabor Jet Local Descriptors. In 9th International Conference, Interdisciplinarity in Engineering, Tîrgu-Mureş; 2015 8-9 October. p. 780-785.
17. Mayr A, Binder H, Gefeller O, Schmid M, others. The evolution of boosting algorithms. Methods of information in medicine. 2014; 53(6): p. 419-427.
18. Cortes C, Vapnik V. Support-vector networks. Machine learning. 1995; 20(3): p. 273-297.

19. Cristianini N, Shawe-Taylor J. An introduction to support vector machines and other kernel-based learning methods: Cambridge university press; 2000.
20. Lefkovits Sz, Lefkovits L. Enhanced Gabor Filter Based Facial Feature Detector. In The 5th International Conference European Integration - Between Tradition and Modernity IETM, Tîrgu-Mureş; 2013 5-7 October. p. 1204-1214.
21. Platt JC. Sequential Minimal Optimization: A Fast Algorithm for Training Support Vector Machines. Tech. rep. ADVANCES IN KERNEL METHODS - SUPPORT VECTOR LEARNING; 1998.
22. Criminisi A, Shotton J, Konukoglu E. Decision forests: A unified framework for classification, regression, density estimation, manifold learning and semi-supervised learning. Foundations and Trends® in Computer Graphics and Vision. 2012; 7(2--3): p. 81-227.

Author: László Lefkovits
Institute: Sapientia University,Tîrgu-Mureş
Street: Corunca 1c
City: Tîrgu-Mureş
Country: Romania
Email: lefkolaci@ms.sapientia.ro

Abnormalities Identification in Mammograms

L.D. Chiorean, M.F. Vaida and C. Striletchi

Communications Department, Technical University of Cluj-Napoca, Cluj-Napoca, Romania

Abstract— **This paper proposes a method for detection of abnormalities in mammograms that could be integrated into a computer-aided diagnosis system. The method is based on segmentation using a clustering method, elimination of small regions, blobs and contour detection and a density analysis. The method was tested on images from screening mammography databases and the results are compared with the selections realized by specialists. The tests show that the method offers good results on images that present well defined abnormalities and by adjusting some parameters it can even detect distortions difficult to be noticed by physicians.**

Keywords— **segmentation, detection, mammography, abnormality, breast cancer**

I. Introduction

A lot of researchers from many domains concentrate their efforts in helping identification and treatment of different diseases. A very serious malady that affects a huge number of people is cancer. Breast cancer is the most common cancer in women worldwide, and the second cause of death all over the world, after lung cancer [1].

Therefore, early detection of any kind of abnormalities in breasts could save lives. At present, X-mammography is the most used screening technique for early detection of breast cancer. Screening mammography presents low reliability on dense breasts of young women, but high sensitivity on fatty breast and good results in microcalcification detection. A lot of examinations are realized every day, resulting in a large number of mammograms that have to be interpreted by radiologists. In order to offer support to radiologists in their work and to improve efficiency of the examinations, computed-aided diagnosis (CAD) systems have been introduced in screening processes. In the last two decades, there has been great progress in the investigation, development and clinical deployment of such systems in screening mammography.

In order to detect breast cancer, some typical signatures of this disease have to be targeted in mammograms: masses and calcifications. Abnormal regions present characteristics that are slightly different from the rest of the image. Although these areas have colors situated in the proximity of the upper level of the grayscale, similar to the glandular breast tissue, they also present their own properties that have to be targeted in the image: higher density or intensity and often relatively circular shape.

Many image-processing methods have been proposed for breast tumor detection. The techniques in the field of computer aided mammography include image preprocessing, image segmentation techniques, feature extraction, feature selection, classification techniques and features for mammograms [2]. Various technologies such as fractal analysis [3], discrete wavelet transform, and Markov random field have been used. In [4] a multiple circular path convolution neural network architecture was proposed that has been designed for the analysis of tumor and tumor-like structures. A two-stage adaptive density weighted contrast enhancement algorithm was also proposed for tumor detection in mammograms [5]. Another paper [6] presents a method of detection and analysis of breast tumor based on texture segmentation. Other methods were also used for tumor detection, such as: Hough transform, marker-controlled watershed segmentation, non-extensive entropy, as is shown in [7]. Another method that offers good results in breast tumor detection is reported in [8] and is based on template matching with mutual information.

In this paper, we propose a method for detection of abnormalities in mammograms, using some preprocessing techniques, segmentation, contour and blob detection and densitometry analysis.

II. The proposed method

CAD systems for breast cancer identification have to realize a separation of the suspicious areas from the rest of the tissues. In other words, they have to be able to distinguish regions that present alteration on density, shape and margins. The cancer cells produce architectural distortions that could be identified in images as masses, asymmetry or calcifications. To highlight these areas, different segmentation techniques have been proposed.

For an accurate segmentation is important to eliminate artefacts that may be present in image, so some preprocessing steps usually precede this process. Digital mammograms may be affected by noise and some of them presents low contrast. Therefore, the first steps of our method are focused on image enhancement, filtering out the noise and increasing the contrast. Figure 1 shows these preprocessing steps.

S. Vlad and N.M. Roman (eds.), *International Conference on Advancements of Medicine and Health Care through Technology; 12th - 15th October 2016, Cluj-Napoca, Romania,*
IFMBE Proceedings 59,
DOI: 10.1007/978-3-319-52875-5_44

For noise removal, we choose to use adaptive median filter. In [9] there is a study that shows that the effects of this filter are better in image mammograms enhancement in comparison with standard median filter, wiener filter and median filter. This filter presents advantages over the standard median filter in terms of reducing the effects of the impulse noise and preserving details, as well as smoothing non-impulse noise. The algorithm is presented in [10].

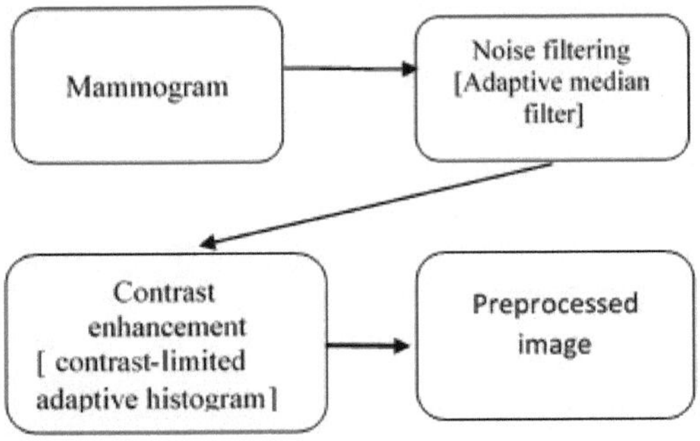

Fig. 1 Preprocessing steps of the mammogram

The enhancement of the image is realized by using contrast-limited adaptive histogram equalization. This method operates on small data regions of the image (tiles). Each tile's contrast is enhanced so that the histogram of each output region approximately matches the specified histogram (uniform distribution, in our case). The resulting neighboring tiles are then stitched back seamlessly using bilinear interpolation, thus removing the artifacts in tile borders. The contrast enhancement can be limited in order to avoid amplifying the noise that might be present in the image.

The next stages of our method are presented in Figure 2. In order to segment a grey scale image on different classes we use K-means clustering. K-means is one of the simplest unsupervised learning algorithms that solve the clustering problem. It is an iterative technique used to partition an image [11], by classifying the given data set through a certain number of clusters fixed beforehand. The main idea is to define k centers, one for each cluster.

The purpose of this clustering is to retain from the image those pixels that have high intensities, therefore we choose to split the image into three clusters. Considering the preprocessed image, we initiate the centroids based on the histogram. A classified image is obtained by applying this kind of clustering. One of the clusters contains only that pixels that have values in the proximity of the maximum value of the greyscale. This is the image that we use in the next steps, because the regions of interest in mammograms are represented by these intensities.

In the next step, a binary image is obtained using thresholding and by complementing the image. This way, pixels that have values greater than the threshold will have 0 value and the pixels that have values under the threshold will be assigned the value 255. Through this, we create a first mask for the image.

The removal of the small parts that could affect the following steps can be realized by applying some morphological operations on the binary image. The erosion deletes small spots and the opening smoothies the remaining ones. A mask is therefore created that contains only those parts of the image that are representative for the following processing.

As cancerous cells tend to form masses or calcifications, a method of identification could be the detection of the blobs in the image. A blob is a region of an image which has some approximately constant properties, all points being similar to each other. We used blob detector method using facilities offered by OpenCV (Open Source Computer Vision) library [12]. This method allows us to detect blobs based on finding contours in the image and to determine their centers. There are some characteristics that can be established for the blobs by setting some parameters related to size and shape. Size specifies the minimum and maximum values for the surface area of the blob and the shape is characterized by the minimum and maximum values for circularity, convexity and inertia ratio.

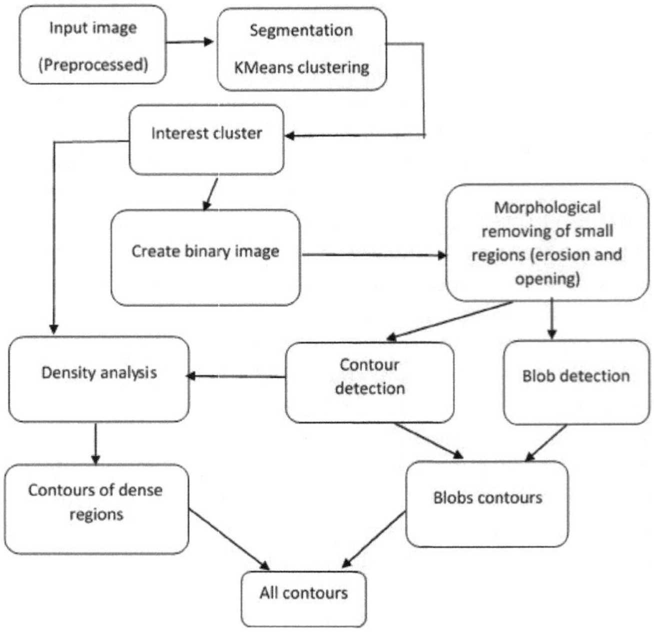

Fig. 2 Structure of the proposed method

Contours of the detected blobs delimitate regions with approximately the same characteristics, so they could be considered as bounds of certain abnormalities in the mammogram.

In some mammograms there appear spots that represent abnormalities, but which are not well defined, their shape is irregular and their margins are not outlined. Therefore, we also propose an analysis of the density of the regions that remain after applying the mask.

In the present stage of our implementation, the density analysis consists in computing the following method: for every detected contour in the image, the mean value of the pixels' values is calculated. If the difference between this value and the value of the pixel situated in the center of the area are close enough, the region is labeled, otherwise this region is not considered to be a region of interest. For future work we will take into consideration methods based on texture parameters proposed by Haralick, and which are used in other studies, as [6] and [13].

III. Tests and Results

This section presents the results of our method in the detection of abnormalities in mammograms. Our selection is displayed in green to separate our results from the selections made by the radiologists (with red).

During our tests, we used images from two databases: DDSM (Digital Database of Screening Mammography) and MIAS (Mammographic Image Analysis Society).

In DDSM [14], information is organized in volumes and cases and every case presents some images. These images are already analyzed, classified and hand-labeled and could be used as references for automatic detection.

The MIAS database [15] contains left and right breast images of 161 patients. It consists of 322 images, which showcase three types of tissues: normal, benign and malignant. It also includes radiologists' truth' marking on the locations of any abnormalities that may be present. The database consists of four different kinds of abnormalities, namely: architectural distortions, suspicious lesions, circumscribed masses and calcifications.

Figure 3 shows images obtained in different steps of the proposed algorithm. The second image is the one obtained by enhancement operations, the third one is achieved after clustering. The fourth image represents the mask and the blob is outlined with a little red circle. The last one is the mammogram, containing the contour achieved with our method and the specialists' selections. For this image our method identified exactly the same region that was outlined by the specialist.

The results obtained using our method can be different, depending on the values of the blob detection parameters. In Figure 4, we present the result obtained using a value of 100 for a minimum surface area of the blob and that obtained for a value of 200. In the first case, we obtain blobs that are not labeled by the radiologist, in the second case these blobs do not appear.

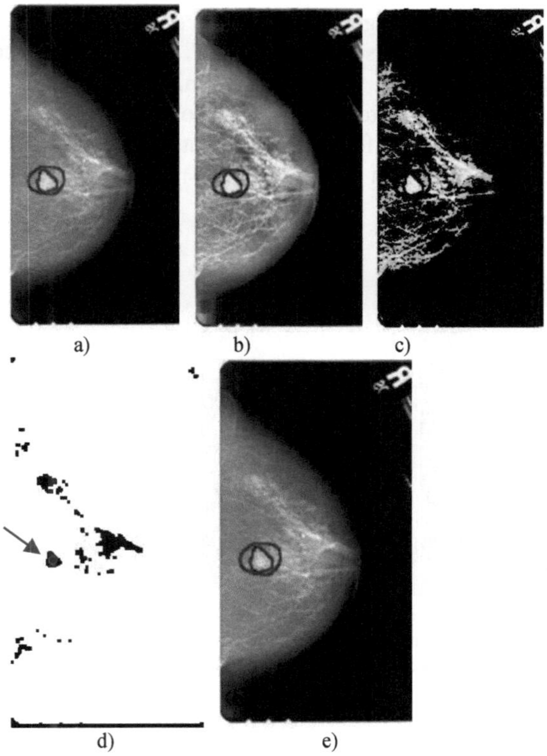

Fig. 3 Our detection phases: a) original image, b) enhanced image, c) selected cluster, d) binary image (mask), e) detection result (green – our result, red – hand-labeled). Volume 10 Case 1574 - Right CC

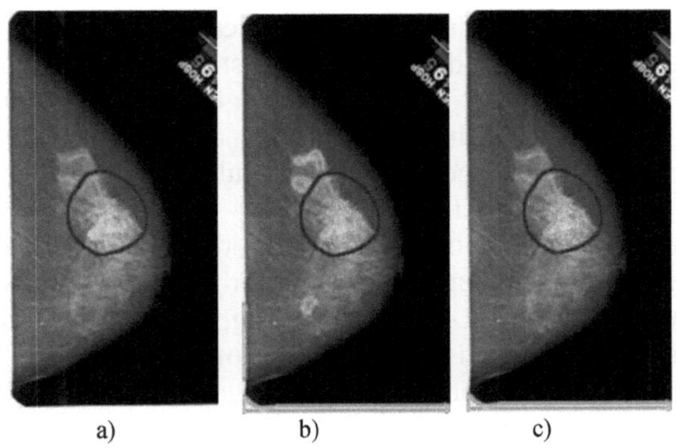

Fig. 4 Results obtained depending on the minimum value of the abnormality surface area. a) original image, b) min area=100, c) min area=200. Volume11- Case 1236 - Right CC

Both images (Figure 3 and Figure 4) present tumors that are reported by specialists to have shapes with architectural distortions.

In Figure 5 there is an image from the MIAS database, which has lower contrast, but presents a tumor with circular shape, well contoured. An analysis based only on intensities could identify other areas as being abnormal, as in Figure

5b), but if the shape is taken into account, these regions will be not outlined (as in Figure 5c)).

In the MIAS database the specialist' selections are not outlined on the image, but for each image, the center of abnormalities coordinates and an approximate radius are presented. Using this information, we outlined the specified area with red. The green color marks our results.

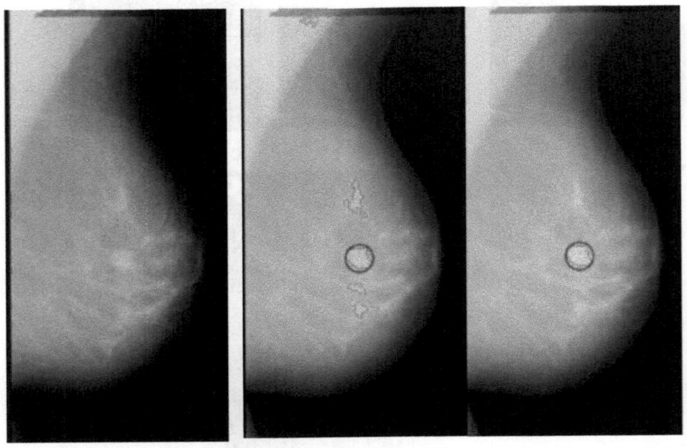

Fig. 5 Selection obtain with our method on image mdb010 from MIAS; a) original image, b) results without shape specifications for the blobs, c) results that take into account the circularity of the blobs

IV. Conclusion and future work

It is well known that cancer is an implacable disease that affects people all over the world. Early diagnosis is very important and is realized mostly by radiologists based on images acquired with different medical modalities. For prevention and early detection of breast cancer, specialists have to examine a lot of mammograms daily. In this situation, CAD systems that could realize a fast detection of abnormalities in images are very useful and can facilitate diagnosis to a great extent.

This paper presents a method for identification of abnormalities in mammogram images. Our method is based on segmentation using K-means clustering, contour detection, blob identification and density analysis of certain regions.

The comparison with annotated images from specialized databases shows that our method offers good results. There are some parameters that are established in the application and which affect the results, like the threshold value used to eliminate some parts of the image, the dimension of the little spots that are removed from the image, circularity and minimum area of the spots. These values could be adapted according to the physician' indications, in order to obtain accurate results.

Future work will integrate texture analysis based on Haralick parameters in order to use more information about the image's structure. Different studies can be made by calculating the correlation between identified areas and the labeled ones.

Conflict of Interest

The authors declare that they have no conflict of interest.

References

1. Breast Cancer Statistics (2016), http://www.breastcancer.org,
2. Yadollahpour A, Shoghi H, (2015), Early Breast Cancer Detection using Mammogram Images: A Review of Image Processing Techniques, Biosciences Biotechnology Research Asia, Vol. 12, pp. 225-234
3. Zheng L, A.K. Chan (2001), IEEE Trans. Med. Imaging 20, 559
4. Li H., Shih-Chung B L, Wang Z, Kinnand L, Freedman M T, (2002), IEEE Trans. Med. Imaging 21, 139
5. Chan H P, Petrick N, Sahiner B, (2000) Computer-aided breast cancer diagnosis, in Artificial Intelligence Techniques in Breast Cancer Diagnosis and Prognosis, Series in Machine Perception and Artificial Intelligence, vol. 39 (World Scientific Publishing Co. Pte. Ltd., Singapore, pp. 179–264
6. Guzmán-Cabrera R, Guzmán-Sepúlveda J R, Torres-Cisneros M, May-Arrioja D. A., et al., (2013),, Digital Image Processing Technique for Breast Cancer Detection, Int J Thermophys 34:1519–1531
7. Mussarat Y, Muhammad S, Sajjad M, (2013), Survey Paper on Diagnosis of Breast Cancer Using Image Processing Techniques, Research Journal of Recent Sciences, Vol. 2(10), 88-98
8. Mazurowski M A, Lo J Y, Harrawood B P, Tourassi G D, (2011) Mutual information-based template matching scheme for detection of breast masses: from mammography to digital breast tomosynthesis, J Biomed Inform, 44(5): 815–823
9. Ramani R., Suthanthira Vanitha N., Valarmathy S., (2013), The Pre-Processing Techniques for Breast Cancer Detection in Mammography Images, I.J. Image, Graphics and Signal Processing 5, pp. 47-54
10. Shrestha S, (2014), Image Denoising Using New Adaptive Based Median Filter, Signal & Image Processing (SIPIJ), Vol.5, No.4, 2014
11. Kanungo T, Mount D M, Netanyahu N S, et al. (2000), An Efficient k-Means Clustering Algorithm: Analysis and Implementation, Proceedings of the Sixteenth ACM Symposium on Computational Geometry, June 2000, pp. 100-109
12. OpenCV Common Interfaces of Feature Detectors (2016), http://docs.opencv.org/2.4/modules/features2d/doc/common_interfaces_of_feature_detectors.html
13. Wibmer A., Hricak H, Gondo T, Matsumoto K, et al., (2015), Haralick texture analysis of prostate MRI: utility for differentiating non-cancerous prostate from prostate cancer and differentiating prostate cancers with different Gleason scores, Eur Radiol. 2015 Oct; 25(10):2840-50.
14. DDSM (2016),http://marathon.csee.usf.edu/Mammography/Database.html
15. MIAS (2016), http://peipa.essex.ac.uk/info/mias.html

Part IV
Telemedicine and Health Care Information Systems

Interconnecting Heterogeneous Non-smart Medical Devices using a Wireless Sensor Networks (WSN) Infrastructure

B. Iancu, R. Kovacs, V. Dadarlat and A. Peculea

Computer Science Department, Technical University of Cluj-Napoca, Cluj-Napoca, Romania

Abstract— **Smart hospitals enhanced through the Internet and related technologies with live monitoring and interconnected devices, using wired and wireless sensors, provide better health services for patients. However, legacy (non-smart) medical devices that are not able to communicate and to be managed by a smart hospital infrastructure are still in use. Patients' data can be collected from a wide range of non-smart medical device. The paper introduces a novel concept, called WSNaaP (WSN as a platform) and a technical solution for interconnecting heterogeneous non-smart medical devices using an existing WSN infrastructure.**

Keywords— **WSN, WSNaaP, e-health, sensors, medical devices.**

I. Introduction

Wireless Sensor Networks (WSN) consist of multiple communicating smart sensor nodes, which are low power devices equipped with one or more sensors, a processor, memory, a power supply, a radio, and an actuator [1].

WSNs are considered to be one of the most promising research and development field in engineering and computer science. The countless number of applications range from logistic, environment or healthcare applications to military applications. A 2015 forecast by Gartner, Inc. [2] shows a massive adoption of wireless sensors in all IoT (Internet of Things) connected applications. By 2020 a number of 20.8 billion devices are predicted to be connected in the IoT.

An important sector, where WSNs can have an influence on people's everyday life is e-health. Ranging from intensive care monitoring to surveillance of chronically ill patients or elderly, wireless sensor networks can improve the quality of life.

Eysenbach [3] provides a comprehensive definition for the e-health term, stating that e-health lays at the intersection of medical informatics, public health and business, and refers to health services and information delivered or enhanced through the Internet and related technologies.

Smart hospitals are designed to fully use the facilities provided by wired and wireless sensor networks, to monitor their patients and staff with the aim of offering enhanced services. Legacy medical devices, also referred in this paper as non-smart devices, are missing network communication capabilities and the ability of being integrated into the smart hospital architecture. Replacing this type of devices, considering that the large majority of them are still in use and in their normal operating and lifetime limits, carries significant costs for a hospital's budget.

The paper proposes to provide a technical solution for interconnecting non-smart medical devices and collecting heterogeneous patients' data using a WSN infrastructure.

The original contributions of the paper consists of:

- the introduction of a novel concept called "WSN as a platform" (WSNaaP);
- the development of a technical solution for interconnecting heterogeneous non-smart medical devices using an Libelium WSN infrastructure.

The paper is organized as follows: Section II provides background information related to wireless sensor networks and research topics in the area of e-health. Section III presents the architecture of the proposed WSN platform for interconnecting e-health systems, with its main modules and communication protocol. The experimental results are described in section VI. Section V presents the limitations of the current study, future developments and concludes the paper.

II. Background

WSNs are designed to gather information about the state of physical world and transmit sensed data to a processing unit.

Generally, a WSN consists of a number of wireless sensors (nodes) which can communicate with other sensors or with a base station (gateway or sink) using a radio connection. The data are collected and compressed at the wireless sensor layer and then relayed to another sensor or sent directly to the gateway [4]. The data is further transmitted from the base station to the core system (local database, cloud, processing system) for storage and data analytics. There are many communication protocols used, most of the nodes using IEEE 802.11 series, IEEE 802.15.1 (Bluetooth) or IEEE 802.15.4 (ZigBee).

Wireless sensors networks can incorporate multiple types of sensors, thus there is a wide range of application areas where WSNs are being used.

S. Vlad and N.M. Roman (eds.), *International Conference on Advancements of Medicine and Health Care through Technology; 12th - 15th October 2016, Cluj-Napoca, Romania,*
IFMBE Proceedings 59,
DOI: 10.1007/978-3-319-52875-5_45

In the environmental area, sensors can monitor precipitations, weather conditions and water levels to provide useful information in flooding detection as seen in USA's ALERT system [5]. Another example is found in [6], where wireless sensors are used to monitor weather conditions, microclimate conditions, air temperature, humidity, leaf wetness and rainfall to predict the spread of grapevine pests and diseases.

WSNs can be part of military command, control, communications, computers, intelligence, surveillance, reconnaissance and targeting systems (C4ISRT) as seen in [7]. The rapid deployment, self-organization and fault tolerance characteristics are some of the reasons why wireless sensor networks are so appreciated, not only for military applications.

Several research projects have studied the use of WSNs in e- health for monitoring of patients using wearable and/or implantable sensors [8] [9] [10]. Several recent research projects [11] [12] are sustaining the development of smart home monitoring of elderly solutions using wireless sensor networks. Body wearable sensor networks solution are being developed to gather patient data and to monitor their daily activities for medical purposes [13].

In the current research the authors propose to make use of the available and unexploited WSN infrastructure processing capabilities, in order to transport data from non-smart medical devices to a central processing and storage system. Classically, a WSN captures and manages data only from the connected sensors at certain time intervals. In the remaining time, the WSN is in idle state, when no processing occurs at sensors' level.

For the proposed goal, a novel concept called *"WSN as a platform" (WSNaaP)* is introduced. WSNaaP is defined as the usage of a WSN infrastructure with the aim of gathering, encapsulating and transporting data generated from different devices other than the sensors that form the WSN. Customers can also develop and manage applications on top of an available WSN infrastructure.

Several constrains can arise when defining and designing a WSNaaP.

Firstly, the energy consumption of the sensors must be addressed. Wireless sensor networks are typically constrained by the lifetime of their batteries. In [14] the authors emphasize that the critical issue in developing WSN applications is the limited amount of energy available at sensors level and present an approach for evaluating the power consumption of wireless sensor networks. In a smart hospital, the majority of sensors are fixed and connected to a continuous power source, rather than batteries. Also, several methods for improving the lifetime of wireless sensor networks exist [15] [16]. Thus, the energy constrains can be overcome for medical applications developed in smart hospitals.

Secondly, a priority scheme must be implemented that will ensure that highest priority traffic and functions - generated by the WSN acquisition sensors, will not be affected by less priority traffic and functions - generated by other devices and systems that will use the WSN as a platform.

Using the proposed WSNaaP concept can bring several economic advantages to customers:

- Lower deployment time and reduced costs - by using an existing infrastructure, instead of developing a new one;
- Development of several innovative services on top of existing WSN infrastructures;
- Easier integration into the Smart City concept.

III. WSN PLATFORM FOR INTERCONNECTING E-HEALTH SYSTEMS

In e-health systems, wireless sensor networks can be used for several purposes: monitoring and tracking patients' health conditions; tracing which medical personnel interacts with certain patients; providing the location of a particular physician, patient or medical device.

Every patient can have attached a sensor or multiple sensors which can track and get data from the medical device that monitors specific health conditions. The sensors process and encapsulate the received data and afterwards send the data to a gateway. The role of the gateway is to process, parse and store the received data into the local database. From this stage it can send all the needed information to an external database or to a cloud storage service.

Considering the classification from [1], used to group the tasks required to enable wireless sensor applications, the proposed WSN platform resolves challenges associated with the system group - responsible for supporting different application software on a sensor system.

The WSN platform proposes the interconnection of non-smart devices using the existing sensor architecture of smart hospital. Non-smart (legacy) medical devices can communicate with other devices using a range of physical interfaces, from RS232 to the modern USB, and usually adhere to CEN ISO/IEEE 11073 Health informatics - Medical / health device communication standards. For interfacing a non-smart medical devices with different types of sensors, intermediary devices can be added to enable communication between different communication standards. Low cost devices (e.g. Arduino, RaspberryPi) and adapters (e.g. USB to RS232 Serial Adapter) facilitate events and data collecting.

A. *WSN platform architecture and components*

For achieving the proposed goals, the WSN platform architecture is composed of six main module:

(i) the *medical device interface module* has the role to interface WSN sensors with the appropriate medical application/device. Sensors will be notified if an event has been triggered in the monitoring process of physiological parameters,

(ii) medical and control data is sent to the physical components using the *network interface communication module,*

(iii) *events and resource management module* detects events from the medical device, log the events and starts the associated tasks.

(iv) *tasks planning service module* is responsible for planning and launching tasks, based on events detected by the events and resource management module.

(v) time service module offers service to all the other module – synchronization, timestamps on the recorded events and data, etc.

(vi) the *storage module* is used to manage the different storage resources (SD card, EEPROM, RAM etc.).

Figure 1 depicts the high-level architecture used for the proposed WSN platform.

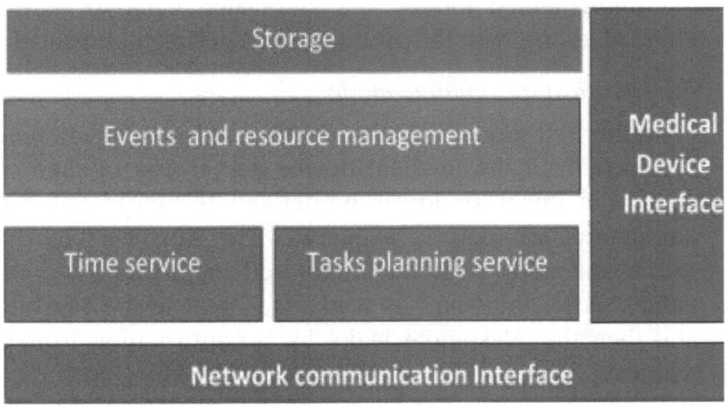

Fig. 1 Proposed WSN platform architecture

For the implementation of the proposed WSN platform, Libelium Waspmote [17] sensors and a Libelium Meshlium [18] gateway were used.

Waspmote wireless sensors, together with intermediary devices if necessary, are responsible with the collection of data from medical devices that monitor patients' health status. Collected data is pre-processed and prepared using Waspmote encapsulation methods. For the forwarding process (sending data to the gateway), Waspmotes are designed to operate in three main modes, modes that are mapped to real-life situations:

- sending data based on patient's health status - data about a patient's health is sent when a worsening of the health status is detected (threshold based),
- regularly sending data – data about a patient's health is sent at predefined time intervals,
- triggered-based sending of data – data about a patient's health is sent when decided by a authorized user (health professional).

After receiving, pre-processing, encapsulating and sending the data, sensors enter in hibernate or sleep mode to conserve energy and to avoid creating interference with other sensors. After the short sleep or hibernate period the cycle is resumed again.

Meshlium router is the gateway for the WSN platform deployment scheme. It has the role of collecting, processing parsing and storing data sent by Waspmotes into the local database. Waspmote encapsulates data in a format that can be sent to and understood by the Meshlium. Received data is saved into a log journal together with the corresponding sensor id, thus every entry can be easily traced. Stored data can be further sent to an external database or to a cloud storing service.

B. *Data sending modes*

Waspmotes receive and pre-process the data from the medical devices and if one of the parameters being monitored by the medical device is over or under a specified threshold, sensors forward the data to the Meshlium. At this point an application can detect the emergency and inform the appropriate medical personnel. In a similar manner, the wireless sensor can detect if a patient is having a convulsion/seizure, using the built-in accelerometer, sends the data and the responsible health professionals are informed.

A second implemented mode is when the wireless sensor, monitoring data received from the medical device, sends them to the gateway at regular intervals according to a predefined time.

The last implemented mode is where Waspmote receives data from the medical devices and stores it locally, to an SD card, therefore every entry is in a ready-to-be-sent form. Whenever a health professional requires the medical data, the Waspmote can be triggered to forward them to Meshlium. In this mode, the health professional decides when to send the data. The described components and sending modes are exemplified in Figure 2.

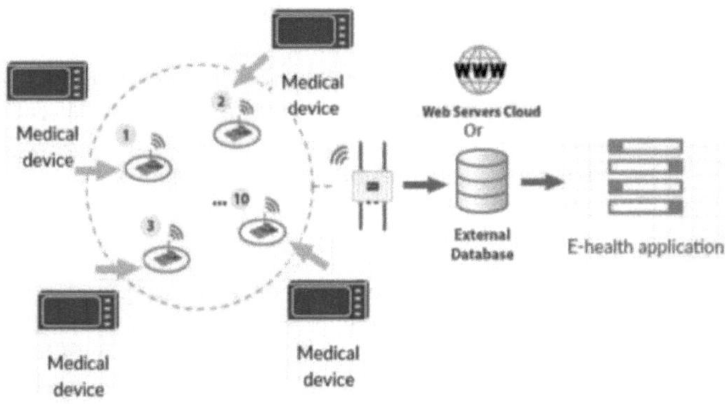

Fig. 2 Data sending modes

C. Collected data format

Received data from medical devices is pre-processed and encapsulated by Waspmotes. After the encapsulation takes place, the data are structured in a frame having the structure depicted in Figure 3.

HEADER						
<=>	Frame Type	Num of bytes	Serial ID	Waspmote ID	#	Sequence

PAYLOAD						
Sensor_1	#	Sensor_2	#	...	Sensor_n	#

Fig. 3 Frame format [19]

The frame facilitates the understanding of the recorded data and also helps Meshlium parse them in an automatic way. The frame structure has two distinct parts. The first part always has the same structure and corresponds to the header. The second part corresponds to the payload and is where data values are included.

The first structure field (<=>) is called *start delimiter* and is necessary to identify the start of each frame. The *Frame Type* field is used to determine the type of the frame (ASCI or binary) and the aim of the frame (event frame, alarm frame, etc.). The *Number of Bytes* field is used to determine the frame length, including the payload. The *Serial Id* field is used to uniquely identify the sensors sending the data. The sensor's identifier is integrated in a specific chip, thus it is different for each device. *Waspmote ID* is a user-defined identifier designed to facilitate sensor's identification in the corresponding network. The *"#"* structure field is used as a separator between the frame fields. The *sequence* field represents the frame sequence number and it is used for ordering the frames and for detecting frame loses [19]. The frame payload is composed by several sensor data. All data sent in this fields correspond to a predefined sensor data type and here is where the parameters received from the medical device and their corresponding values will be placed.

D. Database connection

Meshlium is responsible for processing and parsing data received from the wireless sensors. After this step, Meshlium connects to the local database where a sensor table is available containing the predefined sensor data types. The gateway interacts with the database to inserts the received parameters' values into the corresponding fields, storing the parsed data into the database and making it available to interested applications.

IV. EXPERIMENTAL RESULTS

For the experimental part, the platform was composed of three Libelium Waspmote sensors, a Libelium Meshlium gateway and a MySQL server were used.

Three type of medical data were emulated and stored (both in the RAM memory and also on the sensors' SD cards) at sensors' level: a) heart rate measured as beats per minute (bpm); b) blood pressure measured as systolic and diastolic values (sys, dia) and c) generic data (for further developments). Values were taken from MIMIC II (Multiparameter Intelligent Monitoring in Intensive Care) Clinical Database [20].

According to the implemented data sending modes, Waspmotes behaviors are slightly different. In this chapter the implemented modes and associated behavior will be covered, along with the preliminary experimental results.

E. Health status change mode

In the first mode, the Waspmote monitors the parameters received from the medical device and if one of them exceeds the upper or lower predefined threshold value the communication part is triggered. The sensor creates the frame and adds to it the monitored parameters and their values. After the frame is ready, it is sent to the Meshlium and then the Waspmote waits for a confirmation from the gateway.

Convulsion triggered mode

As a subcategory of health status change mode, a convulsion detection mode was implemented. The wireless sensor waits in an idle mode conserving energy. When the patient's convulsions start (detected by the embedded accelerometers), the sensor wakes up, connects to the gateway, creates the frame with the needed parameters, sends it to the gateway waiting for a confirmation. Afterwards, the sensor clears the interruption flag/pin and restarts the above process. After the patient is taken care of and the situation is under control, the sensor returns to idle mode.

F. Time triggered mode

In the second mode, the sensor receives data from the medical device, creates the frame, encapsulates the parameters and their values, sends the frame to the gateway and waits for an acknowledge frame. Afterward, the Waspmote enters in hibernate mode, conserving energy and keeping the communication medium available for other sensors to send their frames. After a predefined time has passed, the Waspmote wakes up and the entire process is resumed.

G. User triggered mode

In the last mode, the sensor receives and monitors the parameters sent by the medical device, creates the frame and encapsulates them and their values. After the frame is ready to be sent, it is stored on the sensor's SD card. In this way the data is easy to be retrieved and sent when needed. The data retrieval is carried out in a regular manner, and if no data is to be read the Waspmote enters in sleep mode. When new data has to be received, the sensor wakes up and the process starts again. When the responsible health professional considers that the data should be transmitted to the gateway (and the corresponding application), he sends a message to the Waspmote, which retrieves the data frames from the SD card and sends them to the Meshlium.

The created frames and the attached parameters are similar no matter what data sending mode the Waspmote is using and can be observed in Figure 4.

```
<=>?#400582930#WaspNurse1#0#STR:WaspNurse1 here!#BAT:30#
<=>?#400582930#WaspNurse1#1#STR:Bpm:#STR:99.699#
<=>?#400582930#WaspNurse1#2#TIME:Sun, 00/01/01, 01:44:15#
<=>?#400582930#WaspNurse1#3#STR:Id_location:#STR:C7#
<=>?#400582930#WaspNurse1#4#STR:Id_patient:#STR:21011999#
<=>?#400582930#WaspNurse1#5#STR:Id_health_professional:#STR:B
```

Fig. 4 Data frame sent to Meshlium gateway

V. Conclusions

Non-smart medical devices that are not able to communicate and to be managed by a smart hospital infrastructure are still in use. Patients' data can be collected from a wide range of non-smart medical device.

Opposed to the classic use of a WSN infrastructure, where data are captured and managed only from the connected sensors at certain time intervals, the current research proposes to take advantage of the available and unexploited WSN infrastructure processing capabilities (WSN in idle state - when no processing occurs at sensors' level), in order to transport data from non-smart medical devices to a central processing and storage system. Thus, a novel concept called *WSN as a Platform (WSNaaP)* is introduced.

Furthermore, to demonstrate the WSNaaP approach, a technical solution for interconnecting heterogeneous non-smart medical devices (medical devices that are not able to communicate and to be managed by a smart hospital infrastructure) using a WSN infrastructure is described.

Several benefits arise from the proposed solution. Firstly, non-smart medical devices are still in use in many hospitals. The cost of replacing them with smart ones is usually too high, thus providing a way to integrate them into a smart hospital would be a great benefit. By using devices that medical personnel are accustomed with, the operational expenditure cost is also lowered. Secondly, the WSN platform proposes the interconnection of non-smart devices using existing sensor infrastructure of smart hospital, therefore lowering capital expenditures. Only low cost devices (e.g. Arduino, RaspberryPi) and adapters (e.g. USB to RS232 Serial Adapter) are required to be added to the medical devices to facilitate events and data collecting.

The proposed solution has several limitations. It is dependent on the available hospital infrastructure. Not all legacy devices can be redesigned to connect with a smart hospital, due to a lack of any communication interfaces. Several medical devices are not aligned with open communication and interfacing standards, making data acquiring a difficult task. Also, proprietary protocols used for data encapsulation cannot be interpreted by a third party application. All these limitations could be overcome if medical device manufacturers joined open standards and protocols initiatives.

Acknowledgment

This research was supported by the "E-Health WSN Middleware: Middleware for adapting heterogeneous medical equipment and patients' equipment using an existing WSN infrastructure" research project at the Technical University of Cluj-Napoca, under the ClujIT BrainedCity initiative.

Conflict of Interest

The authors declare that they have no conflict of interest.

References

1. Yick J, Mukherjee B, Ghosal D (2008), "Wireless sensor network survey", Computer Networks Journal 52, pp. 2292–2330
2. Gartner Symposium / ITxpo (2015) at http://www.gartner.com/newsroom/id/3165317, last retrieved on May 10, 2016
3. Eysenbach G (2001) What is e-health?, J Med Internet Res. 3(2)
4. Townsend C, Arms S (2015) Wireless Sensor Networks: Principles and Applications, Sensor Technology Handbook, pp 575-589
5. NOAA's National Weather Service (2012) Flood Warning Systems Manual, U.S Department of Commerce, National Oceanic and Atmospheric Administration, National Weather Service

6. Prevostini M, Taddeo A V, Balac K et al (2013) WAMS – an adaptive system for knowledge acquisition and decision support: the case of Scaphoideus titanus, Integrated Protection and Production in Viticulture, IOBC-WPRS Bulletin 58, pp 57-64
7. Salamacha C, Smoot S, Farris K (2000) C4ISRT in an Operational Context, Johns Hopkins APL Tehnical Digest 21:3
8. Jovanov E, Milenkovic A et al. (2005) A WBAN System for Ambulatory Monitoring of Physical Activity and Health Status: Applications and Challenges", Engineering in Medicine and Biology 27th Annual Conference, Shanghai, China
9. Malan D, Fullford-Jones T, Welsh M, Moulton S (2004) CodeBlue: An Ad-hoc Sensor Network Infrastructure for Emergency Medical Care, International Workshop on Wearable and Implantable Body Sensor Networks, Imperial College London, United Kingdom
10. Warren S, Lebak J et al. (2005) Interoperability and Security in Wireless Body Area Network Infrastructure, Engineering in Medicine and Biology 27th Annual Conference, Shanghai, China
11. HELASCoL AAL project at http://helascol.eu/
12. DIET4Elders AAL project at http://www.diet4elders.eu/
13. INTERACTION FP7-ICT project at www.interaction4stroke.eu
14. Damaso A, Freitas D et al. (2013) Evaluating the Power Consumption of Wireless Sensor Network Applications Using Models, Sensors 13, pp. 3473-3500
15. Pantazis N, Nikolidakis S, Vergados D (2013) Energy-Efficient Routing Protocols in Wireless Sensor Networks: A Survey, IEEE Communications Surveys & Tutorials 15 (2), pp. 551- 591
16. Nagarathna P., Manjula R. (2015) Genetic Algorithm with a New Fitness Function to Enhance WSN lifetime in International Conference on Applied and Theoretical Computing and Communication Technology (iCATccT), pp. 95-100
17. Libelium Waspmote at http://www.libelium.com/products/waspmote/
18. Libelium Meshlium at http://www.libelium.com/products/meshlium/
19. Waspmote Data Frame, Programming Guide (2015), Libelium Comunicaciones Distribuidas S. L., Document Version v4.9
20. MIMIC II database at http://physionet.org/physiobank/tutorials/using-mimic

Corresponding Author: Bogdan Iancu, PhD
Institute: Technical University of Cluj-Napoca
Street: 26-28 G. Baritiu
City: Cluj-Napoca
Country: Romania
Email: Bogdan.Iancu@cs.utcluj.ro

Algorithm with Heuristics for Kidney Allocation in Transplant Information System

S. Luscalov[1], L. Loga[2], D. Luscalov[2], A. Lăcătuş[3], G. Dragomir[3] and L. Dican[1]

[1] "Iuliu Haţieganu" University of Medicine and Pharmacy, Cluj-Napoca, Romania
[2] Clinical Institute of Urology and Renal Transplantation, Cluj-Napoca, Romania
[3] Computer Science Department, Technical University of Cluj-Napoca, Cluj-Napoca, Romania

Abstract—**Kidney transplantation from deceased donors is the most popular treatment in our center, Clinical Institute of Urology and Renal Transplantation Cluj-Napoca. Patients affected by end stage kidney disease benefit from this treatment. To get access to a transplant, a patient diagnosed with end-stage organ failure should be identified by a medical team as a possible candidate for transplant. A multidisciplinary team determines whether or not every patient is necessary to be placed on a waiting list. Then a chosen recipient calls for a kidney from a deceased donor. This process is complicated and supported by several criteria. Most of the allocation criteria for kidneys from deceased donors are: blood group, grade of HLA-A/B/DR match, PRA, organ size, duration on waiting list, age, period on dialysis, and also the distance from the donor center. In this paper, we propose a model of a system that benefits from state of the art technology and has at its core the matching module. Selecting the ideal donor-recipient matching pair is a laborious activity and therefore the existence of such a module comes to help both clinicians and patients. A precondition for the functioning of the algorithm is the existence of quality data in the database. This data is collected using web services and distributed agents. To test the algorithm, we used real data from the patients in our clinic.**

Keywords— **HLA, Cross-match, PRA, Waiting-list, Matching-algorithm**

I. INTRODUCTION

Kidney transplantation is usually the foremost effective treatment for patients with end-stage kidney disease.

When an individual dies, the family is asked if they might be willing to give their relatives' organs.

Kidneys from deceased donors are offered to waitlisted candidates in step with a priority score. The priority score depends on donor-patient specific characteristics comparable to [1, 2]:

- Blood-type
- Tissue-type compatibility
- Organ size
- Duration on waiting list
- Duration on chemical analysis
- Age
- Proximity to transplant center
- Level of medical urgency

A. Blood type

Blood type is a crucial factor in the practice of renal transplantation. Blood type influence compatibility between patient and donor blood types. There are four major types-A, B, AB, and O-and every major kind might contain the Rh factor (Rh), in which case it's Rh positive; otherwise, it's Rh-negative blood. People is critical within the organ transplantation method, that depends upon compatibility between recipient and donor blood varieties. Potential patient with blood type O can be given organs only from donors with type O blood. Donors with blood type A can donate to recipients with blood types A and AB. Donors with blood type B can give to recipients with blood types B and AB. Donors with blood type AB can donate to recipients with blood type AB only.

B. HLA (Human Leukocyte Antigen)

The HLA significant in renal transplantation are HLA-A, B (class I antigens) and DR (class II antigens). The subjects (donors and recipients) have two of each HLA -A, B, and DR. These antigens are inherited from each parents. In organ transplantation, these antigens are a decisive measure of tissue compatibility between a donor and a potential patient. In kidney transplantation, for example, six different HLA antigens are typing for a donor and potential recipients; the results of this process are usually expressed in terms of the number of HLA mismatches (MM) between donor and potential recipient. Zero (0) HLA mismatches are indicating a high degree of compatibility and six (6) mismatches indicating complete incompatibility[3, 4].

HLA typing is performed by molecular polymerase chain reaction-sequence specific oligonucleotide (PCR-SSO) or polymerase chain reaction-sequence specific primer (PCR-SSP).

In SSP-PCR, DNA (Deoxyribonucleic acid) is isolated from the subject to be typed, and amplified in multiple wells, every containing specific primers complementary to explicit HLA alleles. The contents of the wells are then pass by electrophoresis through an agarose gel with the amplification product showing as a band on the gel; the HLA typing is appointed by matching the primers of ensuing ampli-

S. Vlad and N.M. Roman (eds.), *International Conference on Advancements of Medicine and Health Care through Technology; 12th - 15th October 2016, Cluj-Napoca, Romania,*
IFMBE Proceedings 59,
DOI: 10.1007/978-3-319-52875-5_46

fication products to the deoxyribonucleic acid sequences of the varied candidate alleles [5].

In SSOP, oligonucleotide probes that are complementary to the distinctive segments of the desoxyribonucleic acid of various alleles are mixed with amplified DNA. The distinctive fluorescent tags recognize those probes that are complementary to the desoxyribonucleic acid, specified the distinctive HLA alleles is also known [6, 7].

C. Cross-match

The lymphocytotoxic cross-match checks detects antibodies within the recipient that react with donor HLA antigens before transplantation. Lymphocytotoxic crossmatch tests are used primarily for transplant candidates to estimate the suitableness of a possible donor. If the the crossmatch is taken into account positive. this suggests the recipient has antibodies “against” the donor’s cells. A positive lymphocytotoxic crossmatch identifies antibodies accountable for hyperacute rejection of kidney grafts and is thus a reason to contraindicated transplantation. If the crossmatch is negative, the pair donor- recipient is taken into account compatible [8].

D. PRAs(Panel reactive antibodies)

Antibodies are molecules made by the immune system in response to a foreign body for example transplanted organ. PRA values are quantities of a patient's level of "sensitization" to human leucocyte antigens. A recipient may become "sensitized" through a previous transplant, a blood transfusion or pregnancy. The patient's serum is screened so as to assess the degree of sensitization, that is expressed as a percentage of PRA: such a proportion will vary from zero to five % (non-sensitized) to 75-100 % (highly sensitized). High levels of PRAs are related to a larger risk of graft rejection and failure. The chance of finding cross-match negative for patients with high PRA values is low; therefore, such patients might wait for much longer and maybe never receive a kidney. Out of concern for equity, such patients are given a relative advantage over patients with low PRA values [9,10].

For assessment of PRA we tend to used LIFECODES class I and class II ID. LIFECODES class I ID Beads are designed to find IgG antibodies to HLA class I glycoproteins. LIFECODES class I ID consists of various Luminex Beads to that affinity pure class I HLA glycoproteins from different people are conjugated. LIFECODES class II ID Beads are designed to notice IgG antibodies to HLA class II glycoproteins. LIFECODES class II ID consists completely of various Luminex Beads to that affinity pure class II HLA glycoproteins from different people are conjugated. An aliquot of the Beads is permitted to incubate with a tiny low volume of test blood serum sample. The sensitized beads are then washed to get rid of unbound antibody. An anti-Human IgG protein conjugated to pigment is then supplementary. After another incubation, the test sample is diluted and analyzed on the Luminex instrument. The signal intensity from every bead is compared to the signal intensity of a negative control bead enclosed within the bead preparation to work out if the bead is positive or negative for bound alloantibody [11].

II. Transplant information system

A. System architecture

The application is based on Cloud Computing technology[12, 13], which topologically consists of distributed clients and distributed data centers as can be seen in Figure 1. Web application can be accessed by a user with role of donor, recipient, physician by means a navigation program (Web Browser) from computers in hospitals and transplant centers, connected via Cloud Computing with the database. With this technology the hospitals benefit from accelerating the implementation of information system, the assimilation of new users, continuity of functionality (automated disaster recovery) and not the last thing, centralized operation of data (consistent information).

Cloud Computing has several advantages over client-server architectures and peer-to-peer. Client-server architecture is similar to Cloud Computing with Central storage, but additionally worrying about Cloud Computing and how a group of computers working together to increase computational power. In the client-server architecture any communication is between clients pass through the server (overload), compared to peer-to-peer architecture that allows each computer to be also client and server, sharing resources and services directly (decentralized control, high complexity).

The software's architecture is modular [14] and uses the MVC design scheme (Spring framework). M (Model) designates data used by the application, V (View) designates the presentation of the application and C (Controller) designates the logic that controls access to data and generate Web pages. The application uses Hibernate framework for ORM (Object-Relational Mapping). The application also contains components for user authentication, generation of messages by email and SMS (Short Message Service), generation of files in different formats, connection to web services needed to access nomenclatures and results of laboratory tests.

For the client (frontend) was used Angular JavaScript framework.

The software language platform used is Java EE. Other used technologies: REST Web services, persistent entities JPA (Java persistence API), EIS (Enterprise Information System), Servlets and JSP (Java Server Pages).

The database management system used is MySql. Conceptual database schema concerning with matching is shown in Figure 2.

The essential elements of the data model entities are: Person, User_Role, Lab_Results_Patient, Parameter_description, HLA_type, Antibody_HLA, Cross_match_direct, Matching, Test_Run, Config_Table.

In Person table personal data of recipients, donors and doctorsare stored. User_Role table contains data about a person's role in the system and to authenticate data. Lab_Results_Patient table contains the results of laboratory tests that are remade every 3 months. The donor-recipient pairs assigned to a run of matching algorithm are saved in Matching table.

Test_Run table is used to know the configuration values that were used by matching algorithm when the doctor decides to make more runs of the algorithm by changing the threshold values in Config_Table.

It is important to note that we assumed that the information system uses distributed agents to collect results of medical tests from dedicated computers and automated enter them in the database.

The advantages of transplant information system come from the ability to automation generate compatibility lists in case of the appearance of donors. Some medical tests should be done on the both presence of actual probe from donor and recipient like cross match.

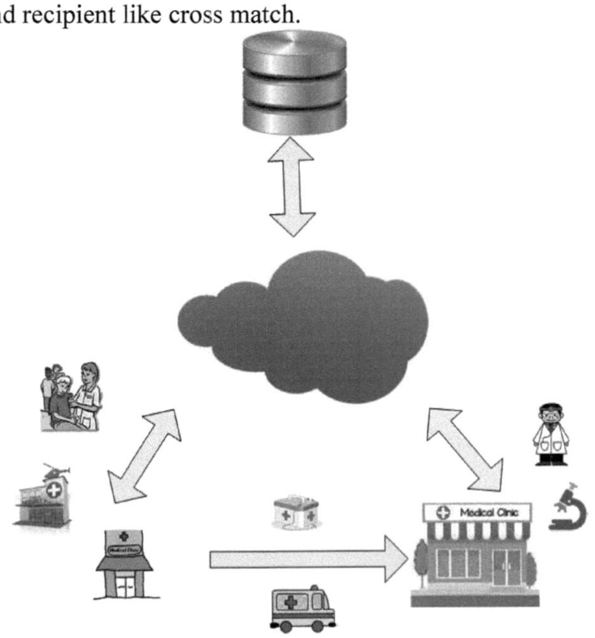

Fig. 1 The architecture of the Transplant Information System

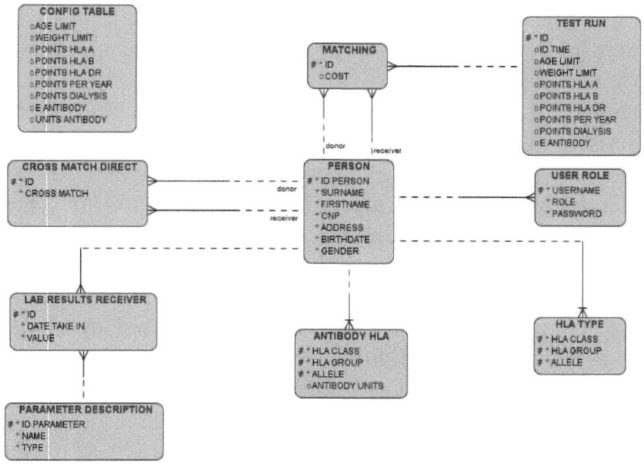

Fig. 2 Logical model of DB

Other information is already known like blood type, age and weight.

The core of the system is the matching algorithm.

B. Matching algorithm description

We denote D the set of persons named donors which is of cardinality n_D.

We denote R the set of persons named recipients which is of cardinality n_R.

From our practice experience n_D is in general below 3 and n_R could be of order of magnitude of hundreds.

The matching problem is to find the set of pairs (d, r) for each d ϵ D and where r ϵ R such as to maximize compatibility.

The set of properties used in determining compatibility consists of two subsets, one with properties that determines the impossibility of matching denoted M (mandatory), the other subset is used in determining compatibility (or cost) matrix S (score).

We denote T.m threshold for m ϵ M, P.s points for s ϵ S and f(d, r, P.s) the function which compute fraction of compatibility between d and r for s.

C_M (Compatibility Matrix) will store 0 for a pair (d, r) if d is not compatible with r.

Figure 3 presents the sub-algorithm which determines the compatibility matrix. Example of mandatory properties are blood type, age, weight and cross match.

The score properties are used as follows: some patients receive bonus points based on presence of dialysis and waiting time (one point per year for both), other points are received based on correspondence of HLA (A-1 point, B-2 points and DR-5 points).

In Table 1 we can see a representative example of C_M where n=5 and m=6. We will discuss matching algorithm based on this example.

Scientific literature describes several matching algorithms as in [15, 16, 17, 18]. One of the most known algorithm is Stable Marriage. There are several major differences between classical algorithm and our algorithm. One difference is that of cardinality of the two sets, in classical algorithm the cardinalities are equals. Based on observations that are presented below we relax condition that maximize compatibility when lockout occurs caused by donor list of recipients used fully before in other allocations. Therefore, we could not guarantee optimal solution but suboptimal.

Definition of Stable Marriage Algorithm adapted to organ transplant application: a pair (d_i, r_i) ϵC_M blocks a matching pair (d_j, r_j) ϵC_M, or is a blocking pair for C_M, if:

- d_i is unassigned or prefers r_j to r_i
- r_j is unassigned or prefers d_i to d_j

A matching allocation M_A is said to be stable if it admits no blocking pair.

Pseudocode of Stable Marriage Algorithm adapted to organ transplant application is showed in Figure 4. We denote D_L Donors List and R_L Recipients List.

Before running the matching algorithm, the clinician will check the report with incompatibilities if it is established that there is a certain threshold by modifying which potential recipients appear on empty donor lists. The application proposes the configuration parameter that should be changed and what be the new value. In example from Table 1, such potential configuration parameter is age, to find recipients compatible with donor 5.

The list of donors D_L is sorted ascending by the number of recipients in R_L_i(for equal number are ordered descending by score).With the data in Table 1 order of donors is don_2 (size = 1 points = 5), don_1 (size = 2 points = 15), don_4 (size = 2 points = 13), don_3 (size = 3 points = 25)).

After a complete walk in D_L the algorithm will found the pairs:(2, 5); (1, 2); (4, 3); (3, 1).

```
input: M, T, S, P, D, R
output: C_M (Compatibility Matrix)

initialize C_M with 0;
for each (d, r) ϵD × R:
 for each mϵM:
  if|d.m - r.m| >T.m then reject (d, r);
 for each sϵS:
  C_M[d][r] += f(d, r, P.s);
.
```

Fig. 3 Sub-algorithm for determining C_M

```
input: C_M (Compatibility Matrix)
output: M_A (Matching Allocation)

order D_L ascending by size of R_L;
each R_L is ordered descending based on C_M;
while D_L is not free do
 d = first donor in D_L;
 r =first recipient on d's R_L list;
 if r is free then
  assign d and r to be allocated;
 else
  if r prefers d to his donor d' and
      not_blocking(d, r, d') then
   assign r and d to be compatibles;
   assign d' to be free;
  else
   d rejects r (and d remains free);
.
```

Fig. 4 Matching algorithm with heuristics

In detail, at first iteration, donor 4 found recipient 2 is assigned to donor 1, points_don_4=8<points_don_1=9 so pair (4, 2) is rejected. At second iteration, donor 4 is paired with recipient 3. At next step donor 3found recipient 2 is assigned to donor 1, points_don_3=10>points_don_1=9 but followed a recursive search which determined blocking (donor 1 has recipient 3 on its R_L, which is paired with donor 4 and donor 4 has recipient 2on its R_L, which is paired with donor 1) so pair (3, 2) is rejected. In a similar fashion pair (3, 3) is rejected. Eventually donor 3 is paired with recipient 1.

Without ordering the list of donors and without relaxing max-points condition at first step pair (1, 2) is found, next pair (2, 5) is found, next pair (3, 2) is found and pair (1, 2) is rejected), next pair (1, 3) is found and because donor 4 is generating blocking algorithm will stop. The solution is worse than the other (we lost 1 donor).

Sub-algorithm not_blocking(donor d, recipient r, donor r') is same like the DFS (Depth First Search) algorithm which find cycles in graph theory.

Table 1 Example of Compatibility Matrix

		Recipient					
		1	2	3	4	5	6
Donor	1	0	9	6	0	0	0
	2	0	0	0	0	5	0
	3	5	10	10	0	0	0
	4	0	8	5	0	0	0
	5	0	0	0	0	0	0

III. Experimental Results

For measure the performance of the Matching Algorithm we used different thresholds tests for different combinations of age and weight (range 10, 25; 5 by 5) with 8 donors and 560 recipients. The results were stored in a table like Matching table, augmented with a Status column. The domain for Status column has four values:

- True positive (TP): Incompatible pair correctly identified as incompatible;
- False positive (FP): Compatible pair incorrectly identified as incompatible;
- True negative (TN): Compatible pair correctly identified as compatible;
- False negative (FN): Incompatible pair incorrectly identified as compatible.

Sensitivity (or true positive rate (TPR)) and specificity (or true negative rate (SPC)) are statistical measures of the performance. The positive and negative predictive values (PPV and NPV respectively) are the proportions of positive and negative results.

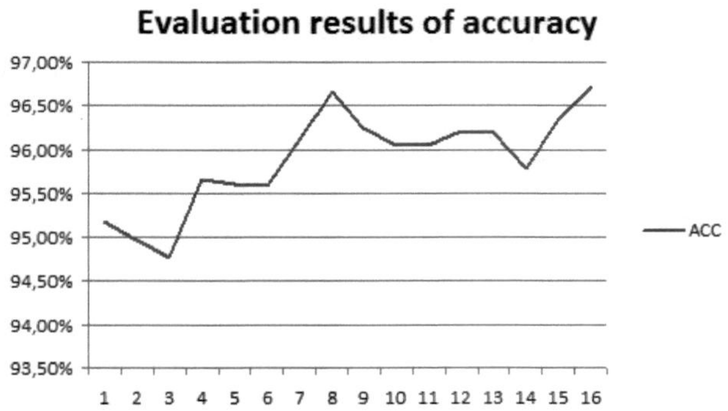

Fig. 5 Accuracy (on X axis 1: t_age=10, t_weight=10 and 16:t_age=25, t_weight=25) ACC = (TP+TN)/(TP+FP+TN+FN)

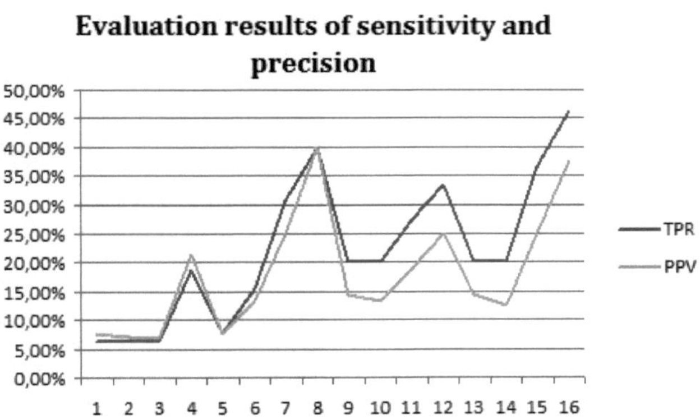

Fig. 6 Sensitivity TPR = TP/(TP+FN), average TPR ≈ 22% and Precision PPV = TP/(TP+FP), average PPV ≈ 18 %

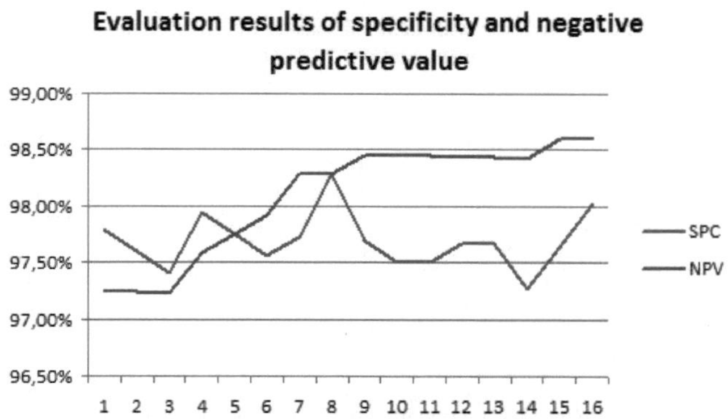

Fig. 7 Specificity SPC = TN/(TN+FP), average SPC ≈ 97% and Negative Predictive Value NPV = TN(TN+FN), average NPV ≈ 98%

Accuracy is a description of systematic errors. We can see in Fig. 5 that best accuracy 96.7% was obtained for age threshold 15 years and weight threshold 25 kg (point 8 on X axis) or age threshold 25 years and weight threshold 25 kg (point 16 on X axis).

From the charts in Fig. 5, Fig. 6and Fig. 7 we can see that matching algorithm is more accurate where sensitivity and specificity are higher (points 8 and 16 on X axis).

IV. Conclusions

In this paper we presented a model for Transplant Information System which has at core a heuristic matching algorithm.

Taking into account the values in experimental tests we can say that where the accuracy indexes are rather low the doctor should not trust indicating combination of configuration parameters.

This matching algorithm for kidney allocation can automation generate the list of a potential recipients for transplantation in case of the appearance of donors regarding two parameters (age and weight). In the next future this algorithm will be improved by adding mandatory proprieties as MM, PRAs and cross-match.

Conflict of Interest

The authors declare that they have no conflict of interest.

References

1. Zenios SA, Chertow GM, Wein LM. Dynamic allocation of kidneys to candidates on the transplant waiting list. Oper. Res. 2000;48(4):549–569.

2. Takemoto SK, Terasaki PI, Gjertson DW, et al. Twelve years'experience with national sharing of HLA-matched cadaveric kidneys for transplantation. N Engl J Med. 2000; 343: 1078-1084.
3. Elsner HA, DeLuca D, Strub J,Blasczyk R. HistoCheck: rating of HLA class I and II mismatches by an internet-based software tool. Bone Marrow Transplant. 2004; 33:165-169
4. Süsal C, Opelz G. Current role of human leukocyte antigen matching in kidney transplantation. Curr Opin Organ Transplant. 2013; 18:438–444
5. Erlich HA, Opelz G, Hansen J. HLA DNA typing and transplantation. Immunity 2001; 14:347–356
6. Mahdi BM. A glow of HLA typing in organ transplantation. Clin Transl Med. 2013; 2:6.
7. Marsh SGE, Albert ED, Bodmer WF, et al. Nomenclature for factors of the HLA system, 2010. Tissue Antigens. 2010; 75:291-455.
8. Taylor CJ, Kosmoliaptsis V, Sharples LD et al. Ten-year experience of selective omission of the pretransplant crossmatch test in deceased donor kidney transplantation. Transplantation 2010; 89: 185–93.
9. Gupta A, Iveson V, Varagunam M, Bodger S, Sinnott P,Thuraisingham RC. Pretransplant donor-specific antibodiesin cytotoxic negative crossmatch kidney transplants: arethey relevant? Transplantation. 2008;85(8):1200-1204
10. Fuggle SV, Martin S. Tools for human leukocyte antigen antibody detection and their application to transplanting sensitized patients. Transplantation. 2008;86(3):384-390.
11. Lachmann N, Terasaki PI, Budde K, et al. Anti-human leukocyte antigen and donor-specific antibodies detected by Luminex post-transplant serve as biomarkers for chronic rejection of renal allografts. Transplantation 2009; 87: 1505
12. J. Liu, T. Zhao, S. Zhou, Y. Cheng, CONCERT: a cloud-based architecture for next-generation cellular systems, IEEE Wireless Communications (Volume:21, Issue: 6), 2014, pp 14-22
13. B. Grobauer, T. Walloschek, E. Stocker, Understanding Cloud Computing Vulnerabilities, IEEE Security &Privacy (Volume:9, Issue: 2), pp 50-57
14. C. Szyperski - Component Software: Beyond Object-Oriented Programming, 2nd Edition, Addison-Wesley Component Software
15. D. Gale, L. S. Shapley, (1962). "College Admissions and the Stability of Marriage". American Mathematical Monthly 69: 9–14. doi:10.2307/2312726
16. D. E. Knuth, (1976). Mariages stables. Montreal: Les Presses de l'Universite de Montreal
17. J. E. Hopcroft, R. M. Karp, "An n5/2 algorithm for maximum matchings in bipartite graphs", Switching and Automata Theory, 1971., 12th Annual Symposium on, pp 122-125
18. H. N. Gabow, R. E. Tarjan, Faster scaling algorithms for general graph matching problems, Journal of the ACM, Volume 38 Issue 4, Oct. 1991, pp 815-853

Author: Gabriel Cristian Dragomir-Loga
Institute:Technical University of Cluj-Napoca
Street: Baritiu St. 26-28
City:Cluj-Napoca
Country: Romania
Email: gabriel.dragomir@cs.utcluj.ro

Exploring Hierarchical Medical Data stored as Multi-trees in a Relational Database

P. Olah[1], I. Movileanu[1], N. Suciu[1], M. Muji[2], M. Marusteri[1], D. Simionescu[3] and C. Avram[1]

[1] University of Medicine and Pharmacy, Tirgu-Mures, Romania
[2] Petru Maior University, Tirgu-Mures, Romania
[3] Clemson University, Clemson, SC, USA

Abstract— **Modern healthcare and medical research increasingly rely on large amounts of medical data stored in complex databases. In our previous work we have proposed a relational database design pattern and a graphical user interface for structuring hierarchical medical data, with the aim to enable researchers to design their own data structures while still benefiting from the advantages of a relational database. In this paper we will present a software tool designed to assist the user in querying hierarchical medical data, represented as custom designed multi-trees in a relational database.**

Keywords— **healthcare information systems, medical databases, data interrogation, design pattern, user interface**

I. Introduction

From an information point of view, modern healthcare and medical research increasingly rely on large amounts of medical data stored in complex databases [1]. These databases are often integrated in larger systems, called Healthcare Information Systems (HIS), which provide a number of functions to the medical practitioner or researcher, as part of the user experience [2]. One particularly important function of these systems concerns data retrieval, a task which may represent a challenge, as both the amount and the complexity of medical data can sometimes become overwhelming. Historical medical data can be retrieved through standard reporting, when the requirements for such reports are well defined. If the data needs to be explored for research purposes, the exact structure of the queries is not always known at the beginning of the process. In order to explore large sets of structured data, medical researchers need appropriate software tools that address this issue. There are two main approaches to this challenge: automated data mining and user-driven, query based, data exploration [3]. In both cases, the goal is to find relevant patterns in the accumulated medical data that will expand the knowledge of medical professionals. Data mining uses a variety of algorithms to discover hidden patterns in the data, whereas custom queries represent a tool for the user to explore the data in an effort to validate a pre-stated hypothesis.

The efficiency of the interrogation mechanisms is in no small part determined by the underlying structure of the data. Loosely structured data collections will have to be interrogated using full-text searches based on keywords, whereas well-structured data can be retrieved with high accuracy using a variety of selection criteria.

In our previous work we have proposed a relational database design pattern and a graphical user interface for structuring hierarchical medical data represented as multi-trees [4] [5]. The specific aim of this approach was to provide medical researchers with a tool that will enable them to design their own data structures, suited to the needs of each research project, enjoying a great degree of flexibility while benefitting from the security and integrity of a relational database. In this paper we will present the techniques used to develop the data interrogation module of this system, a software tool designed to assist the user in querying the data in a flexible and dynamic way, while retaining the advantages of a soundly structured, data centric information system. We have implemented these techniques in a working system that represents, in our view, a proof-of-concept. We have used SQL Server 2008 R2 for the database end and Visual FoxPro 9 as a GUI development environment.

II. Configuring custom interrogations

Building complex custom interrogations can often become an iterative process. The user may start with selecting a small set of data items, filtered according to one or two simple criteria. After analyzing the result, the user may wish to expand the initial selection and/or refine the filtering criteria, perhaps add some ordering criteria or even re-label certain items, in order to obtain relevant information. For instance, a researcher may wish to retrieve all the lab test results of the patients with a certain diagnostic. After reviewing the data, the user may decide to include additional data items for each patient in the query, for example information about previous treatments or exposure to risk factors. The researcher may also require the data to be filtered according to several criteria, like period of time, a threshold for certain lab results, the presence of specific risk factors etc. In the end, the design of the interrogation should be saved for later use or further adjustment.

S. Vlad and N.M. Roman (eds.), *International Conference on Advancements of Medicine and Health Care through Technology; 12th - 15th October 2016, Cluj-Napoca, Romania,*
IFMBE Proceedings 59,
DOI: 10.1007/978-3-319-52875-5_47

A. Selecting the relevant data items from the hierarchy

The data stored in our HIS is represented at the user view level as a collection of trees or multi-trees. Thus, the first step the user must perform in order to configure a complex interrogation on this data is to select which nodes or sub-trees are to be included in the result.

At the Graphical User Interface (GUI) level, we have implemented this functionality using a similar control as the one provided to the user to define the hierarchical structure of the data. This control allows easy navigation trough the structure of each defined tree and offers the necessary functionality to select and configure each item of data to be included in the custom query.

The GUI is presented in Fig. 1 displaying a hierarchical data structure that was developed to support a fundamental research project implemented in a tissue culture laboratory (Fig. 1).

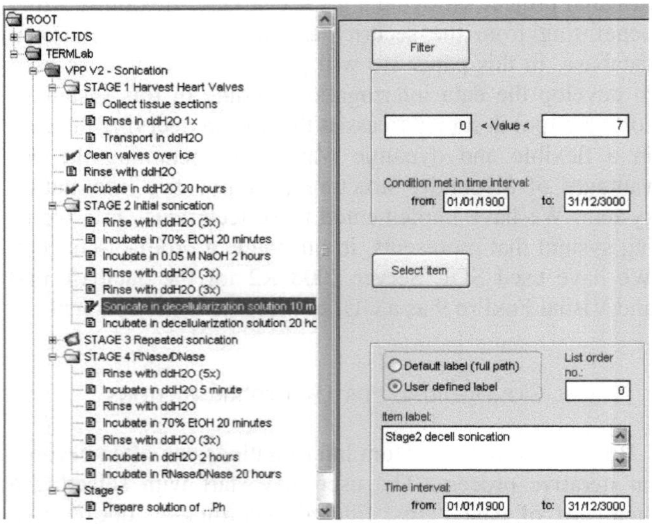

Fig. 1 – GUI displaying a hierarchical data structure

The user can include each desired leaf-node individually in the structure of the query, or an entire sub-tree can be selected for this purpose. In this case the system will automatically mark all nodes of the subtree as being included in the interrogation.

As the structure of the trees can become quite complex, it is sometimes difficult to visualize the entire structure of a defined query in this GUI module. Therefore we have designed a separate control which allows the user to see, at any time, the entire configuration of a query, by presenting only the included nodes and their paths in the tree (Fig. 2).

This viewing tool also informs the user whether there are any filtering conditions associated with a selected node.

To implement this module of the system we have reused the GUI design pattern that we have developed for the module that enables the researcher to build the custom hierarchical structures. We have kept the tree-navigation control on the left side, and re-designed the controls on the right side, using a limited number of objects to provide the needed query configuration functions for the types of data that can be recorded in the leaf-nodes of the trees.

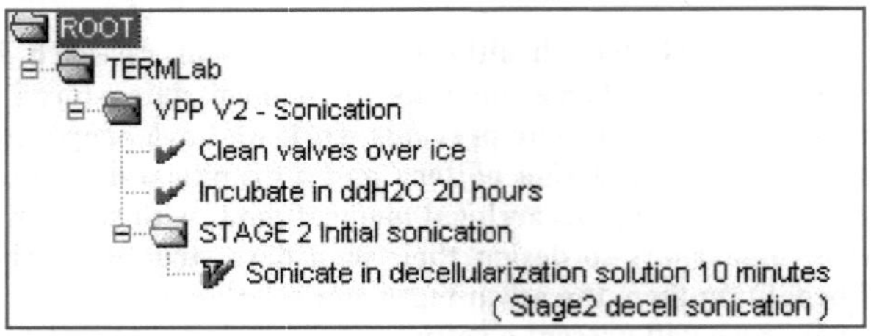

Fig. 2 – GUI control displaying query configuration

At the data level, we have implemented this functionality by extending the structure of the database with a new table, which holds all the necessary query-related data for each node of the user-defined hierarchical structure. This table, shown as exlist_tree_config in Fig. 3, will hold a record for each node that is included in a certain query. The primary key of this table is composed of two foreign keys, migrated from the tables that store the nodes of the user-defined hierarchical structure (CTH_TreeNode_str), on one hand, and the list of custom interrogations (exlist_tree), on the other hand.

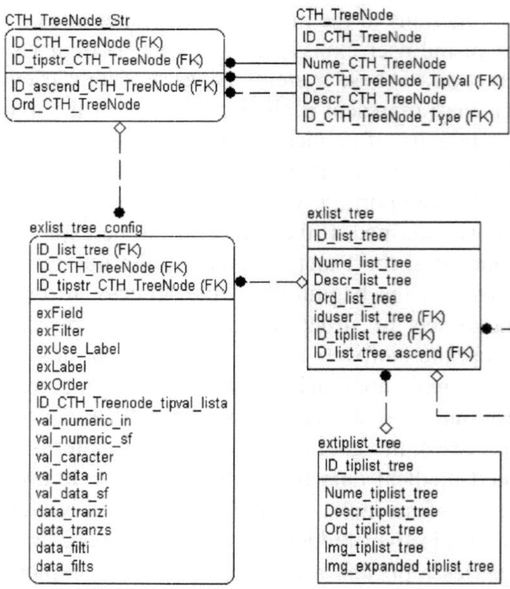

Fig. 3 – Entity-Relationship Diagram representing the key data structures used to implement the system

This design ensures that for each user-defined query all the necessary structural information is recorded correctly, maintaining the integrity of the database. For instance, if a leaf-node is part of two different trees, including it as such in a query will result in two different records in exlist_tree_config. Similarly, including the same node in a number of different interrogations will generate several records in this table, one for each query defined.

B. Filtering the data records

The ability to selectively retrieve data records is an essential characteristic of any database interrogation engine. In order to implement this functionality in our HIS, we have developed a set of specialized GUI controls which allow the user to specify filtering conditions for every selected node of the hierarchical data structure. These controls are selectively activated depending on the data type of each node: text, number, date or predefined list. In addition, as each recorded instance of a tree or node has a time-stamp, we offered the user the possibility to filter the data according to these time-stamps. This may have important semantic value for the medical researcher. For example, a tree structure representing a blood testing protocol could be instantiated several times, for the same patient, to record multiple follow-up investigations. The ability to retrieve only a subset of these instances according to a specified time interval is important from a medical point of view.

At the database level, the filtering criteria specified by the user for each node is recorded in a number of specially designed fields in the exlist_tree_config table (Fig. 3). The stored procedures, which interrogate the relational database to retrieve the actual data requested in the queries, use the values stored in these fields, according to the data type of each node of the hierarchical structure.

III. Querying the Relational Database and Presenting the Selected Medical Data

The actual interrogation of the database is performed, upon the user's request, by the stored procedures implemented on the server side of the system. These rely on the recorded configuration of the selected query. Using this configuration the procedures will parse the instances of the relevant tree or trees, retrieving the specified data from the relational database.

The result will not be a tree-like structure, it will be a plain table listing the values of the selected nodes according to the design of the query, along with the necessary identification and labeling information.

Presenting only the values and the individual labels of leaf-nodes retrieved from a hierarchical data structure could lead to ambiguities, as the semantic meaning of the information is dependent on the context provided by the structure of the tree. Therefore, the system has an in-built default labeling mechanism, which provides for each piece of retrieved information an exact context, i.e. the precise path to the leaf node in a particular tree. However, as the length of these labels depends on the depth of the trees, sometimes these automatically generated expressions can be too long and impractical for everyday use. Thus the medical researcher may choose to label some items in a different way, providing a more concise label to identify each piece of information or providing a specific context for a node, more relevant to the structure of the query. We have implemented this function by including a dedicated field in the structure of the query configuration table (Fig. 3), linked to a set of specialized controls in the GUI which provide the user with the possibility to record a custom label for each node, within a specific query.

By default, the records in the result set are sorted according to the order of the leaf nodes resulting from the parsing of the tree. In certain situations the medical researchers need to alter this sorting method, in order to present the most relevant data first. To accommodate this request, we have implemented a mechanism to record a custom order number for each node within a specific interrogation.

The standard presentation form of the results of the query is a printable report (Fig. 4). Data is grouped according to predefined criteria. If a leaf node from the hierarchical structure has multiple instances included in the query's result, the corresponding values will be listed below the label of the node in chronological order, with the time-stamp visible.

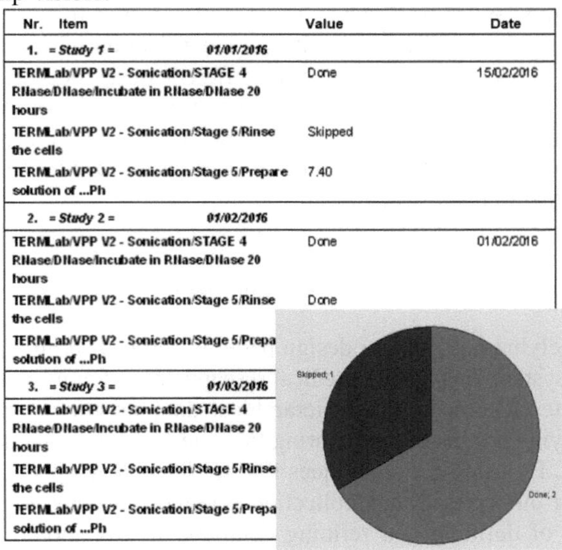

Fig. 4 – Sample cutom report generated by the system

If the selected data is numerical, the system will also provide a graphical representation of the data (Fig. 4). For more advanced processing (i.e. statistical analysis) the results of the queries can be exported into spreadsheet processing applications.

IV. Managing the collection of custom queries

The data exploration tool presented above allows the medical researcher to define an unlimited number of complex interrogations of the hierarchically structured data. In a real environment the number of these queries tends to rise, therefore a tool is needed to keep track of various query designs or group of queries that are meaningfully related.

In order to provide this tool we turned to the same techniques that we used to develop the data structuring and data retrieval mechanisms: database design patterns and object oriented GUI development. As the number and grouping criteria of possible query designs are not known, we designed a tool which allows the user to organize the queries in a custom designed hierarchical structure. This approach allowed us to reuse the GUI classes already developed for the other parts of the system. As for the database structures, we used a well-established design pattern to represent trees: a table which has a foreign key attribute migrated from its own primary key, presented as "exlist_tree" in Fig. 3. We also used a second table to model the different types of nodes needed for this organizing tool: "category", used for grouping purposes, and "report", used to identify the actual queries.

This table also migrates its primary key as a foreign key into the "exlist_tree" table. There is also a third foreign key in this table, which represents the identification of the user. This allows the system to store different query designs for each user who has access granted to this tool. Thus, every medical researcher using the system has the possibility to organize his or her own queries in a customizable folder-like hierarchical structure.

V. Conclusions

Relying on database design patterns and GUI prototypes, our system enables the medical researchers to flexibly interrogate custom designed hierarchical data structures, while enjoying the benefits of storing the data in a relational database. By using the techniques that we have developed, querying this type of data collection becomes an iterative process of defining and refining complex interrogations. The data can be explored with increasingly complex queries, allowing the researcher to validate a hypothesis or to explore newly discovered patterns in the data. The database design pattern used to design the system allows the query engine to translate the user defined interrogations into SQL statements which run against the underlying relational database, thus providing a high level of accuracy for the results. By providing an efficient way to design and manage a large number of custom interrogations, the system has the potential of a data exploration tool suitable for a variety of research purposes.

Acknowledgment

This work was partly supported by a grant of the Romanian National Authority for Scientific Research, CNCS-UEFISCDI, project number PNII-ID-PCCE-2011-2-0036

Conflict of Interest

The authors declare that they have no conflict of interest.

References

1. Bertoni, M; Furlini, G; Gozzoli, G; Landini, MP; Magnani, M; Messina, A Montesi, D (2009) - A Case Study on the Analysis of the Data Quality of a Large Medical Database; The 20th International Workshop on Database and Expert Systems Applications, Proceedings pp: 308-312 doi: 10.1109/DEXA.2009.82
2. Ayumi Takeda, Yosuke Hatakeyama (2016) - Conversion Method for User Experience Design Information and Software Requirement Specification; Design, User Experience, and Usability: Design Thinking and Methods, 5th International Conference, DUXU 2016, Held as Part of HCI International 2016, Toronto, Canada, Proceedings, Part I, pp: 356-364
3. Esther Ge, Richi Nayak, Yue Xu, Yuefeng Li (2008) - A User Driven Data Mining Process Model and Learning System; Database Systems for Advanced Applications, 13th International Conference, DASFAA 2008, New Delhi, India, Proceedings Volume pp: 51-66
4. Olah P, Măruşteri M, Muji M, Bacarea V, Haifa B, Petrişor M, Dobru D (2012) - A Database Design Pattern for Structuring Hierarchical Medical Data; Acta Medica Marisiensis 2012;58(6)pp: 429-432
5. Huang, Y; Pollak, I; Do, MN; Bouman, CA (2006) - Fast search for best representations in multitree dictionaries IEEE Transactions on image processing Volume: 15 Issue: 7 pp: 1779-1793

Author: Peter Olah
Institute: Univ Med & Pharm Tg-Mures
Street: 38 Gheorghe Marinescu
City: Tirgu-Mures
Country: ROMANIA
Email: olah_peter@yahoo.com

Development of a Complex Acquisition and Storage System of Medical Data used in a Clinical Environment

R. Pop Kun, M. Munteanu, D. Rafiroiu, D. Pop Kun and R. Moga

Technical University of Cluj-Napoca, Romania

Abstract— **In the medical field, ample and diverse data related to clinical and logistical processes is produced. In order to facilitate access to this data and ensure secure storage of information, digitization is mandatory. Existing literature shows that integration with medical equipment increases productivity of beneficiaries, facilitates workflow and reduces the prevalence of medical errors arising from incomplete information.**

Up to date, we have no knowledge of any software tailored to meet the needs of the Romanian healthcare system that addresses complex acquisition and storage of medical data. In order to fill this gap, we set out to develop and test components of an integrated solution for this issue using an inexpensive database platform.

Overall, this study has shown that integration of various clinical components in medical software solutions is both achievable and effective in improving the quality of medical care. The low costs of implementation warrant subsequent research on the potential benefits of larger scale pilot studies using this methodology.

Keywords— **Centralized Data Storage, Medical Data Acquisition, Relational Databases, Clinical Informatics**

I. Introduction

Romania is still in the early stages of digitization of medical data. The National Health Card, a platform through which each patient's medical data can be seen by doctors, including the medical services provided by the National Health Insurance Agency (CNAS) was introduced only in 2015.

Digitization in Romanian (where present) is very fragmented, partly due to lack of standardization. There is no centralization of data and usually there are more than three software in each location for various aspects. For example, there are clinics that use a software that keeps track of patients at a basic level (personal information, medical and perhaps history of services that were supplied locally), another software used for management purposes (payments, invoices) and one for appointments. If there is any medical equipment that is used for medical services (usually each equipment has a standalone proprietary software designated for specific use: EKG, ultrasound, spirometer, dynamometer, etc.) it usually does not communicate with other equipment nor a general software which could centralize the medical data. Formative research has revealed cases of some occupational medicine centers that were using even ten different software, due to the large number of medical equipment used to examine patients. The personnel were recording the results from the equipment on paper, then went to another computer where the result was re-entered in order to be able to release the medical file, only so the patient could take it to the reception where all the services had to be entered yet again so a receipt could be issued.

Because there isn't a single software to centralize the data, or the possibility of communication between them, there is a lot of time lost on the administrative side (data entry), thus requiring additional personnel to streamline things. This translates into additional costs for the medical center, due to staff salaries additional workstations, cost for training the staff so they can work with multiple software and less revenue due to the reduced theoretical number of medical services that could be performed in a day's work. Also errors in diagnosis may arise due to lack of data overview, human error in handling medical data between software.

The aim of this study was to develop, implement and test an integrated solution for complex acquisition and storage of medical data that would be cost-effective.

II. Methodology

Although the issue of acquiring and storing signals from patients in a database is a widely discussed topic [1], this system proposes a holistic approach focused on several components of the medical process. It can serve all the demands of a medical center, provide management of patient data, medical services provided in the complex, employed staff and financial management, appointment tracking, marketing of services and interconnecting as many medical devices as possible. The results from medical devices are accessible at any time to the staff, without requiring the use of proprietary software for each equipment. The FileMaker database platform was chosen for the development of this software due to its cross-platform architecture [2]. Because the software allows remote access, patients could send medical data retrieved from portable devices. This system can allow remote

S. Vlad and N.M. Roman (eds.), *International Conference on Advancements of Medicine and Health Care through Technology; 12th - 15th October 2016, Cluj-Napoca, Romania,*
IFMBE Proceedings 59,
DOI: 10.1007/978-3-319-52875-5_48

monitoring of patients, especially the evolution of health for longer periods of time, medical personnel can send recommendations (or alerts as appropriate) to patients, according to the data received. This system is designed with the flow of information presented in the block diagram below (Fig. 1), in which medical data is taken from the patient through sensors, processed and then stored. Also medical investigations made by doctors and patients' personal data are stored in their personal folders.

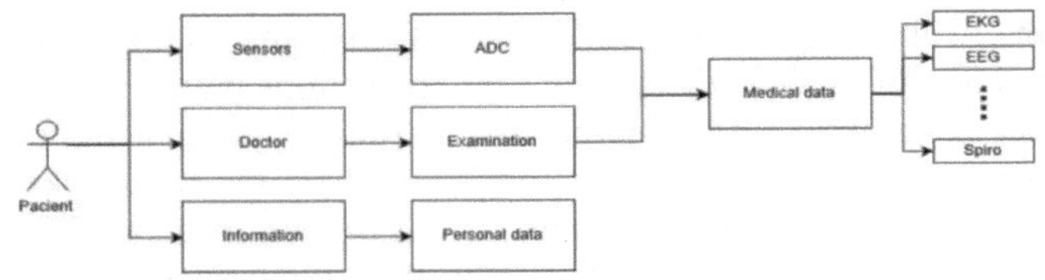

Fig. 1 Patient data flow

Because some medical centers provide fewer medical services than others, a modularization approach was chosen. Thus the basic version provides patient management, financial and administrative management, appointments and marketing. Depending on the medical services they provide locally, different modules can be added such as ultrasound, endoscopy, occupational medicine, etc. and the ability to interconnect various medical devices.

The patient management module is quite complex, being composed of numerous personal and medical data (Fig.2 and 3). They are used to deliver to the medical staff relevant information in order to determine the health of the patient and to provide a correct diagnosis. This can give an overview on the evolution of patient health over time.

Consider the specific case of a complex medical, center where this system is already in place. The medical center was founded due to the desire of the management of a large factory to provide "in house" occupational health services. Later on, the center wanted to provide various medical services, not only occupational medicine for both its employees and factories in the area. Because most patients of this center were also employees of the factories, they realized that it is redundant to use two databases, one for patients and one for HR (Human Relations). Thus a system was created that manages both structures, but because each plant is a separate entity from the administrative point of view, they have access only to its own patients and employees while the medical entity has access to all patients and medical data.

Being a complex system that stores the personal information and patients' medical history, services that have been made, professions they can provide services for (the nomenclature used by the forces of labor) diseases prone for certain professions (nomenclature used by CNAS), various administrative data such as payments and invoices, number of surgeries, etc.; companies, accounts, personnel (restricted by level of access), requires a database that consists of many tables and fields. For this system 40 tables were used, and some of them contain 4281 fields (the list of occupations), 999 fields (disease codes), 330 fields (personal and medical data for patients), 199 fields (medical examinations for occupational medicine), etc. All these fields store information that can be exported in several databases, selecting which information is needed.

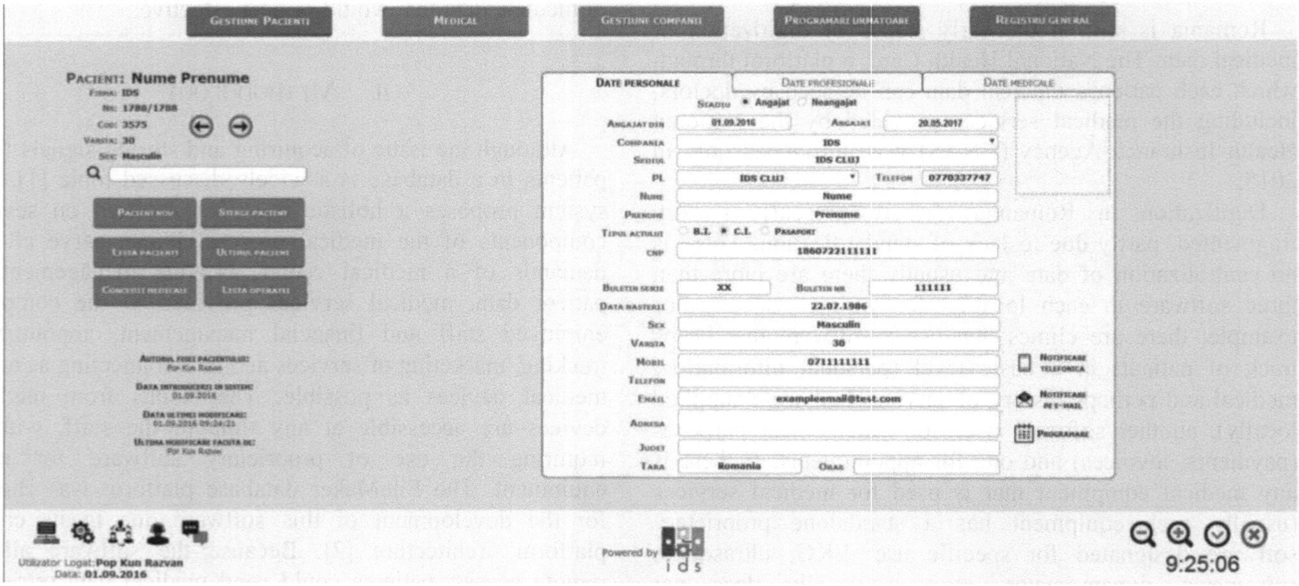

Fig. 2 Personal data file for a patient

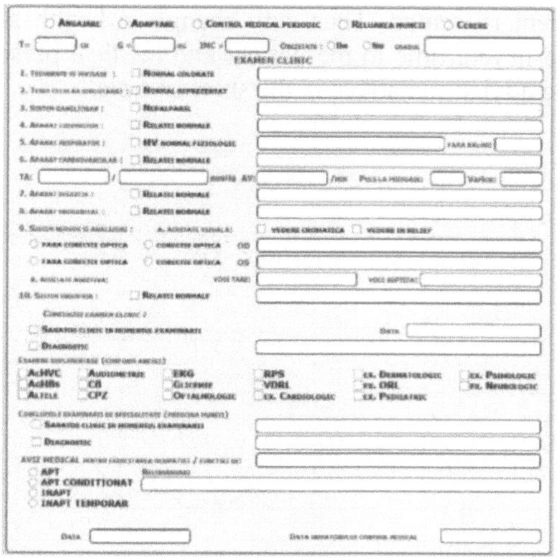

Fig. 3 Medical examination file

But all this information must be linked by relationships, so that medical examinations and data of a patient are related only to that patient [3]. FileMaker databases are non SQL, but due to the complex relations between tables, in some cases it was necessary to use SQL queries (e.g. services that are selected to be paid in a certain bill for a company). This was done by integrating an SQL plugin to the software [4].

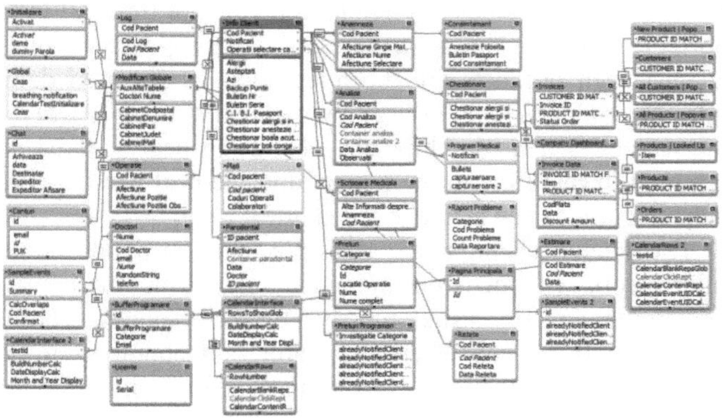

Fig. 4 Tables and relations between them

Because there are so much data and numerous functions in the software, we have to create a workflow to ease the use of it by the staff. It needs to be modularized and compartmentalized, but also all data should be easily accessible at any time. During the research for this paper, it was found that most software that exists on the market today both in Romania and abroad have made the mistake to overwhelm the user with too much data at once. An interface for such a software, especially on the main page, contains dozens of fields that need to be filled and navigation buttons.

Medical personnel who participated in this research has encountered problems in navigating these programs, long periods of time passing until they get used to the cumbersome interface. Many fields and buttons that are rarely or never used, overload the already complex interface. Thus, in this software it was tried to solve these problems by displaying only the interface fields and buttons that are most commonly used at a certain moment by the user, the rest being displayed on other tabs in the interface, or appear only if the workflow the user was following might impose the need to use them. Therefor on the top of the screen there are navigational buttons that lead to the main components of a module. Let's take the particular case of the patient management module. The top buttons lead to the page where personal data for patients can be inputted, occupational medicine files, management of the companies, appointments and financial management. In the bottom of the screen there are navigational buttons that lead to the module selection page, software configuration, accounts, log-in, chat between users, zoom and minimize controls. Also another thing to be taken into account is the need of training the personnel to use the computers and software, a problem which appeared on numerous occasions during research. Thus, the buttons must be as suggestive as possible regarding their function, symbolized by icons or name. Also it was decided to apply some explanatory text above the buttons (tooltips) that offer a more complex explanation of their function when the cursor is over them (hover). To eliminate possible human errors caused by inattention, some buttons such as the deletion of records were provided with a confirmation dialog before executing the function.

Another aspect that was desired to be integrated into the software is automation. Various features, such as sending reminders to patients or doctors based on elapsed time (e.g. remembering the patient to schedule another inspection after passing a fixed period, notices for doctors' appointments, overdue bills that need to paid for provided services) requires no human intervention after the relevant data was entered into the system. Thus, after a patient has passed his regular checkup at an occupation medicine clinic, his next appointment is automatically planned and the patient is warned a few days before that he is supposed to visit the doctor or clinic. Therefore, automation will reduce administrative costs, but also protects against human error which might occur. But automation can still not remove the human factor from the equation. Because of the many variables we cannot hope to automate everything, like interpretation of medical examinations. But using some guidelines, automation can provide information based on the data processed, in order to ease the workflow of the staff. Also, portable devices that will interact with the program, through automation, will take over the acquisition of medical data and storing them in a centralized database, facilitating the interaction between patient and the device and ensuring that the doctor has access to as much data as possible to make an informed decision with regard to the health of the patient. The communication between the respective devices and the platform isn't possible using the functions provided in the basic FileMaker platform. In order to write the code needed for the communication protocols, an additional plugin named TROI is needed to be installed and several custom functions to be created [5].

Data security must be a cornerstone of any program that manages private data (whether personal or medical). The program is built based on three basic principles.

- Limiting access only to authorized users. Authorization can be done only by users who have been appointed as administrators and user credentials are encrypted and stored inside when creating the program.

- Granular control of the data and functionality for each user group. This may prevent visualization of data, such as those that are covered by doctor-patient privilege, by other users or prevent modification of data by others than those who created it.

- Encrypting data is omnipresent. Locally stored data is encrypted using AES-256 standard and remote connections use SSL (AES-256 or AES 128).

III. FUTURE DEVELOPMENT OF THE PROPOSED SYSTEM BY USING SIGNAL PROCESSING OPERATIONS AND CONNECTIVITY TO PORTABLE DEVICES

In recent years, there has been an increased interest from both manufacturers and academic field for portable health monitoring devices [6], [7], [8]. Evolution of technology has enabled miniaturization components of such devices, so they can be worn continuously without affecting daily life. Thus it can perform constant monitoring of vital signs during long periods of time, noting when fluctuations occur and possibly the reason which caused them. With this information, the doctor can correctly diagnose disease the patient suffers from, but it can also track the effects of the prescribed treatment.

The market for wireless medical monitoring devices it is still new and growing but increasingly important. Both major manufacturers of medical devices and startups are investing great resources in developing these technologies and every year there is an increasing number of devices being launched. Products like Qardiocore or BioRadio are able to acquire multiple signals in real time, with the ability to monitor their values through long periods of time, all in a portable system. The advantages of the proposed system against such products are the integration of acquired data into the computer system used by medical structures where the patient is treated. Thus, any change in health status is reported in real time to the patient and medical personnel's help and advice can arrive in the shortest time.

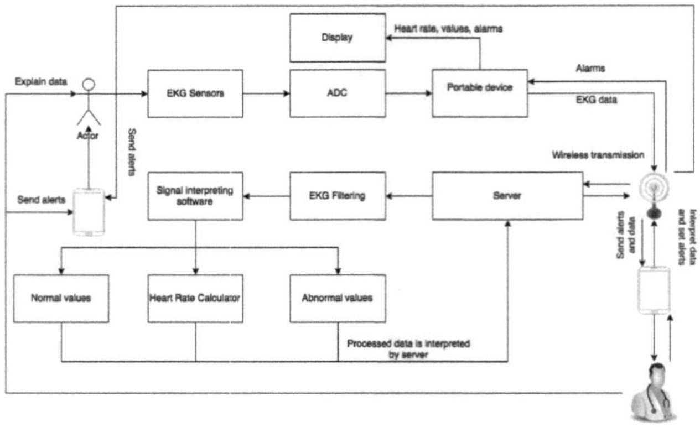

Fig. 5 Workflow Diagram

The market for wireless medical monitoring devices it is still new and growing but increasingly important. Both major manufacturers of medical devices and startups are investing great resources in developing these technologies and every year there is an increasing number of devices being launched. Products like Qardiocore or BioRadio are able to acquire multiple signals in real time, with the ability to monitor their values through long periods of time, all in a portable system. The advantages of the proposed system against such products are the integration of acquired data into the computer system used by medical structures where the patient is treated. Thus, any change in health status is reported in real time to the patient and medical personnel's help and advice can arrive in the shortest time.

The database being realized, as presented in figure 5, the future work will focus on biomedical signal measurements and processing, by using mostly portable devices. These devices will be connected via wireless technology to a server, which will receive all signals sent from different devices. After processing the acquired signals, the server decides if it needs to send alerts towards the patient and/or medical personnel. Both patients and healthcare personnel can monitor the acquired values through an application on a smartphone or browser connected to the server. Thus the medical staff can monitor the health status, inform the patient about treatment progress or alert them if certain values indicate health deterioration. The system is thought to reduce or eliminate completely the interaction of medical staff, provide data as accurate at any time and provide preset recommendations for the patient if values exceed certain parameters, hoping to minimize undesired effects.

IV. Conclusions

The circumstances of the medical centers pre implementation of this system and of those that were interested in implementing it had demonstrated the precarious state of data digitalization in Romania. There is no centralization of data, neither high-level nor locally, a situation which leads delayed health services because of the need of new examinations, less information being available to physicians on the overall health of the patients, but also financial losses due to additional staff and time lost.

The new international trend is to monitor health through various portable devices, doctors having access to the data provided by them without needing the patient to be in proximity. Unfortunately, Romania is still struggling to provide medical data from devices in a fluent way at the centers where the patient was subjected to medical tests, without the need for third party intervention (e.g. personnel) to retrieve data from equipment and manually enter it in a computer software or on paper.

Conflict of Interests

The authors and participating parties disclaim any conflict of interest.

References

1. N. Pampu, M. Munteanu, C. Rusu, R. Ciupa, R. Moga - Integrated System for Monitoring and Storing Biomedical Signals, în Acta Electrotehnica (Special Issue for Meditech 2007), p. 277-280
2. Prosser S, Gripman S (2015) FileMaker Pro 14: The Missing Manual. O'Reilly Media, London
3. Fehily C (2014), SQL Tricks (Advanced Database Programming), Questing Vole Press
4. https://baseelementsplugin.zendesk.com/hc/en-us
5. http://www.troi.com/software/serialdetails.html
6. Ciorap, R., Zaharia, D., Corciova, C., Ungureanu, M., Lupu, R., Stan, A., (2008) "Wireless device for monitoring the patients with chronic disease" Revista medico-chirurgicală a Societății de Medici şi Naturalişti din Iaşi Vol 112, nr.4, p. 1115-1119
7. Mihai Munteanu, Corneliu Rusu, Dan Rafiroiu, Gabriel Chindriş, Radu A. Munteanu, Rozica Moga (2008)– A hierarchical implementation of medical data transmission, ISBN 978-1-4244-2576-1, Cluj-Napoca, Romania, May 22-25, 2008, p. 77-80
8. Pomazan V. M., Petcu L. C., Sintea S. R., Ciorap R. (2009), Active Data Transportation and Processing for Chronic Diseases Remote Monitoring, International Conference on Signal Processing Systems - ICSPS 2009, 15-17 May Singapore 2009

Elderly Fall Risk Prediction System

O. Stan[1], L. Miclea[1] and A. Sarb[2]

[1] Technical University of Cluj Napoca, Faculty of Automation and Computer Science, Department of Automation, Cluj Napoca, Romania
[2]Technical University of Cluj Napoca, Faculty of Machine Building, Cluj, Romania

Abstract— **Preventing diseases of older persons and promoting the lack of necessity in consulting professionals is a priority in the Romanian health system as all these will lead to cost reduction in this important sector of the Romanian economy. Taking these in mind, we propose a new king of medicine, a medicine that is based on connectivity, collaboration, customization and computing. For this kind of medicine to work, we have developed an integrated system that will be used for compulsory planning and for compulsory regularly evaluation of the elder persons. Furthermore, where needed, telemonitoring and assistance will be used.**

Keywords— **e-health, elderly, fall risk prediction, geriatric evaluation tests.**

I. INTRODUCTION

The idea of this project came from the report called "Global Population Ageing" launched by the United Nations in 2013 [1]. According to this report, by 2050, the number of people aged over 60 will triple and for the first time in human history will be exceeding the number of children under 15 years. Moreover, in a report released in March 2010 it is expected that by 2050, the population of people aged over 65 will represent over 40% of Europe's population [2].

The project integrates computing, communication and storage capabilities with monitoring and/or control of heterogeneous entities in the physical world, and must perform these actions dependably, safely, securely, efficiently and in real-time. The present paper addresses the idea of supporting the older adults in order to live longer in their homes with the contribution of ICT based solutions, and is also in concordance with the AAL Call Challenge Programme [3]. The ability of delivering services that can be trusted will increase confidence in these services and improve the quality of life of the elderly.

In the evaluation process and prevention of disability and dependency in elderly people, there are too many factors that go beyond the traditional approach (disease history, pathological and non-pathological personal history, physical examination, laboratory exploration). For this reason, a multifunctional geriatric assessment is vital in assessing the elderly in order to determine which issues are important and also to develop any appropriate intervention plan in order to keep the older people in the community as independently as possible and for as long as possible. This is going to lead to an enhanced quality of life. The paper's innovative outcomes can be used in the exploitation of an elderly's health, disability, dependability, quality of life and also is used for longitudinal data collections and cross-sectional analysis. Its use is not limited by physical boundaries of a country. It can be implemented within European countries and in the non-European ones without changing its initial purpose - identifying and monitoring trends of healthy aging and addiction. The solution will provide well founded and reliable scientific evidence, comparable between different regions of a country or between countries, in order to research and develop policies on aging and dependability.

The proposed solution is based on an integrated system for compulsory planning and compulsory regularly evaluation of the elderly and, where necessary, telemonitoring and assistance. As a consequence, the proposal's scope is to deliver a new kind of medicine, based on connectivity, collaboration, customizations and computing (the 4 C's). This means that it will be a significant change in the patient's and doctor's relationship: more and more of the diagnostic and monitoring functions will be performed by the patient in the comfort of their home and the doctor will just supervise and will react only when necessary. Basically, our solution will provide the transition from the information age to a cognitive intelligence era, where health, for an engineering, is seem as a state variable influenced by the social and economic environment, the physical environment and the characteristics and behaviors of the individuals. In order to fulfil all these, the main objectives are: (1) Assisted planning and evaluation of the necessary geriatric tests through a communication Web platform or mobile application (functional, affective, socioeconomic and cognitive evaluation); (2) Storing and managing the longitudinal data collections and intelligent cross-sectional analysis in a secure and safe environment; (3) Development and implementation of the innovative algorithm to analyze the big data gather through our platform in order to predict the next fall of an elderly.

A major impact of this project will be the fact that will have a significant role in cost reduction within the health system in Romania through preventing diseases of older persons and by promoting the lack of necessity in consulting professionals. Many comprehensive analysis of the current practices presented in literature revealed the necessity to the

S. Vlad and N.M. Roman (eds.), *International Conference on Advancements of Medicine and Health Care through Technology; 12th - 15th October 2016, Cluj-Napoca, Romania*,
IFMBE Proceedings 59,
DOI: 10.1007/978-3-319-52875-5_49

worktime in order to equilibrate the workload ensuring in the same time an adaptation to a predictable, seasonal variability. Taking into account the significant weight of the elderly related with the total number of medical consultations, the present paper proposes a new method which aims to contribute to a better balance of appointments scheduling, by distributing the consultations of the elderly over pre-established periods of time. Several main factors such as: recommended duration between routine consultations (depending on the appropriate periodic review and the adequate monitoring of patients), specific evolutions of patients' states, epidemiological context, holyday periods and particular preferences regarding appointments intervals, expressed by both, patients and medical personnel, are taken into account to elaborate the knowledge base - the set of rules of the expert system.

II. Core Concepts

A. Geriatric evaluation tests

The application contains five geriatric evaluation tests: Mini Nutritional Assessment (MNA)[4][5][6][7], Katz Index of Independence in Activities of Daily Living (ADL)[8], The Mini Mental State Examination (MMSE) [9], Fall Risk Assessment and The Geriatric Depression Scale (GDS) [10]. The Mini Nutritional Assessment (MNA) represents an assessment tool that is used to identify older adults (>65 years) who are at risk of malnutrition. MNA is a clinical completed instrument with two components: screening and assessment.

The Katz Index of Independence in Activities of Daily Living, commonly known as the Katz (ADL), is the most appropriate instrument to assess functional status as a measurement of the patient's ability to perform activities such as independently daily living. Clinicians typically use the tool to detect certain problems in performing daily activities from early stages and to plan the necessary care in accordance with particular needs. The Katz index is able to adequately rank the performance of the six functions: bathing, dressing, toileting, transferring, continence, and feeding.

The Mini Mental State Examination (MMSE) is a tool that can be used to systematically and thoroughly assess the mental status of a patient.

The Fall Assessment Tool includes the patient and the environment as factors that contribute to falls. Additional environmental risks may be present depending on the physical setting. To administer the tool, the user has to circle the score that corresponds with the risk factor listed on the left hand side of the instrument. The tool should be administered on admission to the facility or agency and again at specified intervals and when warren of changes in health status.

Depression is a common disease worldwide, affecting nearly 5 million persons of the 31 million Americans aged 65 and older. Both major and minor depression are reported in 13% of the communities dwelling with older adults, 24% of medical patients of old age and 43% of both acute care and nursing homes dwelling with older adults. Contrary to popular belief, depression is not a natural or desirable part of aging. Depression is often reversible with prompt and appropriate treatment. The Geriatric Depression Scale (GDS) may be used on healthy patients, medically ill ones and mild to moderately cognitively impaired older adults. It has been extensively used in communities that struggle with both acute and long-term care patients. The GDS is not a substitute for a diagnostic issued by a mental health professional, but it is a useful screening tool in the clinical setting to facilitate the assessment of depression in older adults, especially when baseline measurements are compared to subsequent scores.

The results from the tests are sent in real time to the server and then interpreted in order to facilitate a proper diagnosis. The doctor will have the ability to see the evolution of the patient and will take into consideration if an intervention is appropriate. Taking all these measures will avoid wasting time or energy when unnecessary.

B. Semantic interoperability of the medical information

In order to achieve the highest level of semantic interoperability we consider for this project just the EN/ISO 13606 and openEHR standard.

EN/ISO13606 it is a relatively new standard. Its major disadvantage arising from this aspect and there are no still many archetypes on the market that can be used. There is instead a very large community of users who make efforts to develop archetypes. To ensure semantic interoperability using the standard EN/ISO13606 communicating systems must use the same archetypes. The dual model implemented by EN/ISO13606 standard is the biggest advantage of this standard [11][12][13][14].

The main aim of this European Standard is to define a rigorous and stable architecture for communicating part or all of the patient electronic health records (EHR) in care. This is done to support interoperability required in communication process of the systems or of the components (access, transfer, addition or modification) through electronic messages or objects distributed by: maintaining clinical meaning given by the author; coverage confidentiality according to the wishes of the author or the patient.

The key innovation of the EN13606 architecture is the two-level modeling structures obtained by separating record keeping concerns from the clinical data collection using archetypes [15][16]. The first level, i.e. the Reference Model, is used to represent the generic properties of the health record information. It represents the global characteristics of the health record components, the way they are aggregated and the context information required to meet ethical, legal and provenance requirements. [15][16].

The second level, i.e Archetypes and Templates, is the meta-data used to define patterns for the specific characteristics of the clinical data representing the requirements of each particular profession, specialty or service. This level creates a semantic link to the terminologies, clinical guidelines and classifications in the EHRs. The Archetypes are developed by medical staff and, basically, represent a set of constraints on the openEHR Reference Model. [16].

C. Security and safety

In order to create a safe and secure environment, we decide to store separately the medical data from the demographic one. Along the entire application, every elderly patient has two different identifiers. One is used in the medical database and the other one in the database that store demographic information's. The bound between this is carried out in another encrypted database. The core concept of this method is presented in Fig. 1:

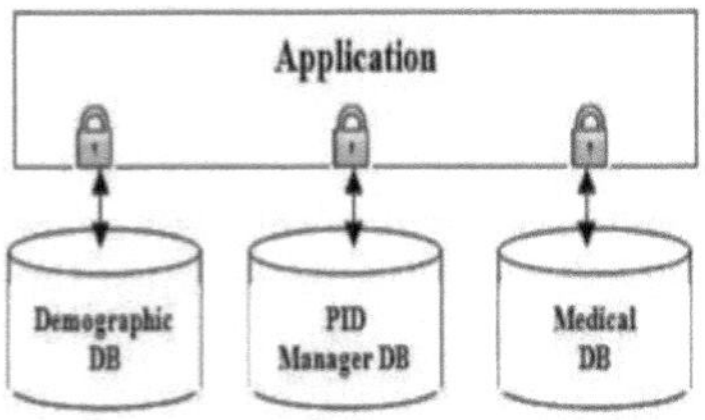

Fig. 1 Information's separation process of the patient

Databases architecture relied on EN13606 and openEHR standards. Archetypes used to express medical and demographic concepts, as well the openEHR templates needed in order to create patient records are store in databases using an XML format.

III. Platform Architecture

The proposed solution can be seen from two points of view. The first is the application for the mobile device used by the elderly patients and the second is the application designed and implemented for specialized medical staff.

A. Mobile devices application (Android)

For mobile applications we use the Android environment due to the fact that mobile devices with Android system are popular and the quality/price ratio is better than the other alternatives (IOS, Windows Phone).

The mobile interface was designed in a simple way in order to target all kind of users, regardless of their degree of disability. According to a recent study, around 10% of the males and 0.5% of the females around the globe have some form of color blindness. This result demonstrates that for every 100 users of the application, up to 10 of them see colors differently than most of the people do. In order help blind and visual impaired people we came up with the following solutions: the application has both colors and symbols, a minimalistic design was used, and there are both pattern and texture to show contrast and bad color combinations were avoided.

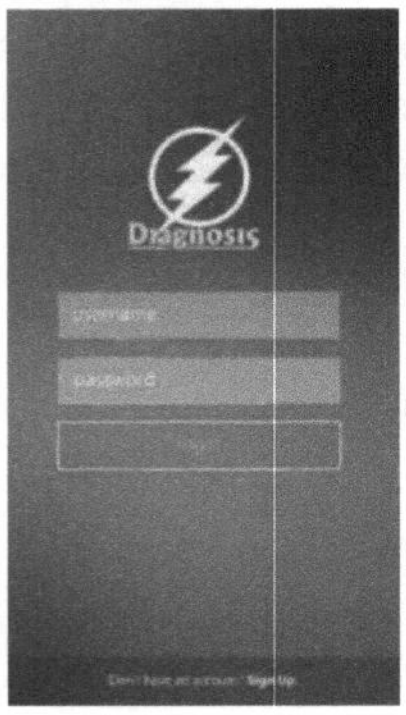

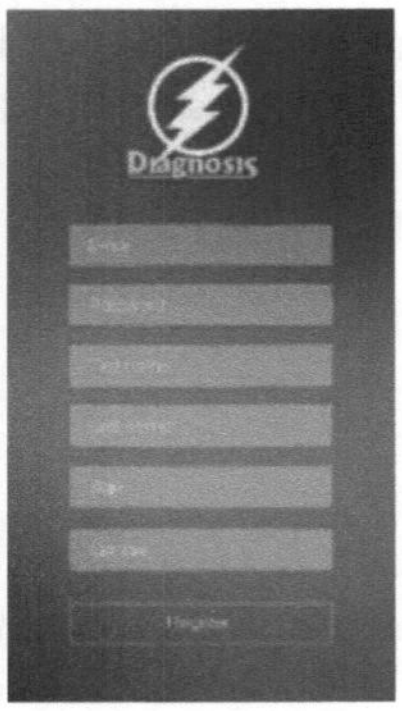

Fig. 2 Login activity Fig. 3 Register activity

The android user interface contains four pages: the login page, the register page, the user's personal page with his background information and the quizzes page. After successfully logging into the application, the user can choose one of the geriatric integrated tests or even to see the push notification from doctors.

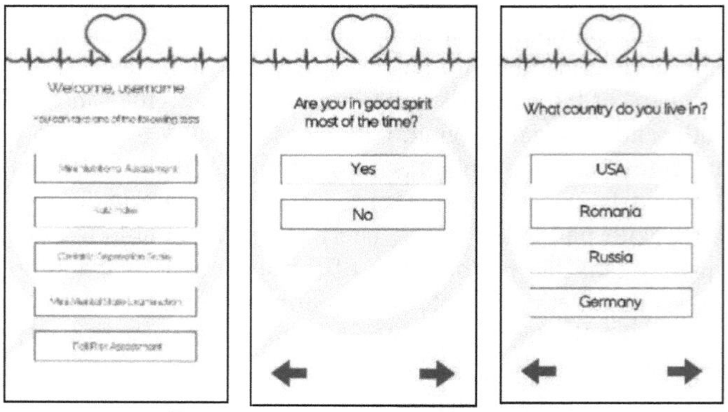

Fig. 4 Main menu and type of questions

B. Doctor's application

The website represents the part of the project that is designed for the doctor. The purpose of the site is to present in real time all the information that is stored on the server about every user of the android application. The doctor can also request additional data about the patients, like history, diseases, treatments and the patient evolution. All the information is presented in an easy readable way: graphics and charts.

The doctor has access to the content received from the server through his/her credentials: email and password. He has the ability to inform the user about the results of the tests, prescribe treatment, give advice and indicate which test should be performed next (Fig 5).

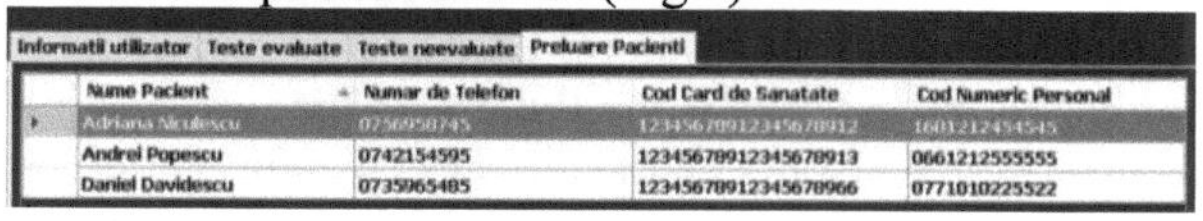

Fig. 5 Assigned new patient to a geriatric doctor

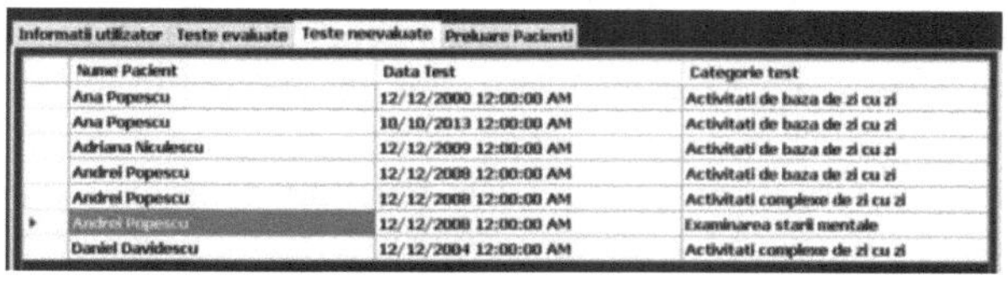

Fig. 6 Unverified test's tab

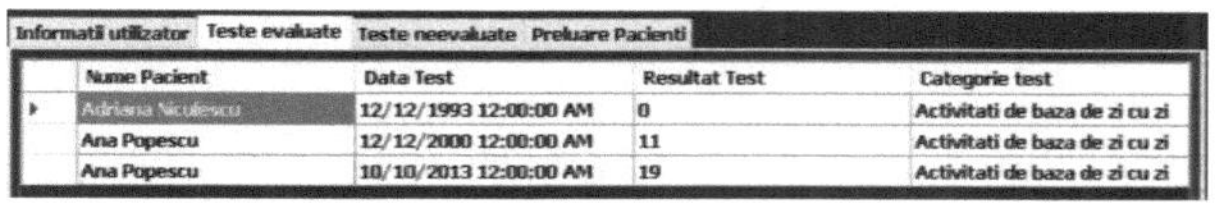

Fig. 7 Test results of the assigned patients

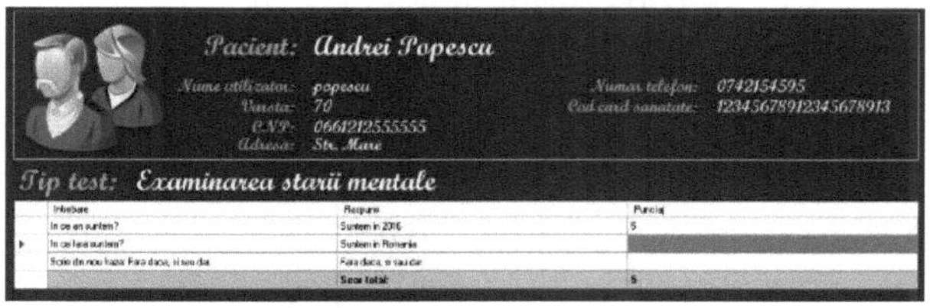

Fig. 8 Manual process of test verification (where is needed)

IV. Conclusions

The project's innovative outcomes can be used in the exploitation of an elderly's health, disability, dependability, quality of life and also is used for longitudinal data collections and cross-sectional analysis. Its use is not limited by physical boundaries of a country. It can be implemented within European countries and in the non-European ones without changing its initial purpose - identifying and monitoring trends of healthy aging and addiction. The solution will provide well founded and reliable scientific evidence, comparable between different regions of a country or between countries, in order to research and develop policies on aging and dependability. Our solution is now used in two elderly center from Alba Iulia, Romania. The prediction algorithm will be implemented after we will have enough data collected through our platform. Basically, the mobile application is used by 64 patients since January 2016 and we have assigned two medical staff. The evaluation geriatric test need to be done on a specific time (for ex. The MMSE is used at every second month), time specified by the medical staff in their dashboard application.

Conflict of Interest

The authors declare that they have no conflict of interest.

References

1. United Nations, Department of Economic and Social Affairs, Population Division (2013). World Population Ageing 2013. ST/ESA/SER.A/348
2. K. M. C. Gassner, "ICT enabled independent living for elderly. A status-quo analysis on products and the research," Institut for Innovation and Technology, Berlin, 2010.
3. AAL Programme, ICT for ageing well, http://www.aal-europe.eu/, accessed in 02.06.2016
4. Vellas B, Villars H, Abellan G, et al. Overview of the MNA® - Its History and Challenges. J Nutr Health Aging 2006, 10:456-465.
5. Rubenstein LZ, Harker JO, Salva A, Guigoz Y, Vellas B. Screening for Undernutrition in Geriatric Practice: Developing the Short-Form Mini Nutritional Assessment (MNA-SF). J. Geront 2001, 56A: M366-377.
6. Guigoz Y. The Mini-Nutritional Assessment (MNA®) Review of the Literature - What does it tell us? J Nutr Health Aging 2006, 10:466-487.
7. Kaiser MJ, Bauer JM, Ramsch C, et al. Validation of the Mini Nutritional Assessment Short-Form (MNA®-SF): A practical tool for identification of nutritional status. J Nutr Health Aging, 2009 13:782- 788.
8. Meredith Wallace, Mary Shelkey, Katz Index of Independence in Activities of Daily Living Try This, Best Practices in Nursing Care to Older Adults, New York University College of Nursing, Issue 2, 2007
9. Folstein MF, Folstein SE, McHugh PR: "Mini-mental state: A practical method for grading the cognitive state of patients for the clinician." J Psychiatr Res 1975;12:189-198.
10. A Biderman, J Cwikel, A Fried, and D Galinsky, Depression and falls among community dwelling elderly people: a search for common risk factors, J Epidemiol Community Health. 2002 Aug; 56(8): 631– 636
11. EN 13606-2, Health informatics — Electronic health record communication — Part 2: Archetypes interchange specification
12. EN 13606-3, Health informatics — Electronic health record communication — Part 3: Reference archetypes and term lists
13. EN 13606-4, Health informatics — Electronic health record communication — Part 4: Security
14. prEN ISO 13606-5, Health informatics — Electronic health record communication — Part 5: Interface specifications
15. T. Beale, S. Heard, openEHR Architecture - Architecture Overview, 12 April 2007
16. T. Beale, S Heard, "Archetype Definitions and Principles", 14 March 2007

Particle Swarm Optimization Based Method for Personalized Menu Recommendations

V. Chifu, R. Bonta, E.St. Chifu, I. Salomie and D. Moldovan

Department of Computer Science, Technical University of Cluj-Napoca, Cluj-Napoca, Romania

Abstract— **This paper presents a Particle Swarm Optimization (PSO) based method for generating healthy daily menu recommendations for elder. In order to apply the PSO method to the case of generating menu recommendations, we have redefined the concepts of particle, position and velocity of the particle, as well as the formulae for updating the position and velocity of the particle. Additionally, to evaluate the quality of a particle (i.e. a solution), we have used a fitness function that has four components: the closeness to a nutritionist dietary recommendation, a price component, a delivery time component, and a diversity component that estimates of how diverse a daily recommendation is. The method proposed has been tested on a set of different user profiles.**

Keywords— **metaheuristics, personalized menu recommendations, fitness function.**

I. Introduction

Aging is joined by physiologic changes that can affect nutritional status in a harmful way. Sensory disability, for example diminished sense of taste and smell, occurs with aging, and it might bring about reduced appetite. Progressive loss of vision and hearing, as well as osteoarthritis, are factors that can constrain mobility and impact the elderly individual's capacity to shop for food and prepare meals. Poor oral health and dental problems are causes for chewing difficulties and inflammation. A monotonous, tedious diet that lacks quality further increases the risk of malnutrition. Alongside physiologic changes, the elderly may likewise experience significant psychosocial, as well as environmental changes, for example, isolation, loneliness, depression, and deficient finances. These influence the admission of the diet negatively, eventually affecting the nutritional status. Even if aging leads to less need for energy, the majority of the nutrients remain necessary. This increases the danger of malnutrition [5]. The interaction between nutrition and the insensible changes caused by aging leads to undernutrition [5]. Malnutrition can weak the mobility, the cognitive function, and the self-care ability [5]. The problem of healthy lifestyle recommendations has been approached by many researchers in their work [1, 2, 3, 4].

In this paper, we propose a Particle Swarm Optimization (PSO) based method for generating healthy daily menu recommendations for elder people according to the nutritional needs, the price, and the time of delivery specific for each older adult. The PSO based method creates a tailored nutritional menu recommendation for each user by gathering personal health information about the user. This includes information such as personal characteristics (weight, height, age, gender), information regarding the elder's health (previous diseases, chronic illnesses, family health history), and also personal dietary preferences (what types of food the elder likes or dislikes). Moreover, any allergies the user might have towards certain types of foods will be taken into account in order to avoid generating such recommendations, which would be harmful for the user. Extrinsic factors such as current dietary habits, level of physical activity and other lifestyle information will also be taken into account. The healthy daily menu recommendations will be generated based on a set of food offers available from different providers.

The paper is structured as follows. Section II presents the PSO based method for generating the personalized healthy menus, while Section III illustrates the experimental results. We end our paper with conclusions (Section IV).

II. PSO Based Method for Generating Personalized Healthly Menus

This section presents a short overview of the PSO metaheuristic as well as our PSO based approach for generating healthy personalized menu recommendations for older adults.

A. Overview of the PSO Metaheuristic

PSO [8] is a population based bio-inspired metaheuristic that iteratively tries to improve the population of particles (i.e. solutions) with regard to a given *measure of quality*. Each *particle* is moved around in the *search space* according to a set of mathematical formulae for updating the particle velocity and position. These formulae consider the local best position encountered by the particle until the current moment in time as well as the best position encountered at the level of swarm. Accordingly, we can say that the PSO metaheuristic has a learning component, since each particle is a self-organized agent, that learns from its previous successes and from the successes of the other particles.

The mathematical formula for updating the *position* of a particle is defined as follows:

S. Vlad and N.M. Roman (eds.), *International Conference on Advancements of Medicine and Health Care through Technology; 12th - 15th October 2016, Cluj-Napoca, Romania,*
IFMBE Proceedings 59,
DOI: 10.1007/978-3-319-52875-5_50

$$x_i^{t+1} = x_i^t + v_i^{t+1} \quad (1)$$

where x_i^t is the current position of the particle, and v_i^{t+1} is the new velocity of the particle.

The formula for the *velocity* of a particle is defined as:

$$v_i^{t+1} = a * v_i^t + b * (x_i^p - x_i^t) + c * (x_j^g - x_i^t) \quad (2)$$

where (i) v_i^t is the current velocity of the particle, (ii) x_i^p is the best position encountered so far by the particle, (iii) x_i^t is the current position of the particle, (iv) x_j^g is the best position encountered so far by a particle at the swarm level, and a, b, and c are scalar constants that weight the importance of each component part of the velocity formula.

B. Mapping the Concepts from PSO onto the Question of Generating Healthy Menu Recommendations

In the context of generating healthy meal recommendations, the *search space* consists of the entirety of meals offered by different providers. In our approach, the *search space* will be represented as an n-dimensional space, where meals will be points with n coordinates. Each coordinate will indicate the value of one of the n nutritional features that will be taken into consideration.

A point (i.e. a meal) in the *search space* is defined as:

$$P(x_1, x_2, ..., x_n) \quad (3)$$

where x_i represents the numeric value of nutritional feature number i as contained in the meal.

Moving on, we consider the representation of a particle (i.e. a solution) as a set of meals corresponding to the main meals of the day (breakfast, lunch, and dinner) and the two snacks.

$$Sol = \{meal_B, meal_{S1}, meal_L, meal_{S2}, meal_D\} \quad (4)$$

where $meal_B$ represents a meal containing a set of food items specific to the breakfast, $meal_L$ is specific to the lunch, $meal_D$ is the dinner, and $meal_{S1}$ and $meal_{S2}$ are meals containing a set of food items specific to the snacks.

A solution is also a point in the above-defined search space. It is specified as:

$$Sol(S_1, S_2, \ldots, S_n) \quad (5)$$

where $S_i = \sum_{M \in Meals} Mi$, i is the coordinate for nutritional feature number i, with M_i as the value on the ith dimension of meal M. Taking advantage of this n-dimensional space, we defined the distance between two points as a Euclidean distance between points in an n-dimensional space.

Also, the operators of *addition*, *subtraction*, and *multiplication* have been defined for this n-dimensional space, as they are used in Formulae 1 and 2. The differences and sums are simple vector differences and sums, and the multiplications are simple scalar-vector multiplications. More specifically, Formula 2 updates the velocity vector. This vector contains the information that is learned from the past and will guide the search onwards.

The *quality of a particle* (i.e. solution) is evaluated with a fitness function, FF, we previously introduced in [7], that takes into account four components: the closeness to the nutritionist dietary recommendations, the price component, the delivery time component, and the diversity component:

$$FF(sol) = c_1*FF_{REC}(sol) + c_2*FF_{PRICE}(sol) + c_3*FF_{TIME}(sol) + FF_{DIV}(sol) \quad (6)$$

The lower the numeric fitness function value the better, since it represents a deviation from standard, desired measures for the four different component criteria. In the formula above, c_1, c_2, and c_3 are constants representing the importance of the corresponding components of the fitness function, and $c_1 + c_2 + c_3 = 1$. The last component is not weighted by any constant, as it is designed like a penalty. Below we describe shortly each of these components.

The nutritional component of the fitness function evaluates the deviation of a solution from the diet recommended by the nutritionist. The price component will give a deviation of the total price of the solution from the amount the user is willing to pay. The time component will give a deviation of the total time necessary to prepare and deliver a daily menu (i.e. a solution) from the time during which the user is willing to wait for the menu.

The diversity component has been introduced now as an additional component to our previous definition of the fitness function in [7], in order to give an estimate of how diverse a daily recommendation is. This component has a range of [0, 1], where 0 means diverse and 1 means not diverse, and it takes into account three groups of foods that have proved to cause diversity issues:

$$FF_{DIV}(sol) = \text{Min}(1,\ VegDiv(sol)+FruDiv(sol)+OthDiv(sol)) \quad (7)$$

This component uses the number of times the three ingredients (mentioned as terms in the sum in Formula 7) occur throughout the solution, and not whether ingredients from each group occur in the solution or not.

$VegDiv(sol) = \text{Min}(1, \sum_{i=2}^{5} \text{NVO}i(\text{sol}) * \text{PNVO}i\,)$ gives an estimate for diversity from a vegetable point of view. $NVO_i(sol)$ gives the number of vegetables that occur i times in the solution, and $PNVO_i$ is the penalty for a number of vegetable occurrences equal to i. The terms $FruDiv(sol)$ and $OthDiv(sol)$ have a similar definition. They give an estimate from a fruit point of view and from a point of view of other ingredients that would make the user not want to accept the recommendation given (pasta, cheese, or eggs). Each of these three components is normalized to take values between 0 and

1, and so does the final result. No weights are used, because if a solution were not diverse for any of the components, the first impression the user would have is that the solution is not diverse overall.

C. The Particle Swarm Optimization Based Algorithm for Generating Healthy Menu Recommendations

The implementation of the PSO based Algorithm deviates a bit from the standard definition of the algorithm, as it is adapted for the needs of generating meal recommendations (see Algorithm 1). Each particle of the swarm has a solution attached (a recommendation of meals, which are correlated to the *position* attribute of the standard PSO). These particles move in an 11-dimensional space (one dimension for each nutritional feature). This movement is defined through the *velocity* attribute of a particle in the standard PSO. These two standard PSO attributes (position and velocity) have been adapted to our needs, and they are vectors of 11 values. Every dimension in the position vector represents the sum of the values of one distinct nutritional feature as collected from all the meals (see Formula 5). The values of the velocity vector help in changing the position vector and consequently in generating a new solution for the particle. At first, a swarm of particles is generated randomly, meaning that for each particle a random solution is generated. This generation process has five steps: for each meal of the recommendation (i.e. meal of the solution), a random meal is selected. After having the complete solution generated randomly, it is possible to compute the position vector by summation of the nutritional information on all the meals, according to Formula 5. The velocity vector is at first generated to hold random values. However, these random values are nutrient-specific, so each nutrient has to have its own possible starting range of values. The values were chosen high enough to ensure that the search space is explored (the particle presents inertia), but small enough not to search in areas that are too far away from what would be expected to be optimum. Each solution has a fitness value, computed by using the fitness function defined in Formula 6. The algorithm runs for a predefined number of iterations. At every iteration, each particle of the swarm updates its position. First, the velocity vector is updated according to Formula 2. Initially, the velocities are generated randomly: for each of the 11 components in the vector, a random value within a predefined interval is chosen. The values for the three weights (*a*, *b*, and *c*) are initially the same, namely 0.33. The meaning of the velocity vector is the information a particle can learn from its *personal best* and from the *swarm level best* (or *global best*). This information then has the ability to improve the solution of the particle and its position. At first, when the solution is far from the global best, this velocity vector will have greater values, and yet simply adding them to the position vector (see Formula 1) is not expected to bring the solution quickly towards the global best. After several iterations, the values of the velocity vector will decrease, as the particle gets closer, and this will help better search the space around the best solution.

Algorithm 1: Adapted Particle Swarm Optimization

Input: *searchS*, *popSize*, *noIt*, *velCompRanges*, *diffT*, *RestLimit*
Output: Solution
begin
Pop = **RandomPop**(*popSize*, *searchS*, *velCompRanges*)
BestOfIndividuals = *Pop*
sol_{opt} = **GetBestFitnessSol**(*Pop*)
i = 0
while(*i* < *noIt*) **do**
  foreach *p* **in** *Pop* **do**
    UOptimRandRestart(sol_{opt}, *RestLimit*, *noIt*, *p*, *diffT*, *searchS*)
    ULocalRandRestart(*p*, *RestLimit*, *noIt*, *searchS*)
    p = **Update_Velocity**(*p*, *BestOfIndividuals*[*p*], sol_{opt})
    p = **Update_Position**(*p*)
    p = **Find_Closest_Meal_To_Position**(*p*, *searchS*)
    p = **Update_Position**(*p*)
    if(**Fitness**(*p*) < **Fitness**(*BestOfIndividuals*[*p*])) **then**
      BestOfIndividuals[*p*] = *p*
      if(**Fitness**(*p*) < **Fitness**(sol_{opt})) **then**
        sol_{opt} = *p*
      endif
    endif
  endfor
i++
endwhile
return sol_{opt}
end

After the new velocity is computed (by Formula 2), a new menu recommendation (i.e. solution) must be generated. By knowing the fitness of each meal, we replace only the worst meal of the current recommendation, keeping the other four. Thus, each particle keeps information from the previous iterations and simply replaces only what it considers to be the worst. By adding the velocity to the position of the worst meal of the current recommendation (using Formula 1), a new reference point is generated. After computing this new reference position, a new meal must be generated to replace the worst one. This meal will be a meal of the type (breakfast, lunch, dinner, or snack) of the one to be replaced, it must not contain foods that the user is allergic to, and it will be the one which is the closest (in the search space) to the newly computed reference position. The distance in the search space will be judged as a Euclidean distance between two points in the n-dimensional search space, as mentioned in section II-B. After finding this new meal, the worst meal is replaced with it. However, the position point of the new meal does not coincide with the previously computed reference position. Consequently, the position of this new meal and the new position of the complete solution (containing all the five daily meals) are computed, and a new fitness is generated. In case the new recommendation (solution) is the best recommendation (i.e. having the lowest fitness value) at particle or swarm level, then it is necessary to update the data structures that keep the currently best solution.

By examining traces of the algorithm, it has been noticed that more often particles improve their solutions in the first half of the iterations of an algorithm run, and not only do they not find better solutions later on, they can remain stuck with a recommendation for a long period (stuck in a position of the search space). This usually happens for the solutions that do not hold the global best, so as from the velocity formula they are encouraged to change their solution and find a better one in their vicinity. By having a number of solutions stuck, the algorithm effectively loses computing power, sometimes by as much as half. There are two steps that have been taken to solve this issue. First, in order not to lose the computing power of the algorithm and still keep all the particles relevant, it was decided to perform a random restart on particles that are stuck in the search space. Random restart is inspired from Hill Climbing, where when a solution cannot seem to be possible to improve it is tried to generate a new random solution and improve on that one in order to find a better solution than the one discarded. This can apply greatly to our implementation as the algorithm keeps track of every particle best position encountered, so even if a worse position is generated and even with all the modifications applied to it a better solution would still not be found, the best position would still be known. The random restart has proven to be of help in this issue, as more than half of those particles that receive a random restart eventually improved their personal best positions. Improving personal bests of some particles that have been stuck does not directly result in improving the best solution found at swarm level, only that a better search is performed through the space. Another restarting step has been chosen, additional to the first one, this time a conditional random restart. This restart is performed only after a number of iterations has passed without the global best to be updated (exactly like in the case of the first random restart step, see parameter *RestLimit* in Algorithm 1). And this usually also happens in the later part of the algorithm run (like in the case of the first random restart step). This second random restart step is conditional as it potentially applies to all particles, with the condition that their fitness differs from the best fitness with a value greater than a certain threshold (see parameter *diffT* in Algorithm 1). This conditional random restarting step (i.e. the second restart step) has proved to be also helpful in better searching the space for solutions, and it frequently improves the personal best position of the individual particles and even the swarm level best.

III. Experimental Results

Testing and tracing the algorithm has proven a difficult task, because of the number of individuals in the population, their complex data, and the general non-determinism of the algorithm. The purpose was to check how individuals in the population react to each other, to see if they improve their solution, the frequency and power of the improvements, the correctness of the fitness function judged from the values of the individual fitness, the algorithm running time and possible causes for it, and the best configuration of the pair population size and number of iterations, so as to find a good balance between running time and quality of solution offered.

In order to analyze the best configuration of the pair population size and number of iterations, the values of both of them were varied and several runs were made in order to try and average out the randomness and unlikely behavior (either unusually good or unusually bad). For these tests, certain constants were left unchanged and changing them could also change the test results. The PSO specific constants used were: *vLowEnergy* = –100, *vHighEnery* = 100, *vLowProteins* = –10, *vHighPhroteins* = 10, *vLowCarbs* = –10, *vHighCarbs* =10, *vLowFats* = –10, *vHighFats* =10, *vLowCalcium* = –10, *vHighCalcium* =10, *vLowIron* = –0.5, *vHighIron* = 0.5, *vLowSodium* = –75, *vHighSodium* = 75, *vLowVitamin_a* = –10, *vHighVitamin_a* = 10, *vLowVitamin_b* = –0.5, *vHighVitamin_b* = 0.5, *vLowVitamin_c* = –5, *vHighVitamin_c* = 5, *vLowVitamin_d* = –0.5, and *vHighVitamin_d* = 0.5, representing the ranges for initial values of the velocity vector, *RestLimit* = 0.2, *diffT* = 0.35.

In what follows, we present how the population size and the number of iterations affect the fitness value as well as the execution time for the case of a user with allergies and a user without allergies.

For the user with allergies, the personal profile contains the following information: *age* = 61; *sex* = male, *height* = 180 cm, *weight* = 79 kg, *physical activity* = sedentary life-style, *diseases* = knee arthritis, *allergies* = dairy products. Also, he is willing to pay up to 50 lei for an entire day, he is willing to wait 45 minutes for meal delivery and 20 minutes for snack delivery. The most important aspect for this user is the time, followed by price. The recommended nutritional values as proposed by the nutritionist for this user are: 49.2-172.19 g proteins, 98.39-172.19 g lipids, 221.39-319.78 g carbohydrates, 1967.86 kcal, 1200 mg calcium, 8 mg iron, 1500 mg sodium, 900 mcg vitamin A, 15 mcg vitamin D, 90 mg vitamin C, 6.095 mg vitamin B6.

For analyzing the behavior of PSO, the population sizes considered were 15, 25, 35, and 50, with 20, 30, 40, and 50 iterations. For each of these combinations, a number of 50 tests have been run.

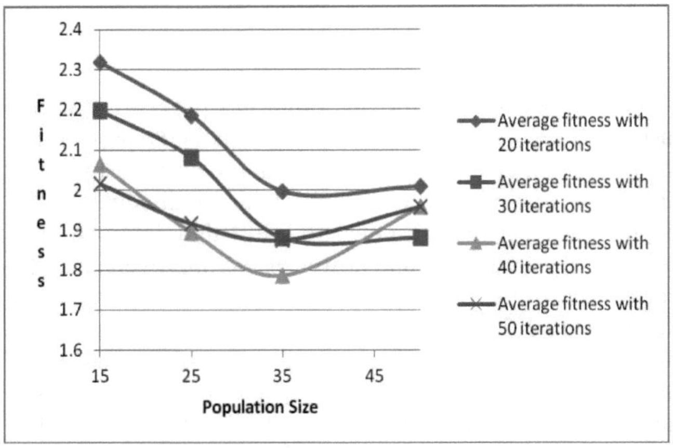

Fig. 1 Average fitness for the user with allergies

From Figure 1, it can be seen that increasing the population size generally improves the fitness of the solutions generated. However, this improvement tends to attenuate, or stop after reaching a certain population size (here approximately 35). This was consistent with all the numbers of iterations taken into consideration. Also, increasing the number of iterations generally improves the quality of solutions, as it is seen in the graphic above (Figure 1). However, there is still a level of randomness and indetermination present, as for the tests with 50 iterations the averages of solutions were not always the best. The best average from the graphic in Figure 1 has been found with a population of 35 and a number of 40 iterations. From Figure 2, it is noticeable that all the values of the execution time are approximately linearly variable with population size, and that increasing the number of iterations always increases the running time. For the first configuration, with only 20 iterations, the resulted values are remarkably smaller, and the level of random restarting is much smaller (particles do not get the chance to perform many time-consuming random restarts). Values under 20 seconds are only generated for a population size of 15 for all configurations, and up to a population size of 35 for 20 iterations. Values of up to 30 seconds also include all the configurations with 25 individuals and a population size of 35 with 30 iterations.

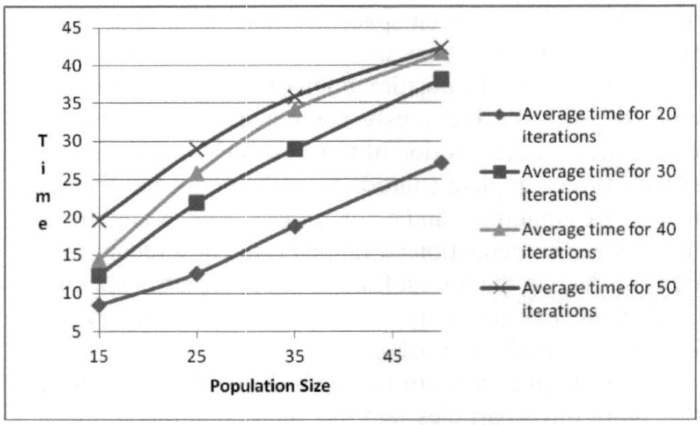

Fig. 2 Average execution time for the user with allergies

As a conclusion for user 1, the user with allergies, from a fitness point of view a population of 35 with 40 iterations yields the best results. However, this is done in an average time of 34 seconds. The second best configurations from a fitness point of view were 25 individuals with 40 iterations and 35 individuals with 30 iterations. Since the first of the two gave a better average time with almost 5 seconds better, this configuration would seem the best (25 seconds and 1.88 fitness).

For the user without allergies the pesonal profile contains the following information: *age* = 68, *sex* = female, *height* = 167 cm, *weight* = 62 kg, *lifesyle* = mild physical activity level, *diseases* = no disease. Also, she is willing to pay up to 45 lei for an entire day, she is willing to wait 30 minutes for meal delivery and 15 minutes for snack delivery. The most important aspect for this user is the price followed by the delivery time. The recommended nutritional values as proposed by the nutritionist for this user are: 43-149 g proteins, 85-149 g lipids, 191-276 g carbohydrates, 1702 kcal, 1200 mg calcium, 8 mg iron, 1500 mg sodium, 700 mcg vitamin A, 15 mcg vitamin D, 75 mg vitamin C, 6.095 mg vitmin B6. From Figure 3 we observe that the average solutions generally improve with the increasing population size. However, there is a certain level of randomness, as seen in the series for 30 iterations, where the average actually got worse. This is caused by the fact that, from time to time, the algorithm may remain stuck in a worse part of the search space, and not get out even with random restarts. So, one bad run actually made the average worse. It can also be seen that from a point, the population size is not relevant anymore, as it happened with the first two series. However, the last two series actually improved almost linearly. Also, it can be noticed that increasing the number of iterations generally improves the quality of the solutions. The values for 40 and 50 iterations were consistently good, with those for 50 iterations remarkably good. For this set of tests, the values for a combination of 50 individuals with 40 and 50 iterations clearly stand out as the best.

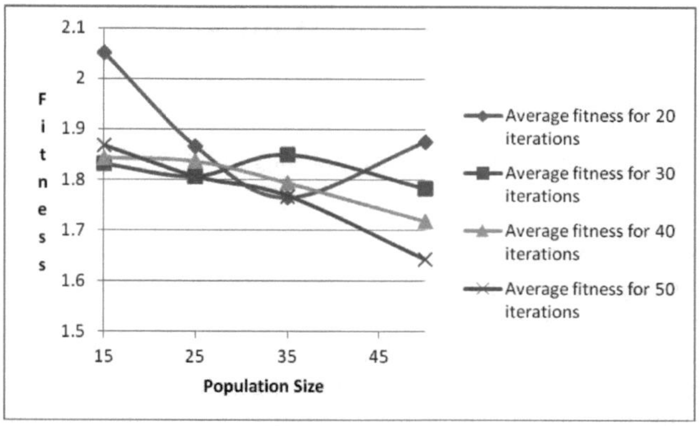

Fig. 3 Average fitness for the user without allergies

It's worth noting that the behavior is pretty much in line with that of the PSO used on a user with allergies, but the average fitness is a bit better.

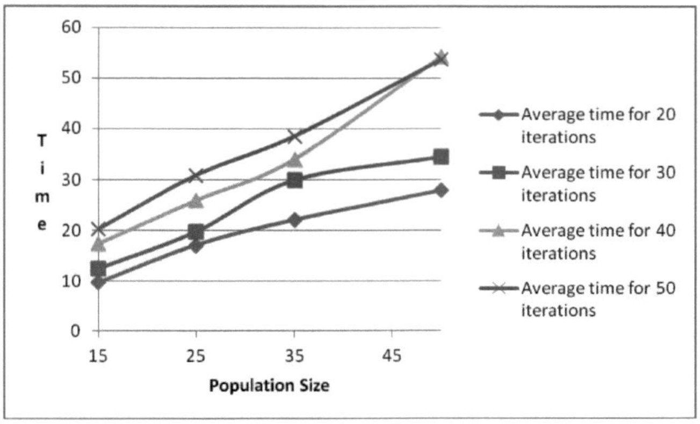

Fig. 4 Average execution time for the user without allergies

The first thing that is immediately noticeable is that increasing the number of iterations for a population size always results in a higher execution time (see Figure 4). Also, increasing the population size for a certain number of iterations always yields an increased execution time. The configurations that give an execution time of under 20 seconds are all configurations for a population of 15 individuals and 20 and 30 iterations for a population of 25. If the user is willing to wait 30 seconds generating a result, then all configurations for a population of 25 are viable and also the combination of 35 individuals with 20 and 30 iterations. It's worth noting that the average behavior is in line with that of PSO for a user with allergies, but with running times a bit worse. So, when it comes to choosing the best configuration, by taking into account both time and fitness of the result, this one would be with a population of 35 individuals and 30 iterations. Although the fitness was worse for that average, it was caused by an anomaly. The time for it is roughly 30 seconds. However, with 34 seconds, there is the much more reliable configuration with 40 iterations. As it can be seen from the graphs, even though using 50 individuals with at least 40 iterations gives significantly better results, they come with the cost of a significantly higher running time, over 50 seconds, mainly because of the higher number of random restarts. And even though the running time of a 20 iterations configuration is attractive, the results have shown to be rather poor.

IV. Conclusions

In this paper we have presented a PSO based method for generating healthy daily menu recommendations for elder people. In order to apply the PSO metaheuristic to the question of menu recommendation, we have redefined the concepts of particle, position, and velocity, as well as the formulae for adapting the position and velocity of a particle. Our method creates a tailored nutritional menu recommendation for each user by gathering personal health information about the user and by considering a set of food offers available from different providers.

Conflict of Interest

The authors declare that they have no conflict of interest.

References

1. J. Hoill, C. Kyungyong, Knowledge-based dietary nutrition recommendation for robese management, Information Technology Managemetn Journal, vol. 17, pp. 29–42, 2016.
2. L. Chang-Shing, M. Wang,and Shun-Teng Lan, Adaptive Personalized Diet Linguistic Recommendation Mechanism Based on Type-2 Fuzzy Sets and Genetic Fuzzy Markup Language, IEEE Transactions on Fuzzy Systems, vol. 23, no. 5, pp. 1777 – 1802, 2015.
3. M. I. V. Segismundo and B. Eleonor V. Comendador, Prenatal Nutrition Diet Generator Utilizing Modified Genetic Algorithm for Smartphone, Journal of Automation and Control Engineering, vol. 3, Issue 1, 2015.
4. S. F. Sufahani and Z. Ismail, Planning a Nutritious and Healthy Menu For Malaysian School Children Aged 13-18 Using "Delete-reshuffle Algorithm" in Binary Integer Programmin, Journal of Applied Sciences, vol. 15, pp. 1239-1244, 2015
5. http://www.mna-elderly.com/causes_of_malnutrition.html
6. http://www.mna-elderly.com/the_problem_malnutrition.html
7. C. Pop, V.R. Chifu, I. Salomie, D. Racz, R. Bonta, Hybridization of the Flower Pollination Algorithm – A Case Study in the Problem of Generating Healthy Nutritional Meals for Older Adults. Book Chapter in Nature Inspired Computation and Optimization, 2016, accepted for publication.
8. J. Kennedy, R. Eberhart, Particle Swarm Optimization, Proceedings of IEEE International Conference on Neural Networks. pp. 1942–1948, 1995.

Diet Generator for Elders using Cat Swarm Optimization and Wolf Search

D. Moldovan, P. Stefan, C. Vuscan, V. R. Chifu, I. Anghel, T. Cioara and I. Salomie

Technical University of Cluj-Napoca, Department of Computer Science, Cluj-Napoca, Romania

Abstract—**This paper addresses the problem of the generation of a recommendation of five healthy meals for the elders for an entire day by taking into consideration their nutritional constraints and their dietary restrictions. This problem is modeled as an optimization problem and is solved by using the Cat Swarm Optimization (CSO) and the Wolf Search (WS) algorithms. These two algorithms were integrated in an experimental prototype that allows the elders to order foods daily. Finally, a series of experiments were conducted in order to determine which algorithm leads to a combination of food packets that best matches the nutritional constraints imposed by the nutritionist and the older adult's preferences for nutrition, price, time and aspect.**

Keywords— **meals, diets, elders, Cat Swarm Optimization, Wolf Search.**

I. Introduction

One of the main problems related to the older population is represented by malnutrition [1]. Some of the features that influence the improper nutrition of the elders are the food's security, the ease of the food's acquisition, the nutritional status and the food intake. Malnutrition describes the state of being poorly nourished and some of its causes are the lack of some nutrients or the excess of other nutrients [2]. There is a correlation between malnutrition in elderly and some factors such as the impossibility to use public transportation, the inability to shop, and the distance between the markets and the elders' houses [3]. In the majority of the cases, malnutrition represents a direct consequence of the imbalance of the nutrients.

In order to prevent malnutrition, we want to solve the following problem: given the ideal nutritional values that an elder should consume during a day and his food preferences, we want to determine which combination of meals from a predefined set of meals that can be consumed during breakfast, brunch, lunch, snack or dinner, is closer to the ideal nutritional values recommended by the nutritionist and to the food preferences of the elder. An exhaustive approach which generates all the possible combinations of meals is impossible in real time and an alternative approach is to use bio-inspired algorithms that find a near optimal solution faster.

In this paper we propose the use of two algorithms CSO [4] and WS [5] for the generation of a recommendation of five meals for an entire day for an elder. The motivation for applying these algorithms is represented by the fact that they present many similarities as they belong to the same class of bio-inspired algorithms (e.g. the swarm intelligence algorithms) and they are the only swarm intelligence algorithms that use the characteristics of the quadruped predator mammals according to the classification of the algorithms presented in [6].

The rest of the paper is organized as follows. Section II presents related work. Section III presents the definition of our problem. Section IV describes the mapping of the CSO algorithm to the proposed optimization problem, while Section V describes the mapping of the WS algorithm to the proposed optimization problem. Section VI describes the experimental prototype used for experiments as well as the experimental results. We end our paper with conclusions.

II. Related Work

This section presents the state of the art in the field of generating healthy lifestyle recommendations.

One approach for the generation of the diets for the elders is presented in [7] and it consists in the use of Genetic Algorithms (GA). The approach uses a database of foods and generates a recommendation of five meals for each day of the week.

A method for the composition of diets for patients suffering from kidney and urinary tract diseases is presented in [8]. The method uses a genetic fuzzy approach which combines fuzzy logic and genetic algorithms.

Another proposed method for the optimization of the diets is represented by the Quantum Genetic Algorithm (QGA) [9]. In their experiments, the authors show that the diet optimization method based on QGA gives better results than the traditional algorithms and the Genetic Algorithm (GA). Some of the advantages of the QGA are the small size of the population, the excellent diversity of the population and the high searching efficiency.

The Bayesian Optimization Algorithm (BOA) was applied by the authors of the paper [10] to the problem of nutrition for breakfast. Compared to other approaches such as Linear Programming and Genetic Algorithm, the BOA gives better results. The Bayesian Optimization Algorithm repeats four steps until the termination criteria are met. First, using a GA selection method, the good solutions are

S. Vlad and N.M. Roman (eds.), *International Conference on Advancements of Medicine and Health Care through Technology; 12th - 15th October 2016, Cluj-Napoca, Romania*,
IFMBE Proceedings 59,
DOI: 10.1007/978-3-319-52875-5_51

selected from the current population. Second, a Bayesian network is built based on these solutions. Third, the new candidate solutions are generated using the Bayesian network built at the previous step. Fourth, the new candidate solutions are integrated in the old population by replacing some of the old solutions.

III. Problem Definition

The structure of the problem is described next. The *optimal solution* is uniquely determined by the preferences of the elder and the nutritional constraints and in most of the cases it is not present in the search space. The set of all *feasible solutions* is represented by all combinations of five meals, one for each part of the day, from a finite set of meals which contains 101 breakfast meals, 112 brunch meals, 2001 lunch meals, 112 snack meals and 429 dinner meals. The number of *feasible solutions* is equal with the product of the cardinalities of these sets which is equal with 1087581470976. For each of these feasible solutions, a fitness score is computed based on the distance from the *optimal solution*. The fitness function will be detailed in the next paragraphs. The *near optimal solution* is a solution from the set of the *feasible solutions* which is the closest to the *optimal solution*, or in other words which has the best fitness score. The objective of the problem is to determine a solution from the set of *feasible solutions* which is close to the *optimal solution*. The solution representation and the solution evaluation are adapted after the ones presented in [11].

A brief description of a solution is presented in Figure 1. A solution consists of five food packets, one for each part of the day: breakfast, brunch, lunch, snack and dinner.

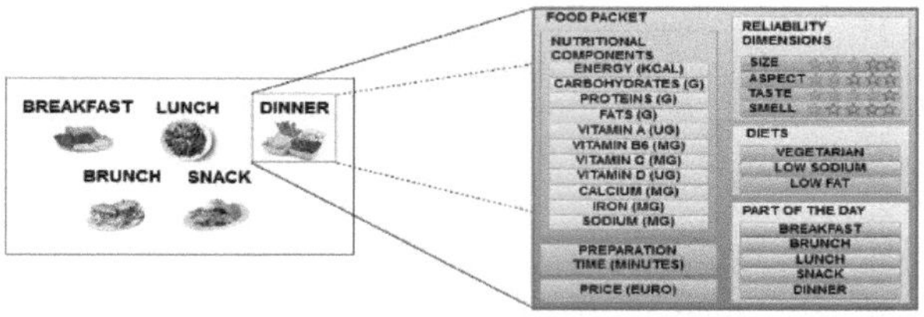

Fig. 1 A visualization of the concepts that are involved in the representation of a solution

A baseline solution, or an *optimal solution*, is uniquely determined by the preferences of the elder for several dimensions such as price, preparation time and reliability and by the nutritional restrictions that describe how many macronutrients the elder should consume during a day. In our approach we propose a fitness function that is proportional with the distance between the *candidate solution* and the *optimal solution*. By minimizing the distance between the two solutions, we aim to obtain an optimal solution.

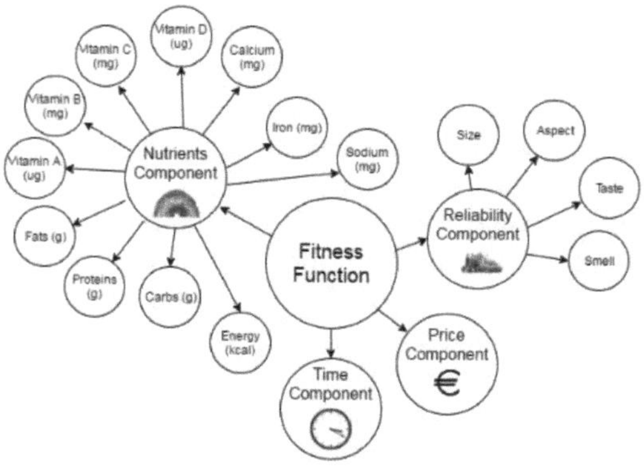

Fig. 2 Solution evaluation

A visual description of the components considered in the evaluation of a solution can be seen in Figure 2. The fitness function for a solution is computed as a weighted average of the fitness functions of the following four components: time component, price component, reliability component and nutrients component.

The interpretation of the fitness function used to evaluate the quality of a solution is the following: if the value is small then the solution is closer to the optimal solution and if the value is large then the solution is farther from the optimal solution. The weights assigned to the components are proportional with the importance of the components in the overall computation of the fitness function.

The mathematical equations used for the determination of the optimal values of the nutrients that an elder should consume during a day are taken from [12], [13] and [14]. The formulas take as input the gender, the weight, the height and the Physical Activity Factor (PAF) of the elder and return the optimal values for each of the eleven nutrients that describe a food packet that the elder should consume during a day.

IV. Mapping of the Cat Swarm Optimization Algorithm to the Proposed Optimization Problem

This section presents the mapping of the Cat Swarm Optimization algorithm to the proposed optimization problem for the generation of a recommendation of five healthy meals for an elder based on his preferences and on the nutritional restrictions. The proposed optimization problem is presented in the previous section. The first subsection maps the concepts of the CSO algorithm to the proposed optimization problem and the second subsection presents the adapted version of the CSO algorithm to the proposed optimization problem.

A. Mapping of the CSO Concepts to the Proposed Optimization Problem

The CSO algorithm [4] models the behavior of the cats into two modes: the seeking mode and the tracing mode. In our model, the cats have been replaced by menus. The *seeking mode* models the cat during the rest and the *tracing mode* models the cat in tracing targets.

Seeking mode – This mode has four main parameters which are mentioned as follows: seeking memory pool (SMP), seeking range of the selected dimension (SRD), contents of dimension to change (CDC), and MR which is a random number from [0,1].

Tracing mode – This mode is the second mode of the algorithm. The parameters of the tracing mode are:

1. r_1 – a random variable from [0,1]
2. c_1 – a constant which has the value 2 in the experiments

Table 1 presents the mapping of the main concepts of the CSO algorithm to our optimization problem.

Table 1 Mapping of the Cat Swarm Optimization Algorithm to our Optimization Problem

CSO Concepts	Concepts from our Optimization Problem
Cat	A menu that consists of five meals
Position	An 11-dimensional vector with values for each nutrition component
Velocity	An 11-dimensional vector with values for each nutrition component
Seeking Mode	A sequence of procedures that imitates the slow and conservative movement of the cats
Tracing Mode	A sequence of procedures that imitates the movement of tracing the prey

B. Adapted Version of the CSO Algorithm to the Proposed Optimization Problem

The adapted version of the Cat Swarm Optimization algorithm (see Algorithm 1) determines the best combination of five meals that meet the preferences of an older adult and the nutrition restrictions imposed by the nutritionist.

The algorithm takes as input the search space which is represented as a set of food offers, the personal profile of the elder, the number of cats that compose the swarm, the number of iterations to run the algorithm, the mutation ratio which specifies how many food packets are in the seeking mode and how many food packets are in the tracing mode and the dietary recommendations for the eleven nutrients that characterize the food packets. Initially, the swarm of cats is generated randomly. For each menu from the swarm, the position and the velocity are initialized randomly. Then, while the number of iterations is less than a specified value, some menus from the swarm are set to tracing mode and the others to seeking mode. If the menu is in seeking mode then based on the previous visited positions, its position and velocity are updated by replacing the worst meal from the five meals that compose the menu with another meal. Else, if the menu is in tracing mode then the velocity is updated using the constants r_1 and c_1 and then the menu updates its position using the new velocity.

Algorithm 1: Cat Swarm Optimization

```
Input: foodOffers, personalProfile, noOfCats,
  noOfIterations, MR, dietaryRecommendation
Output: dailyMenu_optimal
begin
  swarm = GenerateCatsRandomly(noOfCats,
    foodOffers, personalProfile,
    dietaryRecommendation)
  foreach menu in swarm do
    InitializePosition(menu)
    InitializeVelocity(menu)
  end foreach
  dailyMenu_optimal =
    GetMenuWithMinFitnessValue(swarm)
  do
    SetModeAccordingToMR(swarm)
    foreach menu in swarm do
      if menu.SeekingMode() then
        ComputeSeekingModeFlags(menu)
        copies =
          MakeSMPCopiesOfWorstPacket(menu)
        foreach copy in copies do
          RandomlyModifyPos(CDC, SRD, copy)
          ComputeFS(copy, personalProfile)
          ComputeProbabilityToChoose(copy)
        end foreach
        ReplaceWorstPacketByProbability(menu,
          copies)
        ComputeMenuFS(menu, personalProfile)
        ReplaceSolOptIfItIsBetterOne(menu,
          dailyMenu_optimal)
      else if menu.TracingMode() then
        packet = GetWorstPacket(menu)
        UpdateVelocity(packet, menu, searchSpace)
        UpdatePosition(packet, menu, searchSpace)
        ComputeMenuFS(menu, personalProfile)
        ReplaceSolOptIfItIsBetterOne(menu,
          dailyMenu_optimal)
      end if
    end foreach
    noOfIterations = noOfIterations - 1
  while noOfIterations > 0
  return dailyMenu_optimal
end
```

V. Mapping of the Wolf Search Algorithm to the Proposed Optimization Problem

This section presents the mapping of the Wolf Search algorithm to the proposed optimization problem for the generation of a recommendation of five healthy meals for an elder based on his preferences and on the nutritional restrictions. The proposed optimization problem is described in Section III. The first subsection maps the concepts of the WS algorithm to the proposed optimization problem and the second subsection presents the adapted version of the WS algorithm to the proposed optimization problem.

A. Mapping of the WS Concepts to the Proposed Optimization Problem

Table 2 presents the mapping of the main concepts of the WS algorithm [5] to our optimization problem.

Table 2 Mapping of the Wolf Search Algorithm to our Optimization Problem

WS Concepts	Concepts from our Optimization Problem
Wolf	A menu that consists of five meals
Position	An 11-dimensional vector with values for each nutrition component
Hunter	If the value generated by a random numbers generator exceeds a threshold then the menu is replaced with a menu outside of the visual range
Prey initiatively	The current menu is replaced with a better menu from the visual range centered in the current menu
Prey passively	The current menu "moves" towards the best neighbor menus from the visual range
Escape	The current menu is replaced with a new menu which is outside the visual range

B. Adapted Version of the WS Algorithm to the Proposed Optimization Problem

The adapted version of the Wolf Search algorithm (see Algorithm 2) determines the best combination of five meals that meet the preferences of an older adult and the nutrition restrictions imposed by the nutritionist.

The input data for the algorithm is represented by the search space which contains a set of food offers, the personal profile of the elder, the number of wolves, the number of iterations to run the algorithm, the hunter's threshold which is used to determine whether a menu enters the escape mode or not, the visual range of the menus and a minimum value used if the wolf enters the escape mode. First, each menu is initialized to a random location. Then, while the number of iterations is less than the threshold of the iterations, for each of the menus a new location is generated. If the fitness of the new generated menu is better than the old fitness value then the current menu is updated. If there are neighbors in the visual range that have better fitness values than the fitness of the menu then the menu is moved towards the neighbor with the best fitness. Finally, if the number generated by the number generator is greater than the hunter's threshold then the menu is moved to a random position outside the visual range.

Algorithm 2: Wolf Search

```
Input: foodOffers, personalProfile,
  noOfWolves, noOfIterations, visualRange,
hunterThreshold, minValue
Output: dailyMenu_optimal
begin
 wolves =
  GenerateWolvesRandomly(noOfWolves,
   foodOffers, personalProfile,
   dietaryRecommendation)
 foreach wolf in wolves do
  InitializePosition(wolf)
 end foreach
 dailyMenu_optimal =
  GetMenuWithMinFitnessValue(wolves)
 time = 0
 while time < noOfIterations do
  for i = 1 to noOfWolves do
   wolf_i = GenerateNewLocation(wolf_i)
   if ComputeMenuFS(wolf_i, personalProfile)
    < ComputeMenuFS(dailyMenu_optimal,
   personalProfile) then
    dailyMenu_optimal = wolf_i
   end if
   wolf_j = GetNeighborWithBestFitnessValue(
    wolf_i, wolves)
   if Distance(wolf_i, wolf_j) < visualRange and
     ComputeMenuFS(wolf_j, personalProfile)
     < ComputeMenuFS(wolf_i, personalProfile)
    wolf_i moves to wolf_j
   end if
   randomNumber = GenerateRandom(0,1)
   if randomNumber > thresholdNumber then
    ChangePositionRandomly(wolf_i)
   end if
  end for
  time = time + 1
 end while
 return dailyMenu_optimal
end
```

VI. Experimental Results

This section presents the architecture of the experimental prototype used for our experiments as well as the experimental results obtained by running the proposed algorithms.

A. Experimental Prototype

The architecture of the experimental prototype in Figure 3.

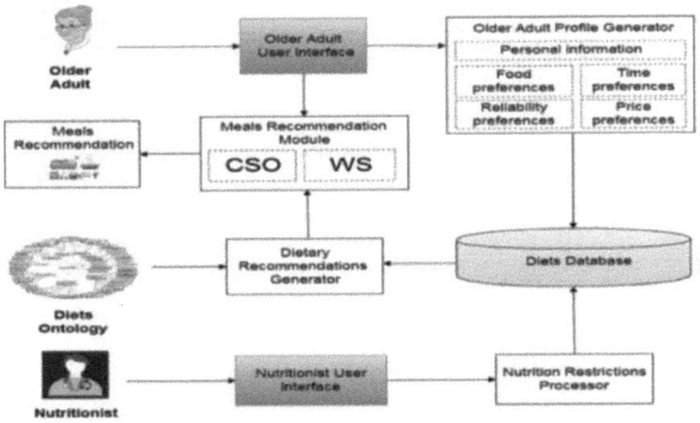

Fig. 3 The architecture of the experimental prototype

The two main actors of the system are the nutritionists and the elders. The *Diets Database* contains around 2755 food packages which are classified according to the part of the day to which they correspond (e.g. breakfast, brunch, lunch, snack, dinner). The nutritionist uses the *Nutritionist User Interface* to insert nutritional recommendations for the older adults.

B. Experimental Prototype

In order to test our proposed algorithms we used the profiles of ten users which are described in Table 3 and Table 4. The search space is composed from around 2755 food packages which correspond to the different parts of the day. The weights used in the fitness function are the following: breakfast weight (0.2), brunch weight (0.1), lunch weight (0.35), snack weight (0.1), dinner weight (0.25), nutritional weight (0.5), price weight (0.3), time weight (0.15) and reliability weight (0.05). For the reported results five repeats are considered for each combination which consists from a user profile and an algorithm configuration. The input parameter values of the two methods (e.g. the number of iterations, the number of wolves, the number of cats, etc.) are hardcoded and thus the end user of the application cannot change them. In this approach the users cannot express their approval or disapproval as concerns the results and there is no correlation between their opinion and the way the fitness function is defined.

Table 3 User profiles used for the testing of the algorithms

User	Gender	Age	Height (cm)	Weight (cm)	PAF
user1	male	74	176	79	1.2
user2	female	74	167	62	1.375
user3	female	69	163	78	1.55
user4	female	65	166	65	1.2
user5	male	69	179	85	1.375
user6	male	75	180	78	1.55
user7	male	68	195	97	1.2
user8	female	44	167	67	1.3
user9	male	74	170	66	1.2
user10	female	68	157	71	1.375

Table 4 User preferences used for the testing of the algorithms

User	Time (minutes)	Price (euro)	Aspect	Smell	Taste	Size
user1	65	70	1	2	4	3
user2	90	50	3	2	4	1
user3	60	70	2	3	4	1
user4	50	30	2	3	4	1
user5	45	35	4	2	3	1
user6	60	42	2	4	3	1
user7	40	25	2	4	1	3
user8	40	30	4	3	1	2
user9	65	70	1	2	4	3
user10	90	50	3	2	4	1

Next, by running a series of experiments we try to determine which combination of adjustable parameters such as the number of iterations, the number of cats, and the MR (Mutation Ratio) gives the better average results for the CSO. We used ten different possible configurations described in Table 5. Table 6 presents the average execution time and Table 7 presents the average score which are obtained after running the CSO algorithm five times for each user.

Table 5 CSO Parameters Configuration

Configuration ID	Number of iterations	Number of cats	MR
1	25	50	12%
2	25	50	25%
3	25	80	20%
4	25	80	40%
5	25	80	60%
6	50	50	12%
7	50	50	25%
8	50	80	20%
9	50	80	40%
10	50	80	60%

Table 6 Average execution time (milliseconds) obtained after running CSO five times for each user for each configuration

	C1	C2	C3	C4	C5	C6	C7	C8	C9	C10
U1	284	548	439	773	1042	387	776	502	993	1637
U2	214	426	279	460	886	298	574	456	976	1435
U3	170	280	257	517	847	305	581	353	1101	1508
U4	201	321	269	573	789	309	622	475	810	1349
U5	130	345	227	585	1000	276	624	421	858	1521
U6	201	408	283	536	767	252	656	354	992	1107
U7	142	402	258	475	853	286	605	405	783	1469
U8	139	376	251	592	663	211	573	422	943	1198
U9	149	300	225	516	734	275	529	339	1045	1152
U10	136	339	266	434	1159	249	535	338	668	1385

Table 7 Average fitness score obtained after running CSO five times for each user for each configuration

	C1	C2	C3	C4	C5	C6	C7	C8	C9	C10
U1	.34	.30	.33	.35	.36	.43	.34	.33	.40	.31
U2	.26	.30	.31	.32	.32	.27	.24	.29	.25	.24
U3	.41	.47	.43	.40	.37	.34	.41	.42	.28	.31
U4	.76	.65	.64	.63	.63	.67	.66	.64	.61	.61
U5	.59	.59	.66	.45	.43	.51	.47	.60	.51	.47
U6	.50	.38	.38	.29	.47	.43	.36	.38	.26	.41
U7	.91	.83	.82	.74	.69	.77	.85	.72	.87	.64
U8	.70	.67	.73	.65	.83	.78	.71	.74	.62	.63
U9	.41	.40	.41	.41	.37	.76	.37	.36	.27	.31
U10	.35	.26	.31	.36	.19	.33	.28	.32	.34	.30

The following tables show which combination of parameters such as the number of iterations, the number of wolves and the hunter's threshold (HT) gives the better average results for the WS algorithm. Table 8 presents the configurations used in the experiments, Table 9 presents the average execution time and Table 10 presents the average score which are obtained after running the WS algorithm five times for each user.

Table 8 WS Parameters Configuration

Configuration ID	Number of iterations	Number of wolves	HT
1	1000	2	25%
2	1000	2	50%
3	1000	5	25%
4	1000	5	50%
5	1000	5	75%
6	5000	2	25%
7	5000	2	50%
8	5000	5	25%
9	5000	5	50%
10	5000	5	75%

Table 9 Average execution time (milliseconds) obtained after running WS five times for each user for each configuration

	C1	C2	C3	C4	C5	C6	C7	C8	C9	C10
U1	450	541	701	572	584	498	516	823	703	642
U2	408	420	545	558	573	387	406	549	535	580
U3	395	404	593	552	511	421	355	559	535	496
U4	391	351	558	532	520	335	363	509	512	520
U5	476	348	542	507	471	392	356	555	516	550
U6	358	352	629	526	538	390	357	617	523	530
U7	400	324	523	475	543	350	338	506	476	507
U8	376	349	511	556	502	367	343	487	496	492
U9	377	356	515	502	481	347	337	534	518	464
U10	368	402	575	484	427	361	334	450	456	531

Table 10 Average fitness score obtained after running WS five times for each user for each configuration

	C1	C2	C3	C4	C5	C6	C7	C8	C9	C10
U1	.64	.68	.70	.69	.68	.81	.16	.58	.52	.59
U2	.88	.90	.65	.79	.79	.96	.80	.66	.79	.65
U3	.96	1.0	.64	.80	.81	.77	2.1	.77	.67	.83
U4	1.5	1.4	.98	1.1	1.1	1.0	1.2	1.1	1.0	1.1
U5	1.5	1.1	.93	.99	1.0	1.0	1.1	1.1	1.1	.97
U6	1.0	1.1	.72	.83	.81	.88	.98	.66	.74	.62
U7	1.3	2.1	1.2	1.2	1.3	1.4	1.4	1.4	1.3	1.2
U8	1.6	1.1	1.0	1.1	1.3	1.6	1.4	1.3	1.2	1.2
U9	.62	.82	.73	.63	.75	.81	.92	.64	.69	.61
U10	.94	.75	.77	.67	.61	.83	.82	.62	.81	.70

VII. Conclusions

We presented two algorithms to solve the problem of the generation of healthy meals for the elders by taking into consideration their nutritional constraints, dietary restrictions and preferences. The two algorithms are the Cat Swarm Optimization (CSO) algorithm and the Wolf Search (WS) algorithm. Compared to other methods such as the exhaustive search and the random search, these algorithms provide a near optimal solution in less than two seconds. As can be seen from the experimental results, the adapted WS algorithm has an overall better execution time while the adapted CSO algorithm provides better results in terms of the fitness function.

Conflict of Interest

The authors declare that they have no conflict of interest.

References

1. Hoddinot J, Rosegrant M, Torero M (2012) Hunger and malnutrition. Global Copenhagen Consensus 1-69
2. Hickson M (2006) Malnutrition and ageing. Postgrad Med J 82(693):2-8
3. Donini L, Scardella P, Piombo L, Neri B, Asprino R, Proietti A, Carcaterra S, Cava E, Cataldi S, Cucinotta D, Bella G D, Barbagallo M, Morrone A (2013) Malnutrition in elderly: Social and economic determinants. The Journal of Nutrition, Health & Ageing 17(1):9-15
4. Tsai P W, Istanda V (2013) Review on Cat Swarm Optimization Algorithms. 3rd International Conference on Consumer Electronics, Communications and Networks (CECNet) 564-567
5. Tang R, Fong S, Yang X S, Deb S (2012) Wolf Search Algorithm with Ephemeral Memory. 2012 Seventh International Conference on Digital Information Management (ICDIM) 165-172
6. Fister I, Yang X-S, Fister I, Brest J, Fister D (2013) A Brief Review of Nature-Inspired Algorithms for Optimization. Elektrotehniski vestnik 80(3):1-7
7. Catalan-Salgado E-A, Zagal-Flores R, Torres-Fernandez Y, Paz-Nieves A (2014) Diet Generator Using Genetic Algorithms. Research in Computer Science (75):71-77
8. Hartati S, 'Uyun S (2011) Computation of Diet Composition for Patients Suffering from Kidney and Urinary Tract Diseases with the Fuzzy Genetic System. International Journal of Computer Applications (0975-8887) 36(6):38-45
9. Youbo L (2009) Multi-Objective Nutritional Diet Optimization Based on Quantum Genetic Algorithm. 2009 Fifth International Conference on Natural Computation 4:336-340
10. Gumustekin S, Senel T, Cengiz M (2014) A Comparative Study on Bayesian Optimization Algorithm for Nutrition Problem. Journal of Food and Nutrition Research 2(12):952-958
11. Pop C B, Chifu V R, Salomie I, Racz D S, Bonta R M (2016) Hybridization of the Flower Polination Algorithm – A Case Study in the Problem of Generating Healthy Nutritional Meals for Older Adults. Nature Inspired Computation and Optimization (NICO), 2016, accepted for publication
12. Wikipedia at https://en.wikipedia.org/wiki/Dietary_Reference_Intake
13. "Macronutrients: the Importance of Carbohydrate, Protein, and Fat", McKINLEY HEALTH CENTER University of Illinois at Urbana Champaign at http://mckinley.illinois.edu/handouts/macronutrients.htm
14. DIET4Elders AAL Project at www.diet4elders.eu

Author: Dorin Moldovan
Institute: Technical University of Cluj-Napoca
Street: 26 Baritiu
City: Cluj-Napoca
Country: Romania
Email: dorin.moldovan@cs.utcluj.ro

Telemonitoring Systems and Technologies for Independent Life of Elderly

S.B. Sebesi, H.L. Groza and D. Mândru

Faculty of Mechanical Engineering, Department of Mechatronics and Machine Dynamics,
Technical University of Cluj-Napoca, Cluj-Napoca, Romania

Abstract— **The population aging is tending to become one of the most significant social challenges of the 21st century. In this ageing period maintaining independents and good health for as long as possible is essential. Using telemonitoring technologies in home environment is still under development, but this method appears to be one of the most promising approaches to facilitate independent living for elderly. With the current technology, it is possible to implement solutions that until recently seemed to be a distant vision of the future and it provides new opportunities for diagnosis, prevention, education, treatment, rehabilitation, and also improve the quality of life. This paper brings an overview of some solutions presented in literature as well as our own concept of telemonitoring system.**

Keywords— **telemonitoring, elderly, independent life, safety technologies**

I. Introduction

The word population is growing by 1.18% per year (ten years ago this growing rate was 1.24 % per year) that means an additional 83 million people annually. The aging of the word population is a noticeable fact in every country in the world. Between 2015 and 2030 globally, the projected grow of the number of people with age 60 years or over is 56%. That means an increase from 901 million to 1.4 billion, and this number is projected to reach nearly 2.1 billion by 2050.

According to the predictions in 2050 the 44% of the world's population will live in aged countries, with at least 20% of the population aged 60 years or over [1].

The trend mentioned above suggests that there will be less people to care for elderly. This problem is aggravated by the fact that elderly place proportionally greater demands on health services than any other population group (outside of newborn babies). Based on the above mentioned information we can predict that the use of technology will be required to create an efficient and safety healthcare delivery systems [2].

There are many issues associated with ageing that societies need to develop strategies for, and the healthcare systems are already under pressure in most countries. Such a solution to solve this issue can be a real-time monitoring system, which allow monitoring elderly people in the environment of their choice and can provide the possibility of independent living. Telemonitoring systems also can lead to a significant healthcare cost reduction, by avoiding unnecessary hospitalization and ensuring that those who need urgent care can receive it in time [2].

Under the above presented circumstances, it is obvious that the elderly population will at some point face the incapacity of society to offer them decent living and medical conditions.

II. Characteristics of Telemonitoring Systems and Technologies

First time the telemonitoring technology was utilized in 1960 by NASA when physiological parameters were monitorized from the astronaut's space suits [3].

The most commonly used technologies for telemonitoring systems are: sensors (vital and other type), motion detectors, wireless technologies to detect changes in behavior, safety monitoring devices etc.

One of the biggest advantages of using telemonitoring systems are that allows the elderly to remain both independent and autonomous. While they are remaining on their own homes valuable information regarding the vital signs, falls, motion etc. can be recorded and passed to the "caregiver" who can take immediate action if needed.

The current telemonitoring technology has the potential to provide the elderly a better access to information, support, care and other services.

According to our research, the current technologies are classified in two big subcategories: active and passive systems and both have significant advantages and drawbacks.

One of the biggest difference between the passive and active telemonitoring systems is the human interaction with the system. The active systems require "user knowledge" how to use and in some situation interact with the system while the passive systems don't require this type on knowledge/interaction.

A passive telemonitoring system refers to embedded sensors in the home environment. The main purpose of the embedded sensors is to provide information regarding the elderly people's activities of daily life, fall detection, bed monitoring, etc. The recorded information is passed to a data manager in which analysis is done automatically to determine if medical attention is needed or not [4].

S. Vlad and N.M. Roman (eds.), *International Conference on Advancements of Medicine and Health Care through Technology; 12th - 15th October 2016, Cluj-Napoca, Romania*,
IFMBE Proceedings 59,
DOI: 10.1007/978-3-319-52875-5_52

One of the biggest disadvantages of using passive sensors is, at times may lead to potentially false alerts or may fail to alert a medical professional when needed.

An active telemonitoring system refers to the elderly's interaction with technology that records, information regarding their vital signs (ex. blood pressure, pacemaker parameters, heart rate, etc.), blood glucose level, pulse oximetry, spirometry, and respiratory rate etc. and send this information to a care-giving center. The active telemonitoring systems can also serve as an interface between caregivers and elderly peoples.

Among the advantages of using active telemonitoring, systems can be mentioned: the possibility to remind the elderly of such tasks as when to take their medicine, the need to keep legs elevated while sitting and also daily monitoring of critical signs.

The use of telemonitoring systems, either through active or passive technologies have been shown extremely useful in improving the quality of life and the possibility of reducing hospitalization.

For elderly peoples living with special health issues (congestive heart failure, diabetes, pulmonary disease, etc.) the use of telemonitoring systems can transfer data on real time basis and identify plus treat problems by triggering adjustment in care before they reach the critic stage [5].

III. Telemonitoring systems

Telemonitoring systems give us new opportunities for diagnosis, treat, educate, and take care of users from distance, besides ensuring their independent and autonomous life.

According to our research for elderly generation independent and safely living is essential:

(1) to track vital signs;

(2) to detect non-medical emergencies;

(3) to track activities of daily living (safety and security point of view)

(1) Tracking of vital signs

As a result of the technology development nowadays many vital signs can be "telemonitorize" successfully. According to our research currently, one of the most investigated area for vital signs monitoring is measuring cardiovascular activities. Research has been performed into monitoring: heart rate, blood pressure, pacemaker parameters etc.

Another well-researched area of vital signs tracking is to measure aspects of metabolism like: blood glucose, blood temperature, blood ethanol, blood lactate, physical exercise, stage of sleep etc. Also has been developed measuring equipment to telemonitorize hematologic systems as well as respiratory systems like: pulse oximetry, spirometry, respiratory rate, etc [6].

(2) *Detecting non-medical emergencies*

With non-medical emergencies we refer to situations which require immediate care but which occurrence cannot be anticipated forwardly, and of which required care does not concern special medical knowledge (as an example falling and wandering incidents fall into this category).

(3) *Monitoring activities of daily living*

As it has been mentioned earlier as a results of technology development numerous systems have been developed for gathering data on activities of daily living: vision systems, systems based on accelerometers, localization systems, infrared motion sensors, other network of sensors etc. Once the data on the activity of daily living has been gathered, the information is subsequently utilized by pattern recognition methods for classification of the activity that was observed (any deviation to the recognized pattern can be a sign of a risky situation) [7].

IV. Contribution for elderly independent and safely life

In the following pages we are going to presents a telemonitoring system concept based on our research on this domain. The main objective of this project is to develop a universal, user-oriented telemonitoring system to allow elderly to extend the time in which they can live at home, surrounded by their own comforts and their loved ones.

As it has been mentioned, according to our research for the elderly independent and safety living is crucial the surveillance of: vital signs, emergency situations, and daily activities.

The communication between the modules is planned to be based on standard protocols and coding systems.

Emergency module- the signals/datas are transferred to the local server via cable connection. In case of unexpected situation appearance, an emergency notification is sent to the Central Monitoring Station where the supervisor can take a decision regarding the next step.

Monitoring activities module-the safety/security signals are transferred directly to the Central Monitoring Station via mobile network (3G/4G where is possible and via GPRS on other cases). Based on the received signal type (if is gas/smoke alert, or flood detection alert etc.) the supervisor on the Central Monitoring Station can take a decision regarding the next step (e.g.: notify the proper organization: ambulance, firemen, policemen, etc.).

Vital signs module - due to the size, complexity and security of information the data transfer from this module to the Central Monitoring Station is disbanded in two phases. In the first phase from the sensors to the local server is performed via WIFI networks, depends on the devices communication protocol.

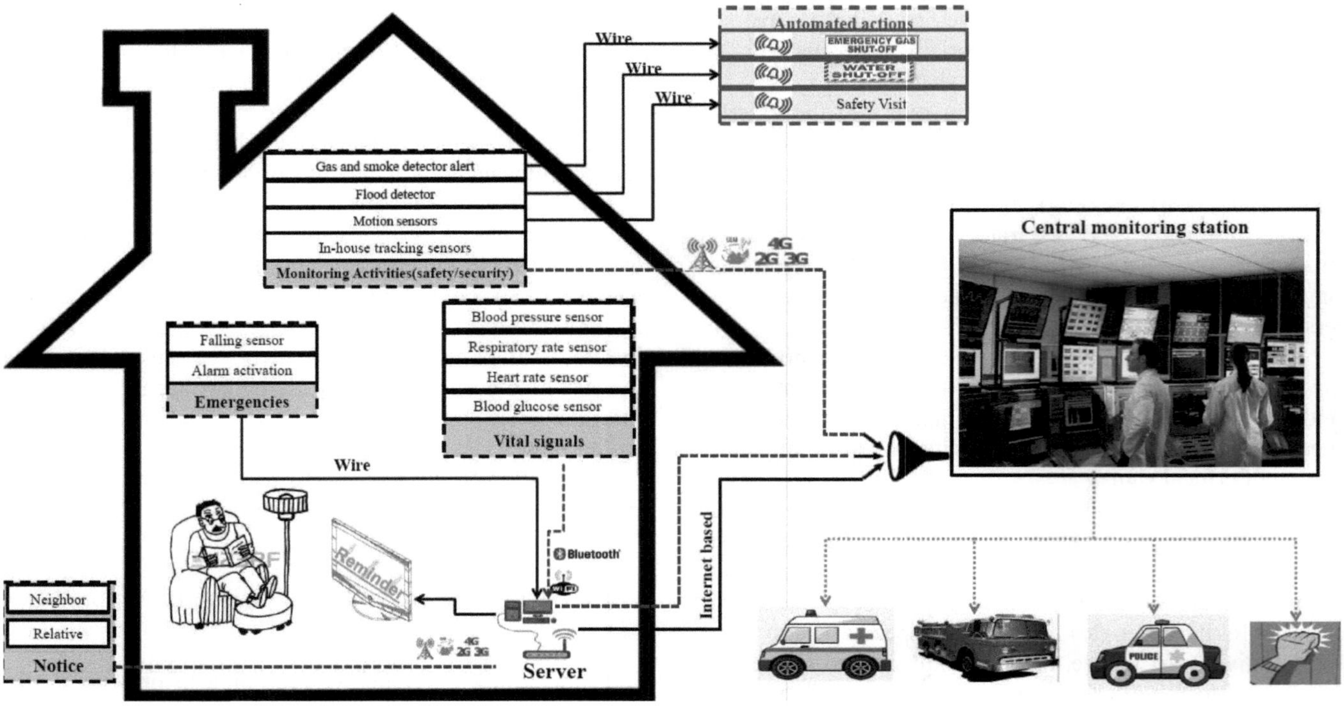

Fig.1 Telemonitoring system architecture

In case of unexpected value appearance (e.g.: the blood pressure value is above or under a pre-set limit) an emergency notification is sent directly to the Central Monitoring Station and the supervisor can take a decision regarding the next step (e.g.: call the supervised elderly to check his/her status etc.).

In the second phase from the local server to the Central Monitoring Station the grouped data transmission is performed via cable internet connection (at least twice a day).

To obtain a higher safety and security level, the presented system also has embedded three automated action beside the above-mentioned tasks:

In case of gas smoke alert: warning tone and the main gas valve shut-off .

In case of flood detection alert: warning tone and the main water tap shut-off.

In case of unexpected motion alert: warning tone a security member safety visit.

Another important part of the presented system is the intelligent remaindering function. Based on a pre-set schedule it can remind the elderly people about important activities such as eating meals, taking the medicine, visiting the bathroom etc.

We need to highlight that the presented concept (Figure 1) is just the beginning of a research. As future actions we are going to analyze and test each module individually. The communication technology between the presented modules is it in a general form (the most common used-based on our research), and it will be specified in the next phase (the modules individually analyses phase). In the next section we will concentrate only for the emergency module but in the upcoming papers we will analyze the rest of the modules too.

V. EMERGENCY MODULE

There are many issues associated with ageing, but one of the most widespread emergency situation for elderly is the falling incident. Approximately 30% of the people over 65 years of age, face an accidental fall each year. Fortunately, less than 10% results in fracture and approximately "only" 20 % of fall accidents required medical attention. [8]

In order to reduce the consequences of falling accidents, varoius technological solutions have been studied. Wearable systems are tipically based on accelerometers, gyroscops or a combination of these. However, there are questions regarding the optimal placement on body and the number of neccesary sensors to obtain accurate results. The desing of wearable systems are also complicated beacuse of the size, weight, and power consumption requirements.

Embedded devices certainly provide more confort to users than wearable devices. Our scope with the emergency module was to find solutions for falling incidents detection and alarm user-activation without any wearable system usage. In order to solve these issues we will use the sensors from Microsoft XBOX Kinect. Through a set of sensors that cach image, audio and depth infromation the Kinect is able to detect movements, identify faces and recognize spech of users. The Microsoft Kinect imput device with the internal components is presented on figure 2a.

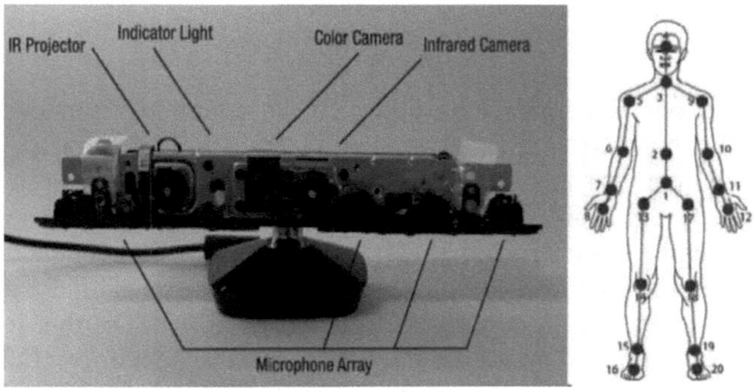

a) b)

Fig. 2 Internal components and Skeleton joint positions relative to the human body of Kinect sensors

To detect the falling incidents we are going to use the Kinect Natural User Interface (NUI) Skeleton tracking module, connected to the local server via USB connection. After the user detection, his/her skeleton is modeled in 3D. For an accurate model the Kinect identifying specific parts of the body as head, feet, knees, shoulders, etc. using in total 20 joints point (figure 2b). For each joint point there are information related to the tracking position in space (x, y, z coordinates). The Kinect can detect simultaneously at most six skelethons.[9][10]

The Kinect device connected to the local server via USB connection through a special application is capable to detect the user falls and sending an alarm to the Central Monitoring Station and also sending notices to preconfigured persons. The users can "manually" generate the alarm signal in case of necessity with voice command by the usage of special pre-set words (for example: HELP).

VI. Conclusions and Future Works

The overall approach of the presented system is enabling extremely powerful strategies for preventing dangerous situations and improving health and the overall quality of life for elderly. The modular design of the presented system allows a high degree of customization as per user's needs.

The elderly can feel secure knowing that the assistance is available anytime even if they are unable to request it themselves, and the relatives/friends can have a peace of mind knowing that the Central Monitoring Station will be alerted when assistance is needed.

The main objective of the presented telemonitoring system is to allow elderly to live in the environment of their choice and avoid institutionalization for as long as possible.

As it has been mentioned, this paper presented the early work of a research based on telemonitoring systems and technologies for independent life of elderly. As future tasks we are going to build, test and improve our emergency module as well as the rest of the modules.

Acknowledgment

This work is partially supported by PCCA Project, no. 180/2012, A Hybrid Fes-Exoskeleton System to Rehabilitate the Upper Limb in Disabled People (EXOSLIM).

Conflict of Interest

The authors declare that they have no conflict of interest.

References

1. Report from Department of Economic and Social Affairs (2015) World Population Ageing 2015 ST/ESA/SER.A/390
2. Scanail N C, Carew S, Barralon P, et. al. (2006) A review of Approaches to mobility telemonitoring of the elderly in their living environment, Annals of Biomedical Engineering Vol.34 No.4 April 2006 pp.547-563, DOI 10.1007/s10439-005-9068-2
3. Bushur R, Lovett J (2010) Assessment of Telemedicine, results of the initial experience. Aviation and space environment medicine
4. Golwater J, Harris Y,(2010) Using technology to enhance the aging experience: a market analysis of existing technologies,Springer Science+Business Media, LLC 2010, DOI 10.1007/s12126-010-9071-2
5. Litan R (2008), Vital signs via Broadband: remote health monitoring transmits savings, enhances life. Available via Better healthcare together: http://betterhealthcaretogether.org
6. Sander B, Richard M, and Ben K (2011) Int. conf on Pervasive Computing Tech. for Healthcare, 152-159
7. Bujnowska-Fedak M, Grata-Barkowska U, (2015) Smart homcare technology and TeleHealth 3 91-105
8. Hussain S, Erdegon Z E, (2008) Monitoring user activities in smart home environments, Springer Science + Business Media, LLC 2008, DOI 10.1007/s10796-008-9124-1
9. Vitale P,(2012) Evaluation and measurements of kinect movement detection in physical therapy, Master degree project in Informatics, University of Skovde
10. Chiuchisan I, Costin H N, Geman O,(2014) Adopting the Internet of Things Technologies in Health Care Systems, Int. Conf. and Exp. On Electrical and Power Engineering, Iasi, Romania

Automatic Learning of Medical Text Annotation Rules – a Case Study on Endoscopies

R.R. Slavescu[1], M.N.Oltean[1], A.P. Torok[1] and K.C. Slavescu[2]

[1] Computer Science Department, Technical University of Cluj-Napoca, Cluj-Napoca, Romania
[2] 2nd Pediatrics Clinic, Iuliu Hatieganu University of Medicine and Pharmacy, Cluj-Napoca, Romania

Abstract— **We present a method for automatic learning of text annotation rules which relies on association rules mining, in particular on a modified version of Apriori algorithm. The method starts from a set of texts written in natural language, each of them having associated one manually established label and aims to mimic the way human experts have established those annotations. The rules learned are basically pairs of words combinations and labels. They are further stored as JAPE (Java Annotation Patterns Engine) rules and can serve to annotating new texts. No natural language processing tool is employed. The method has been applied on a set of descriptions of endoscopies in Romanian language, with promising results.**

Keywords— **automatic text annotation, association rules mining, natural language processing, Apriori algorithm**

I. Introduction

Many Electronic Health Records (EHR) typically include information written in natural language about the patient's medical condition (e.g., anamnesis, oral examinations) and investigations (e.g., endoscopies) which can not be processed directly by a computer. In order to support EHR automatic processing and/or statistical analysis of this information, translating it into a machine readable form becomes of high importance. The progress made in the last decades in the field of Natural Language Processing (NLP) could offer a solution to this. Unfortunately, performant NLP tools are not available for each language, which makes the mentioned task both difficult and challenging.

This paper investigated an alternative way to mitigate the aforementioned problem. It relies on the observation that, in the technical fields like medical records, the texts are written in a more or less standard language, which many times comprises a relatively small vocabulary and set of linguistic structures whose length does not exceed 6-8 words. In order to extract structured data from this kind of texts, we employed a modified version of the Apriori algorithm [1] for rule mining. This algorithm is used in the following manner: it starts from a set of records which incorporate a humanly established label (taken from a standard set of labels) and a sequence of words in natural language and tries to discover relationships between the label and some word sequences / linguistic structures in the texts. The idea was applied to learning the way human experts annotate endoscopy descriptions written in Romanian. As an example, from the following two sequences of words "VGI volvulus gastric incomplet partial" and "VGI volvulus gastric incomplet", our system is able to infer the rule VGI $\leftarrow$ volvulus gastric incomplet, which tells that every time one sees the sequence "volvulus gastric incomplet" in a text, that text should be labeled as VGI. One major advantage of this idea is that it does not depend on the availability of a set of NLP tools. Of course, making use of such tools would highly improve the performance of the annotation rule set. Nonetheless, the preliminary experiments we conducted showed a reasonable performance could be obtained even in the absence of the tools mentioned above, especially in the filed of technical/scientific texts where one can expect to meet rather standardized expressions.

The work presented in this paper continues the approach introduced in [2,3]. The main contributions are twofold. First, an algorithm for ranking generated rules is presented and evaluated on a number of experiments supervised by a medicine specialist. Second, we employ a modified version of Apriori which allows restricting the form of the rules to be generated. Following the ideas in [4,5], the rule form is specified via regular expressions and is taken advantage of in the process of early pruning the generated bunch of rules.

The rest of the paper is organized as follows. Section II gives a motivating example for our research. Section III briefly introduces the instrumentation behind our solution. Section IV describes the results we have obtained when validating the method. Section V presents the Related Work. Section VI concludes and sketches future developments.

II. A Motivating Example

Our solution aims at generating annotation rules by examining frequent associations between raw text chunks and corresponding human-generated annotations. Without risking to loose generality, we used as an input a set of texts written in Romanian representing descriptions of the patient condition. As an example, these texts could represent the text descriptions of the images obtained by medical doctors during the endoscopic procedures. Every text has associated a set of annotations, each of them consisting of a pair <attribute_value> which depends upon the information

S. Vlad and N.M. Roman (eds.), *International Conference on Advancements of Medicine and Health Care through Technology; 12th - 15th October 2016, Cluj-Napoca, Romania*,
IFMBE Proceedings 59,
DOI: 10.1007/978-3-319-52875-5_53

stored in the corresponding text description. The set of attributes and the respective set of possible values for each of them are standardized. The algorithm must reveal the relations between a specific annotation and a sequence of words in the original text.

To illustrate, we focus on an example similar to that presented in [5]. The raw text we start with is: "antru cateva eroziuni pilor diskinetic" / "antrum few erosions diskinetic pilor". Two of the human-established annotations connected of this text are as follows:

1. S-LezANT_EZZ, meaning the attribute S-LezANT (i.e., Stomach Antrum Lesions) has the value ERZZ (i.e., Erosion). This annotation is due to the presence of the word combination "antru cateva eroziuni" / "antrum few erosions" in the text description of one of the endoscopies.
2. Pilor_DISK, meaning the attribute Pilor has the value DISK (i.e., Diskinetic), as indicated by the "pilor diskinetic" / "diskinetic pilor" fragment of the text description.

The algorithm aims to come up with one or more rules revealing the underpinning rationale for these human annotations. For instance, one of the rules for the first example above would be:

S-LezANT_ERZZ ← for some erosions

After generating a bunch of rules of this type, the proposed algorithm performs a heuristic ranking of them, in order to give higher scores to those having the highest likelihood to be confirmed by a human annotating expert. This makes the learning process semi-automatic. We show in the following sections that after just 3 iterations of this type, a set of rules covering as much as 90% of the text instances are obtained. We consider this a valuable result as it greatly simplifies the task of annotating texts: these rules could be further use in automatically annotating new texts and the more general the set of rules, the more chunks of texts could be dealt with in an automatic manner. To this end, our system translates each rule which is generated and approved into a JAPE rule, as used by the General Architecture for Text Engineering (GATE) tool [6].

A GATE JAPE grammar consists of a set of phases, each of which using of a set of pattern/action rules, separated by an implication sign (<-). The phases run sequentially and constitute a cascade of finite state transducers over annotations. The left-hand-side (LHS) of a JAPE rule actually represents an annotation pattern description and could be regarded as a set of conditions. The right-hand-side (RHS) consists of annotation actions, such as adding the appropriate label to a text, to be performed in the situation when the conditions contained in the rule's LHS hold.

As an example, the JAPE code obtained when choosing the rule above is:

```
Rule: ERZZ
Priority: 40
(
{Token.string=="antru"}
({Token.kind==word})?
{Token.string=="eroziuni"}
):erzz
-->
:erzz.ERZZ={rule="ERZZ"}
Phase: firstpass
Input: Token
Options: control=brill
```

III. Mining Meaning as Association Rules

For extracting the text-label associations, we chose a version of the Apriori algorithm [7]. This section describes the basics of this task. For more details on the topic, we refer the reader to one of our previous papers [5].

Apriori algorithm originate in market basket analysis and is designed to operate on databases containing transactions like collections of items bought together by customers. It can produce as output rules in form of implications $X \rightarrow Y$, meaning that "whenever we have X, we also have Y".

The quality of a rule is typically assessed by its support and confidence. The support is the probability that the LHS X of the rule holds (so the rule is applicable):

$$supp(X\text{->}Y) = \#transactions\ with\ X\ /\ \#transactions$$

The higher the support, the more general the rule.

The rule confidence estimates the probability $P(Y|X)$ of finding RHS Y in transactions where its LHS X is known to be present:

$$conf(X\text{->}Y) = \#transactions\ with\ X\ and\ Y\ /\ \#transactions\ with\ X$$

The higher the confidence, the higher the probability of the rule to predict correctly Y given X.

In our scenario, the association rule mining proceeds on two steps. The first step is to find all item sets with adequate supports and the second step is to generate association rules by combining these frequent or large item sets. In the traditional association rules mining, minimum support threshold and minimum confidence threshold values are assumed to be available for mining frequent item sets, which is hard to be set without specific knowledge.

In line with the approach developed in [4], we decided to modify the Apriori algorithm in order to restrict the form of the rules produced by specifying a regular expression the rule must observe in order not to be pruned along the rule generating process. In [5] it is shown that this could drastically reduce the time needed for rule generation. As an example, the rules we want to be generate might have the following form:

S-LezANT_EZZ ← *wrd wrd+*

where *wrd* is any word that may appear in an endoscopy description. To achieve this, we introduced the category Word and put the whole vocabulary in it, then specified the general form of the rule we were interested in.

In order to rank the rules, a rule contest algorithm has been designed. Each rule accumulates a number of points and the winner (i.e., the rule to be displayed on top of the rule stack) is the rule which has the most points in the end. Ties are broken by the rule length: the rule with the highest number of words (i.e., the more specific rule) is the winner. The algorithm is summarized as Procedure *RuleRank*

```
Procedure RuleRank
Input: rules, a set of rules generated by Apriori
           simstep, a similarity threshold, for now 0.05
  Output: ranked_rules, a sorted set of rules

  foreach A in rules
    points(A)  = 0
  endfor
  foreach A in rules
   foreach B in rules
    if (A <> B) then
      sA = set_of_examples_covered_by_A
      sB = set_of_examples_covered_by_B
      cA = cardinality(sA)
      cB = cardinality(sB)
      difBA = set_difference(sB,sA)
      cBA = cardinality(difBA)
      if (cB < cA) and (cBA = 0) then
         points(A) += 2
      else
        if (cB < cA) and (dAB / cB < simstep) then
          points(A) += 1
        else
          points(A) -= 1
        endif
      endif
    endif
  endfor
  endfor
  ranked_rules = sortbykeys(rules, points)
```

The procedure compares all pairs of rules A and B by considering the difference between the set of examples covered by A and those covered by B. If rule A supersedes rule B then A gets 2 points. If rule A covers more examples than rule B and the cardinality of the set difference between the sets of examples covered by B and A respectively is lower than a settable threshold (for now equal to 5%), then A gets one point. In all other cases, rule A loses one point. At the end, a rule hierarchy based on points is obtained. The topmost rule is displayed first in the rule stack. This algorithm represents one of the novelties of this paper. Its accuracy is evaluated in the next Section.

IV. Experimental Setup

For testing, we used a corpus of 979 pieces of raw text descriptions of endoscopies [8], manually annotated by a human expert. The corpus contained about 9847 word occurrences (644 distinct words). Prior to running the algorithms, in a pre-processing phase, the system replaced the abbreviations which were present in the original texts, using the words from the text supplied as input against a dictionary embedded into it.

For the experiments, we employed an in-house implementation of the Apriori algorithm [4] which allows pruning rule by specifying the general pattern they must obey. For example, we can ask the Apriori algorithm to generate rules having solely S-Lum_VGI in the RHS. Thorough the experiments, a value of 0.3 for the support and 0.8 for the confidence were used.

The rules are filtered in order to eliminate those comprising prepositions only, those consisting of just one word and one preposition and those ending in a preposition. After this filtering step, the set of rules is presented to the user. S/he can stick with the rule suggested by the system or choose another one(s). After picking and saving such a rule, the examples covered by it are flushed from the input and new rules are generated over the remaining set of examples.

Table 1 summarizes the percentages of examples covered by the rules generated in the first 3 iterations of the algorithm. Values marked with a star represent percentages obtained by the rules selected manually by a human medical expert, who decided to overrule the automatically suggested ones. All other values are obtained by applying the rules proposed by the algorithm and confirmed by the human expert. As the results show, in nearly 73% of the cases, the rules suggested are confirmed by the human expert.

Table 1. Percentages of examples covered by the rules generated in the first 3 iterations of the algorithm

Rule head	Iteration 1 coverage (%)	Iteration 2 coverage (%)	Iteration 3 coverage (%)
S-Lum_VGI	80.37	90.65	97.20
S-MucANT_NO	65.12*	89.70	93.69
SlezANT_ERZZ	82.29*	88.54*	94.79*
S-Lum_RDG	82.35	94.12	100.00
S-MucCORP_PA	84.00	94.00	98.0

V. Related Work

Paper [9] presents a Natural Language Processing software internally developed at a clinic which was used to identify and extract information within clinical narrative text. The goal was to identify patients with prostate cancer and to retrieve pathological information from their Electronic Medical Record. The results were of high quality, but the system relied on NLP tools which was not available for Romanian when the work for the present paper started. Paper [10] describes different solutions designed to automatically extract medication information from clinical records, but it is mainly concerned with drug name recognition. It relies on rules capturing the document structure and the syntax of each kind of information.

An approach very similar to the one we presented could be found in [11]. It combines association rules mining and decision tree learning in order to build information extraction rules. Similarly to our approach, their system was able to learn rules from a relatively small training set.

ECLAT [12] and FP-growth [13] are among the successors of Apriori in the association mining field. From our perspective, their downside is the difficulty of integrating regular expressions based pruning .

VI. Conclusions

We described a solution based on an algorithm for mining association rules which can extract structured information from raw natural language texts. To this end, the algorithm takes advantage of a set of previously annotated texts and tries to discover associations between some typical language structures in the text and the corresponding structured annotations. Experiments conducted on a set of texts in Romanian describing endoscopies showed remarkable similarities between the manually annotated texts versus the automated process. This is particularly the case for technical/scientific texts, with a relatively small vocabulary and language structure.

The solution is implemented as a standalone application with no need for other Natural Language Processing tools. Once the rules are generated they are presented to the user who confirms them. If necessary, the process could be repeated until a convenient set of rules is built. The tests show 3 iterations are usually enough to obtain 90% coverage. Portability is further insured due to their translation into JAPE rules which can be further more imported into an external application.

As further work, we want to exhaustively explore the whole set of attribute_value pairs and compare the rule sets generated automatically with the human validated ones. The length of the word combinations relevant for a specific annotations should also be investigated.

Acknowledgment

Publication of this work was supported by the Computer Science Department at the Technical University of Cluj-Napoca, Romania.

Conflict of Interest

The authors declare that they have no conflict of interest.

References

1. Agrawal R, Srikant R (1994) Fast algorithms for mining association rules in large databases, in Proceedings of the 20th International Conference on Very Large Data Bases, VLDB '94, 1994, pp. 487–499.
2. Slavescu R R, Bali A, Slavescu K C (2015). Building Annotation Rules for Text Description of Endoscopies in Romanian – an NLP-free Approach, in Proceedings of the 2015 IEEE 11th International Conference on Intelligent Computer Communication and Processing (ICCP), Cluj-Napoca, Romania, 2015, pp. 19-25
3. Oltean MN (2016). Learning Annotations for Medical Texts: Combining Apriori and GATE, in Proceedings of the Computer Science Students Conference, Cluj-Napoca, Romania, 2016.
4. Persa R A (2015) Pruning Based on Regular Expressions and Categories for Association Rules Mining. License thesis, Technical University of Cluj-Napoca, Romania, 2015
5. Slavescu R R, Persa R A, Slavescu K C (2015). Association Rules Mining with Categories and Regular Expressions Based Pruning, in Proceedings of the 2015 IEEE 11th International Conference on Intelligent Computer Communication and Processing (ICCP), Cluj-Napoca, Romania, 2015, pp. 5-12
6. Cunningham H, Tablan V, Roberts A et. Al (2013) Getting More Out of Biomedical Documents with GATE's Full Lifecycle Open Source Text Analytics. PLoS Comput Biol 9(2): e1002854. doi:10.1371/journal.pcbi.1002854
7. Srikant R (1996) Fast algorithms for mining association rules and sequential patterns, PhD. dissertation, University of Wisconsin, Madison, 1996.
8. Slavescu KC, Margescu C, Pirvan A et al. (2013). Atrophic Gastritis: Helicobacter Pylori versus Duodenogastric Reflux. Clujul Medical 86(2), 2013, pp. 138-143.
9. Thomas A, Zheng C, Jung H, et al. (2014) Extracting data from electronic medical records: validation of a natural language processing program to assess prostate biopsy results. World Journal of Urology, 32(1), pp. 99-103, 2014.
10. Deleger L, Grouin C, Zweigenbaum P (2010) Extracting medical information from narrative patient records: the case of medication-related information. JAMIA 17(5), pp. 555—558.
11. Agrawal R, Ho H, Jacquenet F et al. (2005) Mining Information Extraction Rules from Data sheets Without Linguistic Parsing, in Proceedings of the 18th International Conference on Industrial and Engineering Applications of Artificial Intelligence and Expert Systems, 2005, pp. 510—520.
12. Zaki M.J, Parthasarathy S Ogihara M et al. (1997), New Algorithms for Fast Discovery of Association Rule, in Proceedings of the 3rd ACM SIGKDD Int. Conf. on Knowledge Discovery and Data Mining (KDD'97, Newport Beach, CA), pp. 283-296
13. Hah J, Pei H, Yin Y. (2000) Mining Frequent Patterns without Candidate Generation Proceedings of the Conference on the Management of Data (SIGMOD'00, Dallas, TX), 1-12 New York, NY, USA, 2000

Author: Radu Razvan Slavescu
Institute: Technical University of Cluj-Napoca
Street: G. Baritiu nr. 28 room 21
City: Cluj-Napoca
Country: Romania
Email: radu.razvan.slavescu@cs.utcluj.ro

Use of Machine Learning for Improvement of Similarity Searches of Patients

B.Petrovan[1], B.Orza[2] and A. Vlaicu[2]

[1] Laitek Medical Software, Software Engineer, Cluj-Napoca, Romania
[2]Technical University of Cluj-Napoca/Telecommunications, Cluj-Napoca, Romania

Abstract—**Due to various factors (human error, broken communication links) patient information within a healthcare enterprise varies for a given patient. Medical personnel and technicians are often faced with the problem of searching similar patients within the hospital information system. The heterogeneity of attributes on which the search is performed increases the difficulty of retrieving conclusive results, thus simple search rules are unsatisfactory in this case.**

The work presented in this paper compares different machine learning algorithms for improving the similarity rating based on a set of human decisions.

Keywords— **machine learning, similarity search, attributes heterogeneity.**

I. Introduction

With the continuous increase of digital medical documents usage, more data gets stored into healthcare systems. That data needs to be retrieved and shared across the systems within a healthcare institution to ensure proper patient care.

Errors do occur, either human or software that make the retrieval of documents difficult or even impossible. When a patient's folder needs to be retrieved the patient needs to be found in the system and the documents related to that entry are retrieved. When errors occur, some of the patients documents are related to an erroneous entry and the operator can easily miss that. First point for correcting such an issue is to determine the correct patient entry and move the documents in the correct patient folder.

In the early years errors missing documents were either missed or identified by clinical personnel. Improvements have been made and alerts were implemented that would notify the system's administrator that there are issues with the data within that system. Still, human errors (like creating another patient entry with other data) are hard to spot and involves manual intervention.

Even if the error rates within a system kept quite constant, due to the increased volume of data stored, finding and correct data errors in a system becomes difficult and unmaintainable.

Operators and system administrators need means to be able to perform searches in a system based on similarity and not on exact data. Such searches are needed for example by an operator when a patient is admitted, the patient says that he/she has been previously registered, but the operator cannot find his/hers records. A similarity search would yield a list of similar entries (eg patient's name is SMITH^MARY^JANE and there is a patient entry within the system with name SMIHT^JANE^M) from which the operator might choose the corresponding previous records and correct the patient demographics. Operators are faced with same issue during data cleansing, where same patient appears with different demographics in different systems and the operators need to match the entries between systems.

Systems need to evolve and adapt to the users' input to output more relevant search results. Also, alerts must be "smarter", like an alert saying "there is another patient in the system with similar information" to a system administrator when an operator has created a new patient entry similar with an existing one.

The work presented in this paper searches a way of scoring the similarity between two patient entries.

II. Problem statement

Various issues within a hospital network and human error generate differences between information stored in different systems for the same entity. System errors can be: missing informational links for propagating changes to an existing entity, broken communication links that lead to filling up the queues for data propagation, different approaches in implementing the standards, use of different coding schemas, bugs in the software that led to data loss or leaking information from one entity to another, etc. Human error is more straightforward: typographical, confusing last/ first/middle names, misspells of foreign or uncommon names, not filling in optional fields.

In this paper we focus on patient entities, analyzing their common attribute differences that appear between systems and how to compute a similarity ranking value based on a dataset of user decided matches.

The goal is to determine a metric/ranking score between the attributes of two patients that can be used in similarity searches, such that the most relevant similar patients come first in a list.

Difficulty of comparing two patient entities based on their attributes comes from the heterogeneity and scarcity of these

S. Vlad and N.M. Roman (eds.), *International Conference on Advancements of Medicine and Health Care through Technology; 12th - 15th October 2016, Cluj-Napoca, Romania*,
IFMBE Proceedings 59,
DOI: 10.1007/978-3-319-52875-5_54

attributes. There are a few usable attributes common on almost all systems, these attributes have short values (like identifiers or names) and their meaning varies.

By having the means to compare the similarity of two patient entries as accurate as possible, it's easy to develop tools that aid operators to match information from two different systems or to better find a patient's prior electronic records.

III. Methodology

The proposed approach is to analyze each of these attributes according to their meaning and develop specialized individual scoring functions. Then, develop a method of weighing these scores to obtain a correct classification. Due to the variance of the samples and the need to adjust to user inputs, it's proposed to use several machine learning algorithms that are suited for fitting existing data and evaluate their training.

A. The Dataset

The data set used is comprised of 33812 entries containing user decisions between the patient information in a *Radiology Information System (RIS)* system and in a *Picture Archiving and Communication System (PACS)* system [1]. Each entry contains the following attributes: identifier, name, date of birth and sex, from both RIS and PACS.

RIS information is usually considered to be the "source of truth" because it sits on top of the PACS in the propagation chain. The user had to choose if the RIS patient matches the PACS patient or not. An accepted match is considered a positive sample and a rejected match a negative sample within the dataset.

Table 1 shows the initial analysis of the dataset was a distribution of attributes that match perfectly; least significant cases were omitted. Figure 1 shows the distribution of the users' decisions within the dataset.

Samples having last name, first or sex varying (first three rows in Table 1) cover 60% of the dataset.

B. Attributes

Identifiers: are values usually assigned by a system. Differences between identifiers can appear due to:

- prefixes/suffixes appended by some systems; eg. 123 used in PACS and 000123 used in RIS

Table 1 Analysis of the data set

Number of entries	% of data set size	User accepted matches	Matching attributes
7971	23.57%	4475	ID, First, DOB, Sex
6987	20.66%	5571	ID, Last, DOB, Sex
5959	17.62%	5925	ID, Last, First, DOB
5053	14.94%	5019	Last, First, DOB, Sex
2906	8.59%	2618	ID, Last, First, Sex
1774	5.25%	1774	ID, Last, First
1400	4.14%	961	ID, DOB, Sex
286	0.85%	286	Last, First, DOB, Sex

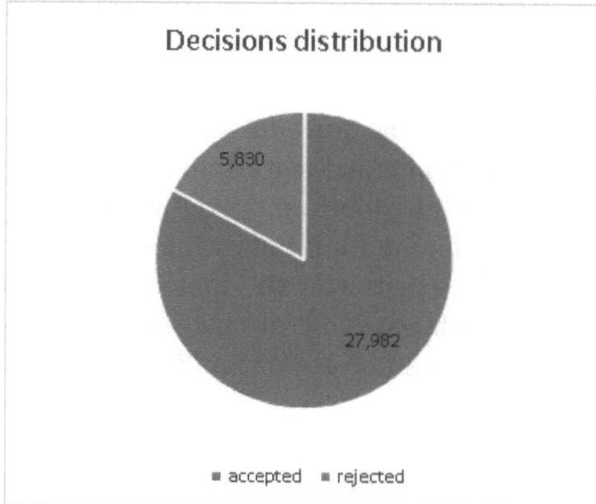

Fig.1 Distribution of user decisions

- different assigning authorities: appear when data is imported from another institution or when there are more than one Master Patient Index within an institution; for example an imaging study from *HospitalA* was imported in the PACS system in *HospitalB*, then the same person will have in the PACS system two identifiers one from *HospitalA* and one from *HospitalB*
- merges not propagated: an operator finds that a person has more than one patient entity registered in the system; performs a merge operation but due to communication or protocol errors the merge operation is not propagated to other system(s).

The comparison score between two identifiers was considered 1 if they matched perfectly and 0.9 if one was included in the other.

Names: the structure of a person name varies between implementation, most common components are first name, last name, middle name, prefix and suffix. Differences of names for the same person can appear due to:

- typographical errors made by the human operator, misspelling foreign or uncommon names;
- last name changes for female patients after marriage or divorce; updates don't get propagated to all

systems or another patient entry is created at the next visit

- •mistaken order of last, first and/or middle name: the operator fills the wrong fields for name components (eg. SMITH^MARY^JANE and SMITH^JANE^MARY)

Score is maximum if the three components match, 0.9 if the name components are swapped and, if still are not matching, the score is computed as ratio of Levenshtein distance [2][3] over the length of the full name.

Date of birth: are date values usually validated upon reception/entry in a system. Differences for the same patient might occur due to:

- •typographical errors, the operator enters wrong digits
- •missing data: it's not a required field in many systems, thus the attribute might be missing;
- •mistaken month and date; date representation varies around the globe, an operator can easily mistake date with month if both values are under 13;

Score is maximum when two dates match, proportional with the Levenshtein distance if the distance is less than 3 (maximum accepted typos) and 0.5 if one of the dates is null (missing data).

Sex: depending on the system it can have multiple value sets, most common are F-Female, M-Male, O-Other, U-Unknown. Differences for the same person might occur due to:

- •missing data because it's not a mandatory field in many systems
- •operator error assuming a value based on the first and last name

Score is maximum if the values match (we considered O and U as matching) or 0.5 if one of them is missing or has value O or U.

Another score was extracted from the sex attribute, maximum for female and 0 in rest, having in mind that last name changes for women are very probable.

C. Scoring function

The search scoring function should take parameters the five scores described earlier and take value from 0 to 1, while trying to fit as best as possible the decisions made by the users.

D. Tested Algorithms

Individual attribute scores were computed on all samples in the evaluation set, resulting a vector of 5 values and a target class (positive or negative).

Average it was used as a baseline for comparing the machine learning algorithms. All the samples used have at least one attribute that varies, thus an absolute comparison would yield zero matches.

K-Nearest Neighbors (KNN) [4] was used with 5 neighbors and Euclidean metric.

Support Vector Machines (SVM) [5] were used with radial basis kernel.

Multi-Layer Perceptron (MLP) [6] with two hidden layers, sizes of 25 and 5, step activation function (Eq. 1) and a stochastic gradient-based optimizer algorithm[7]. This algorithm was chosen because it has good performance, both validation score and training time, for large datasets.

$$f(x) = \max(0, x) \tag{1}$$

IV. RESULTS

The dataset was split in two sets, for training and for evaluation. Size of the training set was varied to assess the improvement of accuracy when increasing the training set size. Training samples were chosen at random from the dataset. After choosing a training set all four algorithms were trained and evaluated.

Figure 1 shows the evaluation results for all algorithms and training set size. In Table 2 is an analysis of the predictions made with each algorithm. Samples for which the user decided they match the same patient are considered positive and the ones that were marked as "no match" as negatives.

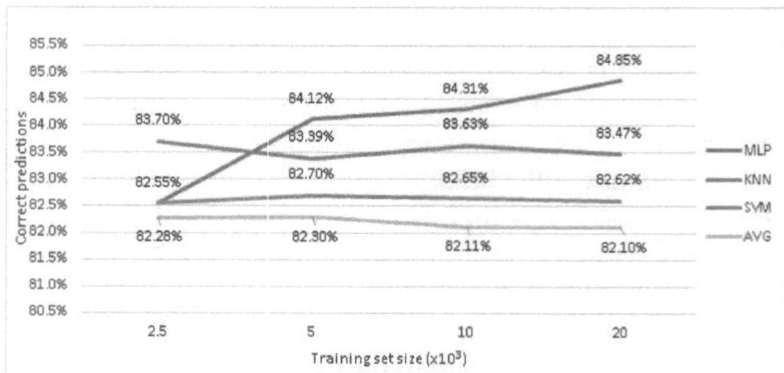

Fig. 2 Accuracy of each algorithm – percent of the evaluation set size

Table 2 Table caption

	True Positives	False Positives	False Negatives	True Negatives
SVM	11411	0	2400	0
KNN	10614	798	1485	915
MLP	11021	390	1701	699
AVG	11338	74	2398	2

It can be seen that the simple averaging of all scores gives pretty good results due to the knowledge that was introduced in the scoring functions. There is no improvement with the increase of the size of training set. Erroneous predictions are for false negatives. It was expected because this algorithm doesn't fit the data.

SVMs have trouble fitting the data because there are a lot of samples close with each other, but with opposing outputs. In Table 1 – first row it can be seen that almost half of the samples having only last name differences (one attribute is varying) were rejected by the users. There is no improvement with the increase of the size of training set. There are no false positives but a lot of false negatives. It can be seen in Table 2 that all negative samples have been incorrectly classified.

KNN have the same issue with the agglomerated samples having opposing expected outputs. Its accuracy is almost constant with the increase in size of the training set.

MLP shows it can fit the training set better, is improving accuracy when increasing the training set size and it has the best specificity of all.

Data tables were stored in PostgreSQL and the individual scores were computed in the database engine. Training and evaluation was implemented using Python and scikit-learn module.

V. Conclusion

We have analyzed the problem of comparing two patient entries that can reside in the same system or in different systems and we evaluated most common machine learning algorithms on a dataset.

Although there is no perfect solution, the approach of using MLP is overall better than KNN or SVM, showing improvements when increasing the training set.

Such similarity metric can be used to determine if there are more than one patient folder in a system, to match entries coming from different systems and in more complex data mining algorithms [8][9].

Conflict of Interest

The authors declare that they have no conflict of interest.

References

1. D. Clooney, DICOM Structured Reporting, Oct 2000, 2000.
2. Levenshtein, Vladimir I. "Binary codes capable of correcting deletions, insertions, and reversals". Soviet Physics Doklady. 10 (8): 707–710.
3. Wagner, Robert A.; Fischer, Michael J. (1974), "The String-to-String Correction Problem", Journal of the ACM, 21 (1): 168–173, doi:10.1145/321796.321811
4. Altman, N. S. "An introduction to kernel and nearest-neighbor nonparametric regression". The American Statistician. 46 (3): 175–185. doi:10.1080/00031305.1992.10475879.
5. Cortes, C.; Vapnik, V. "Support-vector networks". Machine Learning. 20 (3): 273–297. doi:10.1007/BF00994018.
6. Rosenblatt, Frank. x. Principles of Neurodynamics: Perceptrons and the Theory of Brain Mechanisms. Spartan Books, Washington DC, 1961
7. Diederik P. Kingma, Jimmy Ba (2014), "Adam: A Method for Stochastic Optimization", Proceedings of the 3rd International Conference on Learning Representations (ICLR)
8. E. de Fortuny and D. Martens, "Active Learning Based Rule Extraction for Regression," in Data Mining Workshops (ICDMW), 2012 IEEE 12th International Conference on , 10-10 Dec. 2012
9. K. Rameshkumar, M. Sambath and S. Ravi, "Relevant association rule mining from medical dataset using new irrelevant rule elimination technique," in Information Communication and Embedded Systems (ICICES), 2013 International Conference on , 2013.

Part V
Biomechanics, Robotics and Rehabilitation

Motor Imagery Brain-Computer Interface for the Control of a Shoulder-Elbow Rehabilitation Equipment

A. Ianoşi-Andreeva-Dimitrova, D.S. Mândru, M.O. Tătar and S. Noveanu

Technical University of Cluj-Napoca, Faculty of Mechanical Engineering, Department of Mechatronics and Machine Dynamics, Cluj-Napoca, Romania

Abstract— **The aim of this paper is to present a non-invasive brain-computer interface (BCI) with which a patient that suffered cerebrovascular accident (CVA) might have the ability to control a rehabilitation equipment designed for upper limb repetitive passive exercises, namely, for the movement of the shoulder and elbow in the sagittal plane. The rehabilitation equipment, developed previously, was upgraded with a customized BCI interface that uses a motor-imagery control paradigm, translating user movement intent into control signals. Performance of the BCI system is assessed and several further research recommendation are made.**

Keywords— **brain-computer interface, rehabilitation equipment, motor imagery.**

I. Introduction

Medical rehabilitation is one of the fundamental pillars of health services, which enable a partial or, in some fortunate cases, quasi-total function recover that facilitate a significant increase in life quality, better emotional attitude and social reintegration. Modern medical rehabilitation is extensively supported by advancement in rehabilitation engineering which provides technical infrastructure that is advantageous both for the patient as well as for the clinical practitioner. This technical infrastructure is developed in many distinct branches such as rehabilitation equipment design, assistive robotics, etc. that encompass both engineering as well as medical sciences; this interdisciplinary approach must benefit from a good collaboration between specialists with expertise in different fields.

CVA is widely recognized as one of the leading cause of death in the world [1]; for those who survive it, it is the main cause of long term disability, therefore developing new approaches that might have the potential of further increasing the chance of successful rehabilitation in an as higher degree as possible represents a great incentive for research. Another problem is that CVA tends to affect upper-limb functions in a greater proportion, roughly 70% of CVA survivors, a third of them suffering from this condition permanently [2].

In order to strengthen the residual functionality, or merely keep an adequate muscular mass and articular mobility, repetitive exercises are necessary; this might become demanding for a physiotherapist, therefore, robotized exercisers are very useful in this respect. In previous work [3] a shoulder-elbow rehabilitation exerciser was developed, that assist a physiotherapist in repetitive passive exercises of the upper-limb in the sagittal plane. This paper further develops the system by fitting a BCI that translate user movement intent into control signals; its rationale is the fact that an active and motivated participation from the patient side is an important factor that enables a successful rehabilitation [4]. Two electrode placement configurations are investigated in order to find an optimum arrangement that satisfy both simplicity as well as signal robustness.

II. State of the Art

The scientific literature presents several solution of integration of a BCI system with an upper-limb rehabilitation equipment, some of which, considered relevant for the present paper, were selected and discussed below.

Ang and Guan review in [5] the main strategies that make use of BCI for upper-limb neurorehabilitation, determining two main classes: those who rely only on neurofeedback, and those who use in addition physical practice. They note that the second method, through harder to implement (the rehabilitation equipment must have the ability to work simultaneously as an active and passive exerciser, and switch between the two states as needed) it provides the best clinical outcome. Another study [6] compared the results between a group of patients that used standard robotic rehabilitation and those who used in addition a BCI; the results were statistically inconclusive due to the small number of subjects involved, but nevertheless promising due to the fact that among the patients who had positive motor improvement, those who used BCI scored a better result with significantly less motor activity.

The approach taken in the previous mentioned papers was by using a robot that allows movement only in the horizontal plane; another popular approach is the use of a system that has the ability to provide motion path in all three spatial dimensions. Barsotii et all propose in [7] the use of an 8 degree of freedom exoskeleton (4 for the arm, 2 for the wrist and 2 for the hand) that receive via a BCI the

S. Vlad and N.M. Roman (eds.), *International Conference on Advancements of Medicine and Health Care through Technology; 12th - 15th October 2016, Cluj-Napoca, Romania*,
IFMBE Proceedings 59,
DOI: 10.1007/978-3-319-52875-5_55

cue for the start of an exercise that consist of arm movement to reach a target object, gasping of the said object, moving and releasing it in a target area.

An interesting research direction is the use of hybrid interfaces, in order to have more inputs; if there are other viable remaining function, such as eye-movement, these might be integrated as in [8], where a complex system composed of a Kinect sensor, an eye-tracking device and a BCI is proposed. The Kinect sensor is used for surrounding object identification, the eye-tracking device determine which of these objects are of interest for the subject and through the BCI the intent of arm movement is transmitted. In the same line of hybrid interfaces, Rouillard et all present in [9] a system that links both electromyography (EMG) as well as electroencephalography (EEG).

There is a potential disadvantage when combining signals from various sources into a hybrid interface: there are patients with a residual functionality that is so low that such a strategy is inapplicable. A solution to this problem is the use of a hybrid-BCI, that is, a BCI which combines different control paradigms as in [10], where motor imagery is used along steady-state visual evoked potentials (flicker frequency of a visual stimulus that the subject is concentrating upon, is discoverable in the occipital area of the brain).

A relatively new research direction is the combination between a BCI and transcranial Direct Current Stimulation (tDCS) technics [11]; in the cited study, prior to motor-imagery robotic feedback exercises, the subject received 20 minutes of tDCS. Such an approach is closer to real-life post-stroke scenarios, where a patient might need reactivation of brain motor area in addition to repetitive exercise tasks.

III. Material and Method

The proposed system (refer to figure 1) consist of a rehabilitation equipment, a BCI system and a computer which handle data processing, display the BCI-paradigm and allows a physician to supervise the session.

A. The rehabilitation equipment

As stated in the introductory part of this paper, the development of this rehabilitation equipment was the subject of previous work detailed in [3]. It is a semi-portable shoulder-elbow exoskeleton, with a usable amplitude range of motion as follows: -90°...+60° in respect to the transverse plane for the elbow joint, respectively -20°...+95° in respect to the frontal plane for the shoulder joint. It is actuated by two 12 V DC motors, each delivering a maximum torque of 20 Nm; the absolute position is read by resistive goniometers and limit switches provide an extra layer of security. It might also be independently of the BCI-system controlled via its own graphical user interface which enable the adjustment of the exercise parameters, and provides visual feedback for the supervising physician.

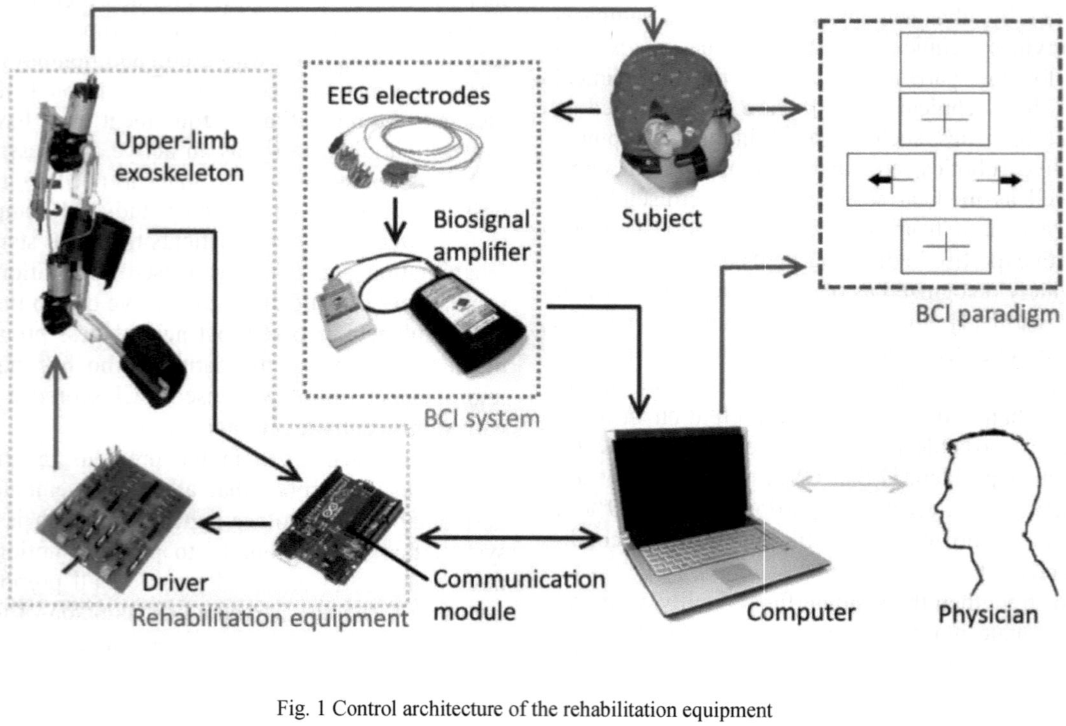

Fig. 1 Control architecture of the rehabilitation equipment

B. The BCI system

In order to test how the system performs with different number of sources, two electrode placement configuration were tested, one with 8 active dry g.Sahara (frequency range: 0.1-40 Hz) electrodes at C3, C4, Cz, CP1, CP2, FCz, C5 and C6, respectively the second with 6 electrodes at: FC3, FC4, CP1, CP2, CP5 and CP6; the location designation is according with the 10-10 international system, and the electrodes were held in place with the aid of a textile cap. Two additional electrodes were used, one for the ground (located at Fpz) and one as reference (located at A2) – this being a requirement for the proper functioning of the electrode driver.

For the test, the EEG was recorded from one consenting 27 year old human male clinically healthy subject in two separate sessions. OpenViBE (by INRIA) and BCILAB (by C. Kothe) were the software used for in-depth signal analysis.

The first session consisted of 80 trials, the subject being asked at random to imagine left, respectively right hand movement. Each trial consisted of presenting in sequence (refer also to figure 1, BCI-paradigm section): a cross for 1 second (s), to capture subject attention, a cue (left/right arrow) for 1.25 s to ask which hand movement to imagine, again the cross for 3.75 s during which time the subject actually imagine performing the indicated movement, and, between trials, a rest period of 4 s.

The second session, performed in another day with the 6-electrode configuration, differed from the previous in the following: it consisted of 70 trials, the cue duration was reduced from 1.25 to 1 s, as well as the time in which the subject had to imagine performing the task from 3.75 to 3 s. The sole purpose of reducing both the number of used electrodes as well as the time in which the subject were asked to perform motor imagery task was to investigate if this is a proper way of optimization (less recording time per stimulation and fewer channels translate in reduced processing power).

IV. Results and Discussion

For each session individually a spectrally weighted common spatial pattern filter was computed (refer to figure 2) and a quadratic discriminant analysis (QDA) was used as machine-learning function. The evaluation of the QDA trained model was done using 5-fold cross-correlation, results being presented next page in table 1.

The machine learning algorithm performed quite well in the first session, with an average accuracy of 70% (66.25% worst case). Computing the confusion matrix based on data presented in table 1, it results a mean sensitivity of 72.6% and a mean specificity of 66.99%. The mean information transfer rate (ITR) was 3.79 bits/min.

In the second session, the algorithm performed surprisingly poor, with an average accuracy (44.84%) worse than random chance (which for this classifier is 50%). It has no significant sensitivity (49.14%) nor specificity (42.74%). The error rate for this electrode configuration suggests that

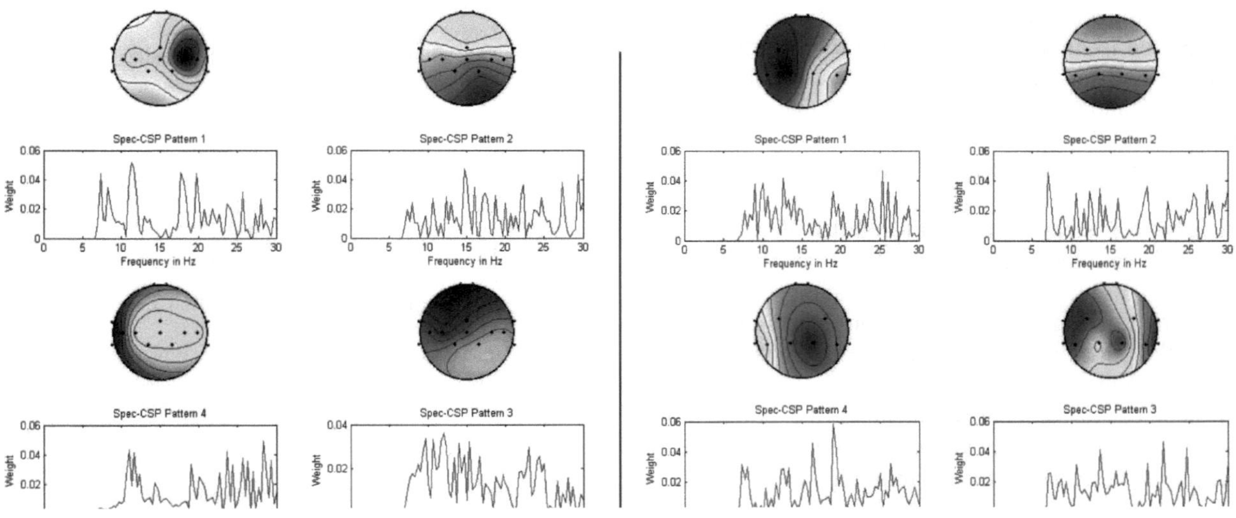

Fig. 2 Spectrally weighted common spatial pattern mapped on the surface of the scalp (as viewed from above the subject) for first and second session; black dots marks electrode position

the reduction of recording channels from 8 to 6 coupled with the cut of 1 second/trial and 10 trials/session greatly deteriorates the performance; for the aim of the current paper, the first electrode configuration is the optimum arrangement.

Table 1 Five-fold cross-correlation for both session

Fold	True Positive	True Negative	False Positive	False Negative	Error rate
Session 1					
1	0,750	0,375	0,625	0,25	0,438
2	0,750	0,625	0,375	0,25	0,313
3	0,572	0,778	0,222	0,428	0,313
4	0,667	0,571	0,429	0,333	0,375
5	0,875	1,000	0,000	0,125	0,063
Session 2					
1	0,286	0,500	0,500	0,714	0,615
2	0,600	0,333	0,667	0,400	0,571
3	0,500	0,500	0,500	0,500	0,500
4	0,500	0,375	0,625	0,500	0,571
5	0,571	0,429	0,571	0,429	0,500

V. Conclusion

The aim of the study was to present a BCI fitted to an upper-limb robotic system, and investigate how two different electrode configuration impacts its performance; as stated, the first configuration performed well, but the second proved to be inadequate: there might be several factors that are supposed to be involved and have to be further investigated: the reduced number of electrodes, the lack of electrodes at C3 and C4 (it was hypothesized that the electrodes placed around this points will pick and interpolate the signal), the reduced trial period, the reduced number of total trials.

A robotic system decrease the burden that relies on a physiotherapist; the presented system has the additional benefit that provides an alternative pathway between the patient mind and his/her rehabilitation equipment, and this fact has the potential to strengthen the engagement into the rehabilitation program from his/her part.

A planned further improvement is the addition of a transcutaneous functional electrical stimulation unit that has the ability to better assist the rehabilitation of CVA patients.

Acknowledgment

Work presented in this paper was partially supported by PCCA Project 180/2012, titled “A Hybrid FES-Exoskeleton System to Rehabilitate the Upper Limb in Disabled People (EXOSLIM)”.

Conflict of Interest

The authors declare that they have no conflict of interest.

References

1. World Health Organization (2002) The World Health Report – Reducing Risks, Promoting Healthy Life, available online at: http://www.who.int/whr/2002/en/
2. Rabadi M H (2011) Review of the randomized clinical stroke rehabilitation trials in 2009. Med Sci Monit 17(2):RA25-RA43, DOI: 10.12659/MSM.881382
3. Ianosi-A-D A, Noveanu S, Tatar O M, Mandru D S (2016) Shoulder-Elbow Exoskeleton as Rehabilitation Exerciser. IOP Conf. Ser.: Mater. Sci. Eng., vol. 147, 012048, doi:10.1088/1757-899X/147/1/012048
4. Timmermans A A A, Seelen H A M, Willmann R D and Kingma H (2009) Technology-assisted training of arm-hand skills in stroke: concepts on reacquisition of motor control and therapist guidelines for rehabilitation technology design. J Neuroeng Rehabil., vol.6, DOI: 10.1186/1743-0003-6-1.
5. Ang K K and Guan C (2015) Brain-Computer Interface for Neurorehabilitation of Upper Limb After Stroke. Proc. of IEEE, vol. 103(6), DOI: 10.1109/JPROC.2015.2415800
6. Ang K K et all (2009) A clinical study of motor imagery-based brain-computer interface for upper limb robotic rehabilitation. 31st Intern. Conf. EMBS, Minneapolis, MN, USA, DOI: 10.1109/IEMBS.2009.5335381
7. Barsotti M et all (2015) A full upper limb robotic exoskeleton for reaching and grasping rehabilitation triggered by MI-BCI. IEEE Intern. Conf. on Rehab. Rob. (ICORR), Singapore, DOI: 10.1109/ICORR.2015.7281174
8. Frisoli A et all (2012) A New Gaze-BCI-Driven Control of an Upper Limb Exoskeleton for Rehabilitation in Real-World Task. IEEE Transactions on Systems, Man, and Cybernetics, Part C (Applications and Reviews), vol. 42, no. 6, pp. 1169-1179, DOI: 10.1109/TSMCC.2012.2226444
9. Rouillard J et all (2015) Hybrid BCI coupling EEG and EMG for severe motor disabilities. 6th Intern. Conf. on Applied Human factors and Ergonomics, vol. 3, pp.29-36, DOI: 10.1016/j.promfg.2015.07.104
10. Horki P, Solis-Escalante T, Neuper C and Muller-Putz G (2011) Combined motor imagery and SSVEP based BCI control of a 2 DoF artificial upper limb. Med Biol Eng Comput 49:567-577, DOI 10.1007/s11517-011-0750-2
11. Ang K K et all (2012) Transcranial direct current stimulation and EEG-based motor imagery BCI for upper limb stroke rehabilitation. 2012 Annual International Conference of the IEEE Engineering in Medicine and Biology Society, San Diego, CA, USA, pp. 4128-4131, DOI: 10.1109/EMBC.2012.6346875

Author: Alexandru Ianoşi-Andreeva-Dimitrova
Institute: Technical University of Cluj-Napoca
Street: Memorandumului 28
City: Cluj-Napoca
Country: Romania
Email: Alexandru.Ianosi@mdm.utcluj.ro

Performance and Efficiency Feedback in Rehabilitation Program with Kinematic Analysis System – a Case Study in Rehabilitation after Lumbar Discectomy

S.A.Moldoveanu[1], D. Şardaru[1], L.Pendefunda[2] and C.Luca[1]

[1] University of Medicine and Pharmacy "Grigore T. Popa" Iasi, Department Biomedical Sciences, Iasi, Romania
[2] University of Medicine and Pharmacy "Grigore T. Popa" Iasi, Neurology Department, Iasi, Romania

Abstract— **This paper presents a case study of rehabilitation program following lumbar discectomy with focus on rapid feedback for program improvement, personalization, efficiency and performance, through a kinematic analysis system. An objective method was proposed to evaluate the performance and efficiency in a case study in post-op of lumbar disc herniation during the rehabilitation program. Method consisted of gait analysis with focus on kinematics in sagittal plane. Data of gait biomechanics were obtained through video processing in a specialized software. Gait analysis showed significant change in patients gait during the rehabilitation program. Change was found in gait phases duration, movement angles in sagittal plane, left to right symmetry during gait in angles and timing of gait phases and basic gait parameters such as stride length and velocity. This method proved to be a positive feedback for both the patient and therapy specialist to further continue the rehabilitation process. It was also an aid to modify the program according to the problems that appeared in the analysis, problems that would otherwise not be obvious.**

Keywords— **rehabilitation, gait analysis, disk, herniation.**

I. Introduction

Lumbar discectomy is one of the most common surgical treatment in lumbar disc herniation [1]. Rehabilitation program that follows has the main purpose to reestablish lower spine movement and strength of the corresponding muscles.

During the rehabilitation program, the physiotherapy specialist follows an already established protocol, making some changes to accommodate the patient's current state and health history.

The main challenge in any rehabilitation physiotherapy type program is that there is no real objective feedback regarding its efficiency and effect on the patients gait other than various measurement and evaluation technics such as, VAS pain scales, Oswestry Disability Questionnaire (ODI), Passive Lumbar Extension Test, Manual muscle strength testing (MMST) and AMA Guides and Criteria - American Medical Association Guides). Gait analysis has been used to quantify change in gait parameters and evaluate certain aspects of the rehabilitation process.[2],[3],[4]

The kinematic analysis offers insight into the patients progress and efficiency of the rehabilitation program assigned.

II. Materials and Method

The study was conducted in the Physiokinetotherapy and Rehabilitation Center of U.M.F. "Gr. T. Popa" Iasi. Patient selection criteria for our case study were age ranging between 30 and 40 years, lumbar disk herniation at level L5-S1, with no prior disk herniation or any kind of surgery history, normal healthy weight and consent for participation. Out of the viable sample we selected one patient to start the study with. The patient was 37 years old, height 1.8 m and weight 70 kg.

Data collection and gait analysis were carried out just after the patient underwent surgery treatment. After a period of 4 weeks of recovery, bed rest and medication, the patient began the rehabilitation program in our facility. The patient was asked to walk at a normal walking speed rate covering a distance of 10 m. Body landmarks were established for trunk, pelvis, hip, knee, and data were collected using a digital video camera and further digitalization and data processing in MATLAB®.

Video analysis was performed using DLTdv3 digitizing toolbox for MATLAB® [5] with the purpose of landmark tracking. General functions in MATLAB® where used for obtaining gait angles for each gait segment, plotting values and data comparison.

The rehabilitation protocol for our patient consisted of a four stage program of active lumbar stabilization (ALS) [6].

The four stages are muscle reeducation, static stabilization, dynamic stabilization and functional activities. The modification of this muscle core stabilization program is that as opposed to standard exercises that directly activate stabilization muscles, we have targeted muscles that activate the thoracolumbar fasciae conditioning the extensor stabilization muscles of the lumbar spine.

During stage one of the ALS program, the oblique abdominals, transvers abdominis and multifidus are facilitated. The technic of abdominal hollowing (AH) is used to differentiate rectus abdominis activity from that of the rest of the abdominal muscles.

AH is performed by pulling the abdomen in without allowing significant lumbar flexion [6]. Lumbar lordosis is monitored through pressure biofeedback which also gives information concerning maintenance of lumbar stabilization [6]. In stage 2, while the subject braces the trunk muscles, load is imposed on the trunk. The lumbar spine is kept in midrange while exercising an alignment which is called "neutral position"[6]. In stage 3 the focus is on reestablishing of correct pelvic tilting. Patients are taught to exercise within

S. Vlad and N.M. Roman (eds.), *International Conference on Advancements of Medicine and Health Care through Technology; 12th - 15th October 2016, Cluj-Napoca, Romania,*
IFMBE Proceedings 59,
DOI: 10.1007/978-3-319-52875-5_56

their pain-free range of motion [6]. Stage 4 consists of functional exercises with proprioceptive training and stabilization activities. Muscle activation exercises aimed the thoracolumbar fascia accessing and transferring forces between the upper and lower body through the thoracolumbar fascia. Train coordinated action chains muscle (a muscle that forms a continuum of functional or kinetic chain) intersection that consists of: latissimus dorsi, erector spinae, multifidus, gluteus maximus and hamstrings muscles. Exercises aimed to activate muscle accessing the thoracolumbar fascia and transferring forces between the upper and lower body through the thoracolumbar fascia.

Also, focus was on training of coordinated action chains muscles (a continuum of muscle that forms a functional or kinetic chain) intersection that consists of: latissimus dorsi, erector spinae, multifidus, gluteus maximus and hamstrings.

In total, for our patient, the rehabilitation program consisted of 30 rehabilitation sessions set throughout a period of 5 weeks. Gait analysis, as described earlier, was performed 3 times. First time, right before the first session of rehabilitation, second time after 15 sessions and then third time after another 15 sessions, marking the end of the rehabilitation program for our patient.

III. Results

Primary focus of the gait analysis was to find the abnormal gait segments and angles in relation to the gait phases.

Second focus was to pin point the changes in the patient's gait during the rehabilitation program. Finding these parameters would enable us to better mold the rehabilitation program to our patient's progress. The exercises that the patient had to do targeted various areas of the body and the analysis helped quantify the effectiveness of the movements and, as needed, to change the intensity or location of the area that was worked.

In Fig. 1 is a comparison made between the three gait analysis of trunk movement angles in sagittal plane. The red line corresponds to the first analysis with the curve marked as T1 L, the light blue line corresponds to the second analysis with the curve marked as T2 L and the dark blue line corresponds to the third and last analysis with the curve marked as T3 L. The primary gait graphs were done for the left side of the body thus "L" stands for left. Gait phases end are marked with corresponding colored arrows.

In Fig. 1 is a comparison made between the three gait analysis of trunk movement angles in sagittal plane. The red line corresponds to the first analysis with the curve marked as T1 L, the light blue line corresponds to the second analysis with the curve marked as T2 L and the dark blue line corresponds to the third and last analysis with the curve marked as T3 L. The primary gait graphs were done for the left side of the body thus "L" stands for left. Gait phases end are marked with corresponding colored arrows.

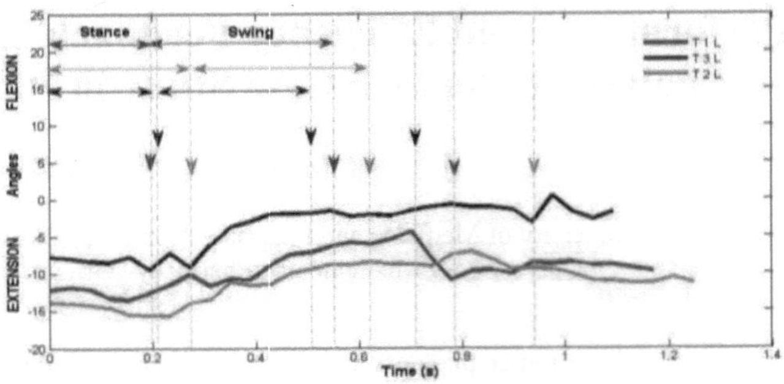

Fig. 1 Comparison between first, second and third gait analysis of trunk movement angles in sagittal plane

In T1 L, values were found, as expected, to not be in normal range[7]. At heel contact, trunk was in a 12° extension, higher than the average normal which is 5° to 6° extension [7]. As an overall characteristic of the curve, the trunk remains throughout the gait cycle in an extension position. This was an unusual finding and did bring a challenge in the rehabilitation process. After the first 15 sessions of kinethotherapy, as can be seen in T2 L, there was some improvement. Movement of the trunk is more stable and balanced. There is still a predominance of hyperextension of the trunk but not as fluctuating in amplitude as before rehabilitation started. Change in gait angles after rehabilitation has become more synchronous with the gait phases. The patient's gait was at trunk level was more balanced and stable. In the last gait analysis, in T3 L, there is a clear improvement in movement angles. Trunk is less extended during gait. At heel initial contact trunk is 7° in extension and then decreases at 2° of extension when reaching end of terminal stance.

The next studied parameter was the hip angles during gait. In Fig. 2 is a comparison made between the three gait analysis of hip movement angles in sagittal plane. For an easy reference we kept the colors corresponding the each of the gait analysis in H1 L, H2 L and H3 L.

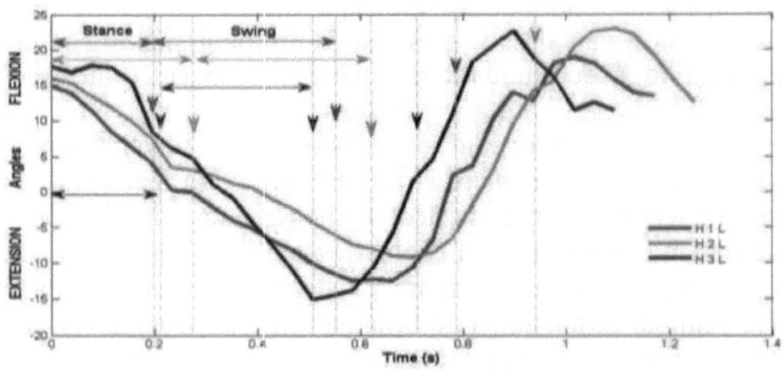

Fig. 2 Comparison between first, second and third gait analysis of hip movement angles in sagittal plane

Before rehabilitation, hip movement was unbalanced. At initial contact the hip flexion was 15°, half the value of the average normal [8]. During terminal stance the hip reaches a maximum of 13° of extension and then continues with flexion of approximately 19° during mid swing, ending the cycle with a decrease in flexion to 18° in terminal swing. The values found are significantly lower than the normal averages [8] and describe a deficit in movement amplitudes during gait. After 15 sessions of rehabilitation, in H2 L, the patient showed a clear improvement in hip movement. Flexion during initial contact was 16°, extension during terminal stance reached 10° and flexion in terminal swing reached 24°, which are normal range values. At that stage in the rehabilitation process it is usually hard to see any major improvement. With the help of gait analysis, the efficiency of the rehabilitation program and the patient's progress were tracked. These positive findings reinforced the program choice. In the third gait analysis, in H3 L, hip extension at initial contact improved even more reaching 17.6°. Extension during terminal stance reached 15° and flexion in terminal swing reached 24°.

In Fig. 3 is a comparison made between the first and second gait analysis of knee movement angles in sagittal plane plotted. For an easy reference we kept the colors corresponding the each of the gait analysis in K1 L, K2 L and K3 L.

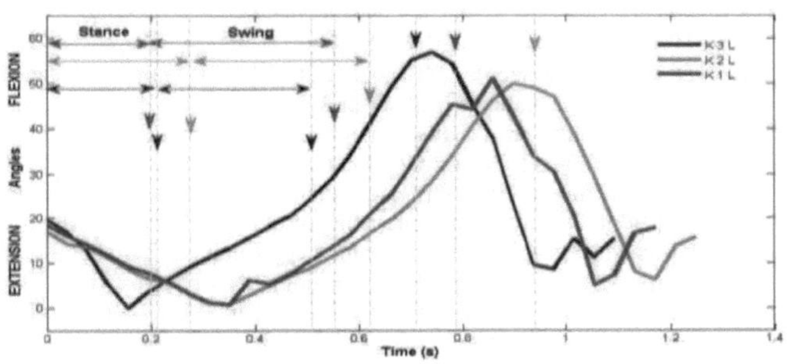

Fig. 3 Comparison between first, second and third gait analysis of knee movement angles in sagittal plane

At initial contact the knee is flexed at 18° which is significantly higher than the normal value which is 5° [9]. Following the onset of stance, the knee flexion decreases under load to an approximate value of 1°. The maximum flexion is reached in the swing phase, reaching 45°. When the swing phase ends, the knee, when reaching initial contact again, decreases flexion to a value of 5°. In K2 L there is some change but the improvement is clearly seen in K3 L where flexion during swing phase reaches 57°.

Through our kinematic analysis we were able to also view gait phases durations and stride length. In Table 1. are values for each duration of each gait phase before and after rehabilitation. In normal gait [10], double stance is 60% of total gait cycle and single stance or swing phase is 40% of the total gait cycle. Our patient had, before rehabilitation, a longer swing phase and a shorter double stance. After 15 sessions, the first gait analysis revealed an improvement in these values. Double stance was 43,7% and single stance was 56,1% of the total gait cycle. In the last gait analysis values do not present a favorable change in terms of gait phases duration.

Table 1 Gait parameters for first, second and third gait analysis

Gait parameter	Before rehabilitation	Gait analysis at 15 sessions	Gait analysis at 30 sessions
Double stance	0,23s (40%)	0,27s (43,7%)	0,2s (34,5%)
Single stance	0,35s (60%)	0,35s (56,1%)	0,33s (65,5%)
Stride length	1,11m	1,37m	1,47 m
Velocity	54,6 m/min	65,7m/min	83,2m/min

According to [11], velocity of gait and stride length reaches normal range value in the last gait analysis.

What is an improvement is timing of gait phases in left vs. right side of body.

In Fig. 4, the dotted curve which corresponds to the right hip for each of the analyses, has corresponding colors to the ones from the left side and are reversed.

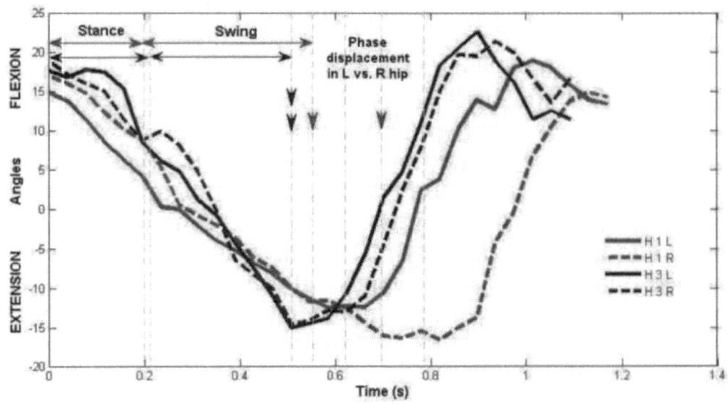

Fig. 4 Comparison between first, second and third gait analysis of hip movement angles in sagittal plane

For a better view we only included the first and last analysis results. Right and left corresponding curves are extracted from the same gait cycle and data was obtained from left and right simultaneous filming. In the first gait analysis, right and left hip do not match in timing of motion, right hip has a delay during mid stance and terminal stance. In the third gait analysis however, rehabilitation program provided symmetry in patient gait phase timing. Curves are similar in phase and amplitude.

The same phenomenon happens at knee level as shown in Fig. 5. Although curves in the first gait analysis are similar in amplitude, they do not match in phase. The two red arrows that mark the beginning of preswing do not overlap. In the third gait analysis, at knee level, curves are similar in phase and amplitude.

Since this was a single case study, the rehabilitation program had a determined length and data was obtained at preset times, there was no sufficient data to develop a relevant statistical analysis.

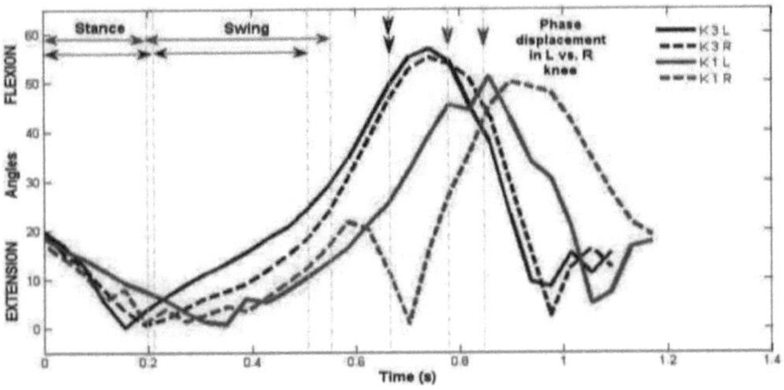

Fig. 5 Comparison between first, second and third gait analysis of knee movement angles in sagittal plane

IV. Conclusions

Performance and efficiency feedback in rehabilitation program was defined and tracked through a kinematic analysis system.

Primary focus of the gait analysis was to find the abnormal gait segments and angles in relation to the gait phases.

Second focus was to pin point the changes in the patient's gait during the rehabilitation program. Finding these parameters, would enable us to better mold the rehabilitation program to our patient's progress. The exercises that the patient had to do targeted various areas of the body and the analysis helped quantify the effectiveness of the movements and, as needed, to change the intensity or location of the area that was worked. Through this gait analysis system, an objective evaluation of the patient during the rehabilitation program was done. Tracking changes and finding problem areas on the gait graphs was possible with correlations made with the real life gait motion.

This method proved to be a positive feedback for both the patient and therapy specialist to further continue the rehabilitation process. It was also an aid to modify the program according to the problems that appeared in the analysis, problems that would otherwise not be obvious.

There is interest in further developing this method by increasing the number of study patients, expanding the analysis for more precise and detail orientated protocol and data collection, improving the precision of the technology used to reinforce the present findings.

Acknowledgment

The authors would like to thank the entire staff of Physiokinetotherapy and Rehabilitation Center of U.M.F. "Gr. T. Popa" Iasi who have contributed with great professionalism to the successful completion of the case study. Also, we would like to thank our case study patient for his patience, hard work and commitment in the rehabilitation program.

Conflict of Interest

The authors declare that they have no conflict of interest.

References

1. Weinstein JN, Lurie JD, Tosteson TD et al. (2006) Surgical vs nonoperative treatment for lumbar disk herniation: the Spine Patient Outcomes Research Trial (SPORT) observational cohort. JAMA. 296(20):2451-9.
2. Pianta L, Cimolin V, Bigoni M et al. (2015) Quantitative evaluation of gait kinematics in post-stroke patients: The effects of a specific integrated upper limb rehabilitation. Gait & Posture 42:S69.
3. Christian J, Kröll J, Strutzenberger G et al. (2016) Computer aided analysis of gait patterns in patients with acute anterior cruciate ligament injury. Clinical Biomechanics 33: 55-60, doi: 10.1016/j.clinbiomech.2016.02.008.
4. Di Marco J, Fraget C, Missaoui B et al (2013) Gait and balance parameters in patients with fascioscapulohumeral muscular dystrophy: A short term evaluation of a rehabilitation program. Annals of Physical and Rehabilitation Medicine 300:e201-e202.
5. T. L Hedrick, (2008) Software techniques for two- and three dimensional kinematic measurements of biological and biomimet-ic systems, Bioinspiration & Biomimetics, Volume 3, Number 3
6. Norris M. C, (1995) Spinal Stabilisation, Physiotherapy 81:32 –39.
7. Perry J., (1992) Head, Trunk and Pelvis, In: Perry J. editor, Gait Analysis Normal And Pathological Function. Slak, New Jersey, pp. 131-134.
8. Perry J., (1992) Hip. In: Perry J. editor. Gait Analysis Normal And Pathological Function. Slak, New Jersey. pp. 111-114.
9. Perry J., (1992), Knee. In: Perry J. editor. Gait Analysis Normal And Pathological Function. Slak, New Jersey. pp. 89-92.
10. Perry J. (1992), Gait Cycle and Phases of Gait Chapter. In: Perry J. edi-tor. Gait Analysis Normal And Pathological Function. Slak, New Jersey. pp. 3-16.
11. Perry J., (1992), Stride Analysis. In: Perry J. editor. Gait Analysis Nor-mal And Pathological Function. Slak, New Jersey.,pp.432-435.

Assistive Technology Product Innovation through Undergraduate Projects

A. Ward[1], I. Grout[2] , L. Grindei[3] and D. Mândru[4]

[1] Department of Electronics, University of York, York, England
[2] Faculty of Science and Engineering, University of Limerick, Limerick, Ireland
[3] Faculty of Electrical Engineering, Technical University of Cluj-Napoca, Cluj-Napoca, Romania
[3] Faculty of Mechanics, Technical University of Cluj-Napoca, Cluj-Napoca, Romania

Abstract— **The final year or capstone individual project undertaken by students in Electrical and Information Engineering programmes is the opportunity students have to demonstrate their ability to integrate all their academic learning and use it appropriately to undertake a significant engineering project in a professional manner. The project not only allows them to demonstrate their proficiency in technical skills but also in a range of generic skills whilst offering potential bonus benefits. This paper proposes that projects that focus on Assistive Technology (AT) solutions to real disability related issues make both excellent project topics from a technical and generic skills perspective but also serve to raise the general awareness of problems individuals with a disability face in their general living and working lives. Such projects also, potentially lead to innovative new commercial product ideas. This paper starts with an introduction to the supply side academic objectives of the student first employment transition in the form of programme learning outcomes and graduate attributes and then describes three AT projects undertaken by students in SALEIE Project partner institutions. It shows that these projects are effective in all the above stated respects and that they provide an excellent topic for student projects. A signpost to a freely available source of disability related project ideas is given at the end of the paper.**

Keywords— **disabilities; product innovation; assistive technologies; final year projects; equality in higher education.**

I. INTRODUCTION

At the time when students graduate and start work for an employer, the "first employment transition" [1] it is important that the graduate has the required graduate attributes for their prospective employer. This alignment is one of the critical parts of the student gaining successful employment in a field professionally related to their academic programme. This paper starts with a review of the supply side expression of the graduate from the three authors' institutions, the University of York, England; the University of Limerick, Ireland; and the TechnicalUniversity of Cluj-Napoca, Romania.

The University of York expresses these attributes in terms of generic programme learning outcomes:

- Subject Knowledge – Assess electronic engineering designs by applying detailed knowledge of algorithms, devices and systems and by consulting relevant documentation and research.
- Eningeering Analysis – Analyse system & component performance through computational methods and modelling.
- Engineering Design – Create designs to address real-world problems by synthesising ideas into engineering specifications.
- Practical Skills – Solve technical problems through employing skills in programming, CAD, construction and measurement and by using safe laboratory techniques.
- Technical Communication – Clearly communicate and explain electronic engineering issues and practice in a technically accurate manner to a variety of audiences, verbally, in writing and using multimedia.
- Management and Personal Development – Coordinate and execute complex projects in electronics, computing and related disciplines, with effective time management, team working, and ethical decision-making.

The University of Limerick is committed to "creating and sustaining an outstanding and distinctive learning environment for all of its students". It's six Graduate Attributes [2], Knowledgeable, Proactive, Creative, Responsible, Collaborative and Articulate form a shared value system across the whole university.

In the Technical University of Cluj-Napoca the skills developed in students are those that help define an engineer. The skills are primarily technical but generic skills such as communication, ethics, working in teams, etc. are also developed. The graduate attributes recognized as being important include:

- A knowledge base for engineering appropriate to the studied program.
- Ability to effectively apply theories into real practical problem solving
- Ability to conduct investigations of complex problems by methods that include appropriate experiments, analysis, interpretation and validation of data

S. Vlad and N.M. Roman (eds.), *International Conference on Advancements of Medicine and Health Care through Technology; 12th - 15th October 2016, Cluj-Napoca, Romania,*
IFMBE Proceedings 59,
DOI: 10.1007/978-3-319-52875-5_57

- Computer skills and ability to use engineering tools for designing new systems, components or processes that meet specified needs with required attention for safety risks and standards
- Team working as an ability to work effectively as a member and leader in multi-disciplinary teams
- Creativity, innovation aspiration and self motivation
- Good communication skills for oral presentation and dissemination of complex engineering concepts within the profession and with society at large.
- Desire for improving knowledge through training and courses
- Ability to apply professional ethics, accountability, and equity
- Foreign language skills

As would be expected there is a high degree of similarity in overall learning objectives between the three institutions. The generic skills included within the graduate attribute statements obviously align with the National and International definitions of graduate programmes [3], [4].

According to the 2015 Skills and Demand in Industry Survey report [5] "*employers still expect "enthusiasm and willingness to learn", but naturally there is a sense that 'higher' technical and interpersonal skills will be presented. "Good level of subject knowledge", "specific industry awareness", "practical experience", "the ability to work in a team and absorb quickly," "confident communications", "problem-solving skills", and ultimately "the ability to hit the ground running" are all on employer checklists. "Commercial awareness", in terms of understanding the importance of their own contribution to the success of the business, was also picked out.*"

Industry surveys such as this together with other sources of intelligence such as job advertisements [6] and research studies [7] all provide windows into the needs of graduates to help them successfully cross the first employment transition.

Within the academic curricula the final year project is an excellent opportunity for students to show what they are able to do and, if the project is specified carefully, this demonstration can include a number of generic skills, see Section III.

The project is also an opportunity to raise awareness of the issues of general living with a disabiltiy and the specific issues of engineers with disabilities have in the general work and laboratory environments. This last idea came from the SALEIE Project, which is introduced next.

II. The SALEIE Project

The "Strategic Alignment of Electrical and Information Engineering in European Higher Education Institutions", SALEIE, Project [8] was a European Union funded project involving 45 project partners and a budget of just over €1m. The financial eligibility period was October 2012 to December 2015. 44 of the project partners came from 26 different European countries, the other partner was from Russia.

The aims of this project were to investigate and explore the challenges HE across Europe is facing, specifically in the EIE discipline areas and to:

- "Build a shared understanding of the skills and competence needs of graduates to help European Companies respond to the current global technical challenges."
- "Enhance current understanding of academic programmes and modules in terms of technical content and level of learner achievement as a means of improving clarity of learner skills and competence for mobility, academic progression and employment."
- "Build a common understanding of current practices and issues associated with marketing programmes and the support of students from unconventional backgrounds and those with special needs. In this context special need are taken to include, but not be limited to students with: physical mobility problems; dyslexia and dyspraxia; visual and audio impairments; Asperger's, autism, depression, anxiety." [9]

Workpackage 4, Widening Participation and Dissabilities, created a significant online resource for the support of students with disabilities, the resource is targeted at three key stakeholder groups, Students, Academic Supervisors and Administrative staff.

All the resources are freely available on the project website and range from International and National Policy and legal statements through summaries of country interpretations; student support models; information on National and Institutional support; mobility; finance; Assistive Technologies for a range of disabilities to advice on making learning materials; and laboratories fully accessible. In addition there are pages with links to other disability related EU and Global projects and a database of "SALEIE Projects".

The "SALEIE Projects" are final year projects that are suitable for final year students in that they will allow a student to demonstrate they have met the required learning outcomes of a final year project whilst also serving to raise awareness of disabilities. Each project has a set of data to a common date set template, comprising:

- Project Supervisor – the original proposer of the project and
- Project Supervisor's Academic Institution – this is

provided soley for the purpose of making contact for additional informaton and discussion.

- Project Title
- Project Duration at the proposer's institution (this can, of course be varied to suit specific needs)
- Project Level (academic level such as Bachelor level of Integrated Masters level)
- Course suitability (this is included as an indicator of academic pre-requisites)
- Project descritpion (the detailed description of the project).

Viewers are free to use the projects as described or as the basis for variations to suit specific local needs.

This paper reports on projects undertaken during the academic year 2015-2016 by undergraduate students from three universities which were involved in the SALEIE project, University of York, UK, University of Limerick, Ireland and Technical University of Cluj-Napoca, Romania. All projects reported on focused on the area of assistive technology. In total 4 undergraduate students from the Deprtment of Electronics, University of York, 2 from the Computer Science Faculty, University of Limerick and 5 from the Department of Electrotechnics and Measurements, Technical University of Cluj-Napoca undertook disability related projects.

This paper gives a description of one project from each University and includes the objective of it and the results achieved. In some cases comments from the students are included. Section III covers the project from the University of York, Section IV the project from the University of Limerick and Section V the project from the Technical University of Cluj-Napoca.

III. Project 1: Emergency Alerting Bracelet

This project was undertaken by a student at the University of York. The 'brief' for this project was: "*The project is aimed at students who cannot hear, and in particular cannot hear the sound of an emergency alarm. The objective of the project is to design an alerting bracelet that vibrates when an alarm is sounding. The circuitry can be sophisticated in that it can be 'tuned' to listen for specific alarm sounds as opposed to just noise above a threshold sound level. This project links into the active EU Lifelong Learning Programme "SALEIE" (Strategic ALignment of Electrical and Information Engineering in European Higher Education Institutions) and the work will be aligned to the area of assistive technologies to support students with disabilities.*"

The project is challenging in that it requires a solution that listens constantly, detects when a fire alarm is sounding and then alerting the user through haptic feedback. The solution challenges the student to undertake research work into alarm signal characteristics, appropriate types of microphones and their required signal conditioning, sampling frequency and resolution, digital signal processing, the concepts of false positive and false negative alerts, vibrating alerting technologies as well as the more general issues of battery powering such a device with a decent battery life and making it small enough to fit into a wearable bracelet.

The three students that undertook this project during the last academic year approached it in quite different ways. One started with a survey of potential users to try to refine the specification. All obviously explored the nature of fire alarm signal characteristic and how they differ from other alarm and general high-level noise signals, such as road construction tools.

Solutions ranged from use of a basic microcontroller chip to a Adafruit Flora (ATmega32U4) programmable board. One solution also embedded an automatic phone messaging system that would, immediately after triggering the bracelet vibrating alert to the wearer, would also send a text message to a preprogrammed ICE (In Case of Emergency) number. In all projects battery power was a concern and, with the best type of battery currently available being lithium polymer, the students were introduced to a new set of genuine Health and Safety engineering considerations, those of charging and storage safety.

Casing design requires the students to learn a suitable 3D design package and them, if they got that far, produce the case using the Department's 3D printing facilities.
Fig. 1 Alerting bracelet case design (left) and completed prototype (right)

1 (left) shows the design of one of the cases that were actually created this year and Fig. 1 Alerting bracelet case design (left) and completed prototype (right)

1(right) a completed prototype.

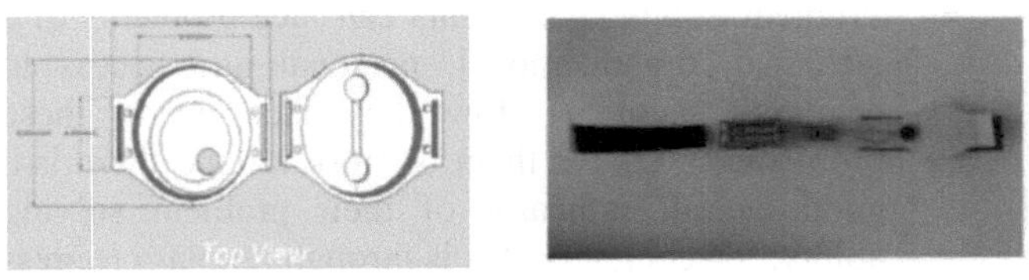

Fig. 1 Alerting bracelet case design (left) and completed prototype (right)

The objective of this project is primarily to provide a 'vehicle' by which the student can demonstrate they have undertaken a significant individual project in a professional manner. This includes the creation of a formal specification for their project, undertaking an appropriate literature review of aspects of the project's scope, undertaking a system design, developing detailed sections of the overall system, designing, building and testing these sections and integrating them all together as a whole system.

Secondly, the project provides a vehicle through which the student can demonstrate proficiency in a number of generic skills including what we require of students in the Department of Electronics and the University of York:

- Communications – students produce an initial and final written report on their work, the initial being a statement of their project, a literature review, formal specification and initial project plan. We have, in the past also required them to produce an advertising Poster of their project and for them to give a Public Presentation on their project. All components carry marks including for structure and layout of their formal reports. They are also required to defend their project after they have submitted their report for 60 minutes against questioning from two academics – this allows us to verify their understanding is truly their own but also to test their active listening and oral communication skills.
- Project Management – students produce an initial project plan and are expected to manage their time and activities to this plan, they are required to include a short section in their final report which discusses the success or otherwise of their management of the project. Included in this is a Risk Register with each risk score on probability and severity and with each having a brief narrative on the recognition the risk is happening and their remedial/corrective actions.
- Personal Organisation and Management – being self disciplined and working to plan in an organized way, maintaining good records of work done and results achieved can be very visible and provides evidence to support ability in this skill. Students are required to maintain a day log of work they do.
- Problem Solving – students can face problems of a technical, organizational, personal and access to resources nature. How they face up to these problems and solve them or work around them is a good overall indicator of their problem solving ability. Oversight of this is through regular progress meetings between the academic supervisor and the student and weekly emailed progress reports sent through the Department's electronic management system to both academic supervisors and the project administrator who will send reminders if the student does not submit a report and if the academic supervisor does not respond each week.
- System thinking – by requiring evidence of a system design the approach taken and the depth of analysis by the student there is assessable evidence of ability in this skill
- Literature Review – again the depth and breadth of the review, the items reviewed, the criticality of discussion and the approach taken to undertaking the review and they way in which it is reported are all indicators of this skill
- Reflective Practice – students are required to include a short reflective section in their final report on their experience of the whole project.

All of the above skills are assessed or inform the marks as part of the overall project marking. Marking is through a formal rubric including word picture descriptors for each category which helps remove differences between markers and the need for wide result marks variation moderation.

Finally, projects such as this one, which are disability related also serve to raise the awareness of the issues of individuals with disabilities face in general living or, as in the case of other projects, such as a soldering aid for one handed individuals, issues engineers with disabilities face in their working life.

A potential side effect of this aspect of the project is that a novel new product idea could easily emerge from the student project.

By way of illustration of the effect the project can have on the student, one of the students who undertook a project to design a talking electronic component identifier said after they had completed the project: "*Undertaking this project has given me a much greater appreciation for both the needs of those with visual impairment and their capabilities. Before the project, I would have considered it impossible for a blind person to work in the electronics industry, particularly with the prevalence of small components with visual markings - even for a colour-blind person, this can cause difficulty. However with the aid of a simple tool such as the talking component identifier, I now believe that a blind person can overcome these difficulties and work effectively. There are already examples of blind people working in the industry, and if a device like this were to become available it would make the industry far more accessible to those with visual impairment - perhaps even helping to address the severe shortage of people in the electronics industry in the UK.*"

IV. Project 2: Assistive Technology for Individuals with Limited Movements in Their Hands and Fine Motor Skill Impairments

The project was undertaken by a student at the University of Limerick. In this project, the ADXL346 3-axis accelerometer was considered to interface to an Arduino UNO microcontroller system and personal computer (PC) in order for head motion to be read by the PC when the accelerometer is attached to a human head. In this arrangement, the sensor would be worn by a student who will control the operation of the PC using head motion and the system would be worn by an individual with a physical disability that would limit their ability to use a keyboard and mouse arrangement.

The purpose of this sensor system would be to act as an assistive technology for individuals with limited movements in their hands and fine motor skill impairments. Hence, an experiment can be run by the individual without touching the equipment or experiment.

Suitable movement of the head would enable the head motion to be measured and sent to the computer. This motion would then be interpreted by the computer application in order to send suitable commands to the equipment used in the experiment. Hence, the head movement would form a non-verbal language.

The student who undertook this project produced a prototype, which partially functioned. More time and a deeper understanding of embedded system design concepts would have been needed to produce a more polished end result.

In part this example helps to demonstrate that the project is a suitable vehicle for discriminating between students of differing ability but also that expecting a fully working prototype for a novel idea or product is beyond the ability of some students.

The student, irrespective of their final result, does however learn from the experience – it is their opportunity to pull together the knowledge and skills they have learned from the entire academic programme and apply them appropriately to their project.

V. PROJECT 3: HYBRID FES – HAND ORTHOSIS SYSTEM

This project was undertaken by a student from the Faculty of Electrical Engineering at the Technical University of Cluj-Napoca. At the University it is recognised that community orientated real-world projects, professionally relevant to the student study programme make good project topics. Student interest and involvement is higher in projects of this nature.

By way of background to this project the grasping function is provided by the bio-mechanism formed by the metacarpal bones, the finger bones and their joints, where the flexion-extension and the laterality movements of the last four fingers are realized as well as the flexion-extension, abduction-adduction and the opposition of the thumb.

Patients with traumatic brain injury, stroke or cerebral palsy lose the ability to control the thumb, with a consequential negative impact on precision grasping and manipulation. This project proposes a hybrid solution to restore the opposable thumb function.

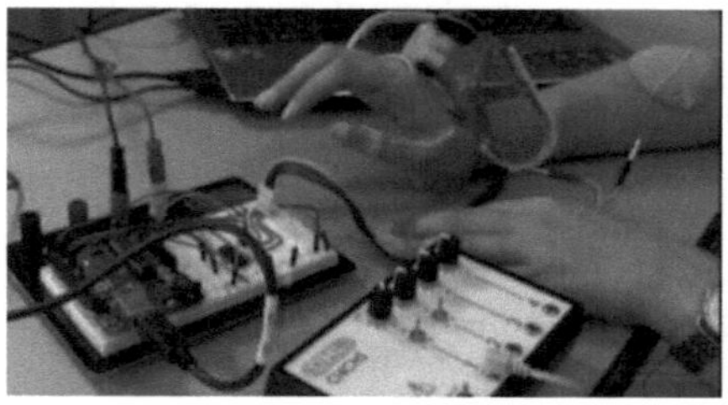

Fig. 2 The hybrid FES - hand orthosis system

It is based both on a functional electrical stimulation (FES) module and an active orthotic device to restore the thumb opposition **Error! Reference source not found.**2.

FES produces contractions in paralysed muscles by the application of small pulses of electrical stimulation to their nerves. The Odstock Four Channel Stimulator was the core of the FES module (**Error! Reference source not found.**3 left). The proper position of the electrodes was experimentally determined. The output can be ramped at the beginning and end of each cycle to give a comfortable sensation and prevent stretch induced spasticity.

The stimulation is controlled in such a way that the thumb is moved toward the index and middle finger.

The thumb orthotic device (3 right) includes a stepper actuator, a pulley and tendon driven mechanism that provides the opposition of the thumb. Based on the anthropometric data, the hardware module was designed and manufactured.

A control system of the orthosis, developed on an Arduino Uno board was proposed. An interface that allows the control of the motor speed and stroke (number of steps) was investigated. The balanced control among FES muscle activation and lightweight active orthosis leads to a better restoration of the grasping ability.

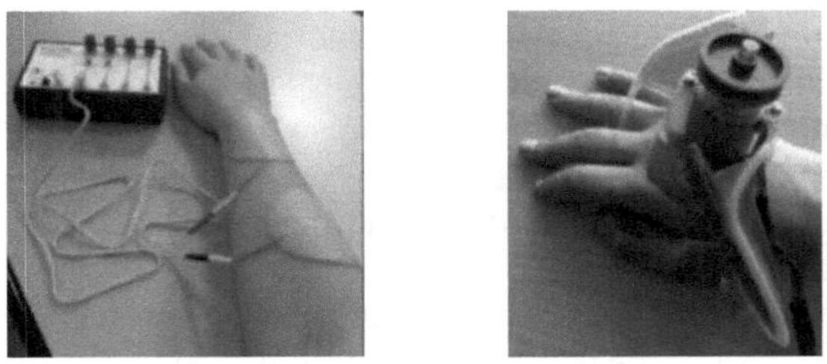

Fig. 3 Odstock Four Channel Stimulator (left), thumb orthotic device (right)

The student that developed this project was very pleased to realise and present the hand orthosis system as a simple engineering solution by using only an Arduino board, a driver and a computer.

For patients that loose certain abilities to control their thumbs for instance, implementation of technical solutions for solving this problem is very important also concerning accuracy of movements and esthetical aspects.

The student who undertook this project produced a functional prototype only based on basic knowledge and skills accumulated during 4 years of studies, and of course with the advice and expertise of his/her project coordinator. Further developments could involve medical specialists and additional efforts and tests to realize a more portable hand orthosis system .

VI. Discussion

Individual final year (or capstone) projects typically follow a generic model irrespective of technical topic or institution. The student is given a statement of the project in the form of a 'brief'. This 'brief' is a high level outline of the project broadly defining why it is important and what the ideal deliverable should be. The brief is a good opportunity to define the project in the form of a problem statement which gives the student freedom to be innovative with the ultimate in this being a solution that is truly novel and potentially commercially exploitable. Being able to demonstrate innovation is another valued generic skill by some employers. Broadly it can be measured on a scale from "truly new and novel solution to the problem" through to "only minor incremental developments over existing or obvious solutions". This scale is far from scientific but is indicative of the students' innovative ability.

This 'brief' forms the starting point for a discussion with the academic supervisor(s) and work undertaken by the student. In these early stages there is an excellent opportunity for the demonstration of professionalism through the development of an engineering specification for the project (requirements capture and specification writing) and a project plan (work breakdown structure, project planning, Gantt or PERT Chart). These are skills that students are somewhat weaker in and specifications are sometimes presented incomplete or without tolerances. Project plans often lack detail and do not focus on all the project deliverables.

The normal project would commence with an overall system design, breaking the system down into component parts that can then be designed in detail. Each system component would then be modeled, simulated, prototyped, tested, built in a more substantial, if not final form, and then retested. Here again, testing is an important generic skill for engineers and gives them the opportunity to understand the role of equipment calibration, measurement accuracy, the effect of the test method on the item being tested, noise and interference.

The overall process mirrors that in industry even to the point, for better students, of understanding tolerance analysis, design for manufacture concepts and the principles of quality assurance.

Once all the components have been designed and tested system integration commences and the build and test cycle repeats. At all stages documentation is vital so the good habits (hopefully) students have been trained in for laboratory record keeping during their earlier study years really have meaning in the final project.

Having the students present their project formally or informally verbally to technical or non-technical audiences is good for the presentation skill section of communication skill. The format report on the project is a test of their written communication skill (at least in terms of a formal report is concerned).

More generically the project exposes the students' ability to solve problems; act on their own initiative; often negotiation skills for resources and help they may need; information searching and management; work ethic; personal time management and organization; and more.

All of these generic skills can be assessed (albeit it usually very qualitatively) in the final assessment. The formal, meaningful assessment of generic skills is, however, still at its infancy with many firmly of the view that meaningful measurement is not practical or even possible. However, advances in the assessment of public speaking, as an example, through the use of word picture descriptor rubrics is improving the reliability of assessments and it is hoped, in the future, may lead to statements of student ability that are truly meaningful to employers [10].

VII. Conclusions

The individual final year (or capstone) project is the opportunity each student has to demonstrate their overall ability to undertake a significant piece of work in a professional engineering manner. The expectations of a student in all three Institutions, as described in section III above, is the same and this applies irrespective of the nature of the project.

Final year projects are usually very closely professionally aligned to the academic programme and hence could be of an analogue electronics, digital electronics, embedded system, music or media technology, computing, medical, control and even engineering management nature. Projects in any sub-discipline of Electrical and Information Engineering fit into the overall generic model described herein.

The addition of projects that raise the awareness of real disability issues is an added bonus for the student, the academic department, individuals with the associated disability and potentially the wider community. Finally, by focusing final year student projects on real world problems the opportunity exists to be innovative and potentially create new products.

There is the issue of who owns the intellectual property in the case of undergraduate student as this is, in some institutions, not as clearly defined as it is for postgraduate students and staff, but this could be addressed through a 'contract'. The bio-medical and BioTech sector could usefully engage with Universities in such developments to either take them forward to real products or as a source of ideas for projects to be undertaken by students.

The projects described in this paper are three from a pool of potential disability related projects freely accessible in the SALEIE "Student Project" page. New projects can be added to this page by submitting a description, using the same data fields as in the description template, to the project webmaster.

We recomment academic staff from technical faculties should encourage students to work on projects in the assistive technology area trying to obtain not only good functional prototypes but also innovation in products, technologies and systems that enable disabled people equal access to life's opportunities and education. The benefits are a challenging and interesting project for the student; a vehicle to truly allow the student to demonstrate and the academic supervisor to see a good range of generic skills; and the potential for a commercially exploitable end result.

Acknowledgment

The authors of this project thank the European Union for the funding to enable this project to be undertaken and to the partners of the SALEIE Project for their contribution of projects to the initial database. We also thank the students who undertook these projects this year for their permission to use quotes from them and photographs of their project work.

Conflict of Interest

The authors declare that they have no conflict of interest.

References

1. T. Ward, "Electrical and Information Engineering Employability Skills: A UK University Perspective," *Submitted for publication*, pp. 1–9, Feb. 2015.
2. "University of Limerick," 03-Jul-2012. [Online]. Available: http://www3.ul.ie/ctl/sites/default/files/GraduateAttributes_03July2012%20(3).pdf. [Accessed: 19-Aug-2016].
3. "The Washington Accord," *washingtonaccord.org*. [Online]. Available: http://www.washingtonaccord.org/Washington-Accord/. [Accessed: 27-Feb-2014].
4. A. Kumar, N. Randerson, and L. Kiwana, "Engineering UK 2013," Engineering UK, Sep. 2013.
5. "**2015 IET skills survey**," 20-Oct-2015. [Online]. Available: http://www.theiet.org/factfiles/education/skills2015-page.cfm. [Accessed: 16-Aug-2016].
6. A. E. Ward, A. Gbadebo, and B. Baruah, "Using job advertisements to inform curricula design for the key global technical challenges," 2015, pp. 1–6.
7. A. E. Ward, "The Alignment of Generic, Specific and Language Skills within the Electrical and Information Engineering Discipline," EIE-Surveyor Project, York, Dec. 2008.
8. http://www.saleie.co.uk/SSSH/text/html/Student_Projects.php, Accessed 27th July 2016
9. http://www.saleie.co.uk, Accessed 27th July 2016
10. N.R. Jackson, A.E. Ward, "Assessing Public Speaking, A trial rubric to speed up and standardise feedback", 13th International Conference on Information Technology based Higher Education and Training (ITHET), York, England, 2014.

Part VI
Health Technology Assessment

Baby Wearing Buying Decision-making - A Focus Group Exploratory Study

A. Constantinescu-Dobra[1] and M.A. Coțiu[2]

[1] Technical University in Cluj-Napoca/Electric Power Systems and Management Department, Faculty of Electrical Engineering, Cluj-Napoca, Romania
[2]Babeş-Bolyai University/Marketing Department, Cluj-Napoca, Romania

Abstract— **With declining birthrates, more and more active mothers and an increasing interest in attachment parenting, baby wearing has become one of the must-haves of modern parenthood, even more so as studies show that it also has important child development benefits. The market is abundant in many different baby carriers, almost every baby goods producer having such an item in their offer. The competition is therefore fierce, aspects considered by parents in their buying decision including not only safety and developmental features, but also traits such as easiness of use, versatility, ability to breastfeed etc. The decision-making process in this regards has not yet though been fully investigated. As such, the aim of this article is to explore the traits mothers consider when deciding on the baby carrier to purchase with the goal of making concrete recommendations for improving sellers' marketing strategy in this regard. Consumers' views are explored using focus groups as they provide the opportunity of eliciting rich quality data through spontaneous interactions. This also permits the uncovering of unanticipated issues that surveys may fail to identify. Results are obtained through qualitative analysis.**

Keywords— **baby wearing, buying decision, marketing, focus group, Y Generation**

I. Introduction

The practice of baby wearing has been on a rise in recent years especially due to an increased interest for attachment parenting, a change in the mentality of mothers who are now more and more active, but also as a consequence of increased interest in preventing hip dysplasia, a developmental condition thought to be strongly connected to the way infants are positioned during their first year [13]. Studies conducted in this domain show that baby wearing has positive effects for the prevention and treatment of hip dysplasia, cultures with a tradition of carrying babies with their hips apart having much lower rates than those culture where babies are kept with their hips extended on a cradleboard or papoose board [13]. Positive effects of baby wearing are also identified with regards to the responsiveness of mothers to their babies' needs and the development of mother-baby attachment, with baby wearing being one of the five elements defining attachment parenting (birth bonding, breastfeeding, bed sharing, baby wearing and belief in the signal value of the baby's cry) [13].

In this context, the industry of baby carriers has developed considerably, the number and variety of types, models, sizes and features of existing baby carriers making the task of choosing one quite overwhelming [11]. This also comes in the context of the Y Generation females (born between 1977 and 1994) now becoming mothers and transferring their shopping patterns to the baby products market [1]. Research shows that Y Generation female shoppers have been socialized into consuming more and earlier than previous Generation, while at the same time benefitting from a higher disposable income than their X Generation counterparts and enjoying thoroughly researching and browsing choices [1]. Y Generation shoppers generally savvy consumers who rely heavily on technology for their buying decision-making process.

For example, Y Generation Canadian mothers used to spend a double amount of time being online on their smartphones in 2014, than they did in 2012, namely an average of 2.2 hours a day [4]. The same study also pointed out that more than half (58%) said that they paid attention to advertisements that were relevant to either their lives or that of their child [4].

Furthermore, the Y Generation tends to be much more involved in raising a baby than their parents who had been mostly job oriented. Studies also show that Y Generation place greater emphasis on family experiences rather than material things, travelling and learning being more important to them than material belongings, aspects which they are also likely to apply in their parenting styles [3][4][14]. As a consequence, they look for houses to be smaller and greener, toys to be fewer and family activities to be more common. Another feature of Y Generation is that they find a median between baby-wearing, organic-life and free-range parents who do not believe in boundaries [3].

From a marketing perspective this means that, on the one hand, baby carriers' producers enjoy a considerable market, but on the other hand they are also facing the difficulties of increased competition in convincing mothers to choose to buy their particular carrier.

Because of all these, it is important that producers know which are the features of the baby carriers mothers are most interested in and how is the buying making decision being made.

S. Vlad and N.M. Roman (eds.), *International Conference on Advancements of Medicine and Health Care through Technology; 12th - 15th October 2016, Cluj-Napoca, Romania,*
IFMBE Proceedings 59,
DOI: 10.1007/978-3-319-52875-5_58

The process of buying decision-making has long been researched in the literature as it is the stepping stone in creating income. The model of consumer buying decision making was developed in 1968 by Engel, Blackwell and Kollat who identified 5 steps: Need recognition (lag between the consumer's actual situation and the ideal and desired one), Information search (seek information about possible solutions to the problem), Alternative evaluation (evaluation of the different alternatives), Purchase decision and Post-purchase behavior (evaluation of the adequacy with his original needs [9],[10].

For the particular case of the Y Generation, [1] identified five segments of shopping behavior: recreational quality seekers (are brand conscious and would pay extra for brand quality), recreational discount seekers (bargain seeking, buy at sale price), shopping and fashion uninterested (quick shoppers, have price/value consciousness), trend setting loyals (fashion and style conscious, shop from the same stores, generally also the same brands) and the confused time/money conserving group (are confused by over choice and have price/value consciousness).

The article builds on these challenges and explores buying decision-making in the case of baby carriers through the use of focus-groups. The added value of this article lies in the fact that such research in this area is scarce in spite of the large number of carriers and fierce competition on the market. The results will therefore allow us to gain more insight into the buying decision of the Y Generation mothers, therefore allowing for concrete suggestions with regards to how sellers can maximize improve their marketing strategies. The article is therefore particularly aimed at scholars and sellers in the baby wearing industry.

II. Materials and Methods

A. Rationale for the use of focus groups

Focus groups represent a form of qualitative research which builds on the interaction between participants to elicit their views, knowledge, perspectives or believes on a certain topic of interest [5] [6]. The purpose of a focus group is that of better understanding the way respondents feel or think about the subject of the analysis (a product, an idea, a service etc.)[8]. As opposed to questionnaires which imply closed-ended questions that might not cover all aspects respondents may consider, focus groups allow participants to discuss open-ended questions thus allowing the researcher to gain a deeper insight into the various experiences and thoughts of the respondents [6]. Furthermore, as a consequence of the discussions generated during a focus group, the researcher has access to spontaneous interactions, participants sharing their views in an atmosphere of openness, where they are encouraged to share different perceptions and points of view without the pressure of reaching a consensus [8]. Results obtained in this way therefore tend to be rich and diverse, often opening new research questions.

B. Focus group participants and protocol

The questions from the focus group guide were grouped in five sections (according to the stages of consumer buying decision process): need recognition/problem recognition, information search, alternative evaluation, purchase decision and post-purchase decision. All questions were tested for clarity and relevance to the objective of the focus group. This resulted in no major changes being made to the initial focus group guide.

A total number of four focus groups (n=22) were conducted. Participants in all focus groups were mothers of children between 0-2 years old, using at least one baby carrier. Focus groups were conducted between 29 May and 30 June in Cluj-Napoca and Bucharest, Romania. All focus groups were homogenous in terms of gender (females) and place of residence (Cluj-Napoca or Bucharest) and heterogeneous in terms of age, income, level of education and field of activity. Out of the 22 participants, 5 were from Bucharest (1 focus group) and 17 from Cluj-Napoca (3 focus groups), with the goal of including participants from major urban areas.

All focus groups were held in quiet areas, appropriate for such discussions. Participants were informed about the purpose of the focus group and of the fact that all their answers will remain anonymous and confidential. They consented to taking part in this study and to their answers being recorded (audio) for analysis purposes and for use in this research. Information saturation has been reached during the four focus groups with regard to the major themes approached. Also, the number of focus groups is considered sufficient for research relevance [7].

Focus group participants were aged between 26 and 39, all coming from urban areas, with a monthly income ranging between 245 and 755 euro (the maximum allowance for maternity leave). Most of the participants were employed (n=20). In terms of the respondents' field of activity, we can observe a predominance of the IT sector in the sample, with 6 persons working in the IT sector or related, 3 in financial services, 3 in educational services and 2 persons in the healthcare sector, the rest working in sales, public relations and other services.

Conversation and open dialogue between participants were encouraged by the moderator at all times. Participants were encouraged to share their ideas, thoughts, suggestions. Qualitative analysis was then conducted on the data obtained.

III. Results

For the first question, need/problem recognition, answers were generally grouped around two main situations: some of the respondents had internal stimuli, while others, much more numerous, were confronted with external stimuli in recognizing the fact that they needed such a carrier. For the first category (n=8), recognizing the need to own a carrier was determined by the physiological needs of the mother (i.e. need to sleep, eat and be independent). Most of the respondents in this category did not buy the carrier until after the baby was born, generally after the first month. This category also comprises respondents now having their second or third baby (5 participants out of the entire sample). For this first category, having an internal stimuli for recognizing the need to own a carrier, the main rationale for the purchasing of such an item was therefore represented by a need to "ease the life" of the mother, "the need to always know how the baby is doing", "helping the baby fall asleep /soothing the baby more easily", "soothing the colicky baby". The main benefit acknowledged by this category was that of reducing their isolation by "increasing the mother's mobility" who can now also walk in areas difficult to access with a pusher. Furthermore, the carrier also enables the mother to have "two free hands", thus allowing her to also tackle different tasks around the house such as cooking, gardening or doing the laundry.

Other respondents in this category, had as main internal stimuli the desire to apply the principles of attachment parenting. They therefore knew that they would be using such a carrier (and had also purchased one) before the baby was born, even if there was a risk that the baby would not like to be put in the system (n=6). Two of the participants even decided to purchase a carrier instead of a pusher as they wanted to "permanently hold their baby". One of the mothers further explained that "I feel we are one person. I know exactly what his needs are and I answer those needs immediately: I feel when he needs his diaper changed, when he is sleepy or when he is hungry.", while the other explained that "The fact that he can hear my heartbeats as it happened when he was in the womb, soothes him."

With regard to the number of carriers held, in the internal stimuli group, five participants have at least two baby carrier systems among which: 4 elastic wraps, 2 slings, 1 woven wrap, universal carrier, SSC.

It is also worth mentioning that these respondents who use the baby carrier most of the time also breastfeed and practice co-sleeping.

The second category (n=14), those mothers for whom the need to have a carrier was determined by external stimuli, comprises exclusively first-time mothers having as primary source of information people in their reference groups: friends, co-workers etc. (60%), pediatricians or specialized personnel delivering Lamaze courses (20%), information provided by online baby goods shops (10%). Out of the 14 mothers included in this group and who were recommended to purchase such an item by someone else, 8 had been more reticent, not being fully convinced by its usefulness from the beginning. However, they did try to see if the carrier could solve the problems that had with their babies, somewhere between a few weeks and three months after delivery. Such problems included: "the baby started crying when I put him in the pusher", "the baby had reflux and had to be held vertically as long as possible", "the baby could not fall asleep because of overstimulation", "the baby had constant stomach pain and keeping them vertically and my warmth helped them feel better", "the baby only regurgitated 30-40 minutes after a feeding and it had become very difficult for me to hold them", "just for discreetly nursing my baby".

Another category of external stimuli for the buying decision was determined by factors not related to the baby, but to the couple's lifestyle: "we go on a lot of hiking trips and the carrier is a comfortable option for both the baby and the one carrying them in this situation", "the carrier protects the baby better than the pusher in case of strong wind", "I had to travel to another city for 2-3 days and I thought it would be easier if I did not have to also carry the pusher", "you can carry your baby while doing your shopping without using a pusher."

Other participants (n=4) declared that they purchased the carrier in order to answer a need for social integration and belonging to various social groups. They explained that in "such a demanding period" in their lives, full of stress, frustration of doing nothing else but nursing the baby, buying a fashionable carrier "shows that you are more than a mother, you are a cool person also". This "is good for the psychic" and also helps raising one's self esteem.

All respondents in this category have more than one carrier. For their last one purchased, they mostly considered fashion and color matching.

The second question addressed the issue of searching for information as a basis for the future buying decision. All respondents had both internal and external information sources. Also, it is worth noting that, with 4 exceptions, all respondents tried to get additional information about the carriers from their friends, family members or other consumers. It was only afterwards that they studied other external sources of information. The most important external sources of information were represented by articles posted by online shops, advertorials, dedicated blogs and social media and were accessed via Internet, mostly from mobile phones (19 participants), palms (2 participants), laptop/PC (1 participant).

For more than half of the participants, advertising is considered important if it provides high-quality, informative content and it also has the power to positively impact the segment. 14 of the respondents declared it could inspire their brand confidence. A key role is also played by the various portrayals used, visuals of a family or a baby generating the most enthusiasm among the focus group participants.

With regard to the type of information mother were looking for, this mostly included the price and various ways for adjusting and fitting the carrier. All respondents declared that the Internet was the main source of information at this point of the decision making process, via Romanian and English language dedicated blogs and online baby carrier specialized shops.

The third step in the buying decision-making process is the alternative evaluation. Here participants identified the different objective and subjective characteristics considered when comparing carriers.

Considerable homogeneity was recorded at this step. All respondents were highly involved in the acquisition process and perceived the purchase as important. They all knew what were the desirable and wanted features, based on the information they had collected previously. They all declared they were interested in three main features: quality, easiness of use and price.

In general carriers quality features were associated with perceived safety and comfort for the baby. Mothers explained that they were looking for carriers which would be "protecting both my and my baby's spinal health", or "with solid fabrics and long-lasting colors", "solid fabrics and strong straps", carriers made from "natural fabrics", or "breathable", "ecological fabrics".

Most respondents were mainly concerned about the well-being of their babies. Half of the respondents also indicated particular interest for a good back support offered by the carrier, as they were looking for a good efficiency of weight distribution. Also, 12 participants indicated they wanted a padded headrest to support the wobbly head and neck of their newborn, while 11 mothers also mentioned that breast-feeding settings were "almost indispensable once the carriers are being used for long periods of time" so this was also an important feature they were considering.

With regard to carriers safety features, four of the respondents mentioned the fact that they were particularly interested in items with a high snugness factor – this indicates how closely a baby or toddler is tied around - mentioning that "I want to be sure that I can diminish any harm that can be caused to the baby if they are moving inside the carrier once I am on the move as a consequence of the constant changing of the baby's cent=r of gravity." Three of the participants also indicated paying attention to the size of leg holes which they indicated should be "small enough to prevent slipping through."

When considering easiness of use, 16 of the respondents indicated flexibility and lightweight. It was therefore important that carriers had multiple buckle adjusters at the top of each should strap to allow for controlling the length of the strap and customize the fit. Furthermore, 20 participants also wanted a compact portable carrier that would be easy to carry around, but would also offer them the possibility of handling babies with ease when using the carrier. One mother mentioned that it should be "easy to pop the baby in and out, for feedings or diaper changing". A number of 6 participants were also interested in extra features such as key rings, toy loops, pockets, while a further two mothers were looking for carriers that with small changes in their configuration could be adjustable for baby growth. They wanted to be able to use the same carrier for wearing a newborn, but to also have the possibility, as the baby grows, to make the carrier taller so it can better support the weight of older babies and toddlers. Furthermore, in the case of newborns, respondents were interested in the "possibility of changing baby's position: vertical when he is awake or horizontal when he is sleeping". Portability was also an important feature for the mothers taking part in the focus groups who mentioned the fact that "The carrier must be convenient to carry, fold quickly in a compact manner so that you can always have it at hand."

Another aspect considered by respondents when evaluating alternatives was the price of such items. This was a very important aspect for all respondents. As such, 10 of the mothers indicated that while all the previously discussed features were important for them, price was the most important trait. An important aspect to mention here is that price was not the most important feature for those purchasing a carrier for travelling purposes or those opting for such an item as a consequence of their desire to apply attachment parenting. They tended to prefer well-known brands such as Boba, Manduca, Fidella or Isara which are renewed both in Romania and abroad and have a price range between 60 and 100 euros. Respondents working in healthcare, education or the public sector were mostly interested in carriers available for a price between 30 and 50 euros, even though these carriers could not be further customized depending on the weight or other characteristics of a growing baby. Brands considered in this case included Marsupi plus, Bertoni or Woomar. Some of the respondents also decided to purchase a no-brand carrier or handmade carriers. In their case, these were generally ordered via Facebook as they believed "the quality can't be so different when the carrier looks very similarly to a Boba or a Manduca, but the price is a quarter". When considering the added value of having such an item, mothers generally also considered purchasing costs.

The fourth step of the buying decision-making process is the purchase decision. In the case of baby carriers, our results show that this is generally a unique and solitary decision. A number of 18 respondents indicated that they took the buying decision alone, while four decided on the carrier together with the baby's father. In this last situation, where the decision was taken jointly, buyers preferred a more simple look, "solid colors will work well if the carrier is intended to be shared among parents". When this was not the case, the carrier was intended to be used by the mothers only, they generally preferred vibrant colors and/or drawings to match different occasions.

Another aspect important when reaching this step was the commercial policy of the online shop where mothers would make the purchase. Among the respondents, 15 participants were influenced by a promotional campaign, with a further seven participants being influenced by the opportunity to test the carrier between three and seven days for free. Other aspects considered included free delivery and the return policy of the shop.

In terms of the post-purchase behavior, the last step of the buying decision making process, this was tested considering the adequacy of the carrier with respect to the original needs expressed by the mothers. Out of the total number of respondents, 15 persons were satisfied with their decision and had a positive review. Mothers in this category said that "The advantages of baby wearing are worth all the money", "My family's peace when putting the baby to sleep is priceless", or "We survived the colicky period very easily". Three of the respondents who had both a more expensive and a cheaper carrier (the latter is not used daily) declared that the premium paid for the more expensive one is not justified as the baby sits just the same in both items. Two respondents chose the wrong carrier in that they opted for one model which was not fit for very thin and not very tall persons, with the straps still being too long although tight to the maximum. Other two persons indicated "back pain when carrying the baby for more than one hour" and were looking for other options.

IV. Discussion

The buying decision-making process in the case of baby carriers is a complex one, strongly influenced by evolving family values and the changing external environment.

Motherhood is viewed by respondents as a life-changing experience which causes a rethinking of priorities, but also influences the buying decision-making process. Such a particularity can be noticed in the need/problem recognition phase where the gap between the desired situation and the real one is quickly noticed and addressed. We note that respondents began their decision-making process form a wide range of needs: physiological or safety needs, the need to belong to a social group or the one for self-esteem.

All respondents in the focus group belonged to the Y Generation and based on the results fit four of the decision-making segments described in the [1].

Based on the results of the focus group and the traits described by [1], the largest group of shoppers among the respondents fit the "quality seekers" profile (41%), being characterized by brand consciousness. They know very well what they want and are willing to put in extra effort in order to finally purchase quality products. In order to accomplish this they set considerable tangible criteria, looking for information on a considerable number of baby products websites. In terms of post-buying behavior, they are also characterized by a tendency to continue to pay attention to decisional alternatives in an effort to seek reassurance that they had made the optimal choice. They tend to be satisfied with the product purchased and loyal consumers to the brand. A particularity of the consumers in our focus group however, is related to their attitude towards discounts. Although, according to the literature, this segment is not generally attracted to lower prices or discounts, mothers in our sample did try to get the best quality, but were, at the same time, also seeking for promotional campaigns. A reason for this could be the high prices of the carriers. Another very interesting finding was the fact that this segment was not interested to online advertisements, even though they were all brand conscious. Only 22% of them paid attention to online advertisements.

The second category is represented by the "discount seekers" (27%), including here mothers with lower disposable income and mothers who already owned a baby carrier so their physiological need was fulfilled, but they were interested in testing other types/brands. This segment is very active on social media, tuning into opinion leaders (66%).

This group is value conscious, while also being seduced by novelty and/or fashion. They are interested in promotions available in order to purchase the latest carrier models on the market. Buying behavior is not affected by their disposable income and post-purchase behavior is only initiated in a few cases.

The next segment is that of the "shopping and fashion uninterested" (18%). Mothers in this segment were generally looking for safe and resistant baby carriers mainly bought for travelling purposes. They are efficient buyers who try to simplify their decision-making process by only referring to two or three technical features in their analysis. They try to save time and energy by purchasing the first product meeting the criteria. While in other studies in the literature they are not at all brand conscious, mothers in our sample differ in that brand is important in their case. They generally tend to be aware of 2-3 brands and only seek information about these ones. In the case of travelling couples, the buying decision is made as a group, information being sought firstly on travelling blogs and then on specific online shopping websites. When evaluating alternatives and selecting where to make the purchase from, they pay attention to convenience and shop responsiveness.

The last segment is represented by the "trend setting loyals" (14%) who are fashion and style conscious. This means that they believe motherhood should not imply no longer paying attention to their wardrobe. Quite on the contrary, they want to be up to date with changing fashions, including baby carrier products. They also have a tendency to visit the same online stores and mainly look for discounts. This segment is very active on social media, displaying all baby carriers used and including comments.

V. Limitations and further research

A limitation of the study was the relatively small number of participants as a consequence of the fragmented free time of mothers, which also limited the duration of each session to 30 minutes. However, we do not believe this to have affected the study negatively with regard to the information obtained as information saturation was reached during the four focus groups.

VI. Conclusions

The focus group we conducted allowed for the exploration of the buying decision-making process of Romanian mothers when purchasing baby carriers. All the respondents in the focus group sample met the features of Generation Y. Results showed that mothers are highly connected to each other and the world, being much more involved in carrying for their families than previous generations. They are also characterized by "smart shopping" meaning that consumers invest time in order to save money. What is quite interesting to note is the fact that mothers do not seem to be confused by the extensive offer of baby carriers on the market. They are able to quickly identify the need and take actions to satisfy it. Also, for our sample, shopping for a baby carrier loses its recreational dimension, mothers engaging in this process in order to satisfy a need, rather than as a leisure activity. The Internet remains the only means for information searching, alternative evaluation and post-purchase behavior, an aspect that could be explained by the short free time mothers have available for these activities. Another important finding was related to the high degree of objectivity they use in assessing alternatives and disseminating their opinions on social media or via other Internet pages.

Conflict of Interest

The authors declare that they have no conflict of interest.

References

1. Bakewell C, Mitchell V W (2003) Generation Y female consumer decision-making styles. Intl J Of Retail &Distribution Management. 2/2003, pp95-106, DOI: 10.1108/09590550310461994
2. Fottrell Q (2015) Step aside Generation X, the Millennials are coming, http://www.marketwatch.com/story/step-aside-Generation-x-the-millennials-are-coming-2015-05-11
3. Boesveld S (2014) Gen Y and Millennial moms having more kids and abandoning helicopter parenting, http://news.nationalpost.com/news/gen-y-and-millennial-moms-having-more-kids-and-abandoning-helicopter-parenting,
4. Canadian report 2015 - State of Modern Motherhood Report, http://www.newswire.ca/news-releases/canadian-millennial-moms-are-spending-twice-as-much-time-online-on-smartphones-vs-2012-according-to-new-babycenter-research-517431891.html
5. Jamieson L, Williams L M (2003) Focus group methodology: Explanatory notes for the novice nurse researcher. Contemporary Nurse 14: 271-280
6. Wong L P (2008) Focus group discussion: a tool for health and medical research. Singapore Med J 49(3):256
7. Rabiee F (2004) Focus group interview and data analysis. Proceedings of the Nutrition Society (0029-6651) 063(004):655 DOI: 10.1079/PNS2004399
8. Krueger R A, Casey M A (2104) Focus Groups: A Practical Guide for Applied Research. 5ed. Sage Publications, Singapore
9. Kotler P, Keller K (2006) Marketing Management. Pearson Prentice Hall, New Jersey
10. Kotler P, Armstrong G (2008) Principles of Marketing. Pearson Prentice Hall, New Jersey
11. Baby wearing International at http://babywearinginternational.org/
12. Granju K A, Kennedy B (1999), Attachment Parenting: Instinctive Care for Your Baby and Young Child. Pocket Books, New York
13. International Hip Dysplasia Institute at http://hipdysplasia.org/baby-wearing/
14. Millennials: A New Generation of Family Values. http://www.millennialmarketing.com/2009/07/millennials-a-new-generation-of-family-values/

Author: Constantinescu-Dobra Anca
Institute: Technical University of Cluj-Napoca
Street: Memorandumului, no. 28
City: Cluj-Napoca
Country: Romania
Email: anca.constantinescu@enm.utcluj.ro

A Critical Analysis of Self-assessment Tools for Improving Workers' Health and Work Performance

S.C. Anca

Babeş-Bolyai University, Faculty of Economics and Business Administration, Cluj-Napoca, Romania

Abstract— **An improved health management increases the performance and productivity of workers, lowers absenteeism and increases presenteeism. Health and productivity of the workers are important issues in the European context of an ageing population in order to maintain economic development. The objective of the study was to critically analyze self- assessment tools in order to obtain information on workers' health and work performance. Three self-report tools were finally selected to be analyzed: Health and Work Performance Questionnaire (HPQ), Work Ability Index (WAI) and Stanford Presenteeism Scale: Health Status and Employee Productivity SPS-6 (SPS-6). Among the observed tools, WAI and HPQ have been considered the most suitable for the proposed use, taking into consideration that they both address health issues in terms of their influence on work productivity, and allow for monetization of absenteeism and presenteeism. Using data collected by this article may allow researchers to improve and develop new tools for health management and health related cost benefit analyses. It may also provide employers with tools for a more complex view on the health status and work capacity of the employee, enabling for actions meant to improve work conditions, health and productivity.**

Keywords— **health, productivity, work ability, absenteeism, presenteeism**

I. Introduction

Europe is facing ageing population as according to Eurostat forecast, by 2060 there will be only two people of working age (15-64 years old) in the EU for every person aged over 65, compared to a ratio of four to one today [1].

It is therefore important to build a healthy and active population in order to maintain economic development, through productivity of the workers [2]. Employee productivity is influenced by direct factors such as workplace conditions or indirect factors related to employee health and wellbeing [3] [4].

An important component in this respect is represented by employers' actions towards improving health management. Therefore identifying assessment tools for worker status on health and productivity may have an important role. Applying of such tools within organizations will allow for information on: the number of workers having health problems; the costs for the employer of such health problems; how work performance is influenced by sickness absence [5][6][7]. Such data being available will enable for actions within the organizations that will contribute to healthier workplaces and increased productivity [8].

This article aims to be a critical and comparative analysis on tools designed to improve age management, referring to the health component at the workplace. These instruments are used to assess the workers' health, their performance at work, and their absenteeism and presenteeism respectively. Using data collected by this article may allow researchers to improve and develop new tools for health management and health related cost benefit analyses. The research may also help employers and occupational health services to build solid information on workers' health and lost performance due to health problems, and therefore to propose measures designed to improve employees' health, as well as to perform better calculations when monetizing sick absence or work productivity.

II. Methodology/Materials

A computerized search was conducted in academic databases in order to identify relevant information on self-assessment tools for evaluating and improving workers health and productivity. The search resulted in 34 articles published in English related to health self-evaluation instruments among workers and their applicability within the organizations. The search was conducted using the keywords: health and occupation, productivity, work performance, absenteeism, presenteeism, work ability. In selecting articles we considered our objective of identifying applicable tools to be used by companies as instruments for evaluating and improving their workers' health as well for providing possibilities to measure the cost of the health problems consequences at work. The selection criteria were: 1. Self-assessment questionnaires completed by employees; 2. Validated tools through studies and internationally tested functionality; 3. Suitability for monetization and cost-benefit analysis. Three self-report tools which met all the inclusion criteria were finally selected to be analyzed.

S. Vlad and N.M. Roman (eds.), *International Conference on Advancements of Medicine and Health Care through Technology; 12th - 15th October 2016, Cluj-Napoca, Romania,*
IFMBE Proceedings 59,
DOI: 10.1007/978-3-319-52875-5_59

III. Results

The following three tools have been retained to be analyzed and compared:

1. Health and Work Performance Questionnaire (HPQ) developed by the World Health Organisation (WHO). Built as a self-report addressing employees with 55 items, HPQ allows for cost evaluation of the worker health problems in relation to work performance, absenteeism and work accidents. Information that can be extracted from the questionnaire involves very detailed health and work productivity related items on three dimensions: 1.identifying health problems and their treatment; 2. assessment of work performance using data related to sickness absence, presenteeism, and critical incidents and 3. basic demographic data. Different scores can be drawn from the self-report as per the needs of the organization. Such scores include values for absenteeism, absolute or relative presenteeism as well as combinations between absenteeism and presenteeism. [9][10]

2. Work Ability Index (WAI), developed by the Finnish Institute of Occupational Health in 1992. With an updated new version since 2012, WAI is a seven item rating scale that grades the present and future work ability of the workers based on a self-assessment questionnaire. The seven items are: 1. Current work ability, 2.Working ability considering the requirements of the work, 3. Current illnesses (accidental injury, musculoskeletal disease, circulatory disease, respiratory disease, mental health disorder, neurological and sensory disease, gastrointestinal disease, urinary or genital disease, skin disease, tumor, metabolic disease, blood disease), 4. Estimated effects of illnesses or injuries at work, 5. Absence from work due to illness, 6.Own estimation of work ability two years from now, 7. Psychological resources. According to the obtained scores it divides work ability into four levels: poor, average, good and excellent. [11]

3. StanfordPresenteeism Scale: Health Status and Employee Productivity SPS-6(SPS-6), is using six items to evaluate presenteeism. While absenteeism measures the number of days missed from the workplace, presenteeism refers at being present at work, but having different levels of performance due to health problems. It consists of six questions on a 5 item Likert scale, addressing the following work situations that may be affected by the health problems: handling stress, ability to finish hard tasks, distraction from taking pleasure in the work, hopeless feelings related to the ability of finalizing work, ability to focus on achieving goals, being energetic to complete all tasks at work. SPS-6 ranges from 6 to 30. The higher the score the less is the amount of lost performance. [12]

The main features of the three tools retained for analysis are presented in Table 1.

Table 1 resumes the features of the three self-report tools based on the criteria they were analyzed for. Both absenteeism and presenteeism may be measured by HPQ and WAI, while SPS-6 allows for presenteeism measuring only. Among the observed three self-reports, HPQ is the only one to include annual income information, which enables direct monetization of the sick absence or of the work performance. As regards the number of items these tools have, with 55 items HPQ includes the most detailed information on the workers' health and work performance, in comparison with WAI and SPS-6, having 7 items and 6 items respectively. This however means that HPQ takes longer to complete. In terms of languages being available, the most widely translated is WAI, with 24 versions. The research also revealed that all tools are mostly used in research studies whereas WAI seems to be the only currently used for practical purposes by occupational health services.

Table 1 Overview of the self-report analyzed tools

Tool name/ features	HPQ	WAI	SPS-6
Allows for measurement of	Absenteeism Presenteeism	Absenteeism Presenteeism	Presenteeism
Allows for direct monetization	Yes	No	No
Items number	55	7	6
Language availability	English and Portuguese	24 languages	English
Use in practice by companies	No	Yes	No

In what follows we are taking a closer look on the three self-report tools in order to have a better view on their utility, based on the proposed objective of this research.

With regards to the assessment tools that enable evaluation of the health problem effects at the workplace by measuring absenteeism, this can be done using WAI and HPQ. Of the two, HPQ results in a more accurate evaluation, by measuring absences from work in the last four weeks, using hours and days, while WAI measures absenteeism in the past 12 months, on days intervals. Thus HPQ can provide precise monetization absenteeism, using hours to calculate the periods of absence from work. Also, unlike WAI, HPQ questionnaire includes information on annual income of the worker, which allows for direct calculation of indirect cost of workplace illness. This would provide cost-benfit analysis a measure of the impact of certain actions meant to improve health or work performance.

To measure presenteeism, all three analysed tools include self-assessment questions, but differently. SPS-6 uses six questions with a Likert scale type with 5 options, providing quick assessment of how various health problems can affect work performance in the past month. It asesses the ability of completing tasks, the stress management, the pleasure to work, the feelings of hopelessness , concentration and energy to work, while WAI measures the perceived current work ability of the employer on a scale from 1 to 10 and scores the effects of illness or injuries at work on the work performance. It provides also an estimation of the future work ability on a 3 point scale. In a similar way HPQ allows for assesing how health problems affect work performance by using scales from 0 to 10 (10 indicating the best performance) . HPQ comprises comparison with other workers and between the usual performance and the recent performance (last four weeks).

Concerning the ease of use through other language version availability, WAI is available in 24 languages and is considered by many authors as a primary tool for evaluation of work ability [13]. HPQ is available in English and Portuguese, short translated versions being available in French, Spanish and Japanese. SPS-6 has been found in English language only.

In terms of their use in actual practice of the companies or occupational health services, of the three, only WAI is a tool effectively used both in research and practice by companies or occupational health services as part of health examinations. The other two register only validation and research studies among different organizations.

IV. Discussion

This article critically analyzed three self-assessment tools used for the evaluation of workers' health and work performance: Health and Work Performance Questionnaire (HPQ), Work Ability Index (WAI) and Stanford Presenteeism Scale: Health Status and Employee Productivity SPS-6 (SPS-6). The study revealed that all three tools could be used as assessment tools for the use of the employers regarding workers' health and their productivity. They allow for monetizing productivity loss due to workers' health problems. As such, these self-report instruments may be useful tools for companies to assess the value of certain actions meant for health or productivity improvement.

Using the above tools may allow employers to have a more complex view on the health status and work capacity of the employee, enabling for actions meant to improve work conditions, health and productivity.

Among the observed tools, WAI and HPQ have been considered the most suitable for the proposed use, taking into consideration that they both address health issues in terms of their influence on the work productivity, and allow for monetization of both absenteeism and presenteeism.

Moreover, the use of these instruments would be of interest to companies in order to analyze the relationship between absenteeism and productivity among older workers, in the context of an ageing population, as empirical evidence reports show that both absenteeism and productivity tend to be lower among older workers [14]. Employee's age would therefore be an important criterion when selecting measures for health and productivity improvement. In the same context of ageing population, the analyzed tools could be appropriate instruments to use for actions in order to restore and maintain work ability of older workers. Proven positive effects of using such tools among organizations might also become a reason for decision makers to grant subsidies in order to support their use on a large scale.

Further research is needed in order to analyze the measures taken in order to improve the health of the workers together with the estimated monetized impact of such actions, based on the results of the self-reports applied to the workers. Furthermore it would be very important to research on case studies regarding the benefits of the taken measures for health improvement, in terms of expected decrease of sickness absence rate, staff turnover decrease, increase of employee satisfaction, cost reduction by productivity improvement, fall of musculoskeletal case level, increase of performance and productivity. In the meantime, for practical purposes it would be also useful to study the necessity of repeating such questionnaires with a certain frequency among workers, in order to assess the positive expected effects of the taken actions.

V. Limitations and further research

There were some limitations to this study. The scientific literature includes a wide range of questionnaires and health related instruments evaluating productivity losses due to health problems, yet we believe that we chose the most representative tools for their ability to be used for monetizing health problems. Our purpose is to further continue the research in this field, to analyze the utility and the characteristics of other existing instruments for health and productivity appraisal. Additionally, we envisage to deepen our research with primary data analysis within the private sector of companies in Romania.

VI. Conclusion

This article provides a comparative analysis on three self-report tools available for researchers and employers to use in studies or practice. The tools allow for comprehensive information on workers' health status as well as for measuring the effects of the health problems on the work performance, using absenteeism and presenteeism data. Among these observed tools, Work Ability Index (WAI) proved to be widely used in practice for health examinations within companies and occupational health services, whereas Health and Work Performance Questionnaire (HPQ) seems to be the most suitable for direct measuring absenteeism and presenteeism. We therefore consider the information gathered in this research useful for actions meant to improve work conditions, health and productivity.

Conflict of Interest

The authors declare that they have no conflict of interest.

References

1. European Commission (2012) Active Ageing Report, Special Barometer 378, at http://ec.europa.eu/public_opinion/archives/ebs/ebs_378_en.pdf
2. Bloom, David E, David Canning, and Jaypee Sevilla (2001) The effect of health on economic growth: theory and evidence. No. w8587. National Bureau of Economic Research
3. Berger, Marc L, et al.(2001) Alternative valuations of work loss and productivity. Journal of Occupational and Environmental Medicine 43.1: 18-24.
4. Schultz, Alyssa B, and Dee W Edington (2007) Employee health and presenteeism: a systematic review. Journal of occupational rehabilitation 17.3: 547-579
5. Collins, James J, et al (2005) The assessment of chronic health conditions on work performance, absence, and total economic impact for employers. Journal of Occupational and Environmental Medicine 47.6: 547-557
6. Hilton, Michael F, et al. (2008) Mental ill-health and the differential effect of employee type on absenteeism and presenteeism. Journal of Occupational and Environmental Medicine 50.11: 1228-1243
7. Martinez, Luis F, and Aristides I Ferreira (2012) Sick at work: presenteeism among nurses in a Portuguese public hospital. Stress and Health 28.4: 297-304
8. Grawitch, Matthew J, Melanie Gottschalk, and David C Munz (2006) The path to a healthy workplace: A critical review linking healthy workplace practices, employee well-being, and organizational improvements. Consulting Psychology Journal: Practice and Research 58.3: 129.
9. World Health Organisation Health and Work Performance Questionnaire at http://www.hcp.med.harvard.edu/hpq/ftpdir/HPQ%20Employee%20Version%2081810.pdf
10. Absenteeism and presenteeism scoring for World Health Organisation Health and Work Performance at http://www.hcp.med.harvard.edu/hpq/ftpdir/absenteeism%20presenteeism%20scoring%20050107.pdf
11. Rautio M, Michelsen T (2014) How to use the Work Ability Index questionnaire. Finnish Institute of Occupational Health, Helsinki
12. Koopman, Cheryl, et al. (2002) Stanford presenteeism scale: health status and employee productivity. Journal of occupational and Environmental medicine44.1: 14-20.
13. European Commission & Warwick Institute for employment research (2006) Ageing and employment: identification of good practice to increase job opportunities and maintain older workers in employment at http://www.ageingatwork.eu/?i=ageingatwork.en.relevantliterature.32
14. Auer, Peter, and Mariàngels Fortuny (2000) Ageing of the labour force in OECD countries: Economic and social consequences. Geneva: International Labour Office

Author: Sanda Crina Anca
Institute: Babeş-Bolyai University, Faculty of Economics and Business Administration
Street: Teodor Mihali, 58-60.
City: Cluj-Napoca
Country:Romania
Email: a_sanda_c@yahoo.com

Promoting a Dental Practice on Facebook

A.I. Iancu and S.D. Cîrstea

Technical University of Cluj-Napoca/ Electric Engineering, Cluj-Napoca

Abstract— **Presence on Facebook can bring additional marketing opportunities to a dentist practice. This preliminary study purpose was to determine which elements of a Facebook page are the most important from a consumer's point of view, how to build an online presence, throw feed-back and to who should we address when conceiving a promotion strategy on social networks. For that, a consumer survey was designed and sent. 161 valid questionnaires were completed, with more than forty percent of respondents indicating that they are searching for his/hers dentist's Facebook page before receiving a dental treatment. Aspects and information found on a Facebook Page can influence more than 43 % of users in choosing a certain dental practice. Most of the people looking for information about a dentists or dentist practices on Facebook are young, with low income, but educated and interested in finding at least a price list, information about contacts and promotions/ discounts, contact number for emergencies and opening hours. Consumers are not interested to see purchased images or photography of auxiliary staff posted on dental practice Facebook Page.**

Keywords— **Facebook, promotion, dental practice.**

I. Introduction

There are numerous studies that show the importance of social networks as tools in the online promotion of dentists and dentist practices [1], [2], [3], [4]. If two-thirds of dentists in Romania are working in their own practices, which means that most of the graduates become managers as well [5] and they will have to work hard to have a solid base patients, social networks just provides the necessary tool to access cheap and easy the type of clients they want. Whether talking about Facebook, You-Tube, Google+ or Pinterest via social networks can build a community with a commitment consistent dialogue between practice and patient [6].

More and more dentists adopt Facebook as a communication tool so that they can forward their messages broadly, so they can pass-along messages (videos, stories, and pictures) with the aim to increase product awareness or brand equity [7], [1]. Benjamin Burris, Jeff Behan, Robert Pickron, Bill Pickard, Kelly Fergus and Mark L. Dake [4] agree that there are huge rewards with a well-thought-out plan that is properly implemented, constantly monitored, and often updated, when talking about the promotion through social networks of dentists. Dentists must consider that Facebook can be a double-edged sword; positive as well as negative reviews are certain to appear.

II. Theoretical Background

Due to the fact that patients choose to spend more time on social media than on any other Internet activity, dental professionals are aware that they must alter their marketing efforts to use social media for reaching patients or potential patients [8]. One of the reasons why social media marketing is such a useful tool, is the high level of interaction and ability to engage consumers [3]. The same authors show that a significant portion of patients (39%) are indicating that they would visit a Facebook page, when making a decision about which practice to use for a dental treatment.

A recent study shows that as of the first quarter of 2016, Facebook had 1.65 billion monthly active users [9], being the most popular network worldwide. In Romania, in 2016 there were over 8.5 million of accounts on social networking site Facebook, a total of 22,241,718 inhabitants [10]. Even without taking into account those 10.77% of Facebook users who are under 18 [11], and the mother is the one who decides [12], data report shows the number of patients that can be reached through social network promotion. Other studies show that the majority of Facebook users are young [13], the number of positive reviews (likes) but also the number of personal friends list decreasing with age [14] [15]. On the other hand, the latest list released by DSV Cluj-Napoca 2012 [16] shows that the number of private dental offices is 648.

One study in US, regarding Facebook Pages shows that the consumers have indicated that the following components of a Facebook page attracts their attention: a link to the practice's Web site, the orthodontist's credentials and before-and-after treatment photographs. There are no national studies to show what Romanian patients want from the dentist's Facebook page. Although the Romanian existing studies that could be extrapolated to the research issue is related to online communication of practitioners in dentistry with their clients. Therefore, the research outcomes exclusively reflect the propensity toward marketing communication of the Romanian websites but with significant disparity between the dental sites from UK in terms of brand awareness content and feedback.[17] On other perspective, the economic crisis has changed the pattern in dental advertis-

S. Vlad and N.M. Roman (eds.), *International Conference on Advancements of Medicine and Health Care through Technology; 12th - 15th October 2016, Cluj-Napoca, Romania,*
IFMBE Proceedings 59,
DOI: 10.1007/978-3-319-52875-5_60

ing, mainly by emphasizing rather on emotion than on rational reason.[18] Finally, Romanian dentists' websites display rational messages, using reasons, by disseminating information rather than images.[19]

Our study aims to cover precisely this niche of online promotion so as to meet the dentists aimed at promoting its services through the social networking site Facebook.

III. METHODOLOGY

We conducted a survey containing 32 items regarding components as: respondents' demographic characteristics, Facebook usage and page content of a private dentist practice. The goal of the survey was to determine which aspects of the Facebook page are most important to the patients from a marketing standpoint.

Except the questions regarding the demographic and socio-economical aspects all items were formatted as a 5 point Likert scale (1 – Not at all important; 2 – Low importance; 3 – Neutral; 4 – Moderately important; 5 – Very important) for determining the Level of Importance for the elements of a Facebook page.

The survey was administered to an unknown number of individuals but it was completed by 172 and 161 were at least 18 years of age. This was a convenience sample; respondents were approached through Facebook and in public locations like the Technical University of Cluj-Napoca. Volunteers were encouraged to forward the link of the survey to their friend and acquaintances. Minors were excluded from the study due to their inability to make oral-care decisions [20], so we didn't consider 11 surveys due to the age of respondents (under 18).

In ranking the importance of elements, the time spent and number of visits on Facebook, we were interested only about the opinions of persons who said that when decide to go to a dentist they are looking for information on his/hers Facebook page (69 respondents).

We emphasize that this study can be considered one of an exploratory nature, the results are specific only to the investigated sample (cannot be generalized to the population).

IV. RESULTS AND DISCUSSIONS

A. Some characteristics of respondents

Of the 161 respondents, 36.65% (59) were females and 63.35% male (Table 1). The distribution of age went from 20 (the youngest) to 41, most of them being 21-25 years old. This is not surprising, knowing that at national level, the most Facebook users are between 18-34 years old (49.9%).

116 live in Cluj-Napoca and the rest of them are from Aiud (1), Alba Iulia(5), Beclean (1), Bistrita (4), Brasov (1), Campia Turzii (3), Carei (1), Dej (1), Dragomiresti (1), Gherla (1), Hateg (1), Ludus (1), Medias (2), Petrosani (1), Satu-Mare (3), Sibiu (1), Tarnaveni (1), Turda (3) si Zalau (4). Most of them were students (82.61%) with a venue of 0-500 lei/month (51.55%) and 500-1000 lei/month (34.78%).

Among the respondents who completed the survey, 43.48% say that when decide to go to a dentist they are looking for information on his/hers Facebook page (69 respondents).

We observe little differences when studding the search pattern of women and men (48.57 % women, 51.43% men) when they are looking for information on his/hers Facebook page. On the other hand, most of the men aren't searching for a dentist's Facebook page (72.53%), when looking for credentials. It appears that with the increase of income, respondents are more likely to search the dentist on Facebook.

Most of the users are visiting their Facebook account more than 8 times a week (68.60%).

Table 1 Characteristics of respondents, searching for a dentists Facebook page

Characteristics	% of Respondents	% of Respondents searching dentist on Facebook	% of Respondents NOT searching dentist on Facebook
Gender			
Female	36.65	48.57	27.47
Male	63.35	51.43	72.73
Age group			
18-25	87.58	87.14	89.01
26-34	8.07	8.57	8.79
Over 36	4.35	4.29	2.20
Income/month			
0-500 lei	50.31	51,43	49.45
500-1000 lei	19,25	17.14	20.88
1000-2000 lei	18.63	17.41	19.78
2000-4000 lei	8.70	10	7.69
Over 4000 lei	3.11	4.29	2.20

B. Importance of a Facebook page elements, in promoting a Dental Practice

Most rated components of a Facebook page (345 points being the maximum and 69 minimum) when looking for a dental practice are: price list (317 points), having contacts (313 points), promotions and discounts (304 points), contact number for emergencies (302 points), opening hours (301 points), real images of the practice (390 points), "before and after" pictures (287 points), link to the dental practice website (283 points), mentions of dentist's credentials (279 points) and stars granted by patients (278 points).

Looking at the first three elements of the top we can observe that two of them are linked to prices. We can explain that due to the number of young respondents (87.14 %) with low income (68.57 % have an income lower than 1000 lei) (Table 1. & Table 2.).

Elements ranked as least important by respondents included: purchased images from a dedicated website (169 points), images of auxiliary staff (184 points), pictures of the dentists working (212 points), links or images towards dental education and hygiene related articles (238 points), number of positive reviews/likes (271 points) and the rapidity of response to messages sent by visitors (275 points) (Table 2.).

An interesting discussion is the low influence of number of reviews or stars granted to the Facebook page by patients. At least one study made in US [3], shows the high level of importance granted to both of them. The explanation of the results could reside in educational factor (most of the respondent of our study are university graduate, so hard to convince) or, even more interesting, in the age of Facebook users (the respondent of our study are over 20's).

Table 2. Rated components on a Facebook page

Elements	Points
The price list	317
Having a contact address	313
The existence of promotions (10% discount for students)	304
The existence of a contact number for emergencies	302
Types of dental work practiced in cabinet	302
The opening hours	301
Real images of cabinet	290
Images of dental treatment "before and after"	287
Link to website	283
Mentions of dentist's credentials	279
Stars granted by patients	278
The rapidity of response to messages sent by visitors	275
The number of positive reviews (like)	271
Links or images towards dental education and hygiene related articles	238
Pictures of the dentist working	212
Images of auxiliary staff	184
Purchased images from a dedicated website	169

When asked if informations and aspect of a Facebook page could influence the decision of choosing a certain dental practice, most of respondents replied yes (43.48%), the rest of them being neutral (23.19%) or said no (33.33%).

Our study shows that users considering important and very important the amount of informations on Facebook page, are interested in finding informations about (Table 3): price list (139 points, from a maximum of 150 points and 30 minimum score), types of dental work practiced in cabinet (136 points) having contacts (135 points), and a contact number for emergencies (134 points). Least important for this patients are: purchased images from a dedicated website (74 points), images of auxiliary staff (87 points) and pictures of the dentists working (98 points).

On the other hand, persons who are not influenced by the informations and aspect of a dental practice Facebook page, consider as important and very important the next elements: price list (110 points), promotions and discounts (108 points), and opening hours (107 points). Like the users considering important and very important the amount of informations on Facebook page, purchased images from a dedicated website (51 points), images of auxiliary staff (56 points) and pictures of the dentists working (71 points) had the lowest score.

Table 3. Most rated components page and level of influence by aspects and informations in choosing a dental practice

Elements	Points (high and very high level of influence)	Points (low and very low level of influence)
Highest scores		
The price list	139	110
Having a contact address	135	
The existence of promotions and discounts	134	108
The existence of a contact number for emergencies		
Opening hours		107
Lowest scores		
Purchased images from a dedicated website	74	51
Images of auxiliary staff	87	56
Pictures of the dentists working	98	71

V. Conclusion

This study shows that Facebook is an efficient communication tool between dentists and patients, more than forty percent of respondents searching their doctor throw this social network. Patients can be attracted to a certain practice based on the image and informations found on a Facebook page.

Based on this study, the managers and the marketers who want to attract patients through a Facebook page must take into consideration some aspects. The people most certain to look for information about a dentist or dentist practices on Facebook are young, with low income, but educated. The ideal Facebook page, from a consumer point of view, has to have at least a price list, information about contacts and promotions and discounts, contact number for emergencies and opening hours.

Consumers are not interested to see purchased images or photography of auxiliary staff posted on dental practice Facebook Page.

VI. Limitations and Future Research

Limited research in promoting a dental practice on Facebook and the number of respondents, are the most important limitation of this study.

A future research could show how and to whom (gender, age, income, education, location etc.) it is best to promote online a dental practice (e-mail, web page, ads, SEO, mobile etc.).

Future research can also address situations in which advertising a dental practice includes users' comments.

Conflict of Interest

Every paper must contain a declaration of conflicts of interest. If there are no such conflicts write “The authors declare that they have no conflict of interest”.

VII. References

1. Shen G, Chiou J, Hsiao C, Wang C, Li H (2015) Effective marketing communication via social networking site: The moderating role of the social tie, Journal of Business Research 69:2265-2270
2. Ozimek P, Bierhoff H (2015) Facebook use depending on age: The influence of social comparisons, Computers in Human Behavior 61:271-279
3. Cox T, Park J (2014), Facebook marketing in contemporary orthodontic practice: A consumer report, Journal of Orthodontist (3)e43-e47
4. Burris B, Behan J, Pickron R et al. (2011), Marketing Directly to Patients, Seminars in Orthodontics 17(4):297-303
5. www.meddent.umfcluj.ro
6. http://ac.els-cdn.com/S0011848612005134/1-s2.0-S001184861200513 4-main.pdf?_tid=294a57b0-41d3-11e6-96d2-00000aab0f01&acdnat= 1467628766_890d7838883 6458c9d85bf8e0ca08c1b).
7. Ho Y, Dempsey M, (2010) Viral marketing: Motivations to forward online content, Journal of Business Research 63:1000–1006
8. Friedman D (2015) Maximize social media presence, Dental economics, 60(5):137
9. http://www.statista.com/statistics/264810/number-of-monthly-active-facebook-users-worldwide
10. http://www.insse.ro/cms/ro/content/popula%C5%A3ia-rom%C3 % A2niei-per-places-to-1-January 2016
11. http://www.facebrands.ro/map.html
12. Walley E, Silberman S, Tuncay O (1999) Patient and parent preferences for orthodontic practices. Clinical Orthodontics and Research 2(3): 110-123
13. http://www.facebrands.ro/Cluj/oras/Cluj-Napoca
14. Lee S (2014) How do people compare themselves with others on social network sites?: The case of Facebook. Computers in Human Behavior, 32, 253-260.
15. Ozimek P, Bierhoff H (2015) Facebook use depending on age: The influence of social comparisons, Computers in Human Behavior 61:271-279
16. http://www.dspcluj.ro/HTML/unitati_medicale/CABINETE%20S TOMATOLOGICE%20PARTICULARE.pdf
17. Constantinescu-Dobra A. (2014) Content marketing in dentist's websites. An empirical comparatively study between Romania and United Kingdom. IFMBE no. 44. pp. 107-112
18. Constantinescu-Dobra A. (2012) The internet marketing and the SMEs". A comparative analisys of dentistry strategy for online and printing advertising. Marketing from information to decision 5-th edition. Cluj-Napoca. Risoprint. pp. 75-88
19. Constantinescu-Dobra A. (2011) Direct response advertising in Romanian dental field. A qualitative analysis, IFMBE no. 36. pp78-84
20. The Merck Manual: capacity to make health care decision-from:http://www.merckmanuals.com/home/fundamentals/legal_a nd_ethical_issues/capacity_to_make_health_care_decisions.html

Generation Z and Online Dentistry. An Exploratory Survey on the Romanian Market

A. Constantinescu-Dobra and V. Maier

Technical University of Cluj-Napoca/ Department of Electrical Power Systems and Management, Faculty of Electrical Engineering, Cluj-Napoca, Romania

Abstract— **The paper aims at analyzing the Generation Z online spending habits for dental services in correlation with the demographic factors. At the same time the paper investigates to which extent the Internet influences their decision in choosing a dental service. Moreover the paper tries to identify which online information related to dental care meets most the expectations of the Romanian Generation Z as well as what kind of information these would desire to find online. The research is designed as a quantitative study based on a questionnaire that has been distributed among 630 students from the universities of Cluj-Napoca. The data was collected using a web based approach and was analyzed using frequencies and correlation models. The findings show us that the Romanian Generation Z does not rely heavily on the information found on the Internet when looking for a dentist, but like to inform themselves online when it concerns specific dental procedures. Moreover, the study shows us that females are easier to be influenced by the Internet when it comes in choosing their dentist, while men are more loyal to their dentists. In what regards the most frequently sought information Generation Z is looking for online we discovered that these are the ones related to dental education, oral hygiene and dental caries and they would also want to find information related to prices, alternative treatments and benefits of the used materials. The discovered results are very useful information for all dental care providers, having an overwhelming importance on dental marketing planning, especially for their online promoting strategies.**

Keywords— **online promotion, Generation Z, Romanian dentistry market, consumer behavior**

I. Introduction

In today's business environment dominated by change, where everything is getting more and more technologized, companies are trying to remain competitive on the market, keeping up with their customers' requirements.
Much so ever we might even state that Schumpeter's "creative destruction" perception is reaching every type of business.

In this contemporary society, which is characterized by a complex dynamic economy, in order to keep up with the constant changes and to be closer to their customers, more and more companies and self-employed persons are making themselves visible on the Internet.

In Romania the number of Internet users has registered a remarkable growth in the past 15 years, namely from 3.6% in the year 2000 to 56% in the year 2015 [1],[2]. One can see that we are speaking here of a growth of more than fifteen times. The increasing availability of Internet has change the decision buying process. What makes the Internet so attractive is not just the possibility to communicate, research and exchange ideas and knowledge, having a global reach, but it also plays a role of selling and advertising channel enhancing the overall interactivity of the businesses today [3]. People look for all kinds of information on the Internet, like news, cooking recipes, health care information, information related to personal development, sports, recreation, fashion, financial investments etc.

According to the Gemius Audience study, one of the main fields that Romanians look for health care information when accessing the Internet [4]. That is also the reason why more and more dental care providers are starting to get reachable via the Internet. Thus their online marketing efforts are just at the beginning as the dental industry in Romanian is just at its starting stage and in a continuous development.

The dental industry is becoming more appealing as the patients are getting more sophisticated and don't attend the dentist only for regular treatment anymore but are opting also for cosmetic dentistry.

According to the latest research reports, the Romanian Dental Market (Euromonitor International, INSE) shows a great potential for future growth, as it offers services at affordable prices, short treatment period, usage of advanced state-of-the-art technology and well-trained professionals [5].

In this respect, in order to elaborate an efficient and effective strategy, the marketers must know the actual situation of the dentistry market, the behavior of their customers as well as all the factors that might influence the patients during the decisional buying process.

The *main goal* of this study is to assess the students' perception and behavior concerning dentistry and their habits in the online decisional buying process. We have emphasized on their actual online actions with regard to their need for recognition/ problem recognition, information search, alternative evaluation and purchasing decision. Moreover

S. Vlad and N.M. Roman (eds.), *International Conference on Advancements of Medicine and Health Care through Technology; 12th - 15th October 2016, Cluj-Napoca, Romania,*
IFMBE Proceedings 59,
DOI: 10.1007/978-3-319-52875-5_61

we intend to analyze in what extent the demographic factors influence the online behavior of the patients, taking into account the information that one can find on dentistry online. Given this, we consider the present study having an overwhelming importance on dentistry marketing planning, especially for the online promoting campaigns. This study can be considered as a starting point for the Romanian marketers and/ or practitioners to be competitive on the local (even on the European) market.

II. Theoretical Background

A. Generation Z

Generation Z refers to the people who were born in the mid-1990s and growing up in the early 2000s. [6] Over the years they were given a variety of names: Generation Z, Internet Generation, iGeneration, because they are mainly characterized by their computer addiction, as well as their addiction to any other type of technology [7].

What makes this generation different from any other previous generation is that these adolescents are the most electronically connected generation in the history [8], they have basically grown up with technology. These adolescents have been growing up with the Internet, mobile phones, laptops, iPads, tablets and other electronic devices, which became part of their daily lives.

Generation Z, individualistic by nature who believe that speaking their mind and expressing their opinion is for the best [9] feel more than any other generation before them the need of belonging to a group [10].

The digital natives dispose of an increased technological intelligence, multi-tasks with online products, variety of electronic devices and processes a large amount of information on the Internet [11]. But even though they process information more rapidly than the generations before them, they are not particularly brand loyal and don't like to be controlled [12], that is why the dental practices today have an even harder job in attracting and satisfying the needs of this uprising generation of patients.

B. Online promotion

Online promotion differs from the traditional promotion channels as it allows publishers and ad networks to learn much more about the online users and allows advertising to be targeted [13], having as such a big effect on the marketing world.

This is the reason why, in this Internet era, practitioners with marketing savvy are spending time and money to get involved within the online world in order to be successful reaching and listening to the their consumers. That is why, today's dental practices see themselves forces to move their advertisement activities to this new media, by creating themselves a web page, making themselves known on social media (Facebook, Twitter, etc.) or even subscribing to news group discussions.

According to a study made by the National Authority for Management and Regulation in Communications (ANCOM), Romanians access the Internet, on average, 24 days per month. 74% of them access it daily or almost daily (90% if we are referring to the Generation Z), while 16% access the Internet 2-3 times a week, and 4% once a week. The majority of Romanians access the Internet from home, 72% of Romanians connect via their PC, 61% via their laptops, while 43% are accessing the Internet via their smartphones and 32% via their tablets. [14]

We can thus conclude that due to the fact that mobile devices have become part of our daily lives, a dental practice that is not connected to the Internet will soon be outdated [15].

III. Research Methodology

A. Research objective

The objectives of the research are as follows:

- assess the influence of various Internet resources that might influence the students' decision in choosing a dental services, a specific procedure or even a practitioner;
- study the Internet information on dentistry that are useful for Romanian student as dental patients as well as the their expectations in terms of dental information;
- analyze the correlation between the purchasing behavior for dental care of the Romanian Generation Z and some demographic factors.

B. Research instrument and sample description

This study employs a quantitative research that was based on a questionnaire administered to a sample of students using a web based approach [16].

The questionnaire contains open as well as closed questions, comprising 37 items, grouped in 4 sections: behavioral section (Likert scale), the typology of the accessed information regarding dentistry (Importance Scale), expectation of patients (Importance Scale) and identification questions (demographic and daily dental care procedures).

The chosen sampling method was the non-random, conventional one, by distributing the questionnaire to groups of students from the following universities of Cluj-Napoca: Technical University, Babes -Bolyai University and the Iuliu Hatieganu University of Medicine and Pharmacy. The respondents are from the Central and North Western part of Romania. We have chosen this region because after Bucharest this is the most dynamic region from an economic point of view and also because the indicator purchasing power/inhabitant are the closest to the country's average.

The sample size

To find out the size of the sample, we used the following formula:

a) $n = t^2 \times p \times \frac{1-p}{e^2}$, where:

n = sample size;

t = probability allowed (1.96 was chosen for a confidence level of 95 %);

p = 0.5(usually);

e = accepted limit of representativeness error (accepted between 1 % and 5% maximum);

e = 4.75 %.

After applying the formula, the resulting sample size is:

$$n = 1.96 \times 0.5 \times \frac{1-0.5}{0.05^2} = 3.8416 \times 0.5 \times (\frac{0.5}{0.002209})$$

n = 434.76

The sample size of the population must be corrected using the following formula:

b) $n_1 = n/[1 + \frac{n-1}{N}]$, where

n_1 = corrected sample size;

n = sample size;

N = the total population.

Therefore, after applying the correction formula we received the following result:

$$n = \frac{434.76}{\left[1 + \frac{434.76-1}{450000}\right]} = \frac{434.76}{1.00096391} = 434.341334$$

According to statistics there were 450,000 students in Romania between the years 2014-2015 [17].

Our sample includes 630 respondents. We have registered 865 responses in our database but have eliminated the ones that were incomplete. Also to mention here is that our survey was conducted during the period of April- May 2016.

According to the identification questions, we have 55% female and 45% male respondents. 41% are students from the Technical University of Cluj-Napoca, 36% are from the Babes-Bolyai University and 22% from Iuliu Hatieganu University of Medicine and Pharmacy. A percentage of 30, 6% of the interviewed students are from the rural area and 69.4% from the urban area. The great majority of respondents (88.2%) are between 21 and 22 years old and 24.5% of them are employed. Their disposable income is as follows:

- under 500 lei/month (111 EUR) – 44%
- between 500-1000 lei/month (111-222 EUR) - 35.2%
- between 1000-1800 lei/month – 15.2%
- more than 1800 lei/month - 5.6%

C. Research results and discussions

The research findings confirm that the Romanian Generation Z generally pay attention to their health and seek to be continuously informed (78%). This result was doubled by the frequency of annually checking their oral health state. In spite of the very poor statistics on national level, which depicted that only 35% of the population go annually to the dentist, Generation Z visit their practitioners more frequently.[18] Even though 19.6% of them are not going to the dentist for a regular check-up, but only when it is absolutely necessary, the majority of them, namely 36.6% visit their dentist twice a year, while 31.5% of them visit their dentist once a year. 43% of the respondents describe themselves as being sensitive to pain, while 37% of them has opted for a procedure of dental cosmetics.

Concerning the prevention, they are brushing their teeth once a day - 16.6%, twice a day - 63.1% and three times a day – 12%. What is interesting to observe here is the fact that the remaining respondents are brushing their teeth just occasionally. We consider these findings as being poor for the Generation Z, because all of the respondents are students, a segment that has access to a higher education and that is better aware of the importance of prevention.

A percentage of 47.3% use as additional mouth care products, besides the tooth brush, the mouth water and 27.1% use the dental floss.

An interesting fact to notice is that 66% of the questioned students are loyal to their dental practitioners, which we consider a significant percentage, taking into account that a character trait of Generation Z is that they are continuously looking for new experiences and are not so loyal in terms of their service provider.

In what regards the frequency with which they are looking for information related to dental care online, we note that the majority of them access such information once a year - 22.7%, while 22.1% of them look up such kind of information twice a year, 18% three times a year and 7.6% never make use of the Internet in finding out such types of information.

The influence of various Internet resources that might influence the students' decision to choose a particular dental services.

This objective was tested in the frame of 15 statements. The respondents were asked to state their agreement regarding these affirmations using a five point Likert scale (1 - Total disagreement, 5 – Total agreement).

The findings that have a mean over 3.5 and under 2.5 are revealing few trends and are displayed in Table 1.

Table1. The results of the influence of the main Internet resources that influences students' decision to choose a particular dental services

Item	Mean	Std. dev.
The Internet is a useful source of information on oral hygiene for patients	3.88	.868
I have check-up an information found on the Internet with my dentist	2.35	1.301
A dentist's website aroused my interest in a procedure, which I have not yet done	2.28	1.342
„Social media" influences my decision in choosing a dentist	2.11	1.159
I read on forums recommendations to help me choose a dentist	2.09	1.219
A dentist's website aroused my interest in a procedure, which I have than done	1.88	1.163
I visited a particular dentist due to an online promotion that I have received	1.68	1.138
I played an electronic game related to dentistry	1.59	1.166

The results reflect a minimum propensity of the Romanian students towards searching information and assessing different decisions concerning dental care. The only statement that has achieved some consensus is that Generation Z (74.5% of the respondents) browse the Internet in order to find information related to oral hygiene. By analyzing the frequency of students that have responded with Totally Agree or Agree (Table 2), we can observe that the Romanian Generation Z is interested only within a small proportion in finding out information related to dental procedures - 26.8% via social media and 35% via forums/ blogs. Moreover the students are not interested to find information related to the person of their dentist on the Internet. They have declared in proportion of 88% that the Internet does not influence their decision in choosing a dentist.

Table 2. The results of the main Internet marketing actions and its influence on students' decision to choose a dental procedure or a practitioner

Item	Dental procedure %	Practitioner %
Social Media	26.8	12.4
Blog	35	15
Site	22	12

Those who are still influenced by certain information found on the Internet about specific procedures discuss them with their dentist only in proportion of 11%. The same percentage of the sample went to the dentist after seeing an online advertising related to a price discount. However, Generation Z wants to 49% to be able to communicate with their dentist via the Internet.

According to the stages that implies the consumer buying decision process we can conclude that the Internet represent an medium-important platform only in seeking dental information and assessing the patients' alternatives. It is also worth mentioning that in dental care, the Internet does not represent a factor in converting the need or desire into action.

The Internet information on dentistry that are useful for Romanian student as dental patients as well as the way in which these meet their expectations

The results are depicted in Figure 1.

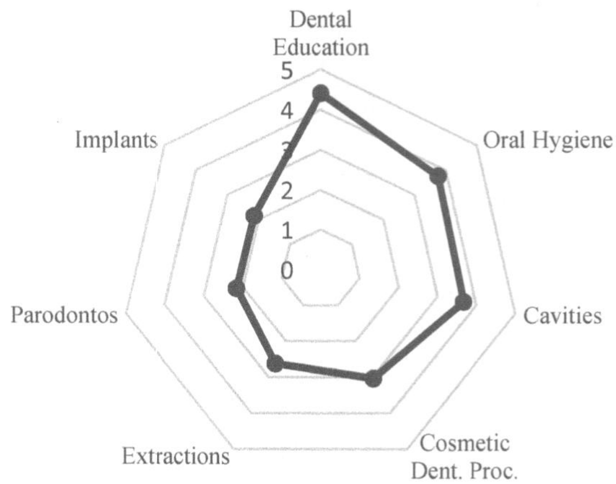

Fig. 1. The importance of dental information on the Internet

In order to be able to analyze the results for our objective we used the importance scale, where 1 stands for unimportant and 5 means very important. The findings reveal that Generation Z is considering important and useful the information available on the Internet concerning the dental education (almost a consensus – mean 4.4 from max. 5), dental hygiene (mean – 3.75) and information regarding cavities (mean – 3.67). The information regarding dental cosmetics like teeth whitening or dental jewelry have only medium importance, just like the extractions. Also, the respondents consider that information related to periodontal diseases or implants are not useful (mean of 2.16, respectively 2.14).

The students expressed also their opinion concerning the desired information regarding dentistry that they want to be able to access on the Internet. The ranking of these information is displayed in Table 3, using the same scale of importance (1 – Unimportant, 5 - Very important).

Table 3 The expectation of the Generation Z in term of the dental information displayed on the Internet

Item	Mean	Std. dev.
Price and Payment Method	4.59	.846
Description of the offered services	4.46	.969
Treatment procedures	4.42	.894
Online patient scheduling	4.38	1.001
Comparison between different treatment methods/ techniques with arguments	4.17	1.056
The advantages of the used materials	4.17	1.048
Prevention	4.07	1.144
Opinions of the existing patients	3.89	1.246
Informations regarding health insurance	3.78	1.302
Patient's personal data sheet	3.77	1.406
News in the domain	3.68	1.235
Online consultations	3.33	1.413
Employees' CV and their personal values	2.93	1.370

Generation Z is expecting to find on the Internet information related to prices and details about dental services and procedures. They also consider the online patient scheduling to be very useful. Practitioners should display on their Internet platforms (website, forum/ blog or social media) also comparisons between different treatment methods, advantages of the used materials as well as information related to prevention.

Medium importance have registered the information related to the patient's own files, patients' testimonials, information regarding health insurance, online consultations and news on the dental field. Last ranked is the information regarding the practitioner (personal information, CV) as these are considered to be uninteresting.

The correlation between the purchasing behavior for dental care of the Romanian Generation Z and the demographic factors

In order to analyze the connections between the features of the dental purchasing behavior and the demographic factors we have used Pearson's bivariate correlation.

The outcomes validate the existence of very few direct strong correlations between some demographic factors and the behavioral features of the respondents in the sample.

The first strong negative correlation is that between the gender and the different types of Internet platforms in influencing the decision of purchasing a particular dental service. Hence, the female respondents seem to be more easily influenced by the information they find on social media and forums in their decisional buying behavior of a dental service (Pearson's Correlation is -.186 respectively - 311). Moreover, a positive correlation has been found between the gender and the loyalty towards a dentist; male respondents are more loyal to their dentist then the female respondents. (.198) The urban /rural factors, the age or the year of study are not determinant variable in analyzing the influence of the Internet.

The last present correlation in the sample is that between the employment status of the respondents and their disposable income on the one hand and the fidelity (.142) and price promotions via Internet (-161) on the other hand. This means that the higher the amount of money the Generation Z earns, the higher their loyalty in opting for dental services. Moreover, the lower their income, the higher their receptiveness to Internet advertisements offering price promotions.

IV. Conclusions

After analyzing the results obtained in our empirical research we can conclude that Generation Z does not rely heavily on the Internet when looking for a dentist or dental practice. Although in a fairly small extent (approximately a quarter of them) make use of the existing information on websites, forums or social media, when searching for information related to specific dental procedures and evaluation of alternatives.

The most frequently sought information they look up on the internet are the ones related to dental education, oral hygiene and dental caries. The respondents to our questionnaire want to find information online that are useful to all segments of the market; information about prices, services, alternative treatments and used materials. Also they would pretty much appreciate if they were given the possibility to schedule their own appointment online. Another particular desire would be that of accessing their own patient folder.

As a result of the correlation analysis the study reveals the existence of links between gender and the influence of different information in choosing a dental service. Women are easier to be influenced by the Internet when it comes in choosing their dentist, while men are more loyal to their dentists.

Even though our study shows that the Romanian Generation Z are not so influenced by dental care information on the internet, not having an online presence as a dental care provider would be a big mistake as they would become antiquated in this technology driven era.

V. Limitations and Future Research

The results of the present study should be seen in regard to the limitations of such a research. One of the first limitations applies to the geographical distribution of our sample. Another limitation is represented by the fact that our sample comprises only students/ adolescents with access to more information, pursuing a higher education.

A future research should try to include all adolescents, representing Generation Z, despite of their level of education. Moreover the study should try to expand to other regions of Romania.

Conflict of Interest

The authors declare that they have no conflict of interest.

References

1. http://www.internetworldstats.com/eu/ro.htm
2. http://www.brat.ro/stiri/comunicat-de-presa-brat-a-publicat-pentru-a-doua-oara-rezultatele-de-audienta-ale-mediului-online-la-nivel.html
3. Kursan, I., Mihic, M. (2010). Business Intelligence : The Role of the Internet in Marketing Research and Business Decision-Making, Management: Journal of Contemporary Management Issues, 15(1), pp. 69-86.
4. http://www.ziare.com/internet-si-tehnologie/utilizatori/ce-informatii-cauta-romanii-pe-internet-1261582
5. Constantinescu-Dobra, A. (2012) The internet marketing and the SMEs. A comparative analisys of dentistry strategy for online and printing advertising. Marketing from information to decision 5-th edition. Cluj-Napoca. Risoprint. pp. 75-88.
6. Kaur, P. (2014). Relationship between social networking sites usage pattern and motivations behind usage: a study of generation Z 'a digital generation'. International Journal of Applied Services Marketing Perspectives, 3(2), pp. 996-1004.
7. adevarul.ro/lifestyle/stil-de-viata/generatia-z--crescuta-internet150aedbfc7c42d5a663a14e3c/index.html
8. C. Geck (2006). The Generation Z Connection: Teaching Information Literacy to the Newest Net Generation, Teacher Librarian, 33(3), pp. 19-23.
9. Euromonitor International. (2011) "Make Way for Generation Z: Marketing to Today's Tweens and Teens", February 2011, http://www.euromonitor.com/make-way-for-generation-z-marketing-to-todays-tweensand-teens/report
10. Williams, K. C., Page, A.R. (2011). Making to the Generations, Jpurnal for Behavioral Study in Business, 3 (Aprilie), pp. 1-17
11. Williams, K.C., Page, R.A., Petrosky, A.R., & Hernandez, E.H. (2010). Multi-generational marketing:descriptions, characteristics, lifestyles, and attitudes cited in Jain, V., Vatsa, R., Jagani, K. (2014) Exploring Generation Z's Purchase Behavior towards Luxury Apparel: a Conceptual Framework, Romanian Journal of Marketing, Issue 2, pp. 18-29.
12. http://www.realitatea.net/cine-este-generatia-z-si-ce-surprize-vor-avea-angajatorii_872467.html
13. Evans, D. S. (2009). The Online Advertising Industry: Economics, Evolution, and Privacy, Journal of Economic Perspectives, 23(3), pp. 37-60.
14. http://www.ziare.com/internet-si-tehnologie/internet/ce-fac-romanii-pe-internet-si-cat-timp-petrec-in-mediul-online-studiu-1382441
15. Kimball, B. (2000). The internet's impact on dentistry: Part I: Will the Online revolution affect your practice? Dental Economics, 90(1), pp. 44-47
16. http://cj.fitsolutions.ro/quest/index.php/262362
17. http://www.insse.ro/cms/files/pdf/ro/cap8.pdf
18. http://www.ziare.com/social/capitala/romanii-europenii-care-merg-cel-mai-putin-la-stomatolog-999244

Author: Constantinescu-Dobra Anca
Institute: Technical University of Cluj-Napoca
Street: Memorandumului, no. 28
City: Cluj-Napoca
Country: Romania
Email: anca.constantinescu@enm.utcluj.ro

Patient Satisfaction with Diabetes Care in Romania – An Importance-performance Analysis

M.A. Coţiu[1] and A. Sabou[2]

[1] Babeş-Bolyai University/ Faculty of Economics and Business Administration/ Department of Marketing, Cluj-Napoca, Romania
[2]Technical University in Cluj-Napoca/ Faculty of Automation and Computer Science/ Department of Computing and Automation, Cluj-Napoca, Romania

Abstract— **The medical care services market is currently confronted with increasing competition in the context of the development of private medical services providers. At the same time patients tend to become much more informed of the various treatment options as a consequence of medical information now being available through a variety of sources. Furthermore, they expect time, information and answers to their questions as well as politeness, empathy and attention from their doctor which brings them very close to the traditional consumer profile. Patients satisfaction is thus increasingly regarded as an important element in healthcare systems, even more so as it is also linked to positive medical and marketing results. It is even more important in the context of chronic illnesses where disease management is extended for a long period of time and treatment success is closely connected to patient compliance. The article aims to identify those attributes medical providers for diabetes care in the ambulatory setting in Romania should focus on in order to maximize patient satisfaction. By using the importance-performance analysis, factors were distributed into four quadrants according to the perceived levels of importance attributed by the consumers and the perceived performance offered by the medical unit. Results show that medical units should maintain efforts for ensuring a high performance level for the availability of the doctors and nurses attribute, engage in more active promotion of auxiliary support services and keep up the good work done with regards to accessibility and clinic facilities. The added value of the article lies in the fact that it presents a starting point for medical units in analyzing their strengths and weaknesses for two criteria used by consumers during the buying decision-making process: the importance of the attributes under analysis and the perceived performance offered by the supplier.**

Keywords— **patient satisfaction, diabetes, importance-performance analysis, Romania**

I. Introduction

Patient satisfaction is one of the indicators of care in the medical sector. Research in this area proves that patient satisfaction influences patient retention, treatment compliance, as well as medical staff satisfaction or patients' intent to seek a second opinion or file for malpraxis [1],[2].

During the past decades, both medical services and healthcare systems evolved considerably especially in the following areas [3]: the development of an increasing number of private healthcare providers offering state of the art technology and procedures, increased availability of medical information on the internet leading to an increase in patients' expectations regarding the medical services received, a much more dynamic and competitive environment in which healthcare providers operate with an increased interest for obtaining high patient satisfaction scores in order to help support differentiating their institution form the competing ones [4][5]. Patient satisfaction and the factors that influence it have therefore come to the forefront of research in an attempt to offer healthcare managers those solutions that can indeed make a difference in maximizing medical and financial results.

At the same time, the past decades have also brought a shift with regard to the role played by the patient in the medical decision. Whereas before patients played the role of a spectator, they are now being brought to the center of this process of decision-making in an attempt to develop a doctor-patient partnership. This means that the relationship is being redefined and brought closer to the consumer goods relationships where all partnership terms are discussed and agreed between the two parties, in this case with the common goal of improving the patient's health [6]. This is also supported by a shift in patients' expectations in that patients today expect time, information and answers to their questions, at the same time as politeness, empathy and attention from their doctor [7] thus coming very close to the classical consumer profile [8]. Because of this, it is important that strategies adopted by the healthcare units for satisfying the needs of this new category of patients benefit from effective marketing plans, as well as policies and procedures targeted to the different consumer groups [9].

When considering strictly medical services for diabetes care, having the patient at the center of the medical activity is even more important. This is because, as diabetes is a chronic disease, diabetes management plays a very important role in preventing the very costly complications associated. Furthermore, the nature and particularities of this disease determine an increased number of interactions between patients and the medical units for a long period of time. With an incidence of 64.000 new cases diagnosed

S. Vlad and N.M. Roman (eds.), *International Conference on Advancements of Medicine and Health Care through Technology; 12th - 15th October 2016, Cluj-Napoca, Romania,*
IFMBE Proceedings 59,
DOI: 10.1007/978-3-319-52875-5_62

each year for a total number of 796.803 patients diagnosed in 2011, Romania only ranked 26 in EU27 with regard to diabetes care, this situation being due more to the problems of the medical system, than to lifestyle issues [10].

From a marketing point of view, patient satisfaction implies positioning the patient as a client of the healthcare providers, be they public or private, thus determining a number of changes. On the one hand, the doctor-patient relationships which had been previously dominated by the former is now changing towards a partnership with the aim of identifying a solution which will then be proposed to the patient, following an informed decision [11][12]. At the same time, the patient-client is also now in a position in which they can ask for certain medical services or procedures for which they can pay a certain fee directly or through the various medical insurance types (e.g. elective medicine services, insulin pump etc.). On the other hand, given the increasing number of private healthcare providers and competition in the area [13], the patient-client now has access to considerable variety when choosing the healthcare provider. Medical services however will remain highly complex [14][15].

From the point of view of medical and marketing benefits, research shows that increasing patient satisfaction levels leads to an increase in staff morale, a decrease in the number of patients seeking a second opinion, an increase in patient compliance with doctor recommendations together with a positive image of the healthcare provider in the community [1][2].

The purpose of this study is therefore to explore patients perceptions regarding the importance of a set of attributes identified as influencing patient satisfaction and the perceived levels of performance of the medical unit. The results will therefore represent a starting point for medical units in identifying their strengths and weaknesses in these areas in order to be able to take the necessary measures for ensuring patient satisfaction. Attributes are analyzed in the context of six dimensions related to patient satisfaction: patients relationship with the doctors, nurses, auxiliary staff, and other patients, clinic facilities and other support services. The article is therefore addressed both at scholars with an interest in patient satisfaction and at medical facilities managers interested in increasing their competitive edge.

The study is conducted at a time when diabetes incidence in Romania is situated at quite high levels. According to data form the National Health Insurance Institute [16], a number of 677.229 patients were undergoing treatment for diabetes in 2013, which led to total treatment costs of approx. 151 mil euro, meaning an average cost/patient of 230 euro/year. At the same time the International Diabetes Federation estimates suggest that the real number of patients with diabetes in Romania is of around 1.5 million [17], almost half of them thus remaining un-diagnosed.

The added value of the article lies in the fact that it offers a concrete starting point for managers in increasing their competitive edge by analyzing two criteria used by patients in their analysis of the medical services they benefit from in the ambulatory setting: the importance of the attributes under analysis and the perceived performance offered by the supplier.

II. Methodology

A. Importance-performance analysis

The importance-performance analysis was first introduced by [18] as a method for identifying those attributes firms should focus on in order to maximize satisfaction [19][20]. Because of its easiness to use and its capacity of presenting data in a way allowing for the formulation of strategic recommendations, the method was shortly after adopted widely in various industries such as tourism, hospitality, environment, educational and medical services [20][21][22]. The method implies the identification of the strengths and weaknesses of the service provider with regard to two criteria consumers use in their buying decision-making: the importance of the attributes considered and the performance of the provider for those attributes [23]. According to this method, we do not examine only the service provider perceived performance with regards to a set of attributes of a product or service, but also the importance of these attributes for patient satisfaction [21]. Based on the respondent evaluations, the averages for importance and performance are calculated which will allow for the creation of four quadrants (Fig.1). The x axis shows the importance associated by the consumers, while the y axis shows the perceived performance for the services or products considered. The four quadrants are: Possible overkill (Low importance/High performance), Keep up the good work (High importance/High performance), Low priority (Low importance/Low performance) and Concentrate here (High importance/ Low performance).

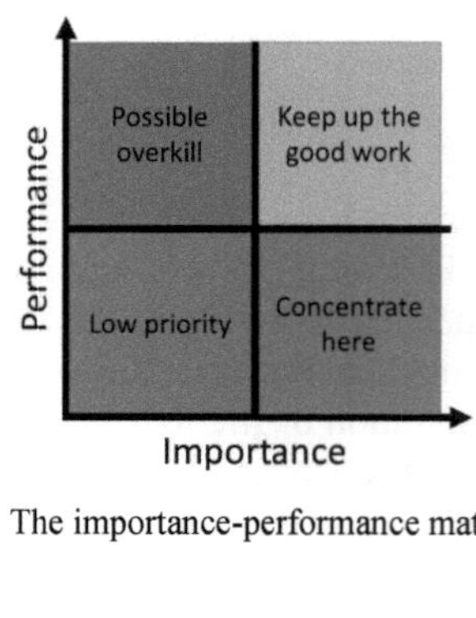

Fig.1 The importance-performance matrix

The Concentrate here quadrant includes those attributes respondents consider as very important in influencing their satisfaction levels regarding the product or service under analysis, but for which the perceived performance is lower. Efforts to increase the performance of these attributes are therefore required. The Keep up the good work quadrant represents the best positioning as it includes those attributes perceived by respondents as very important and for which the organization also offers high perceived performance. With regard to the low priority quadrant, attributes included here are characterized by both a low level of importance and a low level of the perceived performance. Even if perceived performance levels are low, efforts to increase performance on these attributes are not a priority as consumers do not perceive them to be important in influencing their satisfaction levels. Lastly, the Possible overkill quadrant includes high perceived performance attributes which consumers do not perceive as important in influencing their satisfaction levels. This implies that, although consumers are satisfied with the performance level associated to these attributes, it is very likely that the amount of resources allocated to these attributes surpass the benefits obtained, given the low importance levels for the consumers [19], [23], [25].

B. Attributes considered

Attributes considered for this study were obtained following an exploratory factor analysis with varimax rotation using SPSS version 21 conducted on a sample of 339 patients with diabetes with regards to the dimensions describing respondents' perception on the medical services for diabetes care they benefitted from in public ambulatory settings in Romania. The quantitative study was conducted between July 2014 and February 2015. Questionnaires were distributed to patients with diabetes via mail, patients' associations, and special events for patients with diabetes. The sampling method was sampling based on the researcher's judgment. The response rate was 39.5%. The final sample structure was similar to the general structure of patients with diabetes in Romania as shown in Table 1 below.

Table 1: Sample structure as compared to the general structure of patients with diabetes in Romania

	Category	Health Ministry data	Sample data
Age	0-14	3%	0.9%
	15-64	62%	68.5%
	>64	35%	30.6%
Residency	Urban	67%	70.8%
	Rural	33%	29.2%

Source: [24]

The six dimensions considered for this research were: patients relationship with the doctor, nurses, auxiliary staff, other patients, the diabetes clinic as a whole, and other support services.

A synthesis of the six dimensions, the factors under analysis and the respective variables used for the analysis are presented in Table 2 below.

Table 2: Synthesis of factors resulting after the exploratory factor analysis regarding respondents perception on the medical services dimensions in a clinic setting

Dimension analyzed	Factor	Variable name	Description
Patients relationship with the doctor	Doctor's availability	DR_AV	Availability shown by the doctor during the medical exam
	Involvement of family	FAMILY	Attention given and involvement of family members in treatment decisions.
Patients relationship with the nurses	Nurses availability	NURSE_AV	Openness, kindness and attention shown by the nurse towards the patient and their closed ones.
Patients relationship with the auxiliary staff	Auxiliary staff	AUX_STAFF	Responsiveness and kindness shown by the auxiliary staff towards the patient and their closed ones
Diabetes clinic as a whole	Diabetes clinic	CLINIC	Clinic's facilities and accessibility
Patients relationship with other patients	Relationship with other patients	OTHER_PAT	Patients interaction with fellow patients from the point of view of their number and discussions had.
Other support services	Support for diabetes management	SUPPORT	Support through other services: psychologist, support group, patients association
	Access to medicines and treatment	ACCESS	Patients access to medicines and treatment, including GP support.

III. Results

The importance-performance analysis was conducted using the Key Driver Analysis tool in SPSS version 21. Starting from the average values calculated for the perceived performance and importance of the attributes, these were grouped in quadrants as per Fig. 2 below.

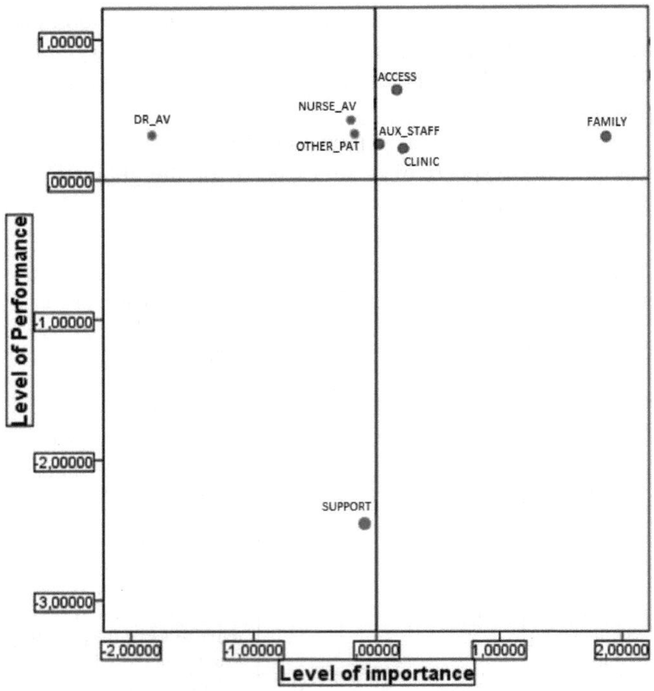

Fig. 2 Importance-performance analysis for medical services in the ambulatory setting

The results obtained show that most factors are grouped in two of the four quadrants: Possible overkill and Keep up the good work, while the factor SUPPORT is part of the Low priority quadrant.

The Possible overkill dimension is characterized by a low level of perceived importance for the patient and a high level of performance offered by the medical services supplier. The following factors are included in this quadrant: doctor availability (DR_AV), nurses availability (NURSE_AV) and patient interaction with other patients (OTHER_PAT). From the point of view of the quadrant grouping these factors, the low level of importance attributed by the patients suggests that the medical unit should not invest further efforts in increasing performance levels for these attributes as they are not perceived as essential satisfaction drivers by patients. However, if we are to consider the nature of the service under analysis, and the description of these factors that mostly refer to the attention and support patients need from the medical staff, together with the influence the experience of other patients can have on themselves, we believe the explanation offered by [25] to be more suitable to this situation. The author suggests that some attributes can be described by consumers as not important as a consequence of the fact that they are considered intrinsic to the respective product or service, so consumers basically expect that each offer, irrespective of the supplier, contains those attributes. This explanation is possible in the context of medical services where patients rely upon the openness and attention/care showed by the medical staff in treating the conditions they suffer from, but also on the experiences of other patients in order to receive different recommendations or opinions. This type of attributes will however play an important role in generating lack of dissatisfaction if absent from the supplier's offer of services or in the case of a low level of performance [25]. We therefore consider that medical units for treating diabetes should support the maintenance of a high level of performance for the three attributes under analysis.

The Low priority quadrant includes the factor SUPPORT regarding the support diabetes patients receive through other services (psychologist, support group, patients association) and is described by a low level of importance and a low level of perceived performance. Given the low level of importance attributed by patients, this service does not represent an issue for the medical services provider. It is however possible that the low level of importance be also determined by the fact that these services are little known and hence not utilized by patients. Given the particularities of diabetes as a chronic disease, but also the results of research showing that psychological wellbeing and acquiring a feeling of auto-efficiency with regards to the management of diabetes contribute to an increase in patient satisfaction [26][27] we recommend a better promotion of this type of services and a further evaluation of their role in generating patient satisfaction.

The Keep up the good work quadrant includes, as shown above, attributes perceived as important by the patients and for which, the medical supplier also offers high perceived performance. The following factors are included in this quadrant: patients access to medication and treatment (ACCESS), responsiveness and kindness shown by the auxiliary staff (AUX_STAFF), clinic's facilities and accessibility (CLINIC), and attention given to family and friends and their involvement in treatment options (FAMILY). The results obtained for these factors confirm a high level of perceived performance with regards to access to medications and treatment as well as to the clinic's services, elements that are also considered important by patients. The inclusion of the FAMILY factor in this quadrant also suggests the fact that a high level of importance is given to the role played by this category in caring for diabetes patients, both by the doctor, thorough their inclusion in the discussions regarding patient's treatment options, and by the patients who consider this attribute of high importance.

It is worth noting that none of the factors were included in the Concentrate here quadrant which would have indicated factors with a high level of importance for the respondents but low performance levels on behalf of the medical unit.

IV. Limitations

The results obtained in this study are particular to patients with diabetes benefitting from medical care in public ambulatory settings in Romania and cannot be extrapolated for describing patients benefitting from medical care for chronic diseases in Romania in general, nor for patients receiving their medical care in private units. Further research could be conducted in order to expand the scope of this study and offer a more comprehensive view on the satisfaction of these categories of patients as well as allowing for a comparison between attributes influencing patients satisfaction in the public and private settings.

V. Conclusions

The importance-performance analysis allowed us to obtain valuable information on how the attributes considered influence patients satisfaction. Factors were grouped according to the average values calculated for the importance attributed by respondents and the perceived performance of the medical unit in three of the four quadrants: Possible overkill, Low priority and Keep up the good work. This shows that differences in perceptions exist both in the case of the importance attributed by patients and in the case of perceived performance. The analysis may represent a starting point for medical services providers for diabetes care in the ambulatory setting in further developing their effort as results showed more promotion for the support services offered by the psychologist, the patients associations and the support group could help in disease management. It is also important that managers consider and analyze patients' perceptions of what is intrinsic to the medical service and aim to attain high levels of availability and kindness towards patients on behalf of their medical staff. The results presented in this paper can therefore be used by managers in detailing different positioning strategies in order to increase their competitive edge.

Acknowledgment

This work was co-financed from the European Social Fund through Sectoral Operational Programme Human Resources Development 2007-2013, project number POSDRU/159/ 1.5/S/142115 "Performance and excellence in doctoral and postdoctoral research in Romanian economics science domain".

Conflict of Interest

The authors declare that they have no conflict of interest.

References

1. Taylor C, Benger J R (2004) Patient satisfaction in emergency medicine. Emerg Med J 21:528-532
2. Boudreaux E D, O'Hea E L (2003) Patient satisfaction in the Emergency Department: A review of the literature and implications for practice. J Emerg Med 26:13-26
3. Prakash B (2010) Patient satisfaction. J Cutan Med Surg 3:151-155
4. Otani K et al (2009) Patient satisfaction: focusing on "Excellent". Int J Healthc Manag 54:93-103
5. York A S, McCarthy K A (2009) Patient, staff and physician satisfaction: a new model instrument and their implications. Int J Health Care Qual Assur 24(2):178-191
6. Haug M R, Lavin B (1981) Practitioner or patient – Who's in charge. J Health Soc Behav 22(3):212-229
7. Shendurnikar N, Thakkar P A (2013) Communication skills to ensure patient satisfaction. Indian J Pediatr 80:938-943
8. Bell R et al (1997) Charting patient satisfaction. Mark Health Serv 17(2): 22-29
9. Chahal H, Mehta S (2013) Developing patient satisfaction construct for public and private health care sectors. J Serv Res 13:7-30
10. Romanian Association of Medicines Producers (2011) Over one million of a half Romanians suffer from diabetes, available at: http://arpim.ro/peste-un-milion-sijumatate-de-romani-sufera-de-diabet/ accessed 14 April 2014
11. Baron-Epel O et al (2001) Evaluation of the consumer model: relationship between patients'expectations, perceptions and satisfaction with care. Int J Qual Health Care 13:317-323
12. Mooney G (1998) Beyond health outcomes: The benefits of health care. Health Care Anal 6:99-105
13. Ahmad A M K et al (2013) The impact of marketing mix strategy on hospitals performance measured by patient satisfaction: am empirical investigation on Jeddah private sector hospital senior managers perspective. IJMS 5(6):201-227
14. Catană Gh A (2009) Marketingul serviciilor de ocrotire a sănătății. Alma Mater, Cluj-Napoca
15. Rădulescu V (2008) Marketingul serviciilor de sănătate. Uranus, București
16. National Health Insurance Institute reports received by the author upon written request – September 2014
17. Federația Asociațiilor Diabeticilor din România (FADR) at http://fadr.ro/
18. Martilla J A, James J C (1977) Importance-performance analysis. J Mark 41(1):77-79
19. Blěsić I et al (2015) An importance-performance analysis of service quality in spa hotels. Econ Res. 27(1): 483-495
20. Pak R J (2013) Combining Importance-Performance Analysis with Analytic Hierarchy Process for Enhancing Satisfaction. JOAMS. 1 (4):368-371
21. Silva F J H, Fernandes P O (2011) Importance-Performance Analysis as a Tool in Evaluating Higher Education Service Quality: The Empirical Results of Estig (IPB), The 17th IBIMA conference on Creating Global Competitive Economies: A 360-degree Approach, Milano, Italia, 14-15 November, pp. 306 -313
22. Tyrrell T J, Okrant M J (2004) Importance-Performance Analysis: Some Recommendations from an Economic Planning Perspective. Tourism Analysis 9: 1-14

23. Wong M S et al (2011) The Use of Importance-Performance Analysis (IPA) in Evaluating Japan's E-government Services. JTAER 6(2): 17-30
24. Ministerul Sănătăţii (2014) Programul Naţional de Diabet Zaharat şi alte boli de nutritive at: http://www.ms.gov.ro/documente/8_51_329_c.htm accessed 27 March 2014
25. Oliver R L (2015) Satisfaction. A Behavioral Perspective on the Consumer 2nd ed. Routledge, New York
26. Diţ L et al (2012) Impactul severităţii bolii asupra satisfacţiei cu calitatea îngrijirii medicale la pacienţii cu diabet de tip 2. Clujul Medical 85: 573-577
27. Redekop W K et al (2002) Health-Related Quality of Life and Treatment Satisfaction in Dutch Patients With Type 2 Diabetes. Diabetes care 25:458-463

Author: Mădălina-Alexandra Coţiu
Institute: Faculty of Economics and BusinessAdministration, Babeş-Bolyai University
Street: 58-60, Theodor Mihali
City: Cluj-Napoca
Country: Romania
Email: madalina.cotiu@gmail.com

Analysis of Factors that Influence OTC Purchasing Behavior

S.D. Cîrstea[1], C. Moldovan-Teselios[2] and A.I. Iancu[3]

[1] Technical University of Cluj-Napoca/Electric Engineering, Cluj-Napoca, Romania
[2] Metro Media Transilvania, Cluj-Napoca, Romania
[3] Technical University of Cluj-Napoca/Electric Engineering, Cluj-Napoca, Romania

Abstract— **Over-the-counter (OTC) drugs are the medicinal products sold directly to a consumer without a prescription from a healthcare professional as compared to prescription drugs which may be sold only to consumer's features with a valid prescription. OTC lately generates increasing revenue in total Romanian drug market. OTC buying decision is triggered by a number of factors out of which the most important seem to be: doctor choice, previous own experience, advice of the pharmacist and the information stated on the prospectus. The analysis was conducted locally on a sample of 324 people. The study wants to see if there are changes in the purchasing behavior when individuals evolve as professional preparation. One of the main conclusions of the article emphasizes that both for students and employed persons with higher education, the purchasing decision of OTC is determined by two important factors: the recommendation of experts (physicians, pharmacists) and their assessment (previous personal experience and information stated on the prospectus). Also, it was noted that the influence of commercial factors (brand, price, promotion) is lower for both categories analyzed.**

Keywords— **OTC, purchasing behavior, consumer behavior, pharmaceutical market**

I. Introduction

The pharmaceutical market can be divided into drugs, that can be bought without prescription, so-called OTC products ("over the counter"), and into drugs that are only available on prescription, so called Rx products. Guido et al. add to the definition of OTC drugs that they are "those medicines that, after being used for a given period subsequent to the date of patent expiration, are judged safe enough to be self-administered by patients" [1].

The landscape in which companies in the pharmaceutical industry operate and compete has changed rapidly over the past few years. According to Pharma & Hospital Report, baseline study in analyzing pharmaceutical market, Cegedim estimated that the value of drugs issued to patients in Romania reached 2.74 billion lei at distribution price in the third quarter of 2015.

Prescription drugs (Rx) issued by pharmacies had reached a value of 1.85 billion, decreasing with 16.2%. Drugs without prescription (OTC) reached a value of 0.54 billion lei, increasing with 11.6% and the hospital segment reached 0.36 billion lei, decreasing with 0.3% compared to the 3rd quarter of the previous year.

OTC are medicines that patients can use in order to ameliorate a series of minor ailments, without visiting the doctor. They may be issued directly from a pharmacy, do not have a special scheme of administration and do not require a prescription.

OTC are part of a group of pharmaceuticals that many countries consider them quite safe and can be used without any intervention of a physician or licensed specialist belonging to this area. Many of them can be purchased from numerous locations, including airport shops, gas stations or grocery stores. Rules vary considerably from country to country.

The enlargement of the range and the increased availability of non-prescription drugs has led to the creation of wrongly perceived ideas by consumers. Many believe that these products can be used in any dose, anytime and by anyone.

OTC medications are widely viewed by medical professionals as both safe and effective when used appropriately. Additionally, OTC medicines provide benefits to consumers in the form of savings stemming from fewer doctors' visits, less time away from work and relatively lower cost than prescription drugs [2].

II. Theortical background

We believe that the purchase decision is influenced by two important factors such as: medical or pharmacist advice and the perceived value of information. As can be observed in Figure 1, the perceived value of information is determined by previous own experience, views of other reference groups, the written information in the prospectus, product price or existing advertising.

When we refer to the views of other reference groups, the most important categories are primarily people who have purchased / used that drug, as well as colleagues, friends or family.

Most factors analyzed in this study were also analyzed by other authors from other different perspectives.

Referring to *previous own experience,* many researchers suggest that previous information or experience provides underlying reasons for repeat purchase or brand switching decisions [3,4]. Also, Shohel et all underline that direct experience with the product, price range and brand reliance

S. Vlad and N.M. Roman (eds.), *International Conference on Advancements of Medicine and Health Care through Technology; 12th - 15th October 2016, Cluj-Napoca, Romania,*
IFMBE Proceedings 59,
DOI: 10.1007/978-3-319-52875-5_63

are important determinants of repetitive purchase behavior on OTC drugs [5].

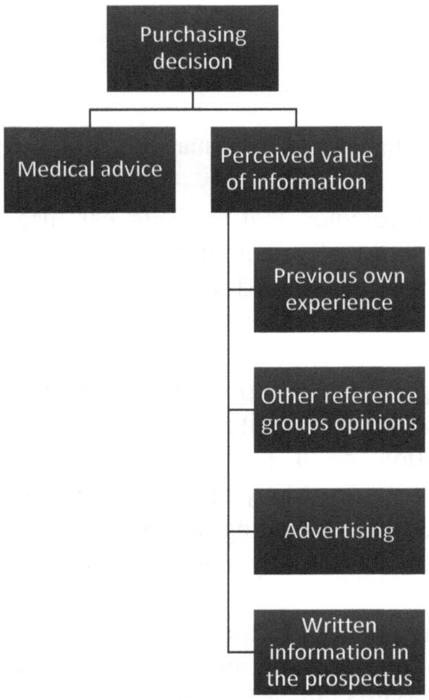

Fig. 1 Factors that influence the purchase decision

Regarding the *price,* studies confirm that a relationship exists between consumers' post purchase experience and subsequent price-sensitivity, and whether before or after, purchase experience will affect price sensitivity [6]. Likewise, customer loyalty to a particular product increases their tolerance for price [7, 8].

Promoting influence on purchase decision is another factor studied. Singh emphasizes that consumer behavioral intentions are nevertheless influenced by a heightened awareness of specific branded drugs. Consumers feel empowered by the information provided in direct-to consumer advertising and they are concerned about governmental attempts to regulate prescription drug advertising [9].

III. Methodology

This study focused on two populations with socio-demographic profile defined as: (1) students, a sample of 183 selected students from the university center Cluj-Napoca (2) persons employed (employees, contractors, freelancers) with higher education, a sample of 141 persons employed in Cluj-Napoca.

The motivation for choosing these people arises from the desire to investigate the purchase behavior of drugs without prescription (OTC) among the most educated categories of consumers and potential consumers, on the one hand and to give a longitudinal dimension to the study, studying how the purchase decision of OTC changes over time. Socio-demographic structure of the two sub-samples is presented in Table 1.

Table 1 Characteristics of gender and age of the two samples

Variable	Category	Students	Persons employed
Gender	Male	56%	35%
	Female	44%	65%
Age	18-24 years	92%	2%
	25-39 years	8%	83%
	40 years and over	-	15%

The questionnaire was online, the selection of subjects being achieved by their voluntary participation, following invitations sent on social sites (Facebook). Therefore, one of the main limitations of the methodology of this study is given by self-selection error, the participation to the study is higher among people more interested in the subject of study.

In order to identify the mechanism of decision making on purchasing drugs without a prescription, we evaluated the importance of 10 factors deemed relevant by the literature. [9,10]. The assessment of the significance was achieved using a four-stage Likert scale (very much, much, least, very little). The Likert scale used is different from the original one, designed with five possible answers, by eliminating median variant, due to the reason to better differentiate the importance given to tested factors and better interpret their role in shaping the purchase decision [11].

If the assessment of each factor based on the Likert scale may not provide a clear hierarchy of these factors, as it may give similar importance to many factors, we asked subjects to rank these factors according to their importance, from 1 - most important factor, 10 - the least important factor. In this case, hierarchies can become clearer and we can better isolate different kinds of buyers, depending on how they agglutinate information received or those held in forming a purchasing decision.

IV. Results and Discutions

A first hypothesis (H1) tested in this study was whether "the importance of rating factors that contribute to making the decision to purchase drugs without a prescription is similar for students and highly educated people employed. " In other words, the way people choose to buy OTC changes throughout time.

As it can be seen from Fig. 2 and Fig. 3, both students and people employed place the same important factors in the decision making on the first four positions: the choice of doctor, their own former experience, the pharmacist's advice and the information stated on the leaflet. Regarding these aspects, the weight of much and plenty importance is one exceeding 60 % in both reference populations.

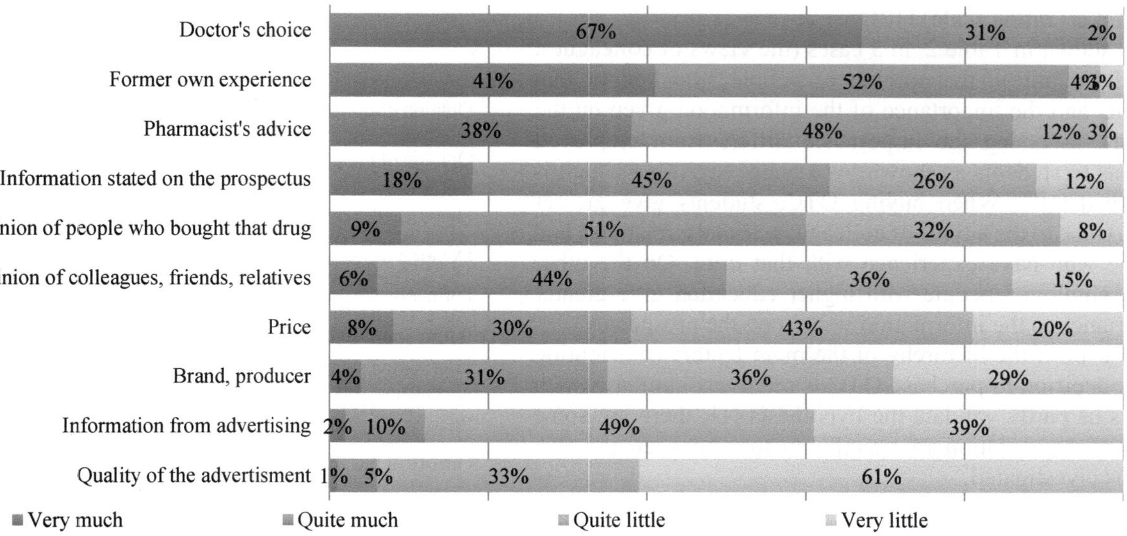

Fig. 2 The importance of factors in deciding to purchase OTC – students

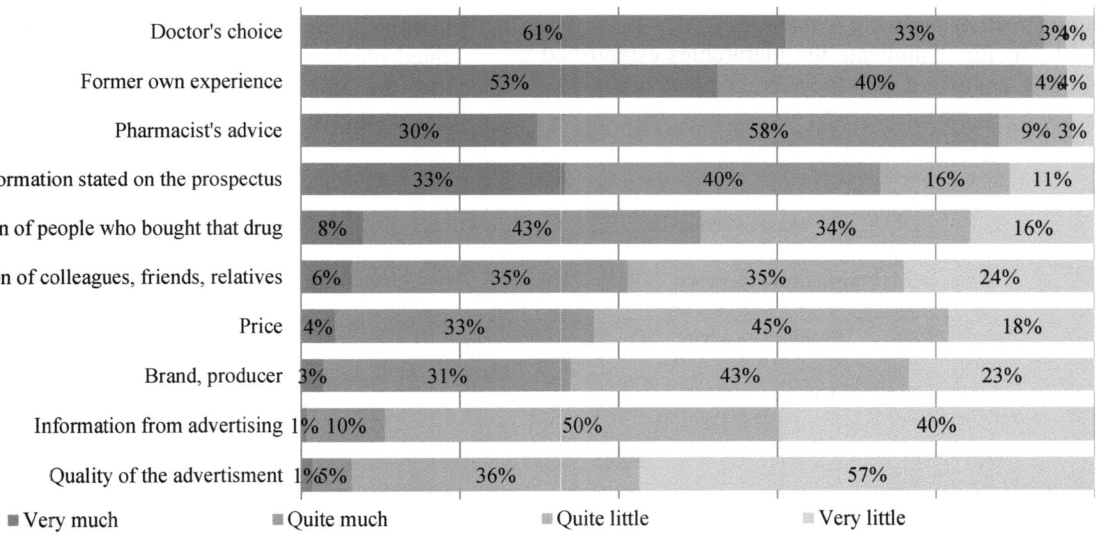

Fig. 3 The importance of factors in deciding to purchase OTC – employed persons

Then there comes a set of four other aspects prioritized differently this time by students and people employed, the views of those who have purchased that product, the views of those close (relatives, friends, colleagues), the price of the purchased product and brand. For these factors, the percentage of those who consider them important and very important falls between 30 % and 60 %. The less important elements that contribute to the formation of the purchase decision are those associated with promoting drug, the information from advertisements and its quality with a weight of much and very much importance of a maximum of 12 %.

So, the decision to purchase OTC seems to depend on factors related mainly to two levels: (1) The doctor's / pharmacist's skill and (2) One's own skill, based on past experience and analyzing information included in the prospectus.

Even if , at first glance , the hierarchy of the main factors is similar , in order to see more clearly how each of these factors is treated differently by students and people with higher education , we tested the association through the method Kruskal – Wallis, a non –parametric test used to compare two or more independent samples that are equal or of different sizes; in our case, we tested the association between a nominal variable (reference group) and an ordinal one (Likert rating scale) [12].

As shown in Table 2, in 3 cases (the views of colleagues, friends, relatives, the opinion of people who bought that product and the importance of the information given on the leaflet), assessing the importance differs from employed persons to students as shown by Asymp. Sig value which is less than 0.05. When buying OTC, students give greater importance to the advice of colleagues, friends, relatives, and people who have experience with that drug. On the other hand, employed people with higher education give greater importance to the information written on the prospectus.

So even if the hierarchy of the main factors contributing to the decision to purchase OTC is relatively similar, which makes us partly validate the hypothesis H1, there are some ways of appreciation of specific factors between the two groups investigated.

The second (H2) hypothesis derives from the intention to check whether *the ranking of factors that determine the buying decision is one similar in the two working models, assessing the significance by using Likert scale and assessing the significance by ordering (ranking).*

Fig. 4 and Fig. 5 indicate the hierarchies established by both groups, compared with the average place occupied.

Table 2 Kruskal-Wallis test, applied in the case of assessing the importance given to tested factors

	Chi-Square	df	Asymp. Sig.
Opinion of the colleagues, friends, relatives	**8,201**	**1**	**0,004**
Opinion of the persons who bought that drug	**3,932**	**1**	**0,047**
Pharmacist's advice	1,054	1	0,305
Doctor's choice	1,547	1	0,214
Former own experience	3,137	1	0,077
Information from advertising	0,025	1	0,874
Information stated on the prospectus	**8,169**	**1**	**0,004**
Price	0,033	1	0,855
Quality of the advertisement	0,321	1	0,571
Brand, producer	1,519	1	0,218

As compared to the previous hierarchy, certain changes occur, but top positions are still occupied by the factors previously identified (with one exception, the information stated on the leaflet for students, is placed on 5th position after the opinion of those who bought the drug). In fact, besides this reversal, the two hierarchies are identical.

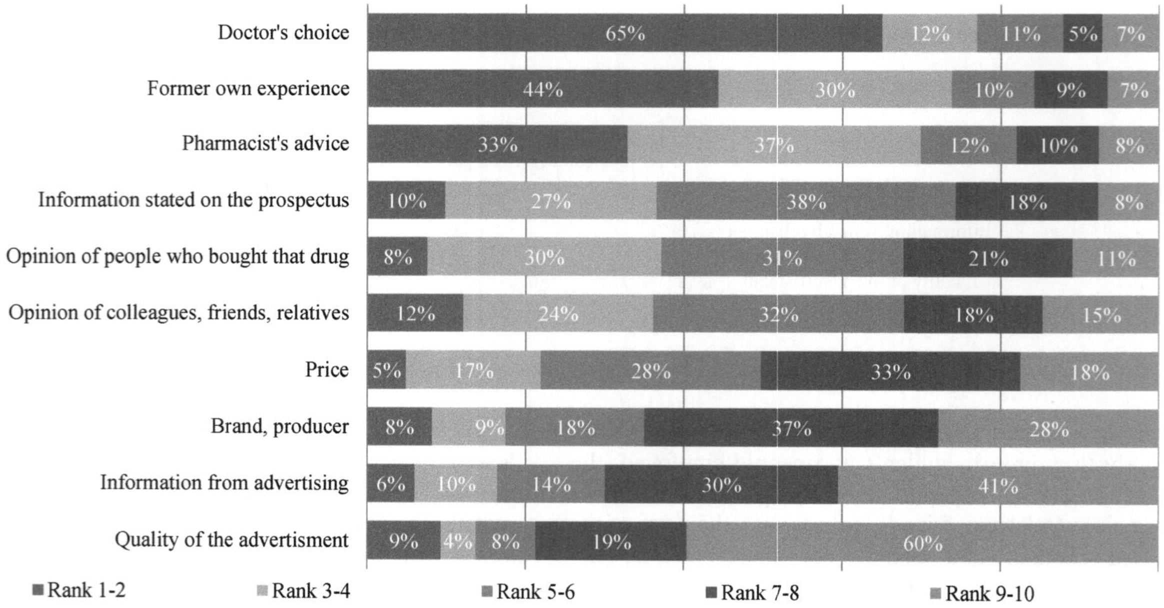

Fig. 4 The hierarchy of factors in deciding to purchase OTC – students

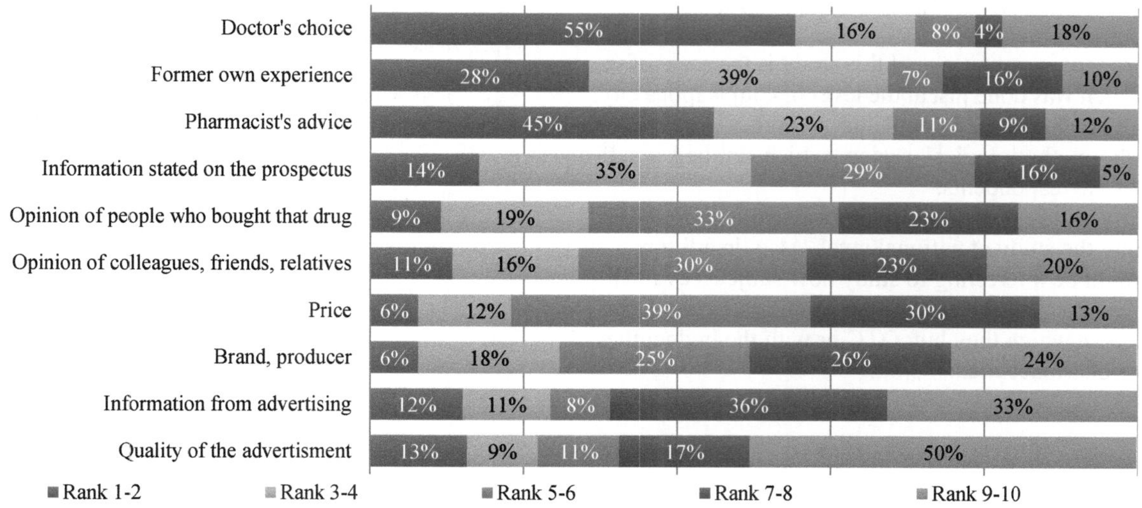

Fig. 5 The hierarchy of factors in deciding to purchase OTC – employed persons

But, although the data indicate a similarity in the hierarchy, an analysis made using Kruskal-Wallis test indicates, however, differences of position in the hierarchy, between students and people with higher education, differences related to the opinion of colleagues, friends, relatives, the opinion of people who bought that product, the information on the leaflet, and doctor choice. If in the first 3 factors prioritized differently we find the same situation as in the previous test (students favor the opinion of those close and those who bought the drug, unlike the employed people, who give greater importance to the information from the prospectus) in the case of choosing the doctor students tend to place it to a greater extent in the first two positions (65%) as compared to those employed (55%).

Table 3 Kruskal-Wallis test, applied in the case of assessing the hierarchy given to tested factors

	Chi-Square	df	Asymp. Sig.
Opinion of the colleagues, friends, relatives	**5,192**	**1**	**0,023**
Opinion of the persons who bought that drug	**6,165**	**1**	**0,013**
Pharmacist's advice	0,029	1	0,864
Doctor's choice	**5,649**	**1**	**0,017**
Former own experience	0,041	1	0,839
Information from advertising	0,919	1	0,338
Information stated on the prospectus	**5,699**	**1**	**0,017**
Price	2,37	1	0,124
Quality of the advertisement	3,491	1	0,062
Brand, producer	3,076	1	0,079

So in this case we can also say that the hypothesis H2 was partially validated as we find a high degree of similarity in the ranking of factors that contribute to the decision to purchase between the two methods, namely the assessment of the importance of each factor and the hierarchy of these.

V. Conclusion

Both for students and employed people with higher education, the decision to purchase drugs without a prescription is one focused primarily on two levels: the recommendation of experts (physicians, pharmacists) and their own evaluation (former personal experience and the information stated on the leaflet). The differences identified are generally determined contextually. For students and those who live and / or spend time with colleagues and friends mostly, the importance of their opinion is higher than for employed persons.

In the case of employed persons, personal competence as a trait of personality leaves its mark on most of their choices.

Since most members of both groups appear to behave rationally before deciding to buy OTC, the influence of other factors (brand, price, reviews from other people) is lower. As a statement, the impact of promotion seems to be minimal (or at least minimized as compared to other factors). Throughout time, this approach appears to be constant, without identifying any major changes.

VI. Limitations and Future Research

One of the main limitations of this study is the scale of the research which was done just at the level of Cluj Napoca city, with a high level educated population. Another limitation is given by the methodological design, which implied a self-selection of the respondents.

One of the future directions of the research is represented by extending the study at national level. Also, in a future paper it would be interesting to study how subjects evaluate their health status and the correlation of this aspect with the frequency with which they buy OTC or with the budget they allocate for pharmaceuticals.

Conflict of Interest

The authors declare that they have no conflict of interest.

References

1. Guido, G., Pino, G. and Frangipane, D. (2011) The role of credibility and perceived image of supermarket stores as valuable providers of over-the-counter drugs. Journal of Marketing Management, 27: 207-24.
2. Bower A , Grau L S and Taylor V A (2013) Over-the-counter vs. prescription medications: are consumer perceptions of the consequences of drug instruction non-compliance different?. International Journal of Consumer Studies 37: 228–233
3. Inman, J.J. and Zeelenberg, M. (2002) Regret in repeat purchase versus switching decisions: the attenuating role of decision justifiability. Journal of Consumer Research, 29:116- 128.
4. Ratchford, B.T. (2001) The economics of consumer knowledge. Journal of Consumer Research, 27: 397.
5. Shohel M, Tasnuva I, Al-Amin M M at all (2013) Investigation of Consumer Attitudes, Intentions and Brand Loyal Behavior on the OTC Drugs in Bangladesh. British Journal of Pharmaceutical Research 3(3): 454-464
6. Hseih, A.T. and Chang, W.T. (2004) The effect of consumer participation on price sensitivity. Journal of Consumer Affairs, 38 (2):282-296.
7. Aaker, D.A. (1991) Managing Brand Equity: Capitalising on the Value of a Brand Name. The Free Press, New York.
8. Samuelsen, B. and Sandvik, K. (1997) The concept of customer loyalty. In Arnott et al., (eds.) EMAC Proceedings, Annual Conference, European Marketing Academy, Warwick pp. 1122-1140. Quoted in: Delgardo-Ballester and Munuera-Aleman (2001).
9. Singh T and Smith D (2005) Direct-to-consumer prescription drug advertising: a study of consumer attitudes and behavioral intentions. Journal of Consumer Marketing 22(7):369 - 378
10. Deborah F. Spake Mathew Joseph, (2007),"Consumer opinion and effectiveness of direct-to-consumer advertising", Journal of Consumer Marketing, 24(5): 283 - 293
11. Boone Jr., H.N. and Boone, D.A. (2012): Analyzing Likert data. Journal of Extension, 50(2): 1-5.
12. Field, A. (2009): Discovering Statistics Using SPSS (3rd edition). SAGE Publications, London.

Wireless Systems with Reduced PAPR Using K-means Modified PTS Implemented for Epilepsy Classification from EEG Signals

Sunil Kumar Prabhakar and Harikumar Rajaguru

Bannari Amman Institute of Technology/Department of ECE, Sathyamangalam, India

Abstract— **Because of unusual discharges in the brain, epilepsy occurs. During epilepsy, the electrical activities become more intense because of the temporary disruptions happening to normal activities and functions of brain. Epilepsy is widely characterized by recurrent seizures and is one of the most common brain disorders. To evaluate the epileptic patients, a non-invasive tool called Electroencephalography (EEG) is used. To examine the patterns of the brain and to assist in the diagnosis of epilepsy, EEG is very helpful. As the recordings of the EEG are too large to process, certain kind of dimensionality reduction technique is required to reduce the dimensions of the EEG data. The dimensionality reduction technique used here is Fuzzy Mutual Information (FMI). The dimensionally reduced data is then transmitted through the Space Time Block Coded Multiple Input Multiple Output Orthogonal Frequency Division Multiplexing (STBC MIMO-OFDM) System. Since the STBC MIMO-OFDM System suffers a high Peak to Average Power Ratio (PAPR), K-means modified Partial Transmit Sequence (K-PTS) is used to reduce the PAPR. At the receiver side, the Linear Support Vector Machine (L-SVM) algorithm is used to classify the epilepsy from EEG signals. The performance metrics includes specificity, sensitivity, time delay, quality values, accuracy and performance index, Bit Error Rate (BER) and PAPR.**

Keywords— **EEG, epilepsy, PAPR, BER, K-means PTS**

I. Introduction

Epilepsy is a very critical neurological disease which stems from the abnormal discharges of the electrical activities of the brain [1]. Epilepsy leads to movements and trembling which are uncontrollable. About 1% of the world population is suffering from this brain disorder [2]. To diagnose the epilepsy, either medicines should be used or surgical treatment should be opted. The electrical activities of the brain are recorded easily with the help of EEG [3]. The EEG gives us a clear understanding into disorders of the activities of the brain. The EEG recordings which are measured in seizure free intervals from the patients who are suffering from epilepsy are considered vital for the diagnosis, analysis and prediction process [4]. The seizures occur unpredictably and so with the help of automatic seizure detection methods and computational models, the classification of epilepsy can be done easily. The block diagram of the prediction tool is given in Figure 1.

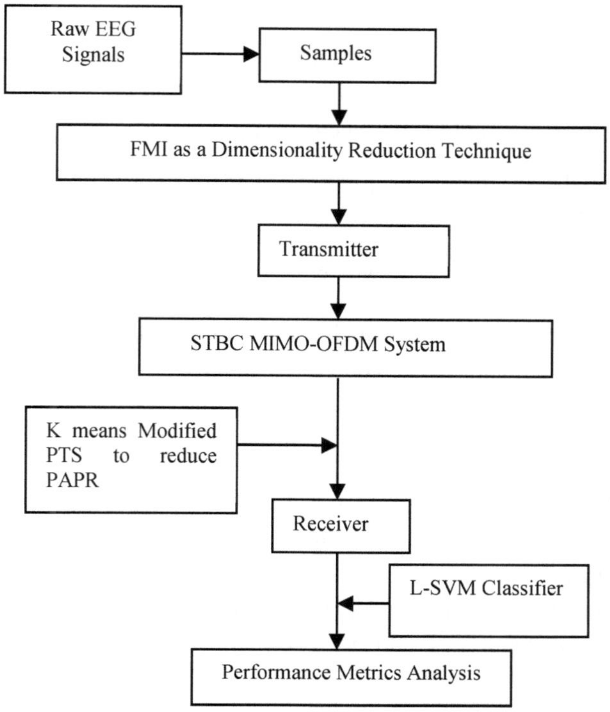

Fig. 1 Block Diagram of the Prediction Tool

II. Materials and Methods

A. Data Acquisition

The EEG data is obtained from Sri Ramakrishna Hospital, Coimbatore, India for totally 20 epileptic patients [5]. The recordings of the EEG data of those 20 epileptic patients were done for nearly 30 minutes each. The recorded signals were in continuous form and so each recorded signal was divided into 2 second epoch duration. For each and every patient, 16 channels are recorded and measured over 3 epochs. The recordings are taken in European Data Format (EDF). The maximum frequency is 50 Hz and so the sampling frequency is about 200 Hz. Ultimately for each and every epoch there are totally 400 values and therefore for all the epochs of the 20 patients the data to be processed is too huge and therefore dimensionality reduction technique is

S. Vlad and N.M. Roman (eds.), *International Conference on Advancements of Medicine and Health Care through Technology; 12th - 15th October 2016, Cluj-Napoca, Romania,*
IFMBE Proceedings 59,
DOI: 10.1007/978-3-319-52875-5_64

required. The dimensionality reduction technique used here is Fuzzy Mutual Information (FMI) [6].

III. STBC MIMO-OFDM SYSTEM AND PAPR

A. System Design

The data sequence with totally N_c subcarriers which is to be transmitted is initially partioned into $'V'$ non-overlapping sub-blocks. These non-overlapping sub-blocks are represented by the vectors $\{X_i^v, v = 1,2,...,V\}$; X_i^v is for the vth sub-block partition at the ith transmit antenna. The vector is then written as

$$X_i = \sum_{n=1}^{V} X_i^v \text{, where } X_i = [X_0^v, X_{1,....,}^v X_{N_{C-1}}^v]^T$$

These sub-blocks which are partitioned are converted to time –domain from frequency domain with the help of N point IFFT. These time domain sequences are mixed or combined with the weighing factors, $b_i^v = e^{j\varphi_i^v}$, where $\varphi_i^v \in [0,2\pi]$ and $v = 1,2,....V$ are used primarily for the phase rotation. To reduce the complexity of the system, the binary phase factors of $\{+1,-1\}$ are utilized thoroughly. The PAPR of almost all the signals which are transmitted simultaneously should be very small. Since the worst-case PAPR governs the performance of the system, MIMO-OFDM is defined as the maximum of all PAPR related to all the N_T MIMO paths [7]. Space Time Block Codes are combined with MIMO-OFDM system to improve the versatility of the system [8].

For the ith transmit antenna, the CCDF of the PAPR of the MIMO-OFDM is given by [9];

$$PAPR_{MIMO-OFDM} = \max_{1 \le i \le N_T} \{PAPR_i\}$$

$PAPR_i$ signifies the PAPR at the ith transmit antenna and hence it is written as:

$$P_r(PAPR_{MIMO-OFDM} > PAPR_0) = 1 - [1 - e^{-PAPR_0}]^{N_T N_C}$$

Since PAPR should be very low for each transmit antenna, the optimal phase vector should be chosen. The simulation parameters are shown in Table 1.

Table 1. Simulation Parameters

Modulation used	QPSK
System analysed	2 x2 STBC MIMO-OFDM
Number of subcarriers	512
No of sub-blocks	4
Maximum symbols loaded	1e5
Symbol rate	250000
No of time slots	2
Window function	Blackman-Haris
HPA Model	SSPA
No of frames	10
No of OFDM symbols/ frame	4
Bandwidth	5 MHz
Oversampling factor	4

B. K-means Based Modified PTS Algorithm

a) As the program initiates, the input bits are generated in random fashion.
b) The conversion of the serial data into parallel data is done and then the sparse $'H'$ matrix for Space Time Encoder is calculated.
c) As the sparse matrix $'H'$ is shifted, the input bits are encoded accordingly.
d) QPSK modulation is used to modulate the input signals.
e) With the aid of N point IFFT also, the parallel data obtained is directly computed.
f) The input data is split into disjoint sub blocks and with the help of IFFT operations, it is transformed into time-domain partial transmit sequences.
g) Phase factors are used to independently rotate the partial sequences [10]. The weighing factor taken here is W=4. To these phase factors, K-means algorithm is applied [11].
h) The suitable and optimal combination of phase factors with a low PAPR is selected and then processed to the next unit.
i) The parallel data is again converted to serial data bits and then decoded using the Space Time Block Decoder and at the end the PAPR value is calculated.
j) The threshold value is computed and checked to find whether PAPR exceeds and is greater than threshold value.

k) Ultimately, the CCDF plot versus probability of PAPR is computed and the plot is drawn.
l) The BER is computed and the program is stopped.

IV. L-SVM AS A POST CLASSIFIER

One of the most popular classification techniques is Support Vector Machine (SVM) [12]. Because of its versatility, it is used in different applications like gene analysis, text classification, facial expression recognition etc. SVM is utilized thoroughly for the construction of a unique rule called a linear classifier, which produces a good predictive performance. A SVM linear classifier can be represented frequently as a function $f(x): R^d \rightarrow R$ [13]. Under a two-class case circumstance, if $f(x) \geq 0$, a point is assigned to the positive class and $f(x) \leq 0$, the point is assigned to the negative class.

A SVM classifier function $f(x)$ is said to be a linear one when it can be expressed mathematically as

$$f(x; w, b) = \langle w, x \rangle + b \,;$$

where parameters of the functions are separated by w and b and $\langle , \rangle$ indicates the inner product of two vectors. A specific set of points (x_i, y_i) is considered, where $i = \overline{1, l}$ are denoted as class labels, is meant to be linearly separable if a linear classifier can be traced so that

$$y_i f(x_i) > 0, \forall i = 1, \ldots. l;$$

Thus the advantage of linear classifier in the field of machine learning is very important nowadays.

V. RESULTS AND DISCUSSION

In this section, the PAPR Results, BER Results and the Classification Results are explained in detail.

A. PAPR Results

The PAPR results and the BER Analysis results are shown here. It is obvious from the careful analysis of the figure 2, that when QPSK modulation is engaged the PAPR is reduced by 1.3 dB with the utilization of K means based PTS technique. The Bit Error Rate is also analysed in Table 2.

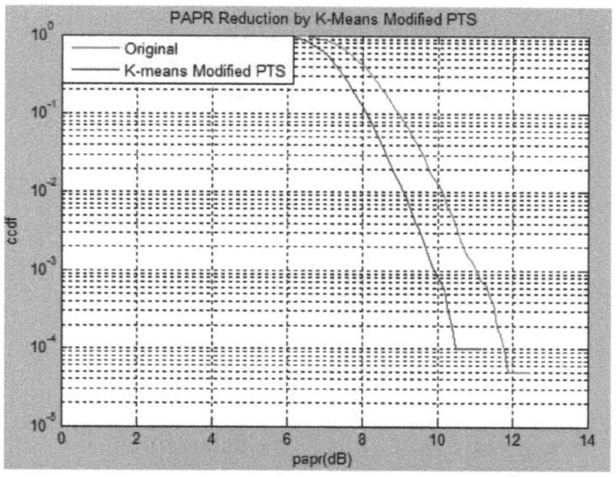

Figure 2 PAPR Reduction Using K-means Modified PTS Technique

Table 2 BER Analysis for the system

SNR	BER
0	0.1130
2	0.0899
4	0.0643
6	0.0318
8	0.0179
10	0.0005
12	0.0001

B. Classification Results

For FMI as dimensionality reduction technique and L-SVM as a Post Classifier, based on the Performance Index, Quality values, Time Delay and Accuracy the results in the receiver side are computed in Table 3. The formulae for the Performance Index (PI), Sensitivity, Specificity and Accuracy are given as follows:

$$PI = \frac{PC - MC - FA}{PC} \times 100$$

where PC – Perfect Classification, MC – Missed Classification, FA – False Alarm,

The Sensitivity, Specificity and Accuracy measures are stated by the following

$$Specificity = \frac{PC}{PC + MC} \times 100$$

$$Sensitivity = \frac{PC}{PC + FA} \times 100$$

$$Accuracy = \frac{Sensitivity + Specificity}{2} \times 100$$

The Time Delay and the Quality Value Measures are given by the following:

$$Time \quad Delay = \left[2 * \frac{PC}{100} + 6 * \frac{MC}{100} \right]$$

$$Quality \quad Values = \frac{10}{\left[\frac{FA}{100} + 0.2 \right] * Time \quad Delay}$$

Table 3 Average Performance Analysis Values of 20 Patients

Parameters	Obtained Values
PC (%)	76.666
MC (%)	21.736
FA (%)	1.597
PI (%)	68.104
Sensitivity (%)	98.402
Specificity (%)	78.263
Time Delay (sec)	2.837
Quality Values	17.044
Accuracy (%)	88.33

VI. Conclusion

When FMI is used as a dimensionality reduction technique and when it is classified with Linear SVM classifier which is implemented for telemedicine applications in this paper, an average accuracy of about 88.33% is obtained. Moreover a perfect classification of about 76.66%, missed classification of about 21.736%, false alarm of about 1.597, Performance Index of 68.104%, specificity of 78.263%, sensitivity of about 98.402%, time delay of about 2.837 seconds and quality value of about 17.044 is obtained. When the PAPR of the STBC MIMO-OFDM System is computed with the help of K-means Modified PTS algorithm, the PAPR is reduced by 1.3 dB with a minimum BER. Future works plan to incorporate various other dimensionality reduction techniques, other types of post classifiers, other types of system design and modifications to be made in PAPR reduction algorithms.

Conflict of Interest

The authors declare that they have no conflict of interest.

References

1. Sunil Kumar Prabhakar, Harikumar Rajaguru (2015), " ICA, LGE and FMI as Dimensionality Reduction Techniques followed by GMM as Post Classifier for the Classification of Epilepsy Risk Levels from EEG Signals", 9th IEEE European Modelling Symposium, October 6-8, Madrid, Spain
2. Tzallas AT, Tsipouras MG & Fotiadis DI (2009), 'Epileptic seizure detection in EEGs using time-frequency analysis', IEEE Trans. on Inf. Tech. in Biomed., vol. 13, pp. 703-710
3. R.Harikumar, P.Sunil Kumar (2015), "Dimensionality Reduction Techniques for Processing Epileptic Encephalographic Signals", Biomedical and Pharmacology Journal, Vol.8, No.1, pp:103-106
4. Sadasivam P.K, Narayana Dutt,(1996) "SVD Based Technique for noise reduction in Electroencephalographic signals", Elsevier Signal Processing, Vol 55, pp 179-189.
5. R.Harikumar, P.Sunil Kumar (2015), "Dimensionality Reduction with Linear Graph Embedding Technique for Electroencephalography Signals of an Epileptic Patient" Research Journal of Pharmacy and Technology, Vol.8, No.5, pp: 554-556
6. Sunil Kumar Prabhakar, Harikumar Rajaguru (2015), "Performance Comparison of Fuzzy Mutual Information as Dimensionality Reduction Techniques and SRC, SVD and Approximate Entropy as Post Classifiers for the Classification of Epilepsy Risk Levels from EEG Signals", Proceedings of IEEE Student Symposium in Biomedical Engineering and Sciences (ISSBES), Universiti Teknologi Mara, Malaysia.
7. H Yang (2005), "A Road to Future Broadband Wireless Access :MIMO-OFDM-Based Air Interface",IEEE Comm, Magazine, pp.53-60.
8. Tarokh V (2000) "Space-time block codes form orthogonal designs", *IEEE Trans. J.Sel.Areas Commun.*, 18, 7, 2000, 1169-1174.
9. Han S.H and Lee J.H (2005), "An Overview of Peak-to-Average Power Ratio Reduction Techniques for Multicarrier Transmission", IEEE Wireless Communication, pp.56-65.
10. Pundir V, Ahmad A, Prasad D (2015), " Study of some PAPR reduction techniques in MIMO-OFDM System", Annual IEEE India conference (INDICON), 1-6
11. Shi Na et al (2010), "Research on K-means Clustering Algorithm : An Improved K-means Clustering Algorithm", Third International Symposium on Intelligent Information Technology and Security Informatics (IITSI).
12. F.F.Chamasemani, Y.P.Singh (2011), "Multi-class Support Vector Machine (SVM) Classifiers – An Application in Hypothyroid Detection and Classification", 6th International Conference on Bio-Inspired Computing: Theories and Applications.
13. Harikumar Rajaguru, Sunil Kumar Prabhakar (2016), "LDA, GA and SVM's for Classification of Epilepsy From EEG Signals", Research Journal of Pharmaceutical, Biological and Chemical Sciences, Vol.7 (3), pp: 2044-2049.

Efficient Wireless System for Telemedicine Application with Reduced PAPR Using QMF Based PTS Technique for Epilepsy Classification from EEG Signals

Sunil Kumar Prabhakar and Harikumar Rajaguru

Bannari Amman Institute of Technology/Department of ECE, Sathyamangalam, India

Abstract— **Seizure is a kind of transient abnormal behaviour of neurons occurring within the brain which disturbs the mental and physical activities of the patient. Due to the synchronized activity of large group of neurons, epileptic seizures occur. These epileptic seizures cause numerous changes in the behaviour and perception of the patient. Even if the epileptic seizures are quite rare in a given patient, the fear of the occurrence of next seizure and helplessness feeling will have a very strong influence on the daily life of a patient. To improve the quality of life of these epileptic patients, a systematic method to predict the occurrence of seizures should be reliable. In biomedical science, EEG signals provide very valid contributions and hence the careful analysis of EEG recordings is required to understand the valuable information. To capture the brain signals of the epileptic patient, Electroencephalography (EEG) is widely used. EEG has a good temporal resolution and is non invasive in nature with a low maintenance cost. Since the EEG recordings are too huge to process, certain form of dimensionality reduction technique is required to reduce the dimensions of the EEG data in order to process the data. In this paper, Power Spectral Density (PSD) is used a dimensionality reduction technique to reduce the dimensions. It is then transmitted through the Space Time Trellis Coded Multiple Input Multiple Output Orthogonal Frequency Division Multiplexing (STTC MIMO-OFDM) System. As the system suffers from a high PAPR, Quadrature Mirror Filtering Based Partial Transmit Sequence (QMF-PTS) is proposed to reduce the PAPR. At the receiver, the classifier engaged here is Polynomial Kernel Based Support Vector Machine (PK-SVM) to classify the epilepsy from EEG signals. The performance metrics is analyzed in terms of performance index, sensitivity, specificity, time delay, quality value and accuracy.**

Keywords— **Seizure, EEG, PSD, QMF-PTS, PK-SVM**

I. Introduction

Rich spatio-temporal dynamics are exhibited in the human brain as it is quite complex in nature. Epilepsy is a very common brain disorder that affects 1% of the world population [1]. The seizures caused by epilepsy are simply the manifestations of epilepsy. When epileptic seizures occur, it is often aided with loss of consciousness. These seizures are viewed as unexpected and sudden abnormal functions of the body with an increase in muscular activity. There are various techniques to probe the dynamics of the human brain in literature but the best and direct way of measurement of cortical activity measurement can be done with the help of EEG. The mechanism which causes epileptic disorders can be easily understood with the help of EEG. The EEG signal is highly complex, non-stationary and nonlinear in nature [2]. An EEG can also easily depict the state of a person in various stages such as sleep, anesthesia, awake state etc. The characteristic patterns of the electrical potentials obtained from EEG differ for each of these states. EEG also holds various applications in detecting the brain tumour, sleep analysis, dementia and to monitor the depth of anesthesia. This paper proposes classification of epilepsy from EEG signals implemented for a telemedicine application. The organization of the paper is as follows: In section 2, the materials and methods are discussed followed by the System Design aspects and PAPR Reduction technique in section 3. In section 4, the post classification scheme is implemented followed by the results and discussion in section 5 and conclusion in section 6. The block diagram of the prediction tool is shown in Figure 1.

II. Materials and Methods

A. Acquisition of EEG data

The recordings of 20 epileptic patients are taken in European Data Format (EDF) from the Department of Neurology, Sri Ramakrishna Hospital, Coimbatore, India. The EEG recordings of the 20 epileptic patients were done for nearly 30 minutes each [3]. The recorded signals were in continuous form and each recorded signal was equally divided into 2 second epoch duration. For all the patients, the total number of channels recorded is 16 and it is simultaneously measured over 3 epochs. As the maximum frequency of EEG signal is about 50 Hz, the sampling frequency taken here is 200 Hz based on the Nyquist criteria. So totally 400 different values are obtained for each and every epoch and for 20 patients, the values of the epochs obtained is too high to process and hence dimensionality reduction is required. The dimensionality reduction technique taken here is Power Spectral Density (PSD). Power Spectral Density as a Dimensionality Reduction Technique.

S. Vlad and N.M. Roman (eds.), *International Conference on Advancements of Medicine and Health Care through Technology; 12th - 15th October 2016, Cluj-Napoca, Romania*,
IFMBE Proceedings 59,
DOI: 10.1007/978-3-319-52875-5_65

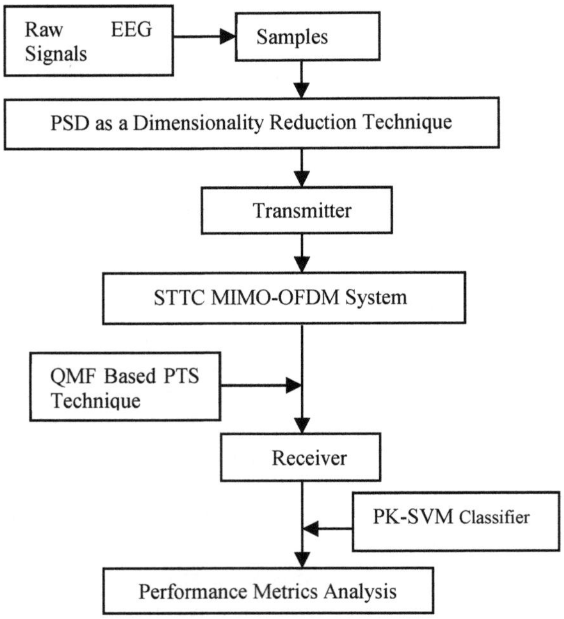

Fig. 1 Block Diagram of the Prediction Tool

B. PSD as a Dimensionality Reduction Technique

Spectral estimation plays a vital role in signal tracking and detection. For the spectral estimation applications like harmonic analysis, time series extrapolation, bandwidth compression, spectral smoothing and beamforming applications, it is widely used [4]. In this paper, the PSD is used to reduce the dimensions of the EEG signals with the help of Bartlett method [5]. Spectral estimation is simply the estimation of autocorrelation sequences of a particular random process obtained from a set of data and then computing the Fourier transform to seek the estimate the power spectrum. Known as Periodogram averaging, this technique is a very simple and most commonly used one. In this technique, the input sequence $x(n)$ of particular length N is partioned into K non-overlapping sequences each of length L so that the following condition is satisfied as

$$N = KL$$

The estimate of the Bartlett is given by

$$\hat{P}_B(e^{jw}) = \frac{1}{N}\sum_{i=0}^{K-1}\left|\sum_{n=0}^{L-1} x(n+iD)e^{-jnw}\right|^2$$

III. STTC MIMO-OFDM SYSTEM

A. System Design

When multiple antennas are utilized at both end of a wireless link, the technology is called as Multiple Input Multiple Output (MIMO) [6]. It holds the strong potential to improve the spectral efficiency in wireless communication systems. A highly promising candidate for next-generation mobile wireless system is the combination of MIMO and OFDM. MIMO OFDM has the capability to provide the highest data throughput. MIMO-OFDM is a special and versatile combination because MIMO does not try to mitigate multipath propagation and OFDM is utilized to prevent the necessity for signal equalization. Space Time Trellis Codes are a specific type of space time codes used in multiple antenna wireless communication. When STTC are combined with MIMO-OFDM the performance of the system is highly enhanced [7]. In this scheme the multiple and redundant copies of a trellis code are distributed over a number of antennas (space) and time. The reconstruction of the actual transmitted data is done by the receiver with the help of those multiple diverse copies of the data. STTC have a better Bit Error Rate (BER) performance and can provide both diversity gain and coding gain. The simulation parameters are shown in Table 1.

Table 1 Simulation Parameters

Modulation used	QPSK
System analysed	2 x2 STTC MIMO-OFDM
Number of subcarriers	512
No of sub-blocks	4
Maximum symbols loaded	1e5
Symbol rate	250000
No of time slots	2
Window function	Blackman-Haris
HPA Model	SSPA
No of frames	10
No of OFDM symbols/ frame	4
Bandwidth	5 MHz
Oversampling factor	4

B. PAPR Reduction Using QMF Based PTS

The PAPR [8] of any STTC MIMO-OFDM signal is defined as:

$$PAPR = \frac{Peak\ \ Power\ \ of\ \ the\ \ Signal}{Average\ \ Power\ \ of\ \ the\ \ Signal}$$

$$PAPR = \frac{\max|x|^2}{E[|x|^2]}$$

where $'x'$ is any signal representation. The steps followed for the PAPR Reduction Using QMF Based PTS is as follows:

Step 1: An input data block comprising of $'N'$ symbols is partitioned into a lot of disjoint sub blocks. Each sub blocks has sub carriers which are weighed by phase factors.

Step 2: The phase factors are selected such that if the pre-requisite condition should be that the PAPR of the signal is minimized [9]. The phase factors should be selected in such a way it should reduce the search complexity also.

Step 3: The phase factors allowed is represented as $P = \{0,1,....W-1\}$, where W represents the number of phase factors which are allowed. The exhaustive search for V phase factors is then found out. Then WV sets of phase factors are thoroughly searched to trace the best and optimum set of phase factors.

Step 4: Once the optimum set of phase factors are found out, Quadrature Mirror Filtering (QMF) is applied to it to make it the best phase factor [10]. As the number of sub blocks V increases, the complexity also increases exponentially.

Step 5: The threshold value is calculated and then it is checked that whether PAPR>threshold value

Step 12: As a final step the CCDF plot Vs probability of PAPR is computed and the plot is drawn and BER is calculated. Thus the PAPR can thus be easily computed using the QMF Based PTS scheme.

IV. Polynomial SVM (Kernel Trick) as a Post Classifier

Kernel trick helps to map the data into a different space called feature space. The Kernel trick also helps to construct a linear classifier in this specific space [11]. According to the Mercer's theorem, which states that any symmetric positive semi-definite function $K(x,z)$ is an inner product in some space. In other contexts, any function $K(x,z)$ implicitly defines a particular mapping into so-called feature space $\phi : x \rightarrow \phi(x)$ such that $K(x,z) = \langle \phi(x), \phi(z) \rangle$. Here the functions K are called kernels. The feature space can have infinite dimension or it can be high-dimensional too. Since kernel functions are used to compute the similarity in the feature space, the necessity to know the actual mapping is not required. A typical example of Polynomial Kernel is

$$K(x,z) = (\langle x,z \rangle + 1)^p$$

Various kernels are developed for special applications in various fields.

V. Results and Discussion

In this section, the PAPR Results, BER Results and the Classification Results are explained in detail.

A. PAPR Results

The PAPR results and the BER Analysis results are shown here. It is obvious from the careful analysis of the figure 2, that when QPSK modulation is engaged the PAPR is reduced by 4 dB with the utilization of QMF based PTS technique. The Bit Error Rate is also analysed in Table 2.

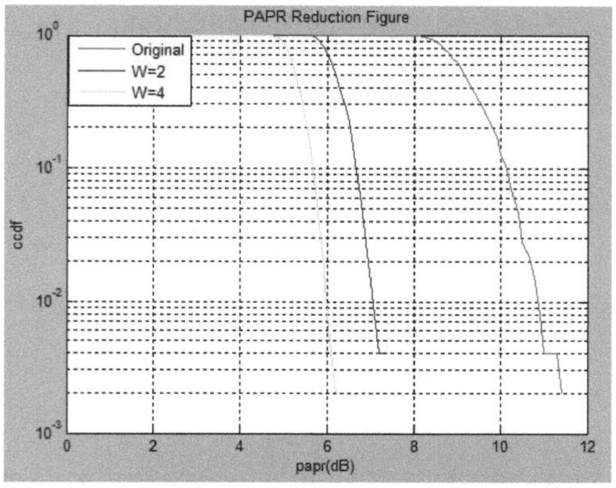

Fig. 2 PAPR Reduction Using QMF Based PTS Technique

Table 2 BER Analysis for the system

SNR	BER
0	0.2478
2	0.1796
4	0.1243
6	0.07478
8	0.01319
10	0.00308
12	0.006452
14	0.001552
16	0.000623

B. Classification Results

For PSD as dimensionality reduction technique and PK-SVM as a Post Classifier, based on the Performance Index, Quality values, Time Delay and Accuracy the results in the receiver side are computed in Table 3. The formulae for the Performance Index (PI), Sensitivity, Specificity and Accuracy are given as follows

$$PI = \frac{PC - MC - FA}{PC} \times 100$$

where PC – Perfect Classification, MC – Missed Classification, FA – False Alarm.

The Sensitivity, Specificity and Accuracy measures are stated by the following:

$$Specificity = \frac{PC}{PC + MC} \times 100$$

$$Sensitivity = \frac{PC}{PC + FA} \times 100$$

$$Accuracy = \frac{Sensitivity + Specificity}{2} \times 100$$

The Time Delay and the Quality Value Measures are given by the following

$$Time \quad Delay = \left[2 * \frac{PC}{100} + 6 * \frac{MC}{100} \right]$$

$$Quality \quad Values = \frac{10}{\left[\frac{FA}{100} + 0.2 \right] * Time \quad Delay}$$

Table 3 Average Performance Analysis Values of 20 Patients

Parameters	Obtained Values
PC (%)	96.04
MC (%)	3.95
FA (%)	0
PI (%)	94.93
Sensitivity (%)	100
Specificity (%)	96.04
Time Delay (sec)	2.15
Quality Values	23.43
Accuracy (%)	98.02

VI. Conclusion

Thus in this paper, the PSD was successfully incorporated as a dimensionality reduction technique and then transmitted through a 2 x 2 STTC MIMO-OFDM System. At the receiver side, when PK-SVM is used to classify the epilepsy from EEG signals, perfect classification of about 96.04% is obtained. A less time delay of 2.15 seconds, quality value of 23.43 and an average accuracy of 98.02% are observed. Future works aim to incorporate various other dimensionality reduction techniques with other system design and post classifiers for the telemedicine application of Epilepsy Classification.

Conflict of Interest

The authors declare that they have no conflict of interest.

References

1. R.Harikumar, P.Sunil Kumar (2015), "Frequency behaviors of electroencephalography signals in epileptic patients from a wavelet Thresholding perspective", Applied Mathematical Sciences, Vol. 9, no.50, 2451-2457
2. Harikumar Rajaguru, Sunil Kumar Prabhakar (2016), " Clinical Health Care for Long Distance using Matrix Factorization and Mahalanobis Based Sparse Representation Measures for Epilepsy Classification from EEG Signals", International Journal of Pharmaceutical Sciences Review and Research, Vol.38(1), Article 24, Pages:144-148
3. Sunil Kumar Prabhakar, Harikumar Rajaguru (2016), "Factorization and Particle Swarm Based Sparse Representation Classifier for Epilepsy Classification Implemented for Wireless Telemedicine Applications", IFBME Proceedings (Springer), 6th International Conference on the Development of Biomedical Engineering, pp: 474-478
4. F.Vernotte (1999), "Estimation of the Power Spectral Density of phase: comparison of three methods, "Proceedings of the 1999 Joint Meeting of the European Frequency and Time Forum, vol.2, pg:1109-1112.
5. Q.Ding et al (2011), "A blind spectrum-sensing method based on Bartlett Decomposition", 6th International ICST Conference on Communication and Networking in China (CHINACOM), pg:639-644.
6. Lozano A et al (2005) , "High-SNR Power Offset in Multiantenna Communication. *IEEE Tr.Comm*", pp.4134-4151
7. Z. Chen, J. Yuan, B. Vucetic (2001), "Improved space-time trellis coded modulation scheme on slow Rayleigh fading channels," Eletronics Lett., vo1.37, pp.440-441
8. Tao Jiang, Chunxing Ni, and Lili Guan (2013) "A Novel Phase Offset SLM Scheme for PAPR Reduction in Alamouti MIMO-OFDM Systems Without Side Information, " IEEE Signal Processing Letters, Vol. 20, No 4.
9. Han S.H and Lee J.H (2005), "An Overview of Peak-to-Average Power Ratio Reduction Techniques for Multicarrier Transmission", IEEE Wireless Communication, pp.56-65
10. D.Esteben, C.Galand (1997), "Application of Quadrature Mirror Filters to split band voice coding schemes", IEEE International Conference on Acoustics, Speech and Signal Processing (ICASSP), pg:191-195.
11. P.Arti, S.C.Deepak (2013), "SVM Kernel Functions for Classification", International Conference on Advances in Technology and Engineering (ICATE), pg:1-9, 2013

The Impact of Dizziness in Life's Quality of Elderly Patients with Vestibular Disorders and Their Caregivers

A. Maniu[1], G.S. Chiş[2], O.E. Harabagiu[1], R. Holonec[3] and A.I. Roman[4]

[1]Department of Otolaryngology-Head and Neck Surgery, University of Medicine and Pharmacy „Iuliu Hatieganu", Cluj-Napoca, Romania
[2] Department of Economics Informatics Faculty of Economics, Babes Bolyai University, Cluj-Napoca, Romania
[3] Department of Electrotechnics and Measurments, Technical University, Cluj-Napoca, Romania
[4]"Octavian Fodor" Regional Institute of Gastroenterology and Hepathology, Cluj Napoca, Romania

Abstract— **This study is proposing a solution to support patients with dizziness who live alone and need medical assistance. The aim of this study was firstly to evaluate the impact of dizziness in the quality of life of the patients and their family members, and to propose a system to assist both them in case of need. The proposed solution is based on a 3-axis accelerometer system (like a wristband) that understands your motions, connects to a smart phone and automatically calls the patient's doctor in case of falls. The wristband is built with Pure Pulse® [12] heart rate and connects via Bluetooth to a smartphone. Additional feature of the wristband includes a panic button. An incident from April 2016, when a patient's normal heart rate of 70 jumped up to 190, and a medical team was sent to patient's home, saving his life, together with medical knowledge regarding the dizziness behavior triggered the idea to develop a system that in case of falls it calls the patient's ORL doctor. In the future, we plan to integrate it with the national health system like 112. We based our study on the assumption that the families of the people with dizziness are prepared to use this kind of system because it is safe and cheaper than other solutions (like nurses for example).**

Keywords— **dizziness, wristband, fails, healthcare, telemedicine**

I. INTRODUCTION

Dizziness is the main symptom of vestibular disorders, frequently met in the older population. Its prevalence reaches 50% in the population over 85 years of age [1], [2]. This symptom appears as a result of losing the ability to achieve a stable gaze, posture, and gait. The deficiency in the spatial orientation and motion perception is perceived by the patient as an illusion of rotatory movement (classical vertigo) disequilibrium, unsteadiness, visual blurring or light-headedness are [3].

The sole presence of dizziness in the elderly is a strong predictor of falls [3], [9] increasing the risk of hip and wrist fractures [4], [9]. Injuries related to falls lead to mobility restriction and loss of independence. It also increases the fear of falling, which also predicts subsequent falls. In addition, falls are the leading cause of accidental death in persons older than 65 years [5]. In addition, many patients suffer an intense emotional distress and symptoms of anxiety and depression [6]. The symptoms limit physical and social activities of patients, and may affect dramatically their quality of life [7]. Patients presenting with associated psychological symptoms are those who are more likely to remain symptomatic and disabled, with the highest levels of disability [7].

Dizziness in elderly may cause another variety of psychosocial problems such as decreased quality of life of the patient's family members as well as increased social distance for the patient and the family caring for the patient. The term presbyastasis has been proposed to encompass the age-related degeneration of different neural structures that affects balance, but many other causes can be added: neurodegenerative disorders, stroke, arrhythmia, postural hypotension, musculoskeletal system disorders etc [8].

The diagnostic and therapeutic approach must be multisystemic and oriented to the visual, proprioceptive, and vestibular systems.

Since the causes of dizziness in older people are multi-factorial, management of this disease should be customized according to the etiology of dizziness in each individual. Management of dizziness includes various approaches, including medical and rehabilitative ones as well as the use of prosthetic devices.

Medical therapy and the vestibular rehabilitation exercises was not the subject of this study.

Ensuring safety for the patients with dizziness is another issue to be achieved for the specialists.

Therefore, research should also focus on preventive efforts to avoid falls and to find a method of signaling in case of falls [3].

There are many methods of monitoring the patients at home like:

- permanent supervision 24/7 (social workers, nurses, family members);

S. Vlad and N.M. Roman (eds.), *International Conference on Advancements of Medicine and Health Care through Technology; 12th - 15th October 2016, Cluj-Napoca, Romania,*
IFMBE Proceedings 59,
DOI: 10.1007/978-3-319-52875-5_66

- supervising all the house with webcams (a little expensive);
- a wristband with connection to a smartphone (our prototype).

Lately, these kinds of systems are widely used and nowadays everybody has a smartphone permanently connected to a mobile network.

A system that is monitoring all patients is Sidly Care [11] – was develop by Edyta Kocyk in Poland for persons with Alzheimer[10] but the system is using also data to collect and send to a portal.

The only two conditions for a proper functioning of the wristband are: the phone needs GSM signal and the wristband, as well as the phone, are charged. Our system is using only the GSM network [20]which, as you can see in the Fig 1. covers more than 95 % of Romania's territory. In this proposed version, the smartphone is used only to call the doctor/112 and no mobile data is needed it for the moment. The patients using the wristband will be connected to the smartphone via Bluetooth, and in the case of falls or dizziness, they will push a button that will trigger in the smartphone the call the doctor/112. In the present days, the telecom industry is growing fast, very soon the mobile data will be covered more and more. Our plan is to use this improved mobile data coverage in order to have the wristband function as a prevention tool also, not just as a saving tool. Regarding the charging of the device, we recommend that the devices are charged overnight. During the night, the patient is sleeping and the wristband can charge on the near nightstand. Another solution would be that the patient has two different wristbands, this way one is always charged.

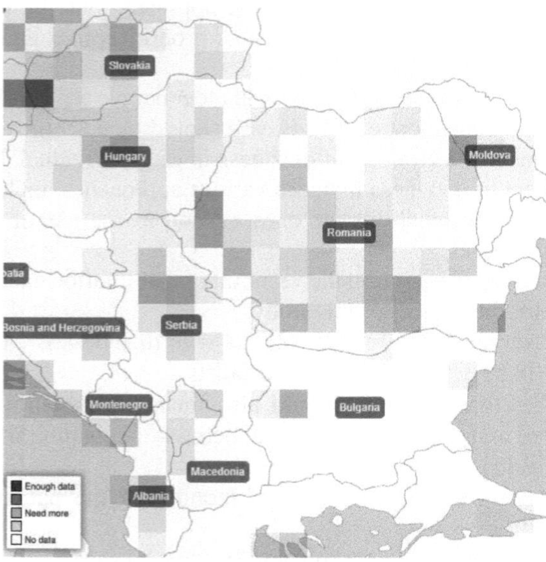

Fig. 1. – GSM cover map Romania[20]

The usual Wristband trackers use a 3-axis accelerometer to understand person's movements. An accelerometer is a device that turns the movement (acceleration) of a body into digital measurements (data). By analyzing acceleration data, our trackers provide detailed information about frequency, duration, intensity, and patterns of movement to determine the steps taken, distance traveled, calories burned, and sleep quality. The 3-axis implementation allows the accelerometer to measure the motion in all three directions, making its activity measurements more precise than older, single-axis pedometers [12].

Until now, we have not found a system that is able to make the difference between sleeping/rest and dizziness, and we added therefore the panic button on the wristband. We are planning to develop in the future a system using genetic algorithms and artificial intelligence that is able to learn all patience's movements and trigger the alarm for help.

The costs of a normal bracelet will be approximately 100 Euro. The rest of the services involved (the doctor, the customer service etc.) would cost around 25/35 euro a month, the equivalent of a private consultation. We have accessed a Research and Innovation Project funded by the European Union that will allow us to fund the prototype for the bracelet.

The aim of this study was to test the impact of dizziness in the quality of life of the patients and their family members, to propose a system of signalization for the relatives, in order to increase the quality of life of the patients' family members, avoiding psychosocial problems such as decreased social distance for the patient and the family caring for the patient. With the help of the wristband, patients will be more and more independent. They will be able to go for example on holiday as long as there is GSM signal. The purpose of this project is to create an e-care call center. This way the wristband carriers can be monitored directly and non stop.

II. Material and Methods

Sixty chronic vestibular outpatient patients aged over 65 years who had been seen at the ENT Department of Cluj-Napoca University Hospital between January 2014 and December 2015 were included in the study. The patients complained of dizziness and had a diagnostic hypothesis of chronic peripheral vestibular syndrome (dizziness for more than 3 months) unresponsive to the medical therapy. The following medical data were collected for the study: were age, gender, psycho-affective complaints (anxiety, depression and insecurity), general health (arterial hypertension, spinal disorders, metabolic conditions, strokes, cranial trauma, problems with vision, and others), audiological evaluation results and Video- Frenzel testing [10] results (classified by otorhinolaryngologist as normal, peripheral, central, mixed or inconclusive). . Patients living together with their family members and/or patients suffering from mental illness were excluded from the study. The patients answered two questionnaires (translated by a bilingual translator): The Vestibular Activities of Daily Living Scale (VADL) [13] and the Handicap Inventory (DHI) [14].

Additionally, for each patient, a family member was asked to fill in a questionnaire consisting of 10 questions regarding their status concerning the patient health.

A. The questionnaires

Vestibular Activities of Daily Living Scale (VADL) [13] is a questionnaire that quantifies the dizziness impairment in daily activity. The patients had to evaluate their own performance regarding each activity. If the performance varied due to the intermittent vertigo and static disturbance, they should have marked the highest level of disability. For each activity, they had to mark the level that best described their performance until the moment when filling in the questionnaire. The questionnaire „Vestibular Activities of Daily Living Scale" has a content of 28 questions. The patients were asked to answer every question with a grade from 1 to 10. The grade given was proportional to the extent the activity influenced their life. In case the patient did not want to answer the question, or he did not perform the activity he could answer the question with no answer „ NA".

The Dizziness Handicap Inventory (DHI) [14] questionnaire was developed considering the most common consequences of dizziness in interviews with people suffering from that condition. The scale has shown reliability and validity. Most of its 25 items concerned the restriction and disruption of a wide range of physical and social activities (daily chores, travel, family affairs, leisure pursuits), but some items investigated the assessment of social support or stigmatization and the emotional distress caused by dizziness. The items were sub classified in three content domains representing functional (9 items), emotional (9 items) and physical (7 items) aspects of dizziness and unsteadiness. To each item, the following scores could be assigned: No=0; Sometimes=2; Yes=4. The total score (0-100 points) was obtained by summing ordinal scale responses, higher scores indicating more severe handicap: 16-34 Points (mild handicap); 36-52 Points (moderate handicap); 54+ Points (severe handicap).

The questionnaires for the family members consists of 10 questions regarding the investigating caregivers' emotional stress and the condition of the patient with dizziness and willingness to purchase a device capable of signaling in case of falls.

III. RESULTS

The group included 28 (46.6%) women and 32 (53.3%) men. The mean age was of 71±6.5 years (95%CI), with a minimum of 65 years and a maximum of 92 years. The etiology of the peripheral vestibular syndrome was established as following: benign paroxysmal postural vertigo (BPPV) (28 patients-47%), vestibular neuritis (11 patients-18%), Ménière's disease (7 patients-12%), viral labyrinthitis (5 patients-8%) and peripheral vestibular syndrome with unknown etiology (9 patients-15%).

B. VADL

From all daily activities performed by the patients, the easiest ones were intimate activity (1.85) and easy household activities (1.89), while reaching the top (mean 3.95), walking on an unsteady surface (mean 3.92) were the most difficult ones (Fig. 2).

C. DHI

Emotionally, the most affecting feeling among our patients was frustration. The median grades given to the questions with emotional impact were 1.35, - to the questions with functional impact were 1.76 and to the questions with physical impact were 1.84. Functionally, patients were mostly affected while reading (mean 2.2) and being at high altitude (mean 2.13). Physically, our patients were most affected by quick movements of the head (mean 2.53), by bending over (mean 2.1) and by looking down (mean 2) (Fig. 3).

D. The total score

The higher the score the more disabling the vertigo for our patients was. Fig. 4 shows the distribution of the patients according to the total score. The maximum sub score of emotional impact was 36. Twenty of our patients got a sub score of 32 (the highest in our case), and four of them got a minimum sub score of 0. Eight patients received 8 points each; seven patients received 12 points, and other seven patients received 4 points (Fig. 3).

Regarding the distribution of our patients according to the functional impact, the maximum subscale score in this case is the same as in the emotional impact (36). Fifty one of our patients marked 36 points and one of our patients received 0 points.

In the case of the subscale aiming the physical impact the maximum score was of 28 points, 43 of our patients marked 28 points and six of them marked 0 points.

The questionnaires for the family members: The responses of the caregivers for 28 out of 60 patients, who were living alone, revealed that the majority of them (89.2%) have considered very useful the purchasing of a signaling device. 96.4 % of responders considered that the device would increase the safety of their relative.

E. Statistical analysis

The medical records were collected using Microsoft Excel 2013 and then analyzed using the SPSS (Statistical Package Social Science) software, version 11.0. Data were codified, digitized and analyzed in SPSS.

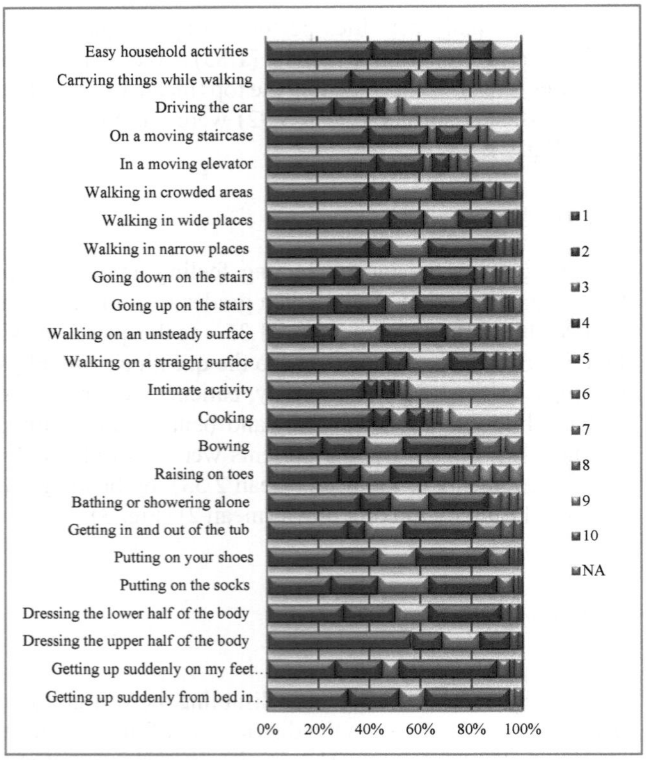

Fig. 2. The score given by the patients to each activity according to the Vestibular Activities of Daily Living Scale (**VADL).**

IV. Discussions

Our study revealed that the vestibular disorders especially in elderly, are causing functional limitations or decreased ability to perform daily activities independently, having a negative influence on the quality of life. Two valuable questionnaires (VADL and DHI) developed by The World Health Organization were used.

The results of this work showed similarities with other studies [15, 16] where physical disability was the most frequent aspect, followed by functional impairment and emotional disability. As regard to the daily activity (the VADL questionnaires) the patient's answers showed basic mobility skills impairment. The DHI responses demonstrated that from the emotional points of view the patients presented frustration, impaired concentration and feelings of depression. These results may indicate that there are difficulties in learning to cope with a vestibular disorder in elderly. The same results were found in the previous studies[17], who confirmed that patients with vertigo present concomitant psychological symptoms in 56.38% of cases, anguish being the most prevalent (47.38%), followed by anxiety, fear, depression and memory disorders, thus stressing the relation between the vestibular disorder and emotional alterations.

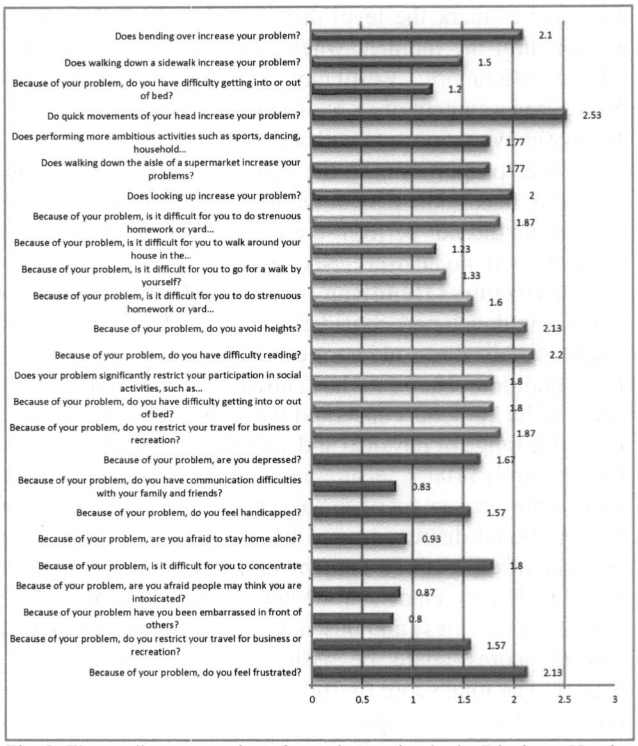

Fig. 3. The medium score given for each question in the Dizziness Handicap Inventory (DHI)

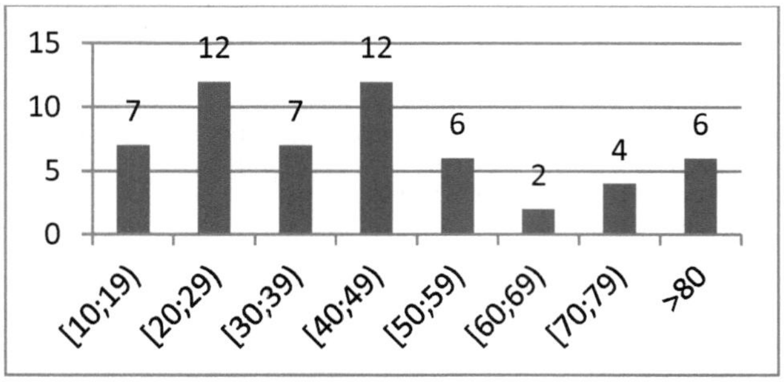

Fig. 4 Distribution of the patients according to the total score

Table 1 The questionnaires for the family members

Questions for the family members	Yes	No
There is between your family member a relative suffering from dizziness living alone?	28	32
Are you concerned about him/her?	26	34
Are you worried when he/she does not answer the phone?	24	36
It has happened to interrupt your activity to pay an emergency visit?	9	51
You feel guilty because you do not spend enough time with him/her?	27	33
Would you be interested to have a signaling device for him/her?	25	35
Would you feel more comfortable with this device?	25	35
Would you agree to pay for the device?	23	37
This device would be easy to use?	13	47
Do you think that the safety for the patients would be increased?	27	33

The questionnaires for the family members emphasised worries about their relative suffering from vestibular disorders, a sensation of incapacity and changes in family relationships. Although in some studies [18, 19], the quality of life for the caregivers of patients with Alzheimer disease, stroke or cancer was investigated, to the best of our knowledge, no study investigated the quality of life for the caregivers of elderly patients with chronic vestibular disorders. Although these questionnaires need further improvement, the questionnaires for the family members revealed that the majority of them consider very useful the purchasing of a signaling device for increasing the safety of their relative.

II. Conclusions

Our system, using the GSM network will be a very useful tool for increasing the safety of the elderly suffering from chronic vestibular disorders. The cost for a month will not be higher than a regular visit to the doctor. The system we intend to create is easy to use, with a high success rate and makes sure that the patients are monitored and supervised all the time. The only condition is that the wristband, as well as the phone are charged all the time.

Conflict of Interest

The authors declare that they have no conflict of interest.

III. References

1. Moraes SA, Soares WJS, Rodrigues RAS, Fett WCR, Ferriolli E, Perracini MR. Dizziness in community-dewelling older adults: a population-based study. Braz J Otorhinolaryngol. 2011;77:691-9.
2. Barin K, Dodson EE. Dizziness in the elderly. Otolaryngol Clin North Am (2011) 44:437–54.10.1016/j.otc.2011.01.013
3. Sloane P, Coeytaux R, Beck R, Dallara J. Dizziness: State of the Science. Ann Intern Med 2001;134 (9) Part 2:823–832.
4. Agrawal Y, Carey JP, Della Santina CC, Schubert MC, Minor LB.. Disorders of balance and vestibular function in US adults: data from the national health and nutrition examination survey, 2001-2004. Arch Intern Med (2009) 169:938–44.10.1001 /archinternmed.2009.66
5. Kannus P, Parkkari J, Koskinen S, Niemi S, Palvanen M, Jarvinen M, et al. Fall-induced injuries and deaths among older adults. JAMA (1999) 281:1895–9.10.1001
6. Staab JP. Chronic dizziness: the interface between psychiatry and neurootology. Curr Opin Neurol. 2006;19:41-8
7. Yardley L. Overview of psychologic effects of chronic dizziness and balance disorders. Otolaryngol Clin North Am. 2000;33:603-16.
8. Lo AX, Harada CN.. Geriatric dizziness: evolving diagnostic and therapeutic approaches for the emergency department. Clin Geriatr Med (2013)
9. Lara Fernández, Hayo A. Breinbauer, Paul Hinckley Delano, Vertigo and Dizziness in the Elderly, Front Neurol. 2015; 6: 144. Published online 2015 Jun 26. Doi:10.3389/fneur.2015. 00144
10. http://www.businessmagazin.ro/actualitate/tanara-care-din-dorinta-de-a-si-salva-bunica-a-inventat-un-dispozitiv-medical-care-va-ajuta-70-de-milioane-de-oameni-15678298
11. SIDLY CARE http://www.sidly-care.eu/en/
12. FITBIT https://www.fitbit.com/eu
13. Cohen HS, Kimball KT. Development of the vestibular disorders activities of daily living scale. Arch Otolaryngol Head Neck Surg. 2000 Jul;126(7):881-7
14. Vereeck L, Truijen S, Wuyts FL, Heyning PH Van de. Internal consistency and factor analysis of the Dutch version of the Dizziness Handicap Inventory. Acta Oto-Laryngologica. 2007;127:788–795
15. Neuhauser HK, Radke A, von Brevern M, Lezius F, Feldman M, Lempert T. Burden of dizziness and vertigo in the community. Arch Intern Med 2008;168,2118-24.

16. Mendel B, Bergenius J, Langius A. Dizziness symptom severity and impact on daily living as perceived by patients suffering fromperipheral vestibular disorder. Clin Otolaryngol 1999;24,286-93.
17. Paiva AD, Kuhn AMB. Psychological symptoms associated to dizziness complaint in neurootological patients of Universidade Federal de São Paulo - Escola Paulista de Medicina. R Bras Otorrinolaringol. 2004;70:512–515
18. Markowitz JS, Gutterman EM, Sadik K, Papadopoulos G Health-related quality of life for caregivers of patients with Alzheimer disease.Alzheimer Dis Assoc Disord. 2003 Oct-Dec;17(4):209-14.
19. Kitrungroter L, Cohen MZ. Quality of life of family caregivers of patients with cancer: a literature review. Oncol Nurs Forum. 2006 May 3;33(3):625-32.
20. https://gsmmap.org/assets/pdfs/gsmmap.org-country_report-Romania-2016-08.pdf

Author: George Sebastian Chiş
Institute: Department of Economics Informatics Faculty of Economics, Babeş Bolyai University,
Street: Teodor Mihali no. 58-60
City: Cluj-napoca
Country: Romania
Email: George.chis@econ.ubbcluj.ro

Prioritization of Medical Devices for Maintenance Decisions

C. Corciovă, D. Andrițoi, C. Luca and R. Ciorap

University of Medicine and Pharmacy "Grigore T. Popa" Iasi, Department Biomedical Sciences, Iasi, Romania

Abstract - **The objective of this study was to define a working method for biomedical engineers/ medical engineers to determine realistic maintenance intervals for medical equipment in hospitals. Maintenance period was analyzed for 145 medical equipment, including monitoring and treatment devices. Some indicators were established on the conditions of use of equipment and taking into account the manufacture year of the equipment; the data were analyzed using logistic regression predictors. The average time between failures was determined and was reported to some categories of relevant indicators.**

Keywords - **failure, medical equipment, procedures, regression, maintenance.**

I. Introduction

Our society expects that competence and efficiency will guide the development of applications and support of medical technology. According to this, biomedical engineers/medical engineers in hospitals face every day the challenge of managing appropriate medical technology with limited resources. To make the most of their resources and assist in delivering high quality health care in most cost effective manner, clinical engineering department in hospitals must develop a system for quantifying risk and integrate this system into a medical technology management program (Fig.1) [1].

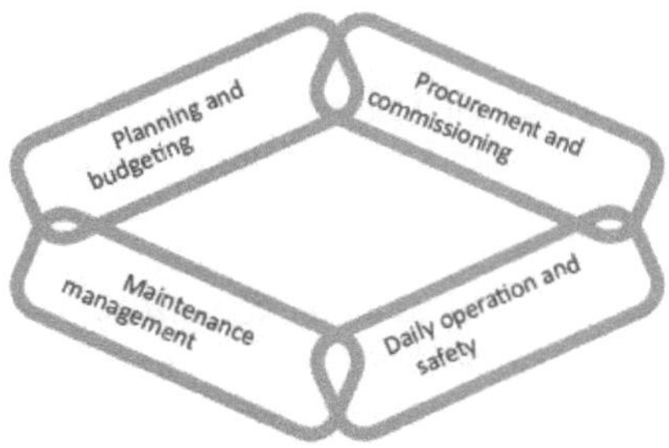

Fig.1 Chain of activities in the equipment life cycle

An early phase of any technology management program involves an assessment of existing technology. Medical technology assessment has been proposed as one way of improving patient care and wellness by providing that only appropriate technology is used in the health care environment. In addition to providing for technical evaluation and clinical trials of equipment, technology assessment attempts to control negative economic consequences by assessing risk throughout the medical equipment life cycle.

Historically risk assessment has been of two types, perceived and quantitative. The perceived style of risk assessment is routinely, qualitative informal, intuitive and generally undocumented. This style is reactive, involving on the spot response to risk events or situation in the hospital [2].

The quantitative risk assessment style is formal, explicit, disciplined, rigorous, generally peer reviewed and always documented. Dynamic risk assessment tools include the possibility to measure the risk of the medical equipment and contain as many quantifiable elements of the environments as possible. Parallel goals include the following:

1. To create a method for classifying medical equipment that would ensure the effective deployment of available resources;
2. To provide a comprehensive and accurate tool for identifying equipment related technical and clinical training needs;
3. To guide triage of repair, preventive maintenance and other service requirements on the basis of their effectiveness at reducing equipment associated risk;
4. To advance the biomedical engineering program beyond a traditional, reactive risk assessment mode, typically based on failure analysis to a more quantitative and proactive one;
5. To develop and implement methods to review large amounts of data easily without losing the capacity to identify equipment details and higher than acceptable incidences of operators errors, unsuccessful repairs, equipments failures and so on [3].

During the study, hospital was performing maintenance contracts for the supplied medical equipment, which included visits for repairs and preventive maintenance. Hospital had no maintenance department or dedicated staff for health technology management.

II. Materials and methods

The original dynamic risk assessment tools consist of four modules paired by their static and dynamic risk characteristics. The two static components, equipment function and physical risk are assigned when the medical equipment is entered into the biomedical engineering equipment database and this category provides the baseline risk level for

S. Vlad and N.M. Roman (eds.), *International Conference on Advancements of Medicine and Health Care through Technology; 12th - 15th October 2016, Cluj-Napoca, Romania,*
IFMBE Proceedings 59,
DOI: 10.1007/978-3-319-52875-5_67

the equipment. The equipment function measure assigns a level risk keyed to the equipments purpose, with life support equipment getting the highest rating because it's potential failure would be accompanied by the highest level of risk. The physical risk measure represents an estimate of the worst case effect if the equipment does not perform as expected, with patient death receiving the highest rating [4]. These two modules are classified as static because their values usually remain the same over the life cycle of an item of medical equipment (Table 1.).

Table 1. Initial assignment of the risk factors provides a baseline risk level for medical equipment

Risk Management Tool				
Static Risk Factors		***Dynamic Risk Factors***		
Equipment Function	*Physical Risk*	*Maintenance Requirements*	*Risk Points*	*Risk Groups*
No patient	No significant risk	Based on equipment type and hour per maintenance	Operator/ Patient injury	
Patient related	Patient discomfort		Equipment failure	High (5 pct)
Monitoring	Patient injury		Exceeds MTBF	
Surgical	Patient death		PM inspection failure	Low (1pct)
Physical therapy			Physical damage	
Life support			Operator error	
+ year of the manufacture of the equipment				

The two dynamic risk factor modules are the maintenances requirements and risk points. The maintenance requirement measure works on the assumption that an increased number of interventions by bioengineer both indicates and causes risk [5]. For instance, if a defibrillator requires high maintenance, this indicates an incident waiting to happen. In addition the repeated testing of the equipment shortens the life of high voltage relays, capacitors and cables and moves the equipment closer to failure.

The risk point measure combines various risk factors such as actual failures, reasons for failure or poor performance with regard to such criteria as mean time between failures (MTBF). The output of each of four modules is algebraically summed, averaged over six month period and rated from 1 (Low) to 5 (High). Because no standard exists yet for assessing risk, the tool uses current practices to establish a baseline. Then a feedback loop permits the clinical engineer to review equipment that shows an increase a risk over a predetermined period of time. If the clinical engineer confirms an increase in the risk factor, action to reduce that risk is necessary.

Table 2. Equipment classification

Variable	Category	Definition	Coding
IMPORTANCE	*Low*	Is not necessary daily routine	0
	Medium	Daily routine is important	0
	High	Is vital for life	1
INTENSITY OF USE (hours)	*Inactivated*	Equipment not in use	-
	Low	Very little use	0
	Medium	Frequent utilization, but not daily	0
	High	Turned on consecutively for 24 hours/day. Repetitive use in a same day	1
USE IN STRESS CONDITIONS	*Normal*	Sporadic use in hospital	0
	Repetitive	Constant use in hospital	0
	Emergency Use	Use in the emergency sector, need for fastest response	1
	Under pressure	Use in hospital sectors with medical staff constantly under pressure	1
TECHNOLOGICAL LEVEL	*Modern*	Recent technologies	0
	Average	Digital technology	0
	Old	Old analogical technology	1
	Obsolete	Very old technology	1

When the hospital's inventory there is a lot of models and types of equipment, it is necessary to designate the categories with high risk. Using these designations, the personnel can focus their attention on the equipment with the greatest potential for injury or damage. Selection is based on repair service reports filled out by engineers. First an item is only included in the high risk category if an engineer has used the "Equipment Failure" code.

Equipment with these ratings would include, for example, monitoring equipment, defibrillators, dialysis equipment, and electrosurgical units. The critical decision regarding risk is based on whether the failure code "Failed PM" is present. If it is, the equipment was discovered to be out of tolerance or in a failed state during PM, that is a clinical engineer discovered the abnormally during PM, not a clinician who was attempting to use the equipment.

This is called a high risk soft failure and is not as serious as when "Failed PM" is not present. If is not present the problem was detected by clinician during the clinical procedure. This is called a high risk failure and is considered a more hazardous condition.

The strategy is to improve procedures in order to reduce the number of failures discovered by clinicians, by having clinical engineers to discover equipment problems during PM and to reduce the total number of failure for high-risk equipment. It is necessary to monitor the ratio of hard failures to soft failures and to compare the ratios for various equipment categories, identifying strengths and weaknesses in PM procedures.

The model was built in the Statistical Package for the Social Sciences (SPSS), version 20. The equation used was designed from first principles described in 2000 by Lemenshow [6].

$$P_F = \frac{\exp^{(b0+b1V1+b2V2+b3V3+b4V4+b5V5)}}{1+\exp^{(b0+b1V1+b2V2+b3V3+b4V4+b5V5)}} \quad (1)$$

where:

P_F - probability of failure;
V_1 – technological level;
V_2 – intensity of use;
V_3 – stress use;
V_4 – importance of the equipment;
V_5 – year of manufacture of the equipment.

After the modeling, the failure rate (R_F) and the mean time between failures (MTBF) were computed for the equipment groups defined by the categories of the identified failure predictors.

$$R_F = n_F \cdot \Delta T \quad (2)$$

where:
n_F – number of failures;
ΔT – duration of failure.

$$\text{MTBF} = \frac{1}{R_F} \quad (3)$$

Failure percents are:

$$\%\text{ failure} = \frac{n_G}{n} 100 \quad (4)$$

where:
n_G - total number of failures;
n – failures in equipment group.

The upper and lower confidence limits of the 95% confidence interval for the MTBF was calculated using next equation determined by Birolini in 2007 [3].

$$\lim_i = \frac{2*T}{\chi^2 A/2;2*n_F+2} \quad (5)$$

$$\lim_s = \frac{2*T}{\chi^2 1-A\ /2;2*n_F+2} \quad (6)$$

where:
$\lim_i$ – lower limit of the confidence interval;
$\lim_s$ – upper limit of the confidence interval;
T – total time of the study;
A – significance level;
n_F – number of failures;

χ^2 - chi square (standardized distribution with 2n+2, 2n or 2 freedom degrees).

III. Results

In Table 3. are presented the number of equipments, the number of equipments in the critical categories and the total number of failures for type of equipment. Twenty one equipments did not have failure during the study.

Table 3. Number of equipment in critical categories

Equipment	Number	Intensity of use	Use in stress conditions	Failures
Monitors	44	32	20	12
Infusion Pump	54	38	21	31
Automated NIBP	10	8	6	6
Oximeters	16	12	10	4
Sensors	-	-	-	11
Monitors cables	-	-	-	19
Total	124	90	57	82

Table 4. presents the results of the regression model. It can be noted that only one variable (intensity of use) may be associated with situation equipment failure (p = 0.002). The initial model contents all the variables. The final model shows only variables that were statistically significant compared to the initial model.

Table 4. Variables comparation between the initial and final model

Variable	Standard errors	p-value	Odds ratio
Initial model			
Intensity of use- low	-	-	1
Intensity of use- high	0.72	0.061	3.2
Use in stress- normal condition	-	-	1
Use in stress- pressure	0.75	0.780	0.80
Technology level- modern	0.83	0.860	1.1
Importance- high	0.43	0.626	0.84
Year of manufacture- new one	0.040	0.314	0.96
Final model			
Intensity of use- low	-	-	1
High	0.48	0.002	4.2
Constant	0.44	0.000	0.12

Table 5. shows the number of devices, number of failures and the MTBF depending on the categories selected by logistic regression identified by the relevant variable.

Table 5. Equipment according to the categories of intensity of use

Intensity of use	Number of equipment (%)	Failures (%)	Failures rate (R_F)	MTBF (days 95 % confidence interval)
Inactivated	2	-	-	-
Low	21.3	2	0.0078	118.3
Medium	19.8	30	0.0895	17.3
High	56.9	68	0.1924	5.8

The results showed how maintenance contracts could be applied taking into account the operating conditions of the equipment, so that equipment with high rates of failure should receive inspections more frequently than preventive maintenance, and those with low rates could have a longer interval between inspections. So the hospital will achieve a higher degree of availability of equipment and maintenance companies would be able to focus on more effective interventions.

Table 6. Maintenance requirements

Grade	Procedures	Ratio
Low	Visual inspection, a basic performance check, safety testing, minimal maintenance	0.15
Medium	Only performance verification and safety testing	0.50
High	Equipment having components like mechanical, pneumatic or fluidics requires the most extensive maintenance.	1.00

Most devices in the study were classified as high-intensity use. It was recommended that for short MTBF equipment, like infusion pump or oximeters, to shorten the maintenance intervals, e.g. 7-9 days. Similarly, for equipment with an average intensity of use (MTBF = 18 days) it was suggested that maintenance intervals should be defined as 15 days.

IV. Conclusions

Clinical engineering department provides the technology related expertise required for safe and efficient integration interventions at the bedside. One strategy is to develop effective programs and to make changes on the basis of performance indicators that measure the efficacy of the medical equipment management program. The results obtained in this study enable a precise and consistent timetable for the maintenance of medical equipment, which will improve the work of clinicians and the patient's comfort and outcomes.

Conflict of Interest

The authors declare that they have no conflict of interest.

References

1. Bronzino J. D., Medical devices and systems (2006), Boca Raton FL, USA: CRC Press.
2. Garrick J. B., Dykes A.A., Kapaln S (2005), Possible roles for quantitative risk assessment (QRA) in the field of health care and health regulation, Proceedings from Role of Technology in Controling Health Care Cost, The International Society for Optical Engineering 2499:205
3. Birolini A. (2007), Reliability engineering, The 5th Ed. New York: Springer
4. Pecht M. (2009), Reliability maintainability and availability Handbook of Systems Engineering and Management, Wiley: pp. 361-396
5. Bevilacqua M., Braglia M. (2000), The analytic hierarchy process applied to maintenance strategy selection, Reliab. Eng. Syst Safe 70(1): 71–83
6. Hosmer D. W., Lemeshow S. (2000), Applied Logistic Regression, 2nd Ed. New York: John Wiley and Sons

Author: Corciovă Călin
Institute:University of Medicine and Pharmacy "Grigore T. Popa"
Street: Universitatii, No 16
City: Iaşi
Country:Romania
Email: calin.corciova@bioinginerie.ro

Development of Wireless Biomedical Data Transmission and Real Time Monitoring System

C. M. Fort[1], S. Gergely[2] and A. O. Berar

[1]Technical University of Cluj-Napoca/Department of Electrotechnics and Measurements, Biomedical Engineering, Cluj-Napoca, Romania
[2]National Institute for Research and Development of Isotopic and Molecular Technologies Cluj-Napoca Romania

Abstract—**The acquisition and remote transmission of patient data is becoming an ever more important topic in medical research. Recent improvements in electronic technology and accessibility can provide interesting solutions for medical diagnostics and therapy. The goal of this paper is to present the development and investigation of a system capable of wireless biomedical data transmission and real time monitoring using off the shelf products. The biomedical data sensors consist of a skin temperature sensor, a heart rate sensor and an accelerometer. The wireless communication provides sensor data to a PC, at which point, real time data monitoring can be performed.**

Keywords— **wireless transmission, biomedical data, real time monitoring, pulse, BPM**

I. Introduction

In recent years, due to technological advances in integrated electronics, new and accessible solutions for data acquisition and transmission emerged. Such solutions could be effectively used in medical research, diagnostics and therapy, as the acquisition and remote transmission of patient data is becoming an ever more important topic, according to [1].
The main goal of this paper is to present the development and investigation of a system capable of wireless biomedical data transmission and real time monitoring using off the shelf products.

For demonstration purposes, real-world patient data was collected and presented.

II. Description and implementation of tools

A. General system description

A simplified schematic of the system described in this paper is presented in Fig 1, and can be divided into three units.

The first unit is a miniature portable unit containing the biomedical sensors, microcontroller, wireless data transmission module and power supply. This can be defined as the data acquisition and wireless transmission unit and a general view of Unit 1 is presented in Fig 2.

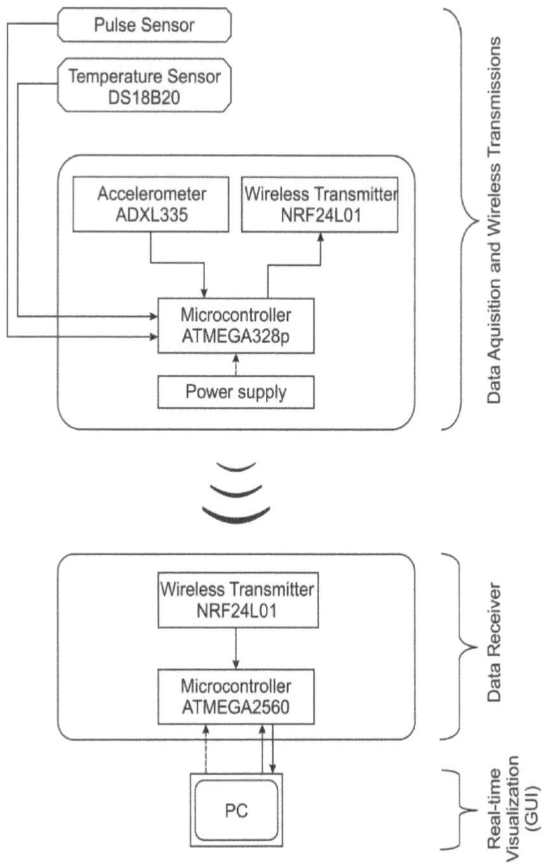

Fig. 1 General System Schematic

The biomedical data sensors are: a skin temperature sensor, a heart rate sensor and an accelerometer for patient fall detection. For convenience, the accelerometer board was placed inside the portable unit enclosure. The microcontroller (ATMEGA328p) receives data from the sensors, computes various parameters such as Heart Beats per Minute and sends the data wireless to the second unit.

The second unit consists of a wireless data receiver module and microcontroller that transfers the data to a Personal Computer (PC) for real time data visualization and data storage.

S. Vlad and N.M. Roman (eds.), *International Conference on Advancements of Medicine and Health Care through Technology; 12th - 15th October 2016, Cluj-Napoca, Romania,*
IFMBE Proceedings 59,
DOI: 10.1007/978-3-319-52875-5_68

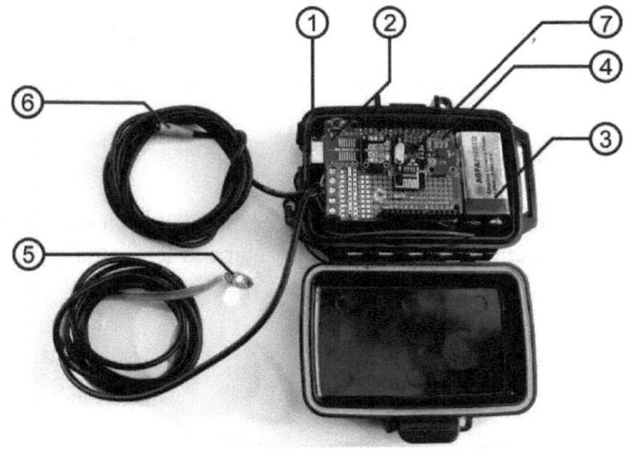

Fig. 2 Picture of the data acquisition and wireless transmission unit: 1-Enclosure; 2-Board Assembly and Microcontroller; 3-Power supply; 4-Accelerometer; 5-Heart rate sensor; 6-Skin temperature sensor; 7-Wireless data communication module.

B. Sensors

a)Skin Temperature Sensor

The DS18B20 digital thermometer provides 9-bit to 12-bit Celsius temperature measurements (-55°C to 125°C at ±0.5°C) and communicates over a 1-Wire interface. This 1-Wire communication interface requires only one data line and one ground connection for communication with a microcontroller. As every sensor is identified by a 64-bit serial code, a large number of sensors can be used on a single data bus, thus giving the 1-Wire communication interface a distinct advantage in the case of measuring temperatures at multiple locations [2].

To initiate a temperature measurement and analog to digital conversion, the master must issue a "Convert T" command and the resulting thermal data is stored in the temperature register.

A block diagram of the DS18B20 sensor is presented in Fig 3:

The scratchpad memory (Fig 3) holds the temperature sensor digital output data. The scratchpad also provides access to the low and high temperature alarm trigger registers (not used for this study). The configuration register can be used toset the resolution of the conversion from temperature to digital to 9, 10, 11 or 12 bits corresponding to increments of 0.5°C, 0.25°C, 0.125°C and 0.0625°C [2].

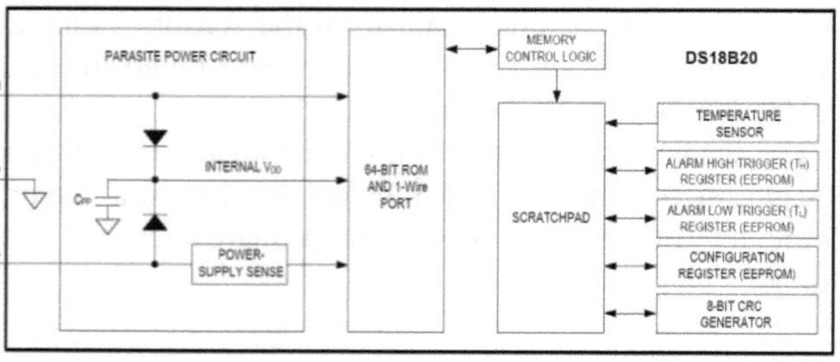

Fig. 3 Block diagram of DS18B20 sensor [2]

	BIT 7	BIT 6	BIT 5	BIT 4	BIT 3	BIT 2	BIT 1	BIT 0
LS BYTE	2^3	2^2	2^1	2^0	2^{-1}	2^{-2}	2^{-3}	2^{-4}
	BIT 15	BIT 14	BIT 13	BIT 12	BIT 11	BIT 10	BIT 9	BIT 8
MS BYTE	S	S	S	S	S	2^6	2^5	2^4

S = SIGN

Fig. 4 Temperature register format [2]

As presented in Fig 4, the temperature register stores the temperature data as a 16-bit number. The sign bits (S) indicate if the temperature is positive or negative: for positive numbers S = 0 and for negative numbers S = 1. If the DS18B20 is configured for 12-bit resolution, all bits in the temperature register will contain valid data. For 11-bit resolution, bit 0 is undefined. For 10-bit resolution, bits 1 and 0 are undefined, and for 9 bit resolution bits 2, 1, and 0 are undefined.

The data transaction sequence for accessing the DS18B20 consists of initialization, ROM Commands and Function Commands. The initialization represents a reset pulse transmitted by the bus master, in our case being the microcontroller. This is followed by a presence pulse transmitted by the slave, in our case being the DS18B20 sensor. The presence pulse signals the microcontroller that the slave device is on the bus and is ready to operate. Then, the master can give a ROM Command to the slave. The master device must issue an appropriate ROM command before issuing a DS18B20 function command. After the bus master has used a ROM command to address the DS18B20, it can issue one of the DS18B20 function commands. These commands allow the master to write and read data from the DS18B20's scratchpad memory, initiate temperature conversions and determine the power supply mode [2].

b) Heart Rate Sensor

The heart rate is the number of heartbeats per unit of time, in our case per minute (BPM). The heart rate can be measured using different technical approaches. The sensor that we have used for this study is based on the Photoplethysmography (PPG) technique. PPG is the optically obtained volumetric measurement of an organ (blood vessel for pulse detection).

At each cardiac cycle the heart pumps blood to the periphery. By the time it reaches the skin, this pressure pulse looses in amplitude, but it is enough to distend the arteries and arterioles present in the subcutaneous tissue [3].

This change in the volume of the blood vessel is then detected by illumination of the skin by means of a light-emitting diode (LED) and measuring reflected light by means of a photodiode. Fig 5 presents the schematic for the pulse sensor used in this study. The subcutaneous tissue is illuminated using the D2 LED (560 nM - green). The reflected light is then detected by the APDS-9008 light photo sensor. The signal is than filtered and amplified by a 1MHz Operational Amplifier (MCP 6001) before being outputted as an analog signal.

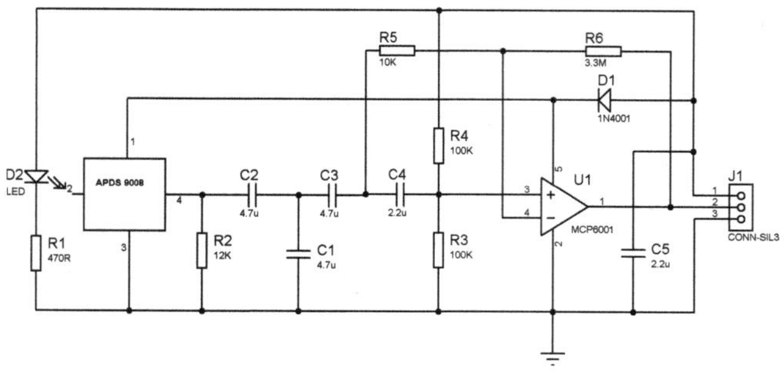

Fig. 5 Heart Rate sensor schematic

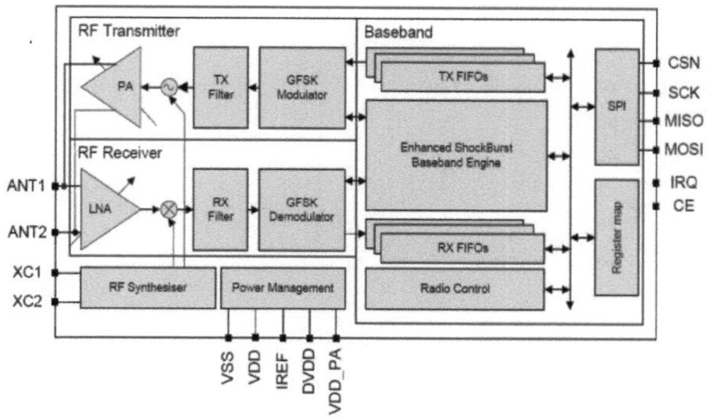

Fig. 7 Block diagram of nRF24L01 module [6]

The analog to digital conversion and pulse detection is handled by the microcontroller. The pulse detection is designed to measure the Inter Beat Interval (IBI) by timing between moments when the signal crosses 50% of the wave amplitude during that fast upward rise (Fig 6). The BPM value is then derived from the average of the previous 10 IBIs [4].

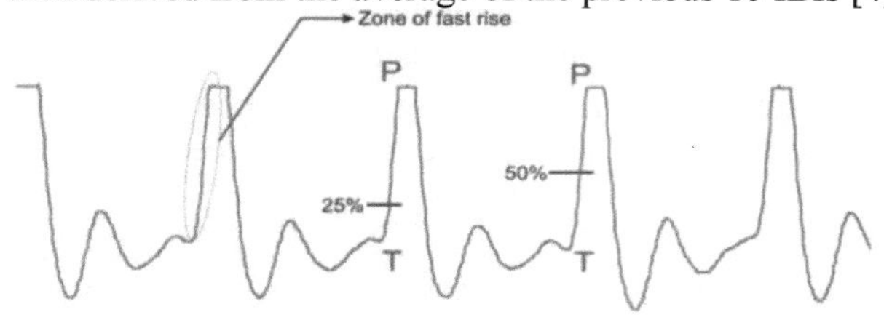

Fig. 6 Pulse signal and BPM detection

c) Accelerometer

The ADXL335 is a 3-axis acceleration measurement device with a measurement range of ±3 g. It contains a polysilicon surface micro machined sensor and signal circuitry to implement an open-loop acceleration measurement architecture. The output signals are analog voltages that are proportional to the acceleration. The accelerometer can measure the static tilt acceleration as well as dynamic acceleration resulting from motion, shock, or vibration [5]. The accelerometer can provide data related to patient body movement or fall detection.

C. Wireless Data Communication

The nRF24L01 is a 2.4GHz transceiver suitable for ultra low power wireless applications. The nRF24L01 is operated through Serial Peripheral Interface (SPI). The SPI interface uses four pins, CSN (SPI Chip Select), SCK (SPI Clock), MISO (Master In Slave Out), and MOSI (Master Out Slave in) for data transmission and reception [6]. The block diagram for the nRF24L01 wireless data transmission module is presented in Fig 7. In this study, the nRF24L01 was employed as both data transmitter (TX mode) and data receiver (RX mode). The nRF24L01 specific module is capable of up to 100m line-of-sight data transmission.

III. Results and Discussion

Using the tools presented in the previous subsection, real-world patient data was acquired and wirelessly transmitted to a PC for real-time monitoring demonstration and data storage. This data consists of: skin temperature measurement; pulse detection together with BPM calculation and three-axis body acceleration.

Fig 8 presents the measured temperature evolution in time, using the DS18B20 temperature sensor. It is of importance to mention that the sensor was placed at skin level and also that Fig 8 presents the temperature evolution from the moment just prior to sensor-skin contact. As can be seen, the moment of sensor-skin contact is approximately at 9s into the data logging process. After this, the temperature evolution is characterized by a logarithmic rise, eventually followed by the stabilization of the measured temperature value. Using this data it is possible to derive the thermal inertia of the sensor, an important term in temperature measurement.

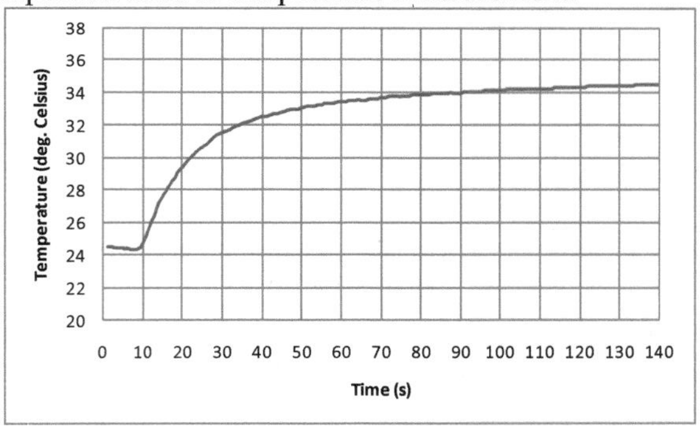

Fig. 8 Measured temperature evolution

Fig 9 presents the pulse signal obtained from the pulse sensor. The signal is acquired as an analog signal (from 0 to 3.3V) by the ATMEGA328p microcontroller, with integer values ranging between 0 and 1023.

In Fig 10, we present the BPM calculated values having as data source the pulse signal previously presented (Fig 9). It was chosen to show the data from 15s onwards, because at this time the calculated BPM value stabilized.

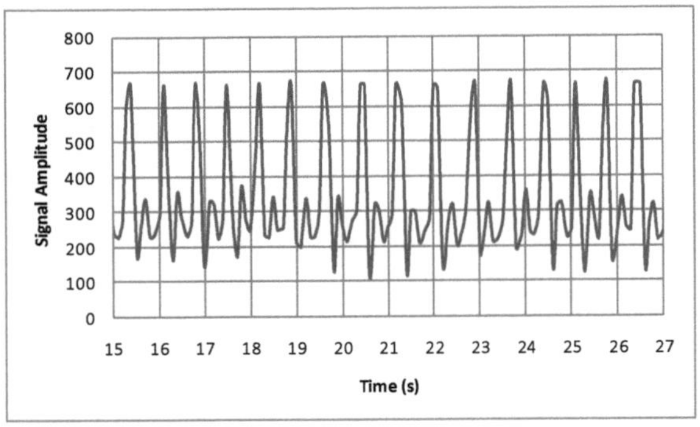

Fig. 9 Pulse signal

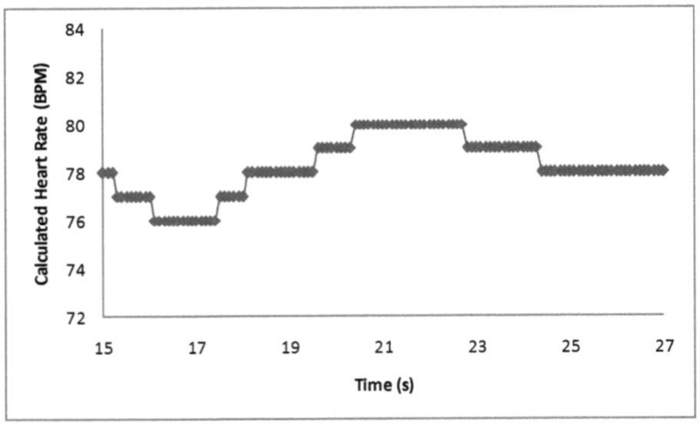

Fig. 10 BPM calculated value

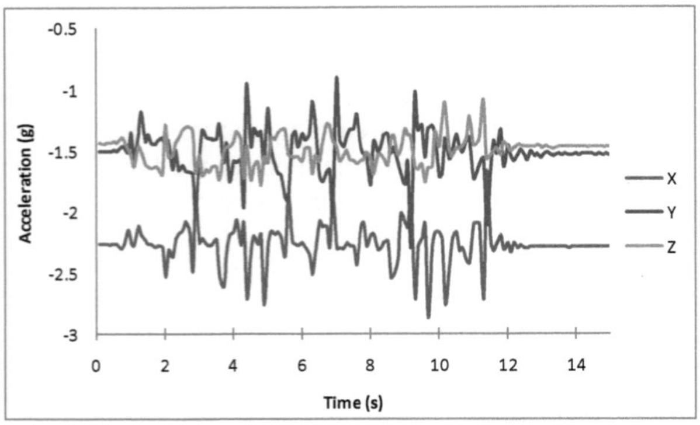

Fig. 11 Patient body acceleration measurements in the case of light physical activity

Fig 11 presents X axis, Y axis and Z axis body acceleration values measured in the case of light physical activity. Although, in this case, the presented values haveonly a demonstrative purpose, fall detection could be calculated from body acceleration measurements.

IV. Conclusions

This paper presents the development and investigation of a system capable of biomedical data acquisition, transmission and real time data visualization and storage using off the shelf products. For reasons of practicality, the hardware unit containing the data acquisition and wireless transmission module has been developed as a miniature portable unit. The biomedical data sensors consist of a skin temperature sensor, a heart rate sensor and an accelerometer. The sensor data are transmitted wirelessly using a 2.4GHz transceiver.

Real-world patient data (skin temperature measurement; pulse detection with BPM calculation and three-axis body acceleration) was acquired and wirelessly transmitted to a PC for remote monitoring and data storage. The results are presented and discussed.

The presented system also represents an evaluation of thenRF24L01wireless transmission solution for medical data applications.

V. Future work

As related future work, we will further investigate and develop this system following the next requirements:

- development of a Graphical User Interface (GUI) that will provide better real time data visualization and storage
- interfacing new biomedical sensors
- a system assessment implying long-term, multiple patient surveillance and professional physician feedback

VI. Acknowledgment

We acknowledge Technical University of Cluj-Napoca for granting us access to the Medical Engineering Laboratory.

Conflict of Interest

The authors declare that they have no conflict of interest.

References

1. Davis C, Bender M, Smith T, Broad J. Feasibility and Acute Care Utilization Outcomes of a Post-Acute Transitional Telemonitoring Program for Underserved Chronic at Telemed J E Health. 2015 Sep; 21(9):705-13.
2. Dallas Semiconductor - Programmable Resolution 1-Wire Digital Thermometer (datasheet) at http://cdn.sparkfun.com/ datasheets/Sensors/Temp/DS18B20.pdf
3. Stephen P. Linder, Suzanne M. Wendelken, et al - Using PPG Morphology to Detect Blood Sequestration -Department of Computer Science, Thayer School of Engineering, Dartmouth College. Hanover, NH, USA. 2006
4. Puls sensor at http://pulsesensor.com/pages/pulse-sensor-amped-arduino-v1dot1
5. Datasheet Accelerometer ADXL335 at http://www.analog.com/ documentation/data-sheets/ADXL335.pdf Rev. B 2009
6. Datasheetn RF24L01 at http://www.nordicsemi.com/eng /Products/2.4GHz-RF/nRF24L01 Revision 2.0 July 2007
7. A. T. van Halteren, R. G. A. Bults, K. E. Wac, D. Kon- stantas, I. A. Widya, N. T. Dokovski, G. T. Koprinkov, V. M. Jones and R. Herzog, "Mobile Patient Monitoring: The Mobihealth System," The Journal on Information Te- chnology in Healthcare, Vol. 2, No. 5, 2004, pp. 365- 373.
8. E. Jovanov, C. Poon, et al., "Guest Editorial Body Sensor Networks: From Theory to Emerging Applications," IEEE Transactions on Information Technology in Bio-medicine, Vol. 13, No. 6, 2009, pp. 859-863.

Part VII
Miscellaneous Topics

Preparation, Characterization and Preliminary Evaluation of Magnetic Nanoparticles based on Biotinylated N-palmitoyl Chitosan

V. Balan, M. Butnaru and L. Verestiuc

Department of Biomedical Sciences, Faculty of Medical Bioengineering, Grigore T. Popa University of Medicine and Pharmacy, Iasi, Romania

Abstract— **Magnetic nanoparticles based on biotinylated N-palmitoyl chitosan and magnetite have been prepared via ionic gelation method. Dynamic light scattering results showed that magnetic nanoparticles average size is dependent on a series of parameters: polymer concentration, weight ratio polymer/cross-linking agent and the stirring speed. In vitro release studies have shown the ability of magnetic nanoparticles to release an antitumoral drug (Doxorubicin) for a period of 6 hours whereas in vitro cytotoxicity tests indicated that the prepared magnetic nanoparticles exhibited anti-proliferative effects on tumoral cells (MCF-7 cell line human breast adenocarcinoma), up to the lowest tested concentration. Fluorescence microscopy revealed that magnetic nanoparticles (BMN6-DOX) were internalized in MCF-7 cells. These properties indicate the potential application as targeted drug delivery system for breast cancer treatment.**

Keywords - **magnetic nanoparticles, drug delivery, biotin, N-palmitoyl chitosan, doxorubicin hydrochloride**

I. Introduction

Magnetic nanoparticles based on natural polymers have a wide range of biomedical applications such as drug delivery systems [1], magnetic resonance imaging [2] or recently, theranostic approaches [3]. Typically, magnetic nanoparticles intented for drug delivery applications refer to a complex nanostructure comprise by a magnetic inorganic material (magnetite, maghemite, etc), a biocompatible surface coating and a specific therapeutic agent [4].

Among natural polymers, chitosan (a linear polysaccharide comprising of glucosamine and *N*-acetyl glucosamine units linked by (1–4) glycosidic bonds) offers the combined benefits of the required properties of biocompatibility, biodegradability and low toxicity with those of functionalization ability due to the presence of -OH and -NH_2 moieties [5]. Moreover, grafting of hydrophobic chains into chitosan structure, could lead to compounds with new physicochemical characteristics that can exploited to improve drug delivery efficiency [6]. With the same aim, a series of active compounds with targeting functions have been developed and used to formulate various drug delivery systems, such as: micelles, nanoparticles, nanocapsules or hydrogels [7-9].

Taking into account that biotin, also known as vitamin B7 or vitamin H is involved in various cellular functions and its receptors are overexpressed on tumoral cells surface, numerous biotinylated compounds has been proposed as suitable vectors for anti-cancer formulations. The interaction between biotin and its avidin type receptors is the strongest known non-covalent biological interaction, very stable and unaffected by a wide range of pH values, temperatures, or other denaturing agents. In addition, recent studies have revealed that biotin-functionalized polymeric nanoparticles encapsulating a chemotherapeutic agent exhibits tumour targeting potential and efficiency drug release into cells subsequent to receptor-mediated endocitosys [9-11].

Doxorubicin (DOX) is an antineoplastic agent of the anthracycline family frequently used in association with other drugs to treat a large number of cancers, and particularly breast cancers[12]. The mechanisms which determine the doxorubicin's cytotoxic effects are: initiation of DNA damage by acting on topoisomerase II, DNA intercalation, interaction with components from membrane, redox cycling leading to the generation of reactive oxygen species (ROS) and subsequent lipid peroxidation and damages at the DNA level.

In this context, this paper presents the synthesis and characterization of magnetic nanoparticles based on biotinylated N-palmitoyl chitosan and magnetite and evaluates the ability of these systems to incorporate antitumoral drugs (Doxorubicin).

II. Materials and Methods

A. Materials

Biotinylated N-palmitoyl chitosan (codified BPCs) has been obtained through the reaction of N-palmitoyl chitosan with biotin, according to our previous report [9]. Doxorubicin hydrochloride (DOX), sodium tripolyphosphate (TPP) and solvents were purchased from Sigma-Aldrich and used as received. Magnetite suspension has been previously prepared in our laboratory [13].

S. Vlad and N.M. Roman (eds.), *International Conference on Advancements of Medicine and Health Care through Technology; 12th - 15th October 2016, Cluj-Napoca, Romania,*
IFMBE Proceedings 59,
DOI: 10.1007/978-3-319-52875-5_69

B.Methods

1. Synthesis of magnetic nanoparticles

Magnetic nanoparticles based on biotinylated N-palmitoyl chitosan and magnetite have been prepared by the method of ionic gelation, described below. Briefly, in a three-necked flask were mixed 100 ml of BPCs solution with various concentrations (5 mg /mL, 3 mg /mL and respectively 1 mg /mL, in 0.1 M acetic acid) and a volume of magnetic suspension (masic ratio polymer/ magnetite was 3/1) at room temperature, under mechanical stirrer for 1 hour. Afterwards, different volumes of TPP were added dropwise (masic ratio polymer/cross-linking agent was 3/1, 5/1 and respectively 6/1) and stirring was continued for other 2 hours. The magnetic nanoparticles prepared (encoded BMNP1-6 as in Table 1) were purified by centrifugation cycles/redispersion in double distilled water and freeze dried.

2. Nanoparticles characterization

Zeta potential and hydrodynamic mean diameter of magnetic nanoparticles were determined by Dynamic Light Scattering (DLS) measurements in water, at 25°C using a Malvern Zetasizer NanoS (Malvern Instruments, UK).

3. Drug released study

In vitro release profile of DOX from the magnetic nanoparticles was studied in phosphate buffered saline (PBS) medium (pH 6.8). A weighed amount of freeze-dried BMNP6-DOX was redispersed in PBS and transferred into a dialysis bag (molecular weight cut-off 12 400 Da) that have been placed in preheated PBS (total volume: 25 mL). The release study was performed in an incubator shaker, at 37 °C, under protection from light, for 24 h. At selected time intervals, the solution outside of the dialysis bag was removed (n = 3) for UV–Vis analysis at 480 nm (UV-1700 Pharma Spec, Shimadzu) and replaced with fresh buffer solution.

4. Cell viability assay and fluorescence microscopy

A MTT cell viability assay was used to determine cytotoxic effects of BMNP6-DOX on MCF-7 cell line. Cells were grown in DMEM medium supplemented with 10% fetal bovine serum and antibiotics. For in vitro study, 5000 cells/well were cultivated in 96-well tissue culture plates (Sigma–Aldrich) at a temperature of 37 °C in a humidified atmosphere containing 5% carbon dioxide, for 48h. The magnetic nanoparticles were suspended in DMEM supplemented with 2% FBS and 1%antibiotics at different concentrations and applied to culture wells in various volumes. A negative test control (growth medium only) was used. At 24h, 48h and respectively 72h the MTT solution was replaced with isopropanol, to solubilize the insoluble formazan crystals formed in the cells. The absorbance of the blue formazan was read at 570 nm (Tecan Sunrise Plate Reader). The results are expressed as a mean ± standard deviation (SD) (n=3). Internalization of BMNP6-DOX in MCF-7 cells was investigated by fluorescence microscopy.

III. Results and Discussions

1. Preparation and characterization of magnetic nanoparticles

In Fig 1 a schematic diagram of magnetic nanoparticles (BMNP) synthesis is depicted. First biotinylated N-palmitoyl chitosan (BPCs) has been obtained through the reaction of N-palmitoyl chitosan (PCs) with biotin, in presence of 1-ethyl-3-(3-dimethyl aminopropyl) carbodiimide hydrochloride (EDAC) and N-hydroxysuccinimide (NHS). Then, magnetic nanoparticles were prepared by ionic gelation mechanism that implies electrostatic interactions between available positive amino groups of BPCs and negative groups of the TPP and hydrogen bonds as well (Fig 1).

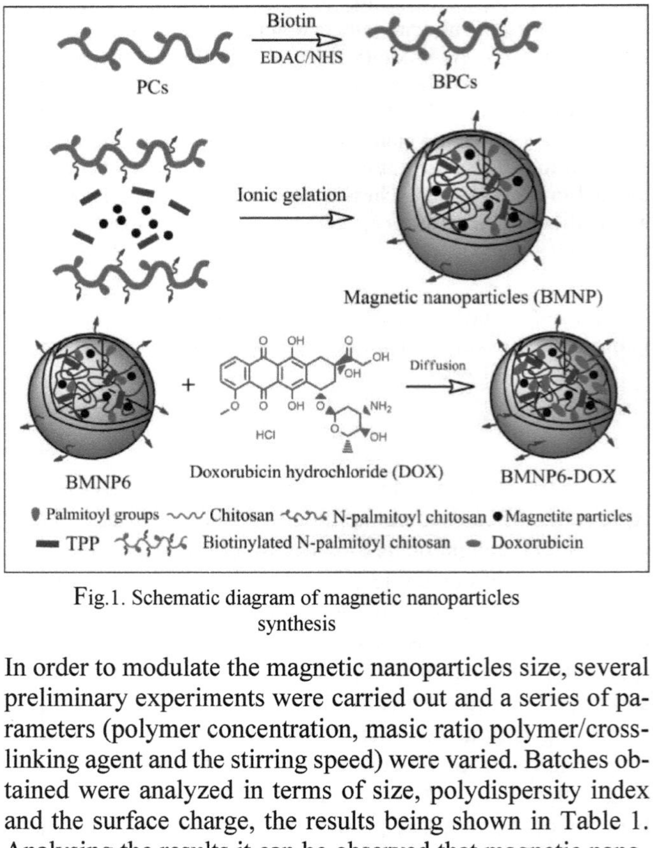

Fig.1. Schematic diagram of magnetic nanoparticles synthesis

In order to modulate the magnetic nanoparticles size, several preliminary experiments were carried out and a series of parameters (polymer concentration, masic ratio polymer/cross-linking agent and the stirring speed) were varied. Batches obtained were analyzed in terms of size, polydispersity index and the surface charge, the results being shown in Table 1. Analysing the results it can be observed that magnetic nanoparticle size became smaller with polymer concentration diminishing and stirring speed increasing. With respect to the ratio polymer/cross-linking agent, the smaller average size was obtained using a ratio of 6/1. All batches exhibited negative surface charges, which confirmed the presence of biotin on the surface of the nanoparticles. The magnetic nanoparticles with smaller size (BMNP6) were further loaded with Doxorubicin and evaluated. In Fig. 2 is depicted the size distribution of BMNP6.

Table 1. Magnetic nanoparticles synthesis parameters and characteristics

Code	PC mg/mL	MR BPCs/ TPP	SS rpm	AS (nm)	PdI	ZP (mV)
1	5	3/1	700	1100	0.54	-11.7
2	3	3/1	700	1030	0.34	-12.3
3	1	3/1	700	877	0.91	-13.2
4	1	5/1	700	566	0.79	-10.9
5	1	6/1	700	382	0.51	-16.8
6	1	6/1	1000	293	0.27	-16.8

PC-Polymer concentration; MR-masic ratio; SS-stirring speed; AS-average size; PdI-polydispersity index; ZP-Zeta Potential

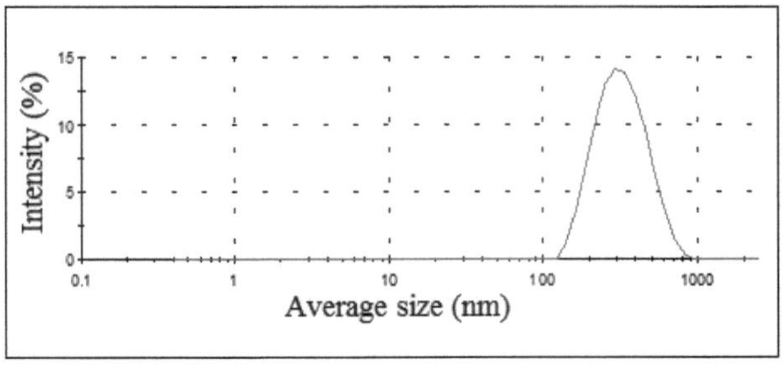

Fig. 2. Size distribution of BMNP6 in water

2. In vitro drug release study

In order to evaluate the potential of BMNP6-DOX to be used as drug delivery systems, in vitro release test was performed in PBS that mimic cancer cells (acidic medium). As shown in Fig. 3, the magnetic nanoparticles exhibited a biphasic drug release pattern: an initial fast released in the first 2 hours, followed by a second phase corresponding to a constant release up to 6 hours.

3. Cell viability assay and fluorescence microscopy

Cytotoxic effects of BMNP6-DOX on MCF-7 cell line were evaluated using a standard MTT cell viability assay. The results presented in Fig. 4 indicated that magnetic nanoparticles exhibited a cytotoxic effect on MCF-7 cells up to the lowest tested concentration. Fluorescence microscopy image (Fig. 5) confirmed that BMN6-DOX were internalized in MCF-7 cells.

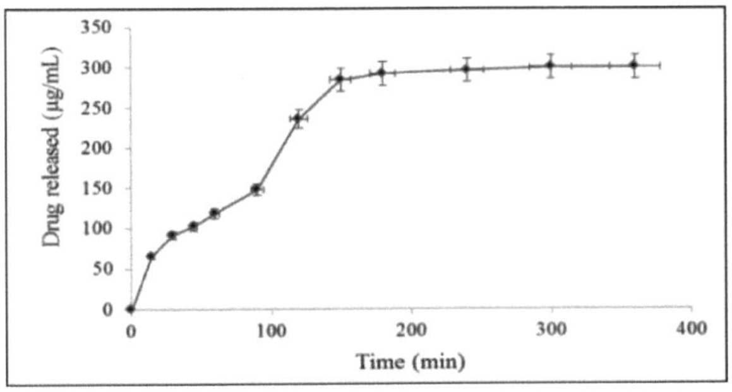

Fig. 3. In vitro release pattern of DOX from BMNP6-DOX

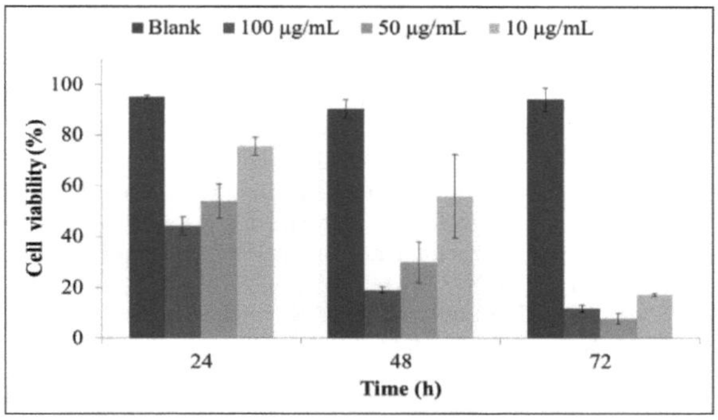

Fig. 4. MTT assay data for BMNP6-DOX

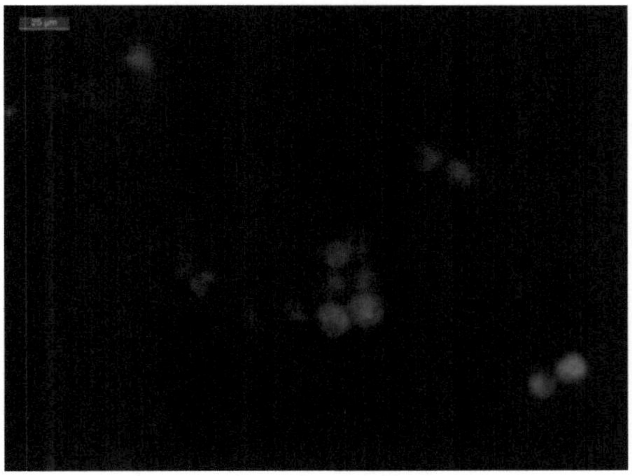

Fig. 5. Fluorescence microscopy image for MCF-7 cell after 72h incubation with BMNP6-DOX

IV. Conclusions

This study proposes a method to obtain magnetic nanoparticles based on biotinylated N-palmitoyl chitosan and magnetite, through ionic gelation mechanism. The obtained systems exhibited submicron size and negative zeta potential. *In vitro* release studies have shown the ability of nanoparticles to release the drug for a period of 6 hours whereas *in vitro* cytotoxicity tests indicated that the magnetic nanoparticles exhibited anti-proliferative effects on tumoral cells. Fluorescence microscopy revealed that magnetic nanoparticles (BMN6-DOX) were internalized in MCF-7 cells. These characteristics encourage future experiments aiming to assess the suitability of proposed magnetic nanoparticles as drug delivery system for therapeutic agents.

Conflict of Interest

The authors declare that they have no conflict of interest.

REFERENCES

1. Namdeo M. Saxena S, Tankhiwale R, Bajpai M, Mohan YM, Bajpai SK. (2008) Magnetic Nanoparticles for Drug Delivery Applications. J Nanosci Nanotechnol 8: 3247-3271.
2. Zhang L., Yu F, Cole AJ, Chertok B, David AE, Wang J,et al. Gum arabic-coated magnetic nanoparticles for potential application in simultaneous magnetic targeting and tumor imaging. AAPS J (2009) 11: 693-699.
3. Shubayev V.I. Pisanic TR, Jin S,. Magnetic nanoparticles for theragnostics (2009). Adv Drug Deliv Rev 61: 467–477.
4. ChomouckaJ., Drbohlavova J.,Huska D., Adam V., Kizek, R., Hubalek J. (2010). Magneticnanoparticles and targeted drug delivering, Pharmacol. Res. 62: 144–149.
5. Dash M., Chiellini F, OttenbriteR.M., ChielliniE.(2011) Chitosan-A versatile semisyntheticpolymer in biomedical applications, Prog. Polym. Sci. 36: 981–1014.
6. Yhee J.Y., Son S., Kim S.H., Park K., Choi K., Kwon I.C. (2014) Self-assembled glycol chitosan nanoparticles for disease-specific theranostics, J. Control. Release 193: 202–213.
7. Yang W., Wang M., Ma L., Li H., Huang L. (2014) Synthesis and characterization of biotin modified cholesteryl pullulan as a novel anticancer drug carrier, Carbohydr. Polym. 99: 720–727.
8. Zhu W., Song Z., Wei P., Meng N., Teng F., Yang F., Liu N., Feng R. (2015) Y-shaped biotin-conjugated poly (ethylene glycol)–poly (epsilon caprolactone) copolymer for the targeted delivery of curcumin, J. Colloid Interface Sci. 443: 1–7.
9. Balan V., Redinciuc V., Tudorachi N., Verestiuc L (2016). Biotinylated N-palmitoyl chitosan for design of drug loaded self-assembled nanocarriers. Eur. Polym. J. 81: 284–294.
10. Heo, D.N., Yang, D.H., Moon, H.J., Lee, J.B., Bae, M.S., Lee, S.C., Lee, W.J., Sun, I.C., Kwon, I.K,. (2012). Gold nanoparticles surface functionalized with paclitaxel drug and biotin receptor as theranostic agents for cancer therapy. Biomaterials, 33(3), 856–866.
11. Bu, L., Gan, L.C., Guo, X.Q., Chen, F.Z., Song, Q., Zhao, Q., Guo, X.J., Hou, S.X., Yao, Q., (2013). Transresveratrol loaded chitosan nanoparticles modified with biotin and avidin to target hepatic carcinoma. Int. J. Pharm., 452(1/2), 355–362
12. Shkilnyy A, Munnier E, Hervé K, Soucé M, Benoit R, Cohen-Jonathan S, et. al. (2010) Synthesis and evaluation of novel biocompatible super-paramagnetic iron oxide nanoparticles as magnetic anticancer drug carrier and fluorescence active label. J. Phys. Chem. C 114: 5850–5858.
13. Hritcu D., Popa MI., Popa N., Badescu V., Balan V. (2009) Preparation and characterization of magnetic chitosan nanospheres. Turk J Chem 33:785–796

Cellular Nanostructures and Their Investigation. History and Perspectives

C. M. Niculiţe[1,2], A. O. Urs[1], E. Fertig[1], C. Florescu[1], M. Gherghiceanu[1], M. Leabu[1,2]

1 "Victor Babeş" National Institute of Pathology, Department of Cellular and Molecular Biology, Bucharest, Romania
2 "Carol Davila" University of Medicine and Pharmacy, Division of Histology, Cellular and Molecular Biology, Bucharest, Romania

Abstract— **Organization of biomolecules inside or outside the cell, at tissue level, proved to respect a micro- and/or nano-morphology and their functions are dependent on the right structuring of these micro- or nano-structures. This short paper summarizes the history of cellular nanostructures' study from their discovery, to current efforts in deciphering their functions, according to the high complexity of live cell organization. We will advocate that the deepening of our knowledge in cell biology has required and will further need a wise combination of efforts made by biologists, chemists, physicists, medical doctors and engineers.**

Keywords— **electron microscopy, STED microscopy, centrifugation, electrophoresis, atomic force microscopy.**

I. Introduction

Cellular nanostructure identification began long before the term was introduced in literature. This happened at the middle of the 20th century through the contribution of George Emil Palade, a Romanian born scientist, who, together with Albert Claude, succeeded in setting up the use of electron microscopy (EM) in cell/organelle study [1-3]. In 1974 the Nobel Prize in Physiology or Medicine was awarded jointly to three scientists (the two mentioned above, together with Christian de Duve), "for their discoveries concerning the structural and functional organization of the cell" [4]. Soon thereafter, the detailed morphological organization of the cell interior was deciphered, membrane bounded organelles were described (micro-structures) and even ribosomes were identified and discovered to be the machine that produce proteins. As a matter of fact, the ribosome was the first identified nano-structure. Nowadays, we may define cellular nanostructures as morphological, complex elements in the living organisms with dimensions in the range of nanometres, in all three spatial directions (e.g. ribosome, proteasome, apoptosome). For more than half a century cell biologists have traditionally described structures, as elements in the organization of a cell seen under a light microscope and ultrastructures as elements that can only be observed by EM. However, the scientific and technological progress at the beginning of the third millennium will change the above mentioned convention. Stefan W. Hell pushed the resolution of light microscopy beyond the limits imposed by Abbe's equation. Again, a Romanian born scientist received, in 2014, the Nobel Prize, this time in Chemistry, but again the distinction was jointly shared with other two personalities (Eric Betzig and William E. Moerner) "for the development of super-resolved fluorescence microscopy" [5]. It is as an arch over time: two Romanian scientists with two significant contributions, by developing approaches for cell study (on fixed and live cells) with a 40 years interval in-between.

In this paper, we will point out some of the cornerstones of progress in cellular nanostructure study obtained through methodological and technological advances due to combined efforts of biologists, chemists, physicists, medical doctors and engineers.

II. History of cellular nanostructure study

We may consider the start for cellular nanostructures investigation to be due to EM use in biology. But EM allows scientists to describe the internal morphology of a cell, with no information about functions. Other methods were necessary to assess the functions of elements in the organization of a cell (e.g. organelles). These methods involved centrifugation to isolate and purify morphological elements of cells and a plethora of biochemical investigations to describe the composition of purified components and to decipher their functions.

A. Electron microscopy

The progress contributed by EM to cell investigation was a morphological one, allowing visualization of the ultrastructure at the nano level. This improvement was due to a specific double fixation procedure, meaning a fixation of the proteins by glutaraldehyde (sometimes mixed with formaldehyde [6]) and a postfixation step using a buffered osmium tetroxide solution [3], targeting unsaturated fatty acids in membrane lipids. Using this double fixation both proteins and membrane lipids are retained in native positions in a spatial relationship very close or identical to that in the living cell. Further on, embedding the tissue sample in a resin, ultrathin sectioning (about 60nm thick sections), and contrasting by lead citrate (for phosphate groups, mainly in membrane phospholipids, sulfhydryl and carboxyl groups in various substrates [7]) and uranyl acetate for phosphate groups in nucleic acids create detailed images of cell morphology under EM. Therefore the conservation of membranes proved to be critical in the investigation of cell mor-

S. Vlad and N.M. Roman (eds.), *International Conference on Advancements of Medicine and Health Care through Technology; 12th - 15th October 2016, Cluj-Napoca, Romania*,
IFMBE Proceedings 59,
DOI: 10.1007/978-3-319-52875-5_70

phology, revealing the trilaminar ultrastructure of the plasma membrane, and membrane bounded organelles. The three laminae of any biomembrane are evidenced as two electron-dense (mainly stained by lead at the polar heads of the membrane phospholipids) defining in-between the third one that is electron-lucent and represents the part of the membrane bilayer containing lipid hydrophobic tails. Simultaneously with the description of the morphological elements, the interest was focused on deciphering their functions. To accomplish this task, it was necessary to isolate and purify the identified ultrastructures.

B. Centrifugation

To isolate and purify the organelles, cells have had to be homogenized and various cellular fractions had to be separated by (ultra)centrifugation. A coarse isolation was done by differential centrifugation obtaining various fractions step-by-step, according to organelle density, but to obtain purified fractions, (ultra)centrifugation in density gradients (discontinuous or continuous) was used [8-12]. The isolated and purified morphological elements (organelles, plasma membrane vesicles, components of the cytoskeleton) were biochemically analysed for (macro)molecular content to deduce and further on to prove specific functions.

C. Biochemistry

Therefore, biochemical analysis of the cellular fractions helped cell biologists in deciphering organelles' functions. The most useful techniques were electrophoresis and chromatography.

Electrophoresis allowed the identification of different charged macromolecules (mainly proteins and nucleic acids) by their various migration speed, led by an electric field, in a viscous medium (usually polyacrylamide or agarose gels). The most used procedure was SDS-PAGE in a discontinuous buffer system [13]. An extension of this technique was represented by the extraction of protein bands from gels and their absorption on various membranes (nitrocellulose or PVDF sheets) followed by specific identification of protein species by immunoblotting [14], a technique later referred to as Western blotting (WB), a term coined by W. Neal Burnette, in 1981 [15]. The method rapidly proved to be a very useful procedure to assess proteins in biological samples, including organelles/nanostructures, and eliciting a great interest for the scientists in cell biology [16].

A more accurate method, in terms of quantitative analysis, was chromatography in a diversity of procedures, exploiting different types of molecular interactions in biological molecule identification and even isolation. Among these, liquid chromatography (with standard or high performance approaches) was highly used, because it allowed separation of (macro)molecules without any chemical degradation. For a better understanding of the liquid chromatography utility in protein investigation, the readers can see [17].

It is noteworthy that all biochemical approaches require equipments that have continuously improved in their performances, by the common efforts of experts in cell biology and engineers.

III. Current approaches

In the past, the progress in our knowledge about the cell was achieved by methods addressing fixed or disintegrated cells. However, the real challenge for scientists has begun to be studying biological mechanisms in live cells. To do this, experts in biology, medicine, chemistry, physics and engineering have to join their efforts in order to find solutions to accomplish this goal. In the next sections, we will consider some of these approaches, which push our knowledge closer to the biological reality.

A. Atomic force microscopy

Atomic Force Microscopy (AFM) is a type of scanning probe microscopy that was developed in the 1980s and has been used to visualize nanoscale cellular structures from living cells. AFM operates by measuring the force between a scanning probe (a sharp tip) and the sample. The tip is located at the end of a cantilever and it scans the surface of the sample, generating a three-dimensional image of the surface. The force imposed on the sample is constantly regulated by a feedback mechanism [18]. Because AFM doesn't require extensive sample preparation – like EM – and it also permits investigation of samples in aqueous solutions, biological structures can be observed in their native environment.

There are three main modes of operation in AFM: (i) contact mode (the tip of the cantilever is in physical contact with the surface of the sample [19]; it is mainly used for rigid samples such as crystals, semiconductors and metals [20], but also for living adherent cells [21]), (ii) tapping mode (the cantilever oscillates at its resonance frequency; as it approaches the surface of the sample, the interaction of forces causes a decrease in the amplitude of the oscillation; an image is produced by measuring the force of the intermittent contacts between the tip of the cantilever and the sample surface; it is used for soft samples, like suspended mammalian cells [22]) and (iii) non-contact mode (the cantilever tip doesn't come in contact with the sample, the image is generated by measuring the distance between the tip and the sample at each data point [23]; it is also used for soft samples).

With the help of AFM, a cellular nanostructure involved in cell secretion was discovered in the late 1990s. Studies on live pancreatic acinar cells showed the presence of circular pits in the apical membrane, which contained smaller depressions involved in cell secretion [24]. The depressions were called porosomes and they have been identified in other secretory cells as well [25-30].

B. STED microscopy

The resolution of conventional light microscopes is limited to approximately 250nm in the focal plane (xy) and 450-700nm along the optical axis (z). In the past two decades however, a handful of so-called super-resolution techniques have emerged to overcome the diffraction barrier, notably: structured illumination microscopy (SIM), stimulated emission depletion (STED), photoactivated localization microscopy (PALM) and stochastic optical reconstruction microscopy (STORM) [31]. Whereas PALM or STORM use sequential activation of fluorophores and subsequent image reconstruction, STED microscopy relies on two synchronized lasers, one for the excitation of fluorophores and a doughnut shaped laser for de-excitation. When superimposing the two lasers, the central region of the doughnut maintains fluorescence, thereby reducing the point spread function (PSF) and increasing resolution beyond the diffraction limit [32].

Since its inception, STED was successfully employed in distinct areas of life-sciences to help resolve the nanostructure and dynamics of molecules, in some cases reaching near-electron microscopy resolution. For example, STED was used to visualize components of the nuclear pore complex at 20nm resolution, revealing the eightfold symmetry of the protein gp210 [33]. STED microscopy was used to study the ultrastructure of endogenous F-actin in living neurons, identifying actin lattices in both dendrites and axons [34]. STED helped understand the fate of synaptic vesicle proteins following their fusion with the plasma membrane [35]. In another study, individual HIV virions could be observed clustering at synapses formed between dendritic and T cells, in culture [36]. With super-resolution systems becoming more accessible and easy to operate, one can expect a surge of studies in the coming years shedding new light on the inner workings of cells, at nanometre resolution.

C. Cryo-electron microscopy

Cryo-electron microscopy in life sciences represents an efficient technique which began to develop in the 1970s and allows the study (at molecular level, under cryogenic conditions) of the architecture of the biological material (e.g. cell suspensions, sedentary cells and tissues) at a resolution of few nanometres [37]. The process of fast vitrification offers the ability to evaluate the configuration of the studied structure in its native state, eliminating the artefacts of fixation. A cryoprotectant medium, such as dextran or sucrose, is needed to inhibit the nucleation of ice crystals. There are two ways of preserving architectural details during sample preparation: (i) plunge freezing in a secondary cryogen for vitrifying small cells in suspension and (ii) high-pressure freezing followed by cryo-sectioning (CEMOVIS), suitable for cell suspensions and for tissue [38]. Before examination under cryo-electron microscope, the sample is transferred in a special holder (cryo-holder) where it is maintained at liquid nitrogen temperature.

Cryo-electron tomography allows the analysis of cellular ultrastructure in three dimensions by acquiring a series of images taken around a tilt axis [39]. The final tomograms used for image processing and reconstruction of the intracellular structures and protein complexes [40]. The direct electron detector device (DDD) cameras with underlying complementary metal-oxide semiconductor (CMOS) technology produce images of extraordinary high-quality that improve the results of digital image processing [41]. High-pressure freezing, combined with CEMOVIS and advanced software processing are the only way to visualize the complex molecular machine inside cells, at atomic scale, with Ångström resolution [42]. Future decades will make possible a molecular atlas of cells at atomic resolution.

IV. Perspectives

In the future, improved communication between scientists in the fields of cell biology and engineers will be needed. The premises are good. Beyond the approaches mentioned under the previous section, other very promising techniques seem to be successfully used in cell physiology and/or pathology studies. For example, investigation of molecular interactions and morphology of cellular nanostructures at a nanometre resolution can be done by small-angle X-Ray solution scattering (SAXS), a technique carrying the advantage that the proteins do not need to be crystallized.

Acknowledgement

Supported by ANCSI under Program NUCLEU, project numbers PN 16.22.02.02 and PN 16.22.03.02.

Conflict of Interest

The authors declare that they have no conflict of interest.

References

1. Palade GE, Claude A (1949) The nature of the Golgi apparatus; parallelism between intercellular myelin figures and Golgi apparatus in somatic cells. J Morphol 85:35-69
2. Palade GE, Claude A (1949) The nature of the Golgi apparatus; identification of the Golgi apparatus with a complex of myelin figures. J Morphol 85:77-111
3. Palade GE (1952) A study of fixation for electron microscopy. J Exp Med 95:285-298

4. "The Nobel Prize in Physiology or Medicine 1974". Nobelprize.org. Nobel Media AB 2014. Web. 30 Apr 2016. http://www.nobelprize.org/nobel_prizes/medicine/laureates/1974/
5. "The Nobel Prize in Chemistry 2014". Nobelprize.org. Nobel Media AB 2014. Web. 30 Apr 2016. http://www.nobelprize.org/nobel_prizes/chemistry/laureates/2014/
6. Karnowsky MJ (1965) A formaldehyde-glutaraldehyde fixative of high osmolality for use in electron microscopy. J Cell Biol 27:137A
7. Karnowsky MJ (1961) Simple method for "staining with lead" at high pH in electron microscopy. J Biophys Biochem Cytol 11:729-732
8. Hogeboom GH, Schneider WC, Palade GE (1948) Cytochemical studies of mammalian tissues; isolation of intact mitochondria from rat liver; some biochemical properties of mitochondria and submicroscopic particulate material. J Biol Chem 172:619-635
9. Blobel G, Potter VR (1966) Nuclei from rat liver: isolation method that combines purity with high yield. Science 154:1662-1665
10. Adelman MR, Blobel G, Sabatini DD (1973) An improved cell fractionation procedure for the preparation of rat liver membrane-bound ribosomes. J Cell Biol 56:191-205
11. Ehrenreich JH, Bergeron JJ, Siekevitz P, Palade GE (1973) Golgi fractions prepared from rat liver homogenates. I. Isolation procedure and morphological characterization. J Cell Biol 59:45-72
12. Bergeron JJ, Rachubinski RA, Sikstrom RA, et al. (1982) Galactose transfer to endogenous acceptors within Golgi fractions of rat liver. J Cell Biol 92:139-146
13. Laemmli UK. (1970) Cleavage of structural proteins during the assembly of the head of bacteriophage T4. Nature. 227: 680–685
14. Towbin H, Staehelin T, Gordon J. (1979) Electrophoretic transfer of proteins from polyacrylamide gels to nitrocellulose sheets: procedure and some applications. Proc Natl Acad Sci U S A 76(9):4350-4354
15. Burnette, W. N. (1981) "Western Blotting": Electrophoretic Transfer of Proteins from Sodium Dodecyl Sulfate-Polyacrylamide Gels to Unmodified Nitrocellulose and Radiographic Detection with Antibody and Radioiodinated Protein A Anal. Biochem. 112:195-203
16. Gershoni JM, Palade GE. (1983) Protein blotting: principles and applications. Anal Biochem 131:1-15
17. Kastner M. (2000) Protein Liquid Chromatography. Elsevier, Amsterdam.
18. Binnig G, Quate CF, Gerber C. (1986) Atomic force microscope. Phys Rev Lett 56(9):930-933
19. Goodman F. O., Garcia N. (1991). Roles of the attractive and repulsive forces in atomic-force microscopy. Phys Rev B Condens Matter 43:4728–4731
20. Pang D, Thierry AR, Dritschilo A. (2015) DNA studies using atomic force microscopy: capabilities for measurement of short DNA fragments. Front Mol Biosci 2:1. doi: 10.3389/fmolb.2015.00001. eCollection 2015.
21. Li M, Liu L, Wang Y. (2015) Nanoscale monitoring of drug actions on cell membrane using atomic force microscopy. Acta Pharmacol Sin 36(7):769-782
22. Li M, Liu L, Xi N, et al. (2013) Atomic force microscopy imaging of live mammalian cells. Sci China Life Sci 56:811–817
23. Jarvis SP. (2015) Resolving intra- and intermolecular structure with non-contact atomic force microscopy. Int J Mol Sci 16(8):19936-19959
24. Schneider SW, Sritharan KC, Geibel JP, et al. (1997) Surface dynamics in living acinar cells imaged by atomic force microscopy: identification of plasma membrane structures involved in exocytosis. Proc Natl Acad Sci U S A 94(1):316-321
25. Cho SJ, Wakade A, Pappas GD, Jena BP. (2002) New structure involved in transient membrane fusion and exocytosis. Ann N Y Acad Sci 971:254–256
26. Cho SJ, Jeftinija K, Glavaski A, et al. (2002) Structure and dynamics of the fusion pores in live GH-secreting cells revealed using atomic force microscopy. Endocrinology 143:1144–1148
27. Cho WJ, Jeremic A, Rognlien KT, et al. (2004) Structure, isolation, composition and reconstitution of the neuronal fusion pore. Cell Biol Int 28:699–708
28. Tojima T, Yamane Y, Takagi H, et al. (2000) Three-dimensional characterization of interior structures of exocytotic apertures of nerve cells using atomic force microscopy. Neuroscience 101:471-481
29. Cho WJ, Ren G, Lee JS, et al. (2009) Nanoscale 3D contour map of protein assembly within the astrocyte porosome complex. Cell Biol Int 33(2):224-229
30. Hou X, Lewis KT, Wu Q, et al. (2014) Proteome of the porosome complex in human airway epithelia: interaction with the cystic fibrosis transmembrane conductance regulator (CFTR). J Proteomics 96:82-91
31. Schermelleh L, Heintzmann R, Leonhardt H (2010) A guide to super-resolution fluorescence microscopy. J Cell Biol 190:165-175
32. Klar TA, Engel E, Hell SW (2001) Breaking Abbe's diffraction resolution limit in fluorescence microscopy with stimulated emission depletion beams of various shapes. Phys Rev E Stat Nonlin Soft Matter Phys 64:066613
33. Göttfert F, Wurm CA, Mueller V, et al. (2013) Coaligned dual-channel STED nanoscopy and molecular diffusion analysis at 20 nm resolution. Biophys J 105:6-8
34. D'Este E, Kamin D, Göttfert F, et al. (2015) STED Nanoscopy Reveals the Ubiquity of Subcortical Cytoskeleton Periodicity in Living Neurons. Cell Rep 10:1246-1251
35. Opazo F, Rizzoli SO. (2010) The fate of synaptic vesicle components upon fusion. Commun Integr Biol 3:427-429
36. Felts RL, Narayan K, Estes JD, et al. (2010) 3D visualization of HIV transfer at the virological synapse between dendritic cells and T cells. Proc Natl Acad Sci USA 107:13336-13341
37. Koning RI, Koster AJ (2013) Cellular nanoimaging by cryo electron tomography, Methods Mol Biol 950:227-251
38. Leis A, Rockel B, Andrees L, Baumeister W (2009) Visualizing cells at the nanoscale. Trends Biochem Sci 34:60-70.
39. Milne JL1 Borgnia MJ, Bartesaghi A, et al. (2013) Cryo-electron microscopy: A primer for the non-microscopist. FEBS J 280: 28–45
40. Harapin J, Eibauer M, Medalia O (2013) Structural analysis of supramolecular assemblies by cryo-electron tomography. Structure 21:1522-1530
41. Cheng Y, Grigorieff N, Penczek PA, Walz T (2015) A primer to single-particle cryo-electron microscopy. Cell 161:438-49
42. Studer D, Humbel BM, Chiquet M (2008) Electron microscopy of high pressure frozen samples: bridging the gap between cellular ultrastructure and atomic resolution. Histochem Cell Biol 130:877-889
43. Kovari LC, Brunzelle JS, Lewis KT, et al. (2014) X-ray solution structure of the native neuronal porosome-synaptic vesicle complex: implication in neurotransmitter release. Micron 56:37-43

Corresponding author:
Author: Dr. Mircea Leabu
Institute: "Victor Babes" National Institute of Pathology
Street: 99-101, Splaiul Independentei, sector 5
City: Bucharest
Country: Romania
Email: mircea.leabu@ivb.ro

Chemical Stability of Vitamin B5

D. Caşcaval[1], M. Poştaru[2], L. Kloetzer[1], A.C. Blaga[1], and A.I. Galaction[2]

[1]Faculty of Chemical Engineering and Environmental Protection/Department of Biochemical Engineering, "Gheorghe Asachi" Technical University of Iasi, Iasi, Romania
2Faculty of Medical Bioengineering/Department of Biomedical Science, "Grigore T. Popa" University of Medicine and Pharmacy of Iasi, Iasi, Romania

Abstract— **The study is dedicated to the kinetics of the chemical degradation of pantothenic acid (vitamin B5). The values of the chemical degradation rate of pantothenic acid have been calculated at different pH-values varying between 2 and 12. Compared to the related pharmaceutical or food products containing this compound, the vitamin stability is considerably reduced in pure aqueous solutions. In the acidic or alkaline pH-domain, within one hour, up to 40% of the initial amount of acid can be degraded, suggesting that the rate of the degradation of pantothenic acid in these systems is considerably higher than those reported in the literature. By using MATLAB software, a complex mathematical kinetic model of degradation was proposed. The model includes the influence of pH-value and offers a good concordance with the experimental results for reaction rate (the average deviation of the calculated values of the inactivation rate from the experimental ones is ±10.21%).**

Keywords— **pantothenic acid, kinetics, chemical degradation, inactivation rate constant**

I. Introduction

Pantothenic acid, also known as vitamin B5, is a water-soluble vitamin involved in the conversion of carbohydrates into glucose needed to produce energy [1]. From the chemical point of view, pantothenic acid is the amide of pantoic acid with β-alanine (Fig. 1).

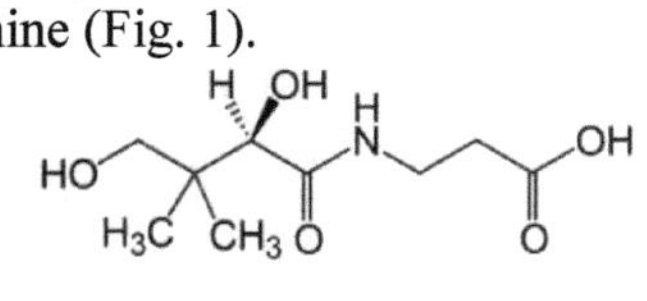

Fig. 1 The chemical structure of pantothenic acid

Vitamin B5 was isolated from yeast in 1933, and few years later from liver, by R.J. Williams [2].

The main role of pantothenic acid in cells is the synthesis of coenzyme A, and the synthesis and metabolism of proteins, carbohydrates and fats. Regarding the human body, this compound is involved in the health of the digestive, nervous, circulatory, and skeletal systems, skin and hair, as well as in the synthesis of hormones (insulin, adrenaline). It also plays an important role in increasing the immunity of human body.

Generally, pantothenic acid is obtained from natural sources (bread yeast, cereals, eggs, peanuts, soybeans, lentil, liver of various animals or birds, etc. From these materials, the compound can be obtained by extraction with aqueous solvents, in weak acidic medium (pH = 4-5) at elevated temperature (80-95°C), with or without prior enzymatic hydrolysis of the natural compounds formed by the acid (usually, the enzymatic complex containing papain is used in this purpose) [3]. Pantothenic acid can be also obtained by chemical synthesis [4]. An efficient alternative is the biosynthesis by microorganisms, due to the reduction of the process steps required and consumption of materials and energy. The biochemical synthesis uses *Brucella abortus*, *Azotobacter vinelandii*, *Escherichia coli*, *Fusarium oxysporum* microorganisms, the main nutrients of the cultivation media being glucose and ammonium inorganic or organic salts [4-8].

The separation of pantothenic acid from natural extracts, chemical synthesis, or biosynthesis media was carried out by crystallization, ion exchange, and chromatography [9-12].

Pantothenic acid is added in various pharmaceutical or food products [13]. A key issue that affects both the operation of separation and purification of this compound, as well as the pharmaceutical and food associated compounds quality is the stability of pantothenic acid. The thermal stability of this acid has been analyzed by a number of researchers, considering the temperature corresponding to the different operations through which the respective products, pharmaceutical or food ones, were processed (sterilization, preservation, cooked, etc.) [14-16]. These studies were carried out in a limited pH range, mainly between 4 and 6. Furthermore, the thermal stability of pantothenic acid was assessed indirectly, being tested either foods containing the acid or pharmaceutical products (e.g., pills containing vitamin complex). Both approaches affect significantly the accuracy of measurements associated with the pure pantothenic acid.

Therefore, the experimental studies are aimed to establish the exact influence of pH on the rate of chemical degradation of pantothenic acid from pure aqueous solutions. In this regard, the influence of pH on the inactivation rate constant was determined, being proposed a more complex kinetic model for this reaction.

S. Vlad and N.M. Roman (eds.), *International Conference on Advancements of Medicine and Health Care through Technology; 12th - 15th October 2016, Cluj-Napoca, Romania,*
IFMBE Proceedings 59,
DOI: 10.1007/978-3-319-52875-5_71

II. Materials and Methods

The experiments on the degradation of pantothenic acid were carried out in the pH range between 2 and 12. The pantothenic acid was dissolved in 100 ml buffer solutions with default pH-value. The initial concentration of pantothenic acid in each solution was 50 mg/l (2.28 x10^{-4} M). The flasks with acid solutions at different pH-values were maintained at 25°C. The unhydrolyzed acid concentration has been determined at different moments of the reaction. In this purpose, from each flask samples of 5 ml solution have been taken, and added in 45 ml of buffer solution of pH = 5, for avoiding the inactivation reaction (the acid stability is maximum at pH = 5-7 [16]). Finally, the concentration of pantothenic acid was determined in the pH = 5 solution. For dosing the pantothenic acid concentration the HPLC with concentration gradient has been used (using Dionex equipment Ultimate 3000, Acclaim Polar Advantage column type II (PA2), with a diameter of 4.6 mm, length of 150 mm, particles diameter of 5 μm). The equipment was provided with UV-VIS detector with diode array DAD-3000. The injection volume was 20 μl. The mobile phase consisted of acetonitrile (A) and phosphate buffer (pH 3.2, phosphoric acid) (B). The gradient was 0-35% A in the first 14 minutes, at a flow rate of 1 ml/min. Analyses were carried out at temperature of 25°C.

III. Results and Discussion

According to the literature data, pantothenic acid stability is maximum in the pH range of 5-7. However, there is no information on the behavior of the acid outside this pH area [16]. At the same time, it was found that the presence of compounds such as nicotinamide and phosphates may exhibit a catalytic effect, by accelerating the acid hydrolysis even in this pH range [16, 17].

Pantothenic acid degradation can be described by a first order reaction [16, 17]. In these circumstances, the reaction rate expression is:

$$v = -\frac{dC_{AP}}{dt} = k_1 \cdot C_{AP} \tag{1}$$

where: C_{AP} - pantothenic acid concentration, mol/l

k_1 - the first order reaction rate constant, min^{-1}.

By solving the integral:

$$-\int_{C_{AP0}}^{C_{AP}} \frac{dC_{AP}}{C_{AP}} = k_1 \cdot \int_0^t dt \tag{2}$$

the equation of a straight line was obtained:

$$ln\frac{C_{AP0}}{C_{AP}} = k_1 \cdot t \tag{3}$$

The constant of the acid degradation rate can be calculated from the straight line slope (C_{PA0} represents the initial pantothenic acid concentration, mol/l).

Initially, the variation of pantothenic acid concentration during the chemical degradation process has been plotted (Fig. 2).

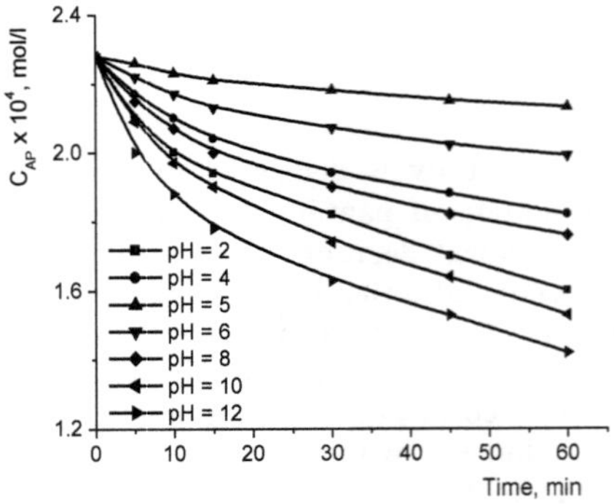

Fig. 2 Variation of pantothenic acid concentration

From Fig. 2 it can be observed that the pH-value of 5 corresponds to the lowest degradation rate of the acid. However, although the acid degradation occurs both in strongly acidic medium (pH < 4) and in strong alkaline medium (pH > 10), figures 2 and 3 suggest that the process is more important in alkaline medium.

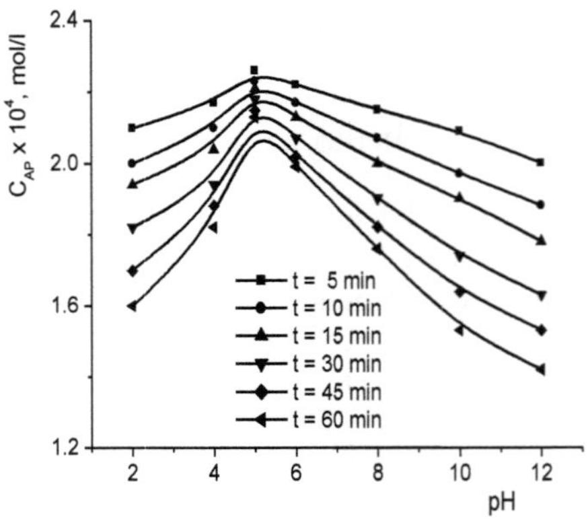

Fig. 3 The influence of pH on the pantothenic acid concentration

As it was mentioned above, the results from literature have been obtained for different food and pharmaceutical products, within a limited range of pH variation [16]. Thus, the degradation of pantothenic acid has been associated with a long period of time, of the order of dozens of days, its stability being improved by the presence of the other compounds in these products and also by neutral pH environmental conditions. However, in the case of pure acid solutions and for pH-values corresponding to its maximum stability, Fig. 2 and 3 indicate that up to 40% of the initial amount of acid could be hydrolyzed within the first 60 minutes. This percent suggests that the degradation of pantothenic acid in these systems is considerably accelerated than has been reported in the studies mentioned in the literature.

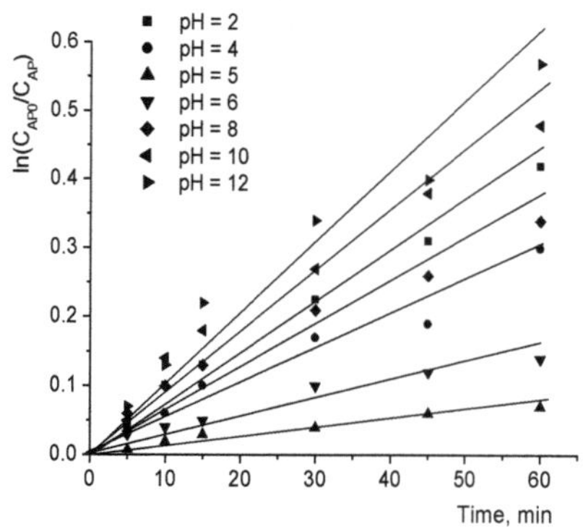

Fig. 4 Graphical representation of equation (3) at different values of pH

By means of Fig. 4, the value of the degradation reaction rate constant of pantothenic acid can be calculated at different pH-values of aqueous solution.

The values of the kinetic constant k_1 are given in Table 1.

Table 1 Chemical degradation rate constant of pantothenic acid

pH	$k_1 x10^3$, min^{-1}
2	7.73
4	5.05
5	1.16
6	2.53
8	5.86
10	8.72
12	9.67

The values of kinetic constant k_1 from Table 1 confirm the above discussed evolution of pantothenic acid stability in function of pH-value, underlining that the increase of pH from 5 to 12 leads to the acceleration of the acid degradation reaction for more than 8 times. By lowering the pH from 5 to 2, this reaction rate increases for about 7 times. The dependence of the kinetic parameter k_1 and pH was plotted in Fig. 5. This dependence suggests the following mathematical correlation between the reaction rate constant and the concentration of H^+ ions:

$$k_1 = \alpha \cdot [H^+]^{\beta} \cdot e^{\delta[H^+]} \quad (4)$$

The values of α, β and δ coefficients were calculated by multiple regression method, using MATLAB software. Thus, the following equation (5) has been obtained:

$$k_1 = 8.78 \cdot 10^{-4} \cdot \frac{e^{3.61 \cdot [H^+]}}{[H^+]^{8.39 \cdot 10^{-2}}}, \ \text{min}^{-1} \quad (5)$$

This equation offers a good concordance with the experimental data, the maximum deviation being 17.72% and the average one ±8.8%.

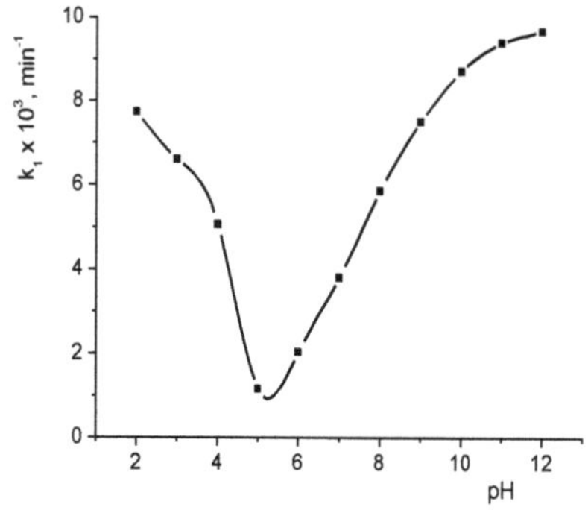

Fig. 5 The influence of pH on the chemical degradation reaction rate of pantothenic acid

In these circumstances, the equation that describes the kinetics of the chemical inactivation of pantothenic acid becomes:

$$v = -\frac{dC_{AP}}{dt} = 8.78 \cdot 10^{-4} \cdot \frac{e^{3.61 \cdot [H^+]}}{[H^+]^{8.39 \cdot 10^{-2}}} \cdot C_{AP},$$

mol/l.min (6)

For establishing the accuracy of the proposed model, the values of hydrolyzed acid concentration calculated with the equation (6) have been compared with the variation on time of the experimental concentration of the degradation products given in Fig. 6. The momentary rate of the reaction is calculated from the slope of the tangent at the point corresponding to the considered reaction time.

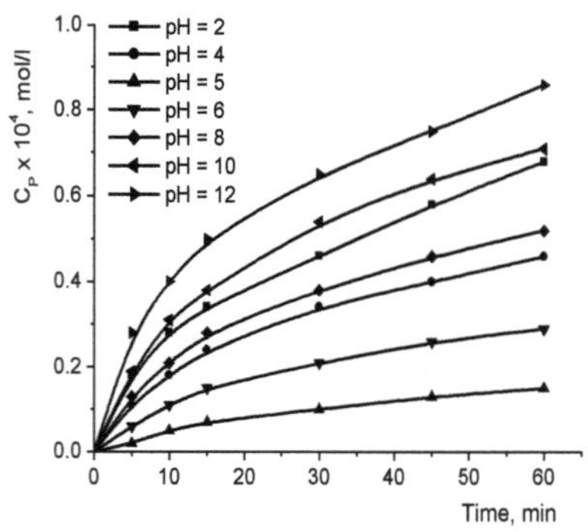

Fig. 6 The variation over time of the concentration of the degradation products

The comparison between the experimental and calculated values of the rate of inactivation of pantothenic acid is presented in Table 2.

Table 2 The experimental, v_{exp}, and the calculated values, v_{calc}, of chemical degradation rate of pantothenic acid

pH	V_{exp} x 10^7, mol/l.min	V_{calc} x 10^7, mol/l.min
2	12.33	13.60
3	9.82	10.12
4	7.66	7.68
5	2.50	1.89
6	4.83	5.36
7	6.01	5.48
8	8.67	9.35
9	10.35	9.46
10	13.82	13.75
11	15.09	16.33
12	16.34	18.56

According to Table 2, the values calculated by the proposed kinetic equation are in concordance with the experimental ones, the standard deviation being ±10.21%.

IV. Conclusions

The experimental studies on degradation of pantothenic acid in pure aqueous solution with pH-value varying between 2 and 12 revealed that the vitamin stability is considerably reduced compared to that of the pharmaceutical or food products containing this compound.

These investigations were the first one which consider a broader pH range and constitutes a completion of the literature reporting the influence of pH on the rate of pantothenic acid degradation.

Based on the original experimental data, a complex kinetic model was developed, which includes the influence of pH on the reaction rate constant. The proposed model provides a good concordance with the experimental results, the standard deviation being ±10.21%.

Acknowledgment

This work was also supported by the Grant of the Romanian National Authority for Scientific Research, CNCS-UEFISCDI, project number PN-II-ID-PCE-2011-3-0088).

Conflict of Interest

The authors declare that they have no conflict of interest.

References

1. Galaction AI, Caşcaval D (2006) Secondary metabolites with pharmaceutical, cosmetic and food applications, Venus Publishing House, Iaşi
2. Richards OW (1936) The stimulation of yeast proliferation by pantothenic acid. J Biol Chem 113:531-536
3. Gonthier A, Fayol V et al. (1998) Determination of pantothenic acid in foods: influence of the extraction method. Food Chem 63:287-294
4. Rawalpally TA (2001) Pantothenic acid. John Wiley & Sons, Inc.
5. Altenbern RA, Ginoza HS (1954) Pantothenic acid synthesis by smooth Brucella abortus. J Bacteriol 68:570–576
6. Kawabata Y, Demain AL (1980) Enzymatic synthesis of pantothenic acid by *Escherichia Coli* cells. Plenum Press, New York
7. Martinez-Toledo MV, Rodelas B et al. (1996) Production of pantothenic acid and thiamine by *Azotobacter vinelandii* in a chemically defined medium and a dialysed soil medium. Biol Fert Soils 22:131-135
8. Drauz K, Groger H, May O (2012) Enzyme catalysis in organic synthesis. Wiley-VCH, Weinheim
9. Kuhn R, Wieland T (1946) Manufacture of the optically active forms of pantothenic acid. Patent US 2407560 A/1946
10. Zhdanovich ES, Kozlova GS, Kibalova NY (1970) Isolation and purification of D-pantothenic acid by an ion-exchange method. Pharm Chem J 4:85-87
11. Hudson TJ, Allen RJ (1984) Determination of pantothenic acid in multivitamin pharmaceutical preparations by reverse-phase high-performance liquid chromatography. J Pharm Sci 73:113-115
12. Moiseenok AG, Gurinovich VA, Lysenkova VA (1987) Separation of pantothenic acid derivatives as precursors for the biosynthesis of the acetylation coenzyme by chromatography on DEAE-cellulose. Chem Nat Compd 23:216-219
13. de Ritter E (1982) Vitamins in pharmaceutical formulations. J Pharm Sci 71:1073-1096
14. Hellendoorn EW, Groot AP, vand der Mijil Dekker LP et al. (1971) Nutritive value of canned meals. J Am Diet Assoc 58:434-438
15. Schroeder HA (1971) Losses of vitamins and trace minerals resulting from processing and preservation of foods. Am J Clin Nutr 25:562-573
16. Hamm DJ, Lund DB (1978) Kinetic parameters for thermal inactivation of pantothenic acid. J Food Sci 43:631-633
17. Frost DV, McIntire FC (1944) The hydrolysis of pantothenate: a first order reaction. Relation to thiamine stability. J Am Chem Soc 66:425-427

Author: A.I. Galaction
Institute: Faculty of Medical Bioengineering/Department of Biomedical Science, "Grigore T. Popa" University of Medicine and Pharmacy of Iasi
Street: Universităţii 16, 700115
City: Iasi
Country: Romania
Email: anca.galaction@bioinginerie.ro

Study upon the Mechanical Properties of Most Used Dental Restoration Materials

D. Cotoros[1], A. Stanciu[1] and M.M. Scutariu[2]

[1] Transilvania University of Brasov, Department of Product Design, Mechatronics and Environment, Brasov, Romania
[2]University of Medicine and Pharmacy "Grigore T.Popa", Faculty of Dental Medicine, Iasi, Romania

Abstract— **Most of the restoration materials should withstand forces during manufacturing or mastication, so the mechanical properties are important in understanding and predicting the material behavior under load. [1] Nowadays there are numerous options in using composite materials for dental restorations, as their exponential development provided multiple choices of combinations with better and better properties. They respond to a large range of requirements making the selection quite difficult for both users (dentists) and beneficiaries (patients). This is the reason why a thorough study of the materials properties might offer wider possibilities for a wise choice according to the situation at hand and also could be the fundament of improving and enhancing the existing properties.**

The present paper aims therefore to performing an accurate study of the mechanical properties for samples of the most used dental materials so that an educated and scientifically based selection of the materials can be made and also new improvements can be proposed.

Keywords— **dental restoration, compression curves, advanced dental materials, composites.**

I. Introduction

It is well known that dental problems do not solve themselves, they need to be approached in due time and very seriously, otherwise the irreversible loss of teeth may occur, also other related disorders.

Caries incidence for example in our country is about 80%, a large number of people avoiding the dentist appointment either for fear of painful interventions or mostly because of financial reasons. A person with dental problems may have pulmonary, renal, cardiac etc. disorders and will never be accepted for an implant, for example. The suitable care for denture may reduce up to 30% the risk of heart attack, stroke but also other cardio-vascular diseases [1].

By neglecting these aspects, especially by the disadvantaged population and even by persons with an average income, the increase of destructive dental diseases incidence is increasing, requiring restorative actions, reconstructions or even prosthetic works with consequences upon social comfort and welfare.

Endodontic treatment is kind of a routine today, more and more teeth being recovered for prosthetic treatment [2]. For these reasons, the correct choice of the dental material becomes an important issue and requires extensive and accurate information, both for the professional users and for the beneficiary represented by the patient.

One of the most important applications in dentistry is the study of the forces applied to teeth and dental restorations. The maximum forces recorded by strain gauges and telemetry devices reach 250 to 3500N. The forces developed in the dental occlusion for an adult subject decrease from the molar area towards the incisors, reaching forces values from 400 to 800N, upon the first and second molar [3].

Obviously the used materials should meet several conditions, the most important one being biocompatibility, meaning that the material is accepted by the surrounding tissues without triggering allergic reactions [3].

But this is not all. The dental material should resist from mechanical point of view to the mastication forces and wear due to abrasion actions, should resist to thermal stress and all kinds of chemical aggressions due to the various types of ingested foods [4].

II. Materials and methods

The oldest type of dental material used for restorations (usually fillings) is the amalgam (a mixture of two or more metals, also containing mercury), which is not very much used lately due to the poor esthetics and suspicions of toxicity.[5,6]

Nowadays, the most used materials are various types of composites (combination between an acrylic resin and some glass-like particles), glass ionomers (combination of acrylic acids and glass powders), resin ionomers, ceramics (porcelain) sometimes on metallic structure, whose resistance is good and they also fit the teeth colour [5,6].

Each type of material has its advantages and disadvantages, several factors are to be considered when selecting one material or another for the restorative work, mostly their mechanical properties, thermal properties, colour, cost, allergic reactions, time of curing, etc.

Obviously the materials manufacturer are making all the necessary testing before releasing the components into production and trading, meaning that all of them are meeting the requirements at some extent but in order to make an educated choice and find solutions for mitigating the shortcomings, a comparison between them is required. For this

S. Vlad and N.M. Roman (eds.), *International Conference on Advancements of Medicine and Health Care through Technology; 12th - 15th October 2016, Cluj-Napoca, Romania*,
IFMBE Proceedings 59,
DOI: 10.1007/978-3-319-52875-5_72

reason the present paper proposes an extended analysis of the mechanical properties for some of the most used restorative dental materials, so that it may offer a tool for their classification from this point of view and providing helpful elements in making a correct choice.

In [7] the authors showed that the most affected area of the tooth is the central area, if the bite is correct and the denture has a normal structure or some eccentric loads may occur if the denture is not normally shaped. In any situation the filling area is subjected to the highest loads and for this reason the filling material should resist to compression in the first place.

The experiments were carried out upon three different samples made of some modern and advanced composite materials used in dental works:

- **Filtek Z 550** is a composite material activated by visible light, designed for the use in anterior and posterior teeth. It is recommended for direct restorations, immobilizations but also indirect restorations [8].
- **Brilliant Flow** is a fluid radio-opaque composite used for repairing dental cavities. It consists of metacrylates, barium silica and hydrophobic amorphous silica [9].
- **Valux Plus** due to its high wear resistance is used in more sustainable works. Bending and traction resistance are the ones providing the growth of durability for this material, but it is not very compression resistant. It consists of BIS-GMA and TEGDMA resins with synthetic minerals involving zirconium or silicon and inorganic elements [10].
- **Biner LC** is a restorative material with fluoride release and radio-opaque characteristics. It is considered to be a basic material specially designed for using with adhesives, composites and conventional restorative materials. For solidification, polymerization light is used [11].
- **NexComp** is a reinforced nano-filler composite used for restoring anterior and posterior teeth [12].
- **Amaris Flow** is a photo-polymerizable fluid composite for special aesthetic restoration works. It has an excellent light dynamics and high color stability [13].

Determination of mechanical characteristics is done following the procedure of testing on special equipment according to the proposed goal. The samples behavior is studied until they break and parameters are recorded, also the manner and aspect of breakage is analyzed.

Compression testing was performed on a LS-100 compression testing machine produced by Lloyd's Instruments, United Kingdom. This has a maximum capacity of 100 kN, accuracy of testing velocity <0.2%, maximum stroke length 840 mm, load resolution <0.01% from the used force cell, extension resolution <0.1 microns, force cell XLC-100K-A1, analysis software is NEXYGEN MT.

The testing precision class is 0.5, the equipment being provided with a digital control device in closed loop and also a computer for data control, acquisition and recording.

The force application point was centric, implying a correct dental occlusion. Malocclusions would require a high number of very expensive samples and will be considered in future researches.

At the critical time, when the first crack occurred, the compression force reached maximum value and started decreasing after the total destruction of the sample.

The experimental data were recorded and the characteristic compression curve was obtained, while the tested sample was fixed in the device.

The crack firstly occurred at the surface as very thin line, then it propagates to the depth of the material leading to spontaneous breakage.

Three samples of each material were used for compression testing, all obtained during the same time of polymerization (3min). The samples could not be manufactured in the exact same size, as they were obtained by courtesy of various dental specialists who were interested in our research. All samples were light-cured.

III. Results and discussions

The compression characteristic curves obtained during the tests are presented in fig. 1 – fig.6.

The Amaris Flow samples have a mean diameter of 6mm, while the area of the sample cross-section reaches an average value of 28,274mm^2.

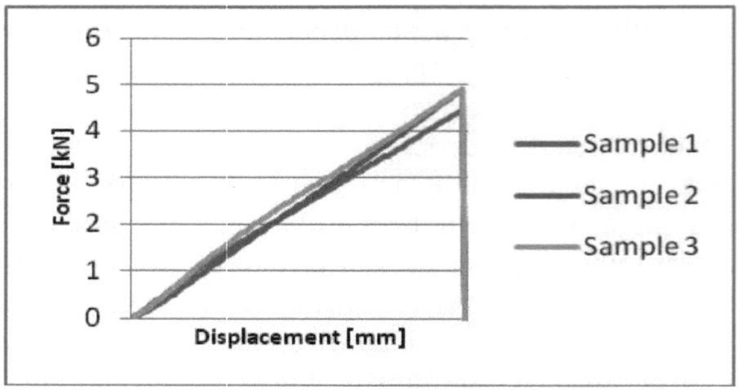

Fig.1 Compression curves for Amaris Flow

As shown in the diagram from fig.1, the first part of the characteristic curve is a straight line, the unit efforts being proportional with deformations. Up to a certain value of the unit effort the material behavior is perfectly elastic. When the unit effort grows higher than the strength at break, the material deformation becomes concentrated in a single point and the sample will crack suddenly in this case.

The Valux Plus samples presented the same diameter and area as the Amaris Flow samples.

But it is obviously a totally different situation for Valux Plus (see fig.2), some of the samples follow the pattern of sudden break, and others go through the plastic phase when the material has the tendency to "flow" before it breaks, showing most likely different concentration of the components.

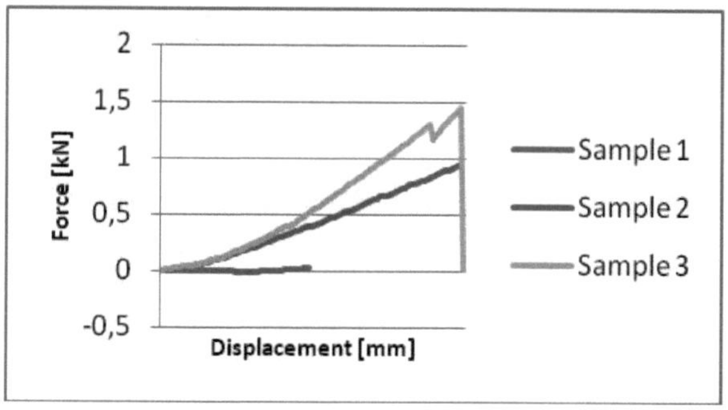

Fig.2 Compression curves for Valux Plus

The Biner LC samples have an average diameter of 9,5mm and the area of the cross-section has a mean of 70,882mm^2.

The samples of Biner LC present an elastic behavior to a certain point, two of them will show a small drop in the force value as the material starts to give in (fig.3).

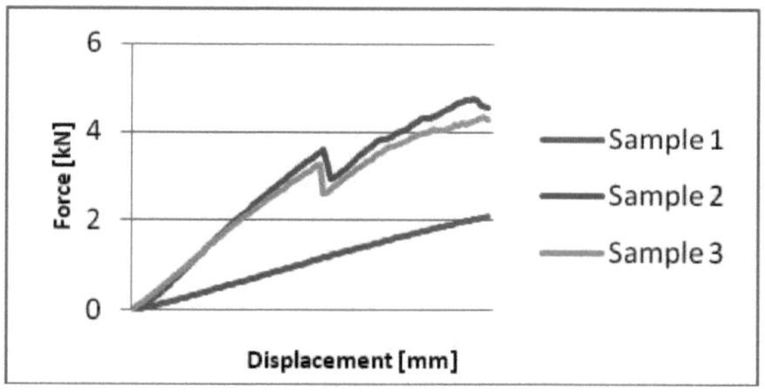

Fig.3 Compression curves for Biner LC

The Brilliant Flow samples have 6mm in diameter and the area 28,274mm^2.

The samples of Brilliant Flow are behaving differently to one another, there is an obvious tendency of sudden break without the plastic flow, which occurs only for sample 3 at a certain extent. The material is more resistant than the others except for Amaris Flow.

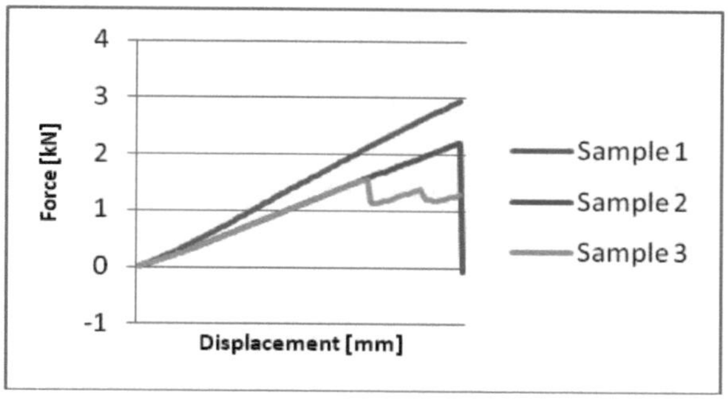

Fig.4 Compression curves for Brilliant Flow

For Filtek Z550 the samples present a mean diameter of 6mm and the area is 28,274mm^2.

Fig. 5 shows the characteristic curves for Filtek Z550 samples. All three behave differently proving the fact that the samples composition is not exactly the same, it is possible to have different concentrations of the components leading to different results. Still the breaking values are high enough by comparison to other materials.

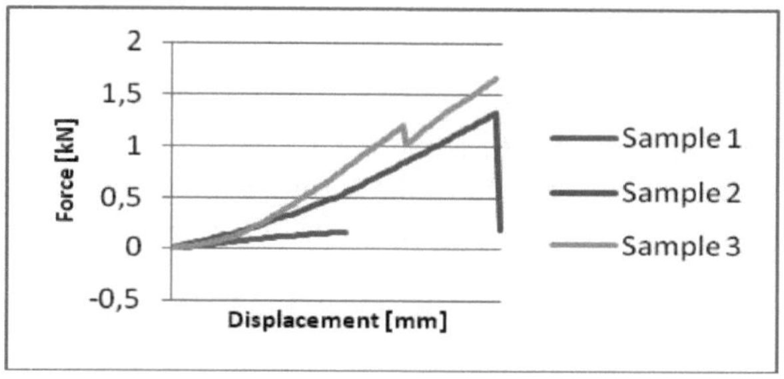

Fig.5 Compression curves for Filtek Z550

The samples of NexComp have the same size as those for Filtek Z550.

In fig. 6 the compression curves for NexComp are displaying a smooth slope in the elastic domain, breaking suddenly at rather average values of the load.

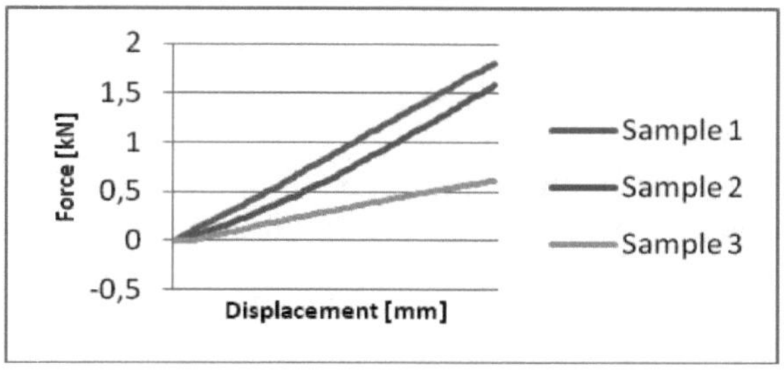

Fig.6 Compression curves for NexComp

The results were summarized in Table 1 in order to facilitate the comparison between the analyzed materials by determining the average load at break.

Table 1 Average load at break for analyzed restorative materials

Materials	Average load at break [kN]
Amaris Flow	4,505
Brilliant Flow	2,606
Valux Plus	0,835
NexComp	1,344
Biner LC	2,093
Filtek Z550	1,067

It becomes obvious that Amaris Flow is the most resistant material to compression as it breaks suddenly for an average load of 4,5kN, while Valux Plus breaks for only 0,835kN (as it was expected, the material being known as wear resistant and not very good at compression). But all the materials are strong enough to resist to the usual forces applied during mastication upon the restorative dental materials, they usually do not increase over 0,8kN.

The experiments allow the determination of many other mechanical characteristics, like Young's modulus, stiffness, stress for different loads, extension for different loads, but in order to achieve a useful and comprehensive comparison to the dental materials requirement, the load at break is the most significant parameter.

Anyway, a direct correlation between the mechanical properties determined in laboratory conditions and the clinical behavior is not very strong yet. Specialists still consider that the laboratory tests take place in ideal conditions; this is why several directions of study of correlating aggressions upon restorative materials are to be considered in order to resist clinical trials.[14]

The visual aspect of the breakage can also provide valuable information concerning the manner of material failure. In order to analyze that, the broken samples were studied by help of a digital microscope (type Keyence) with 20x and 100x magnification. [15]

The images at 20x magnification show the general aspect of the breakage cross-section, followed then by an analysis at 100x magnification in order to highlight the broken structure.

For example, in fig.7 and 8 the breakage cross-section for Amaris Flow (that proved to be the most resistant material for compression load) is shown for both magnifications.

As already shown by the compression characteristic curves the material lacks plasticity, the rupture is abrupt, no visible deformation occurs. But it is the most resistant material for compression, breaking for an average load of approx. 4,5kN.

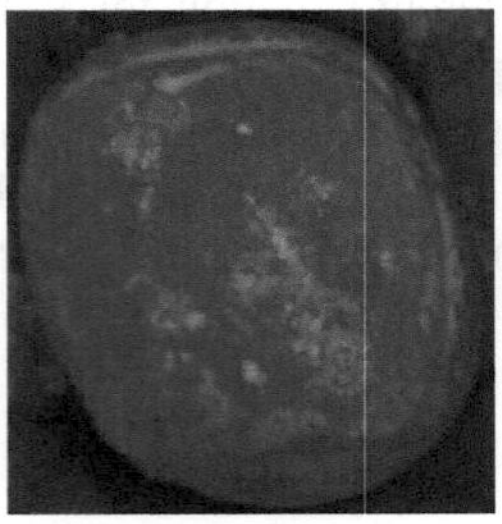

Fig.7 Amaris Flow, cross-section 20x

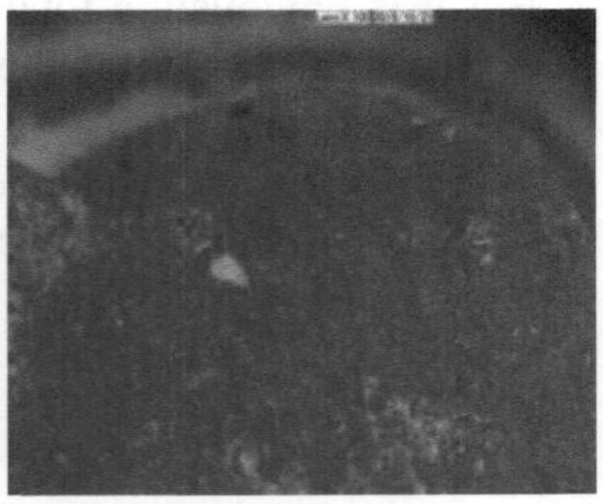

Fig.8 Amaris Flow, detail 100x

Brilliant Flow is the second best material for compression but the average load for breaking drops dramatically at almost half of the value for Amaris Flow, reaching only approx. 2,6kN.(fig.9,10)

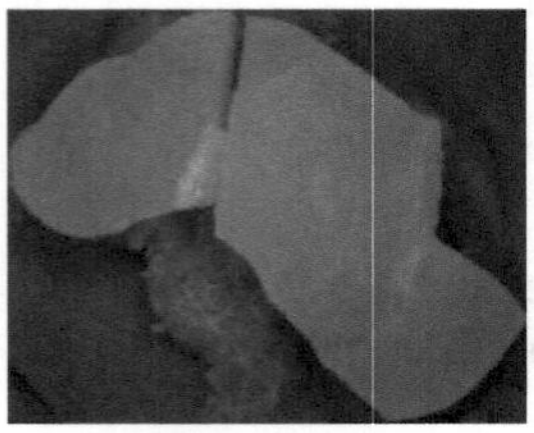

Fig.9 Brilliant Flow, cross-section 20x

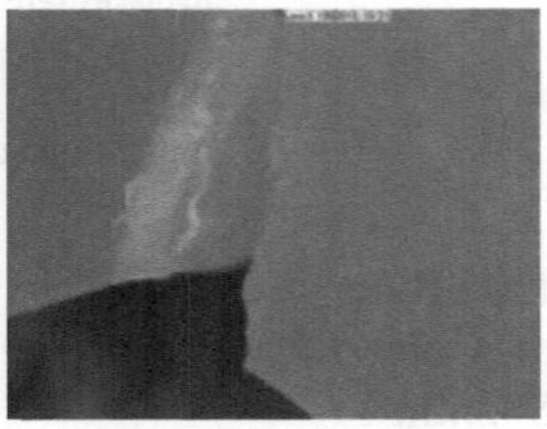

Fig.10 Brilliant Flow, detail 100x

As the characteristic compression curves showed before, there are slightly any plastic deformation (not for all samples), the breakage aspect is clean and cut.

Almost a similar behavior is displayed by Biner LC with an average load at break of 2,09kN. (fig. 11, 12)

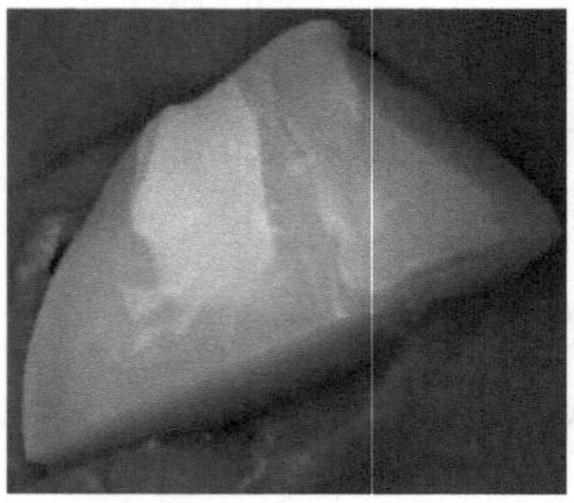

Fig.11 Biner LC cross-section 20x

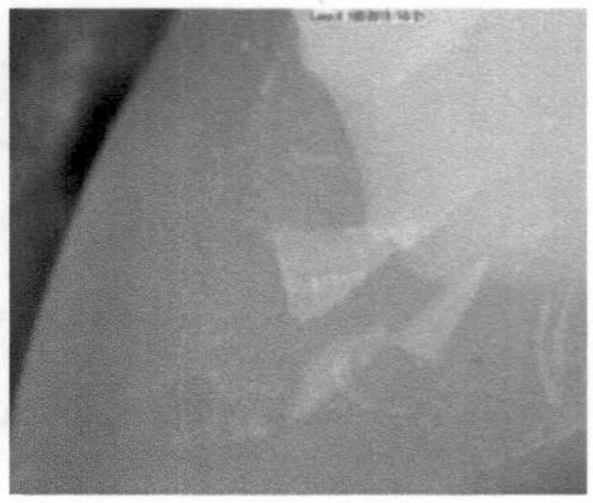

Fig.12 Biner LC, detail 100x

The cross-section is not as smooth as the ones for Amaris Flow and Brilliant Flow, as there are some signs of plastic deformation, which can also be seen in two of the characteristic curves.

The next resistant material proved to be NexComp, the average load at break records another representative drop by comparison to the previous two materials, reaching only 1,34kN.(fig.13, 14)

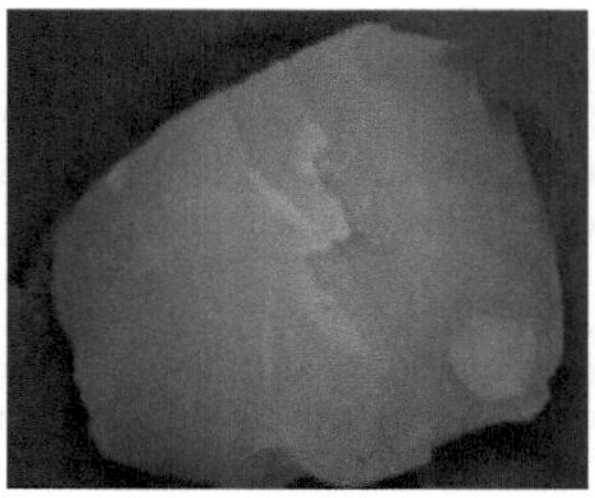

Fig.13 NexComp, cross-section 20x

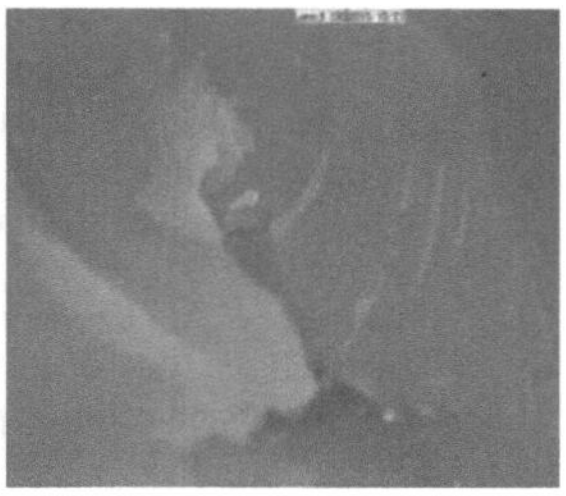

Fig.14 NexComp, detail 100x

The visual analysis shows some sliding lines on the breaking surface proving the plastic deformations already obtained in the characteristic curves.

Filtek Z550 provides an average break load of 1,06kN, the samples behave very different from one another, some show plastic deformations, some do not, and the difference between samples as far as the breaking load is concerned, is very high. The benefit of this material resides in its exceptional wear resistance and ease of processing during restorations (fig.15, 16).

Microscopic analysis shows some sliding lines and also an increased density of material on one side, the breakage is not uniform, the material shows plasticity for some of the samples.

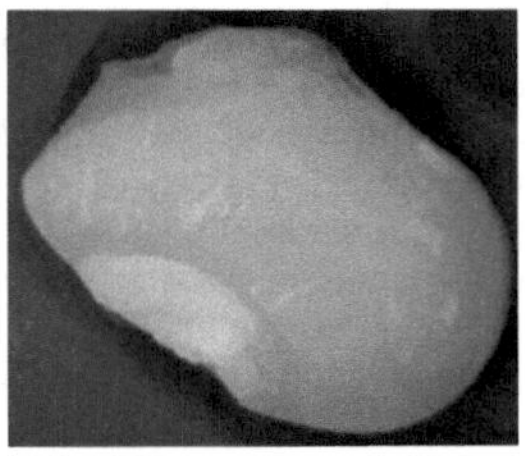

Fig.15 Filtek Z550, section 20x

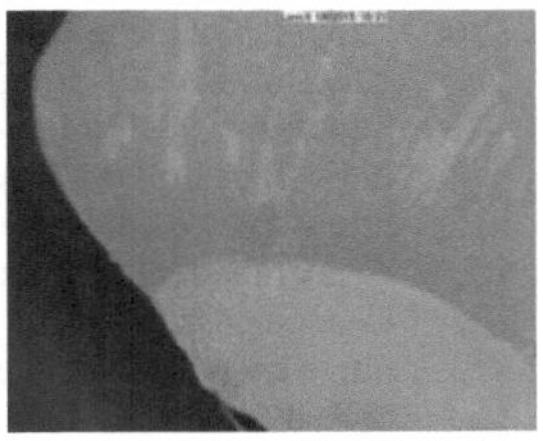

Fig.16 Filtek Z550, detail 100x

Valux Plus proves to be less resistant to compression, but the manufacturers are recommending it for the high wear resistance (fig.17, 18).

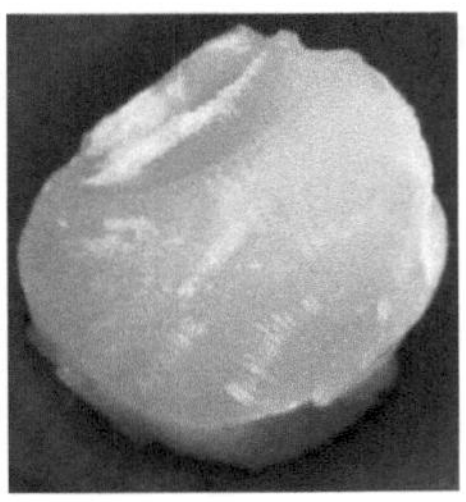

Fig.17 Valux Plus, cross-section 20x

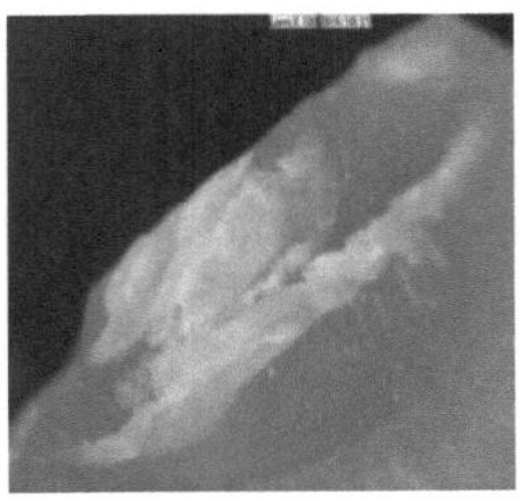

Fig.18 Valux Plus, detail 100x

The average break load for compression determined for Valux Plus is about 0,835kN. Again the samples have behaved very different from one another. Some developed only elastic behavior and some showed slight plastic deformations. The cross section is partially smooth, showing some fine sliding lines and an area of concentrated density.

All tested materials are strong enough to resist to the highest mastication forces that do not overcome 0,8kN.

V. Conclusions

Dealing with the mechanical characteristics of composite materials, especially the polymeric ones may be in a certain way similar to dealing with metals, but it is necessary to keep in mind the fact that they are quasi-anisotropic. Besides, there may be some variations between the properties of different samples of the same material, according to the components concentration and mixture, as the experiments have already proven.

Also, it is a well-known fact that for dental materials whose resistance to compression is much higher than the resistance to tension, meaning they are fragile materials, the differences between the real characteristic compression curves and the conventional ones are insignificant.

The experiments have the purpose of comparing the mechanical properties of various dental composite materials but also for controlling the conformity of different samples of the same materials. This information are usually not provided by the manufacturers and by the dealers but are very important for users, as an educated decision regarding a fair ratio quality-cost is to be considered when selecting a certain material.

Of course, other properties are also to be considered in the long run, like resistance to abrasion; esthetics – color, translucence, opacity; resistance to chemical substances from different nutritional elements; resistance to temperature variations (hot food followed by cold beverages or vice versa), biocompatibility, etc. But the first thing usually considered is: will the restoration be able to resist mastication like a healthy tooth for a reasonable price?

According to the experiments, the diagram in fig.19 offers an expressive classification of the studied materials according to their cost per refill syringe. This would offer the possibility of comparing mechanical properties and evaluate the quality cost ratio.

As far as compression strength, Amaris Flow is much above the other studied materials but is also the most expensive. The lowest values were determined for Valux Plus, while the other materials seem to present slightly decreasing values between those two but costs are not always following the same variation pattern.

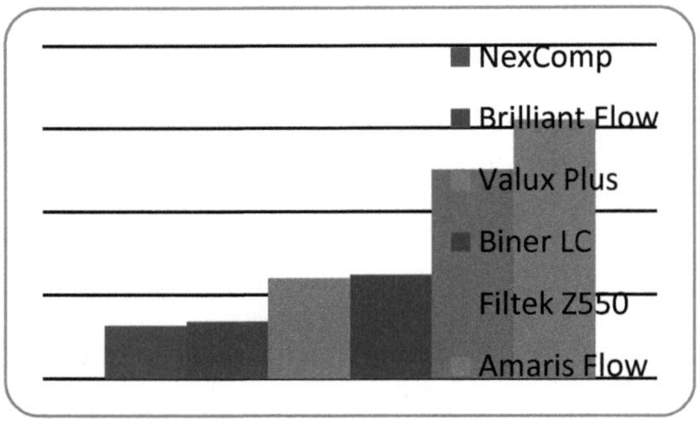

Fig.19 Classification of studied materials according to cost per refill syringe

As a conclusion, modern nutrition is characterized by the presence of very aggressive substances that subject the people's dentition to various aggressions leading at one moment or another to teeth decay. Therefore it is necessary to be able to rely on strong, esthetic and affordable materials in order to restore the damaged teeth.

Due to the explosive development in the field of composite materials several types of dental materials are available, with different properties and also shortcomings making the appropriate selection very difficult.

Both dental professionals and patients need to be informed about the properties offered by this large range of offers in order to be able to make educated choices according to their set priorities.

Acknowledgment

The experiments were performed within the Advanced Mechatronic Systems Research Centre of Transilvania University.

Conflict of Interest

The authors declare that they have no conflict of interest.

References

1. Ionaş M., Sabău M., Ionaş T., Delean A., Toader S., Influence of the Light Curing Source on the Biological Properties of a Self Etching Adhesive, Romanian Biotehnological Letters, 2011: 16 (1): 5063-5970
2. Fokkinga W.A., Kreulen C.M.,Vallittu P.K., Creugers N.H., A structured analysis of in vitro failure loads and failure modes of fiber, metal and ceramic post and core systems.Int.J.Prosthodont., 2004;17:476-482
3. Cotoros D., Baritz M., Combined-correlated methods applied to the analysis of dental prostheses materials quality, Ch.10 in New technologies, trends, innovations and research, InTech Publications, 2012, 209-239
4. Cenci, M.S., Pereira-Cenci, T., Donassollo, T.A., Sommer, L., Strapasson, A., Demarco, F.F., 2008. Influence of thermal stress on marginal integrity of restorative materials. Journal of Applied Oral Sciences 16, 106–110
5. O'Brien W.J., Dental Materials and their Selection, Quintessence Publishing Co, Inc, 2002, 1-12
6. Dental fillings, available at https://www.njda.org/fileLibrary/file_65.pdf [acc. 30 Jan.2016]
7. Cotoros, D., Stanciu, A., Baritz, M., Some Mechanical Characteristics of Materials for Dental Prosthetics, Proceedings 26th European Conference on Modelling and Simulation ECMS, Koblenz, 2012, 212-215
8. http://solutions.3m.com/wps/portal/3M/roRO/3MESPE-CEE/DentalManufacturers/Products/ DentalRestorativeMaterials/DentalComposites/Dental Composite/ [acc. Dec. 2015]
9. http://dentstore.com/composite/126561-brilliant-flow-refill-23g-coltene.html [accessed December 2015]
10. http://cabinet.tehnicaldent.ro/compozite-fotopolimerizabile/1362-valux-plus-refill-seringa.html[acc. Dec2015]
11. http://www.meta-biomed.com/eng/cnt/prod/prod020101.html?uid=37& cateID=2 [accessed December 2015]
12. http://www.medidentexim.ro/cabinet/restaurare-directa-si-cosmetica-dentara/materiale-compozite/nexcomp-kit [accessed December 2015]
13. http://www.voco.com/en/product/amaris_flow/ index.html [accessed December 2015]
14. Ferracane J.L., Resin-based composite performance: Are there some things we can't predict?,Dent Mat. 2013 Jan; 29(1):51–58.
15. Cotoros D., Stanciu A., Baritz M., Cristea L., Microscopic Analysis of Breakage in Materials for Hard Implants, Proceedings of WCE, London, 2011, p.1965-1968

Author: Cotoros Diana
Institute: Transilvania University of Brasov
Street: 29 Eroilor
City: Brasov
Country: Romania
Email: dcotoros@unitbv.ro

Principles to Build a Stochastic Model for a Minimal Biological Cell with Built-in Feedback Reaction Capabilities

D. Stoicovici, A. Cotetiu, M. Banica, M. Ungureanu and I. Craciun

Technical University of Cluj Napoca, North University Center of Baia Mare, Department of Engineering and Technology Management, Baia Mare, Romania

Abstract: **There are two basic approaches used to develop the so called *genetic algorithms*: the deterministic approach, and the second one is the stochastic approach, with algorithms that add randomness to the model. The stochastic model is based on multiple reactions of molecules that can occur in spatially homogenous system, a situation that is characteristic to the natural biological cells. The randomness is a must to have a simulation model behavior that corresponds to the real phenomena. To each simulation model, another problem is to add the feedback reactions that brings the cell model closer to a real one. A cell model built on those principles is describe. The original contribution of this paper is to establish the basic principles that proved to work with that specific cell model.**

Keywords: **Bioinformatics, system biology, stochastic simulations.**

I. Introduction

A. System Biology approach

The cell can be considered as a system. In order to a full understanding of all aspects in the cell life, we cannot consider only the components inside the cell. Instead, we must discover all the interactions between the components, the hole dynamic of what, when and why all that interactions exist. Only after we know all that, we can be sure that we can control them.

A system approach to a cell model requires actions in four possible fields of research [1]:

- **the system structure:** a diagram with all the genes and proteins interactions, their biochemical ways to interact, and the mechanisms of the cell inside structure control;
- **the system dynamics:** the cell reactions over time at the environmental stress. The study can be drive by complex methods, on different areas, such as metabolic analysis, sensitivity analysis and dynamic analysis.
- **the control methods:** building procedures that control the state of the cell in order to minimize the malfunctions. These research can provide new kind of treatments of diseases.
- **the design methods:** building of synthetic biological systems with specific properties, after establishing by simulations the main design principles.

Significant progresses in all these fields were done when computational-based cell models were realized. Even is not possible for the moment to introduce in a model all the components that are present in a real cell, this kind of analysis may provide to the end very useful hypothesis about what can be the real mechanisms that allow a cell to survive and reproduce in a particular environment.

For all computational cell models, we must establish from the very beginning the goal and the level of complexity of our model.

For the goal, we need to decide whether: i) we want to understand the behavior for a very specific process, or ii) we want to find how our model responds to a very wide complex of factors.

To model even a simple cell, new software tools must be developed. Compared with other kind of models, a model of a biological cell combines *the stochastic way of events* with a space with *huge number of reactions* that some of them are feedback processes. All these choices must consider also the availability of biological knowledge possible to be used to build the model.

From the biological point of view, after obtaining the complete genome sequences of some simple organisms, the idea to build a minimal cell model consider also the minimal gene set that can answer at two obvious problems: what was the genome for the very first forms of life, and consequently, what would be a minimum genome necessary to support and reproduce life?

Until now, for example, Mycoplasma genitalium, with 468 identified protein-coding genes is considered as the minimal genome that exists. This organism was compared with that of Haemophilus influenzae (1703 identified protein-coding genes) ([2], [3]). Other micro-organisms were also considered in order to build o minimal cell, such as Ureaplasma urealyticum [4]. The work method was the idea that the genes with same functions and conserved in two different organisms that were compared, must be essential for life. Finally, 256 genes were considered as being essential for life.

S. Vlad and N.M. Roman (eds.), *International Conference on Advancements of Medicine and Health Care through Technology; 12th - 15th October 2016, Cluj-Napoca, Romania,*
IFMBE Proceedings 59,
DOI: 10.1007/978-3-319-52875-5_73

In this case, for so few genes, it is not surprisingly that not all the functions in a normal cell are also present in a minimal cell. For example, there is no amino acid biosynthesis or also "de novo" nucleotide biosynthesis. Also, the lipid biosynthesis is very limited and very few enzymes to be synthesized.

Knowing that from a real living cell, one of the principles used to build the model was that not all the compounds and features present in a complex form of live must be present also in the computer model.

Another central feature of the model is to remain stable, which means to have a tendency to be all the time around the steady-state parameters values, despite the action of perturbations. Another term used for the stability feature of organisms is *robustness* (a definition of robustness is: *the preservation of particular characteristics, despite uncertainty in components and environment* [5]). The most important feature in order to have that is, in the real cell as it is in a model, to have a built-in feedback reaction attributes (positive or negative). A feed-back reaction can bring to a system adaptation to environment, insensitivity to parameter changes, and slow degradation of a function in the case of damages.

B. Examples of computational software tools

Some of the first kind of models created until now follows bellow.

E-CELL is an ambitious project to build a complete computational model for an entire bacteria genome, based on Mycoplasma genitalium organism. The model is realized by the Laboratory for Bioinformatics from Keio University, Japan. The model tries to put together all the features of a real cell. The model has 127 genes and several different kinds of reactions. Many parameters are estimated [16]

Virtual Cell is being developed by the National Resource for Cell Analysis and Modeling (NRCAM) at University of Connecticut Health Center. It has a graphical interface presentation on its own web page. The model can analyze chemical reactions among different substances in the cell and other such spatial locations. It does not appear to be desired to handle complex transcription-translation-transport events in the cell [17]

Bio-Spice is an initiative at Berkeley National Laboratory [18].

These computational tools are all still under development. Thus far them consists of a framework to enable users to add modules that interact with simulation modules from other users. They are all limited in their ability to model complex regulatory interactions between different kinds of molecules inside a cell. Another main limitation is that some software does not account for stochastic reactions, while others does not account for spatial movement of concentrations of molecules. The user-interfaces for all of them are still cumbersome, as is the method for specifying which reaction to include

Another kind of models are made for some very specific interactions. Their only purpose is to propose a possible pathway to occur for these particular interactions.

An example on this regards is a model capable to register the changes in cell composition, cell sizes, cell shape, and the timing of chromosome synthesis in response to changes in external glucose limitation ([6], [7]). So, this model was specifically built for one pathway.

Another example is a model made for a very specific and singular event in a cell: the interaction between cdc2 and cyclin [8]. Even for a whole cell, the model is still based on adding more specific reactions for some of the possible activities in the cell.

II. Methods

A. Steps to create a computational model

The present theoretical biological cell was built considering all these design principles. Other important design principles are also considered, as follows:

- Reducing the inside cellular components to a manageable number of components. Only for gene actions, where the most prominent feature is the binding of transcription factors to the regulatory elements of that gene, the number of states of the complexes grows exponentially with the number of components and their binding sites (a single gene where 10 transcription factor can bind, has $2^{10} = 1024$ different possible states, resulting in the same number of transcriptional rates; also, because each state can have 10 different transcription rates, there are 10,240 potentially reactions to specify).
- Writing the reactions that summarize the stoichiometric relationships within the cell.
- Developing kinetic relationships that reflect the general dependencies of major metabolic pathways or steps.
- Including metabolic control systems using only the concentrations of chemical components as signals.
- Evaluating as many kinetic and stoichiometric parameters as possible.
- The best model should be modular and to permit a continuous increase in complexity by adding new components and must easily admit new functions too [9].

The computational model described below makes the second choice, and has the goal to be available for simulations in all kind of processes inside the cell.

There are two basic scientific methods for analyzing the biological system behavior and that are used to build the models in System Biology:

The first method is *the steady-state analysis*. Knowing the components of a biochemical system of molecules and the reactions rates among them at the steady state, this kind of analysis can reveal how the model reacts when we modify some of the external and internal parameters, in order to simulate the environmental stress.

The second method is *the bifurcation analysis*. This kind of analysis follows the changes in time in the system in a "multidimensional space", where each of these space axes represent a parameter involving evolution in time, shown in correlations with all the others. By this method we can follow the system behavior in its dynamic evolution.

The computational model described below uses the steady-state analysis.

We must introduce all this attributes in the model for having a reliable one, to create a computer model with robustness attribute. We must add to our model features like negative or positive feedback control, modularity and mechanisms to provide structural stability, which is a central feature of a model, that is to have a tendency to be all the time around the steady state parameters values, despite the action of perturbations.

Among them, the negative feedback control is one of the most important, that must provide a stable response to an exterior stress, independent of further internal parameters variations and external disturbances. The most important robustness attributes are: adaptation to environment, parameter insensitivity, slow degradation of a function in the case of damages.

There are mainly two methods to design a cell model:

i. the deterministic method

ii. the stochastic method.

i) The *deterministic approach* builds its model on the basis of a so called *collision volume*: the space around one molecule where we can find the center of a *sphere* of another molecule at the time T (Fig. 1),

where:

- R_1 is the radius of the first molecule;
- R_2 is the radius of the second molecule;
- V_{1-2} is the speed of the first molecule relative to the second molecule;
- $R_1 + R_2$ is the collision volume.

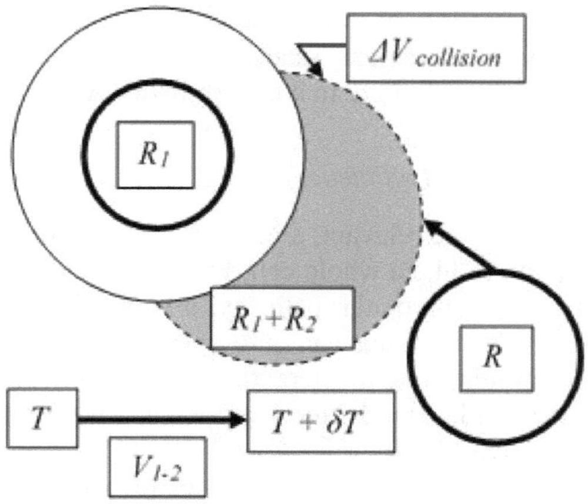

Fig. 1 The collision between two molecules (after [5])

If inside this collision volume there is the center of a second molecule at the initial moment T, then it will take place a collision at the moment $(T + \delta T)$. In order to find the rate of such kind of situations that takes place, we must divide the number of molecules inside the collision volume of one other molecule and divide that number by δT. Then, we can take the limit of the interval $(T, T + \delta T) \rightarrow 0$:

$$Collision\ Rate = \frac{Nr.\ molecules\ in\ \Delta V_{collision}}{\delta T}\Big|\ \delta T \rightarrow 0 \tag{1}$$

The deterministic method is used for example in models based on the evolution of species logical relations ([10], [11], [12]).

But obviously, it might be a problem to find a number for those molecules that come together in the same volume when we consider a very small time, because in that moment this number will be also close to 0.

ii) Instead of the number of molecules, the *stochastic approach* considers the probability that the center of such sphere will be inside the collision volume of another one. This probability is given by the ratio of *collision volume/total volume* and this will have a physical sense even when the collision volume will be closer and closer to 0:

$$Collision\ probability = \frac{\Delta V_{collision}}{V_{total}}\Big|\ \Delta V_{collision} \rightarrow 0 \tag{2}$$

Even that the behavior of only one molecule is "deterministic", the behavior of a complex of molecules in a mixture of different species and different kind of interactions cannot be deterministic. Unless we consider also the influence of the nuclear matrix or other interconnections like this (influence of membrane structures, cytoskeleton, etc.) that reduce the degree of freedom of molecules to each other, the randomness is more convenient because we consider the phenomenon inside the cell more to a probabilistic level.

A. Computational efficiency

In order to be relevant, a model should be more comprehensive, more like a whole cell. Instead of building specific reactions for a particular pathway, it is better to build more general interactions that can fit to a general protein-protein or protein-protein-protein interactions. This kind of approach can bring inside a model the feedback that we need for a dynamic behavior.

From this point of view, in order to build a whole cell model, major computational efficiency problems show up: i). *the minimum number of genes to include inside in a cell model*, and ii). *the most important functions that we need to have in our computational cell model.*

Concerning the functions, we can assume that not all the important functions that are usually present in a normal cell will be also present in a minimal cell. For example, we can assume that some types of the molecules are "imported" from the surrounding media. On the other hand, other functions must be present in all living organism, even in the simplest ones, such as the ability to replicate DNA and to translate the genetic message to produce proteins, also the ability to produce energy, and finally to transport molecules and signals across the cell membrane. So, of course, all these functions we must find also in a computational cell model.

Concerning the number of genes, this is an important matter, because it is a necessity to reduce the inside cellular components to a manageable computational number. Only for the gene activity, for example – where the most prominent feature is the binding of transcription factors to the regulatory elements of that gene – the number of states of the complexes grows exponentially with the number of components and their binding sites. A single gene, where 10 transcription factors can bind, has $2^{10} = 1024$ different possible states, resulting in the same number of transcriptional rates. Also, because each state can have 10 different transcription rates, there are 10240 potentially reactions to specify [13]. But of course that this is only a pure theoretical consideration, because not all the possible reactions can really occur and not all the possible combinations between the compounds are simultaneous. This is the reason that is better from the beginning to approach directly to different possible states for molecules complexes and not for only one compound. Still we need to limit for the beginning to around 100 molecules the number of some of the compound inside the model. Otherwise the running time will last too long.

III. Results

A. Brief summary of the computational cell model

The starting point of the model developed in this thesis was a model created by Dr. Brent Foy, Associate Professor at Wright State University – Dayton Ohio [14]. The original cell model had two genes and a pathway for these genes to produce the corresponding proteins by combined transcription and translation processes. Also, the "cell" was designed to respond to an external chemical compound by increasing the production of one protein while decreasing production of another. The response is possible by having a receptor protein with the capability to bind an external chemical and to generate a signal for a second messenger compound. This second messenger was able to enhance the activity of one of the gene present in the cell and repress the activity of the other gene.

Afterwards, in [14] the capabilities of the cell model were extended beside the previous model by a third gene. So, this model has now three genes, one to encode for the protein that will be produced only as response to the changes in the environment, another that produces a protein all the time but it will be repressed when that changing in the environment occur, and a third new one gene that encodes all the time for the receptor protein (Fig.2). Also, a new important feature is the separation of the transcription and translation into separate events. So, each of the gene will have now a corresponding messenger RNA and proteins (Fig.3). Another important new feature is the presence of some of the metabolism events. The model simulates the taking over of glucose inside the cell and the production of ATP and pyruvate from ADP, glucose and inorganic phosphate (Fig.4).

Also the degradation of all the proteins and messenger RNAs and the presence of the amino acids necessary for building the proteins are other features added to the model.

The model developed analyzes and optimizes the capability to sense and responds the presence of an extra-cellular chemical compound for a whole theoretical biological minimal cell by simulating the regulation of gene expression pathway (Fig. 5), and protein transport (Fig.6).

The final software is even more complex that only simulating all these events. It has also the capability to run a complete experiment with 32 different simulations for different values of some of the parameters and variables.

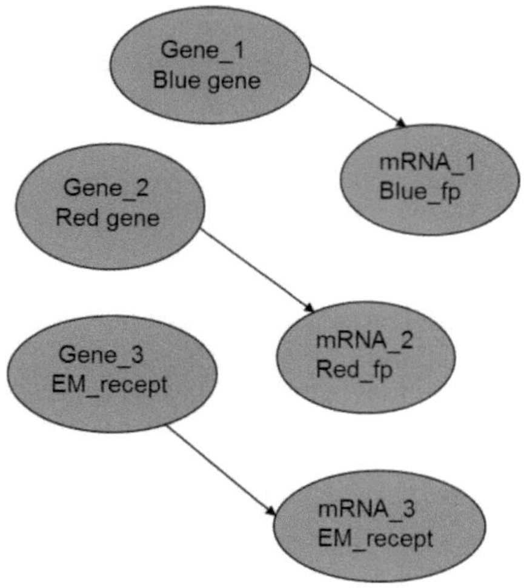

Fig.2 Three genes - transcription

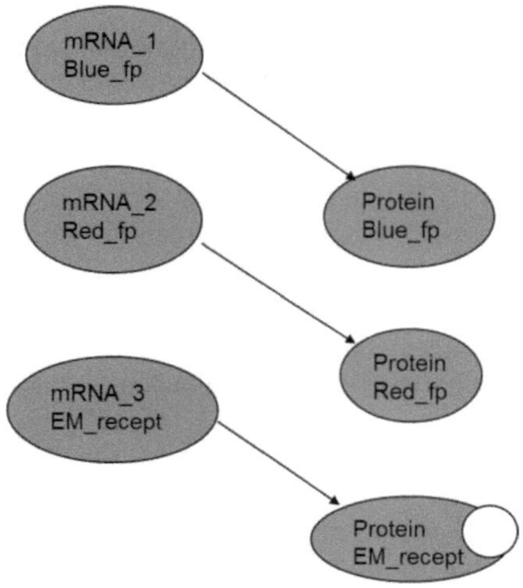

Fig. 3 Three proteins - translation

IV. Discussions

New approaches were improved lately by using the System Biology approach. The design and optimization that were used in this work are built on a system approach to a cell model that requires the actions showed at part I, point *A*.

The first step is to build the system's structure: a diagram with all the genes and proteins interactions, their biochemical ways to interact and the mechanisms of the cell inside structure control. The diagram of this project can be seen in [14].

The second step is to realize the system's dynamics: the cell actions and reactions over time at the environmental stress are simulated in some special files for the case of this project. A best, flexible model should be also modular to permit a continuous increase in complexity by adding new components. Also, it must easily admit new functions [14].

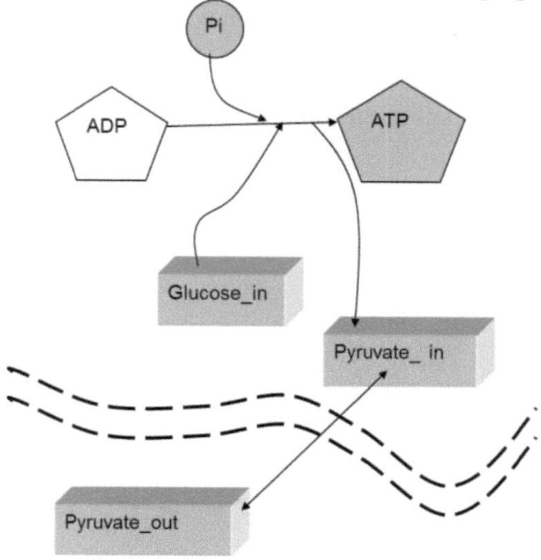

Fig. 4 Metabolism

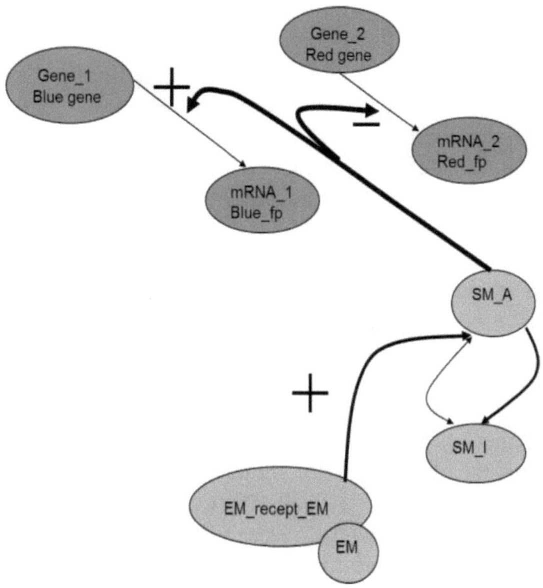

Fig. 5 The regulation of gene expresion pathway

The computer program for this project was conceived from the beginning to insure that. The program has subroutines that simulate one-direction reactions and bi-directional ones. These subroutines can be used to introduce any kind of evolutions inside the cell, because almost any kind of such events can be reduced at these two types of reactions.

A third step would be to study the system: explore the stability, explore the effect of random reactions, explore sensitivity to parameters and optimize system to achieve. In order to do that the present project has used two kinds of experiments, by running 30 times the computer program with the same base line parameters, and by running 32 times but with changing the values of some parameters [13].

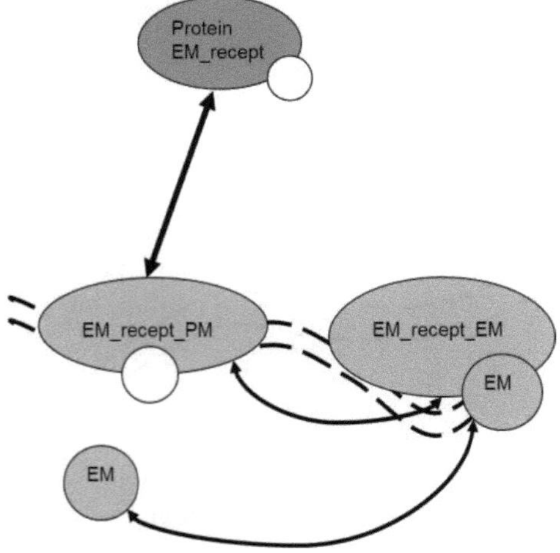

Fig. 6 Protein transport

The fourth step is to conceive the new final synthetic biological systems with specific properties, after establishing the main properties that these models should have. The summary of some of the main model properties that results after the experiments are: i) increasing the amount of Gene_1 produces an increase in the amount of the corresponding protein; ii) increasing the amount of Gene_2 produces an increase also in the amount of the corresponding protein; iii) decreasing the amount of the inactive form of the second messenger (SM_I) from 300 molecules to 30 has produces a decrease in the Gene_1 protein amount and an instability of the response signal, but produces an increase in the Gene_2 signal, because there is no longer repression possible on Gene_2; iv) the amount of the external signaling molecule receptor protein (EM_recept) has a weak effect; v) increasing the protein degradation rates, and the messenger RNAs degradation rates have the most important influence on the cell response, by a very important increase in the protein amount.

The ADP inside the cell is provide by the initial amount, and during the simulation, by the ADP released from the translation reactions. From the fact that the level of ADP is very high all the time we can conclude that the transition rate from ADP to ATP is low and we must consider increasing it in the future.

The chemical sensing capability is the feature introduced to simulate the negative feedback control [15]. The computer cell model function results proved that the negative feedback control provides a stable response to an exterior stress, relatively independent of further internal parameters variations and external disturbances.

V. Conclusions

Even with all these problems and limitations, there are some very important benefits of creating and working with cell models.

The most important help and effect of computational modeling will be in pharmaceutical industries and medical treatments. By creating a complete cell model, with reliable transcription and translation features and also with other important attributes as signal-transduction and metabolism, one can provide new tools for drug discovery.

Another goal is to build a multiple drug system (the simultaneous use of several drugs with different targets on the body) that can bring the state of a sick cell, tissue, organ or organism to a normal shape with minimum side effects.

Creating a cell model can be also a first step in designing a *synthetic* gene network and constructions of integrated biological circuits capable of performing increasingly elaborate functions, such as auto regulatory systems (switches, oscillators, logic gates and so on), or intercellular signaling systems (networks to communicate between cells).

Such a simulation program is a reliable tool in identifying the principles that relate a structural diagram of the genome to the dynamic functioning of all the compounds inside a cell. [9].

Creating models for interactions in some well-studied organisms (where it is easier to do that because all the network of compounds and events is better understood) can be an advantage in explaining other interactions for the less known organisms. Researchers that have used this approach relay on the idea that the evolution toward optimal systems generate similar way to solve the control processes. This is the reason that simple models that are conceived and improved using as pattern some living organisms can explain the functioning of others, often very different, organisms [14].

Finally, to build a data base with all different types of solutions found during their evolution by the organisms in order to better adapt to the environmental stress will be a great achievement for this kind of modeling.

Finally, one can say that this paper brings a contribution in order to establish the basic principles in order to build-in that specific cell model of a living minimal biological cell, and that proved to work with that specific cell model.

Conflict of Interest

The authors declare that they have no conflict of interest.

References

1. H. Kitano System Biology: a brief overview. Science. Vol. 295. March 2002
2. Garrett, R.H., Grisham, C.M. 1999: Biochemistry (Second Edition). Pacific Grove, CA: Thomson Brooks/Cole.
3. Setubal, J., Meidanis, J. 1997: Introduction to Computational Molecular Biology. Pacific Grove, CA: Thomson Brooks/Cole. ISBN 0-534-95262-3.
4. Krane, D.E., Raymer, M. L 2002: Fundamental Concepts of Bioinformatics. San Francisco: Benjamin Cummings.
5. Gillespie, D. T. 1977: Exact Stochastic Simulation of Coupled Chemical Reactions. The Journal of Physical Chemistry, Vol. 81. No25.
6. M. M. Domach, S.K. Leung, R.E. Cahn, G.G. Cocks, and M.L. Shuler (Computer Model for Glucose-Limited Growth of a Single Cell of Escherichia Coli B/r-A. Biotechnology and Bioengineering, Vol. 26, Issue 3, Pages 203-216. 1984
7. (J.J. Tyson – Modeling the cell division cycle: cdc2 and cyclin interactions. Proc. Natl. Acad. Sci. USA, Vol. 88, pp. 7328-7332, August 1991).
8. (Samuel T. Browning and Michael L. Shuler – Towards the Development of a Minimal Cell Model by Generalization of a Model of Escherichia Coli: Use of Dimensionless Rate Parameters. Biotechnology and Bioengineering, Vol. 76, Issue 3, November 2001)
9. [M.E. Csete, J.C. Doyle – Reverse Engineering of Biological Complexity. Science, Vol. 295, March 2002].
10. Bănică, M., Coteţiu, R. 2006: Dynamical Optimization of the Tip Relief Parameters for an Involute Spurs Gearing with Impose Center Based on Computer Simulation, 7th International Conference "Automation in Production Planning and Manufacturing", Zilina, Slovakia, May, pag. 11-16.
11. Chira, F., Bănică, M, Coteţiu, R. 2008: Optimization of the asymmetric gear design for some different mono-objective function using genetic algorithms, Proceedings of 9th International Scientific Conference "New ways in manufacturing technologies 2008", ISBN 978-80-553-0044-3,pg.379-386,19.-21.6., ,Presov, Slovakia.
12. Tudose, L., Pop, D. 2002: Proiectare optimala cu Algoritmi Genetici. Editura MEDIAMIRA, Cluj-Napoca Foy, B.D. 2005: Simulating the Interactions of Genes, Proteins, and Metabolites in Cell-Like Entities. Final Technical Report. Wright State University.
13. Stoicovici, D.I. 2004: Design and optimization of the chemical sensing capability of a theoretical biological cell using a stochastic simulation. Master Thesis, Wright State University.
14. Foy, B., Specification of Molecular complexes in Cell Simulations. International Conference on System Biology, Stockholm, Sweden, 2002.
15. Stoicovici D, Banica M, Ungureanu M, Chira F, Crăciun I: Establishing the Parameter Behavior at a Simulation Program Based On a Stochastic Approach. SCIENTIFIC BULLETIN, Serie C, Fascicle: Mechanics, Tribology, Machine Manufacturing Technology ISSN 1224-3264, Volume 2013 No. XXVII.
16. E-CELL on http://www.e-cell.org/about/
17. Virtual Cell on http://www.nrcam.uchc.edu/index.html?current=one
18. Bio-Spice on http://biospice.sourceforge.net/

Author: D. Stoicovici
Institute: Technical University of Cluj Napoca, North University Center of Baia Mare
Street: 430083 Dr. V. Babes, Nr. 62A
City: Baia Mare
Country: Romania
Email:dinu.stoicovici@cunbm.ro

Microarray Gene Expression Analysis using R

I. Petre and C. Buiu

Politehnica University of Bucharest/ Dept. of Automatic Control and Systems Engineering, Bucharest Romania

Abstract— **Developing effective cancer therapies has been a major focus in biomedical research. This paper proposes an integrated gene analysis procedure, with the purpose of finding differentially expressed probe sets which will lead to a better understanding of cancer molecular basis and hopefully to future drug development. In other words, based on public data sets, we will identify gene expression signatures of cancerous diseases in order to continuing finding new approaches in understanding and controlling tumoral cell signals.**

Keywords— **Gene expression, microarray analysis, clustering, normalization.**

I. Introduction

Over the last years, more and more studies are made on organization, analysis and interpretation of biological data, in order to better understand the mechanisms of life at different levels. Cancer is one of the leading cause of mortality worldwide and is a generic term for a large range of diseases characterized by alterations of normal cells [1].

The motivation for choosing this theme is the major implication that cancer still stands in public health; technology, although advanced, has been failing so far in providing precise treatments to eradicate any type of cancer.

II. Background

A. Genes expressions analysis

Gene expression or genetic code represents triplets of nucleotide sequences (RNA) which form amino acids, activating protein synthesis [2, 3].

Regulating gene expression means all the mechanisms used by the cells to decrease or increase production of specific products genes (RNA/protein) for the proper functioning of the body.

An important step in understanding progression of various diseases is the transcription step, where transcription factors bind in specific places from DNA and promotes or inhibits the expression of a gene. Correct transcriptions phases are vital for maintaining proper functioning and reproduction of cells. Interrupting the gene tuning or problems in genes transcriptions into mRNA can lead to some variety of diseases, such as cancer [3].

Analysis of time series gene expression aims to better understand the dynamics related to transcription and thereby the progression of disease. Gene expression analysis refers to finding different patterns in the genes expressed under specific situation or in a specific cell and to look for associations between regulation of gene expression levels and phenotypic variations [4, 5].

A very useful method for genes expressions analysis is DNA microarray - DNA points collections attached to a solid surface used to measure gene expression levels of two different samples: normal versus pathological, in order to identify chromosomal imbalances [5].

III. Approach

In this paper, using R software for statistical computing and graphs, we will identify, analyze and interpret gene expression signatures of cancerous diseases (Figure 1), according to the following steps:

- **Data acquisition and transfer**

➢ Consult Gene Expression Omnibus database. GEO is an international public repository that archives and distributes different kinds of functional genomics data sets submitted by the research community. Data in GEO represent original gene expression studies generated from microarray or high-throughput sequence technologies, investigating a wide range of biological and medical themes [7].

While the main goal of GEO is to serve as a public genomic data archive, the resource also provides user-friendly mechanisms that allow users to review, analyze and visualize gene expression profiles of interest. Today, GEO archives data for approximately 40.000 studies comprising a million samples, for over 2.200 organisms, submitted by 15.000 laboratories from around the world [6].

➢ Download publically available microarray data (Affimetrix Gene Chip Arrays or CEL files containing Afymatrix data);

- **Data preprocessing and quality control checks**

➢ Loading, reading, normalize and quality control of a large dataset of microarray samples

➢ Method: RMA normalization;

- **Noise filtering and dimensionality reduction**

➢ Selecting genes that pass some criteria to arrive at a reduced set of features;

S. Vlad and N.M. Roman (eds.), *International Conference on Advancements of Medicine and Health Care through Technology; 12th - 15th October 2016, Cluj-Napoca, Romania*,
IFMBE Proceedings 59,
DOI: 10.1007/978-3-319-52875-5_74

- **Hierarchical clustering**

➢ In order to discover novel relationships among samples in a given dataset;

➢ Finding differentially expressed probe sets/genes to identify those with similar expression profiles;

- **Annotating probe sets to gene symbols**

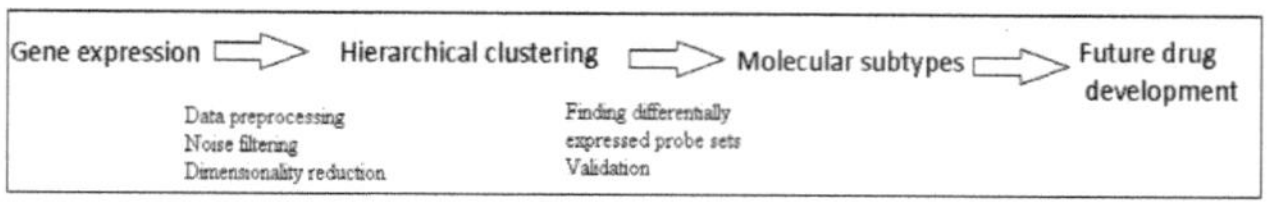

Fig. 1. Overall view of the integrated gene expression analysis

We started the first step: **Data acquisition and transfer,** by downloading seven sample .CEL.gz file for breast cancers from GEO.

After the data is read and uncompressed, the next step is **Data preprocessing and quality control checks.**

Microarray data normalization is necessary to ensure that differences in intensities read by the scanner are due to differential gene expression and not due to printing, hybridization or scanning artifacts. There are several methods to normalize data based on quantile normalization or log-median centering, such as MAS5.0, GCRMA or RMA. If MAS5 is Affymetrix's older probe level normalization algorithm due to the fact that normalizes each array independently and sequentially based on mismatch probe value, in present, most CEL file data in literature are being normalized with one of RMA or GCRMA algorithm [7].

Compared to MAS5, the RMA (Robust Multiarray Averaging) method ignore the mismatch values (fact that increases precision by reducing noise) and scale all the chips to the same mean and fit all to the same distribution using a multi-chip model. GRCMA is similar to RMA, but calculates background differently by making use of mismatch intensities to correct background [7].

In this article, we will normalize all of the microarrays together using RMA, followed by an annotation of those probe sets to gene symbols (e.g., Entrez Gene ID and Symbol), see Figure 2.

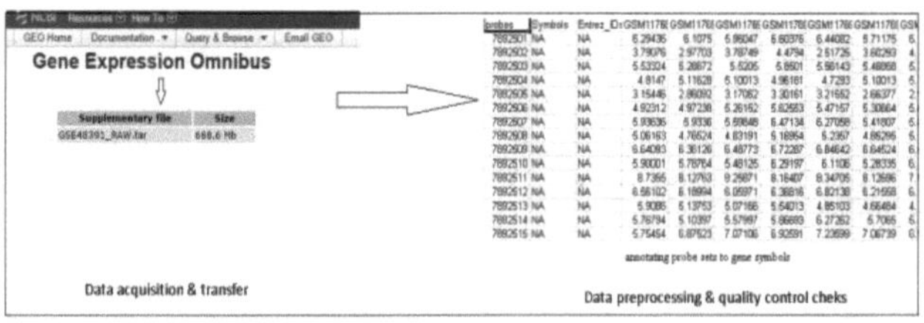

Fig. 2. From downloading to annotating microarray gene expression

To check the effects of RMA normalization, we can plot a boxplot of probe intensities before and after normalization (Figure 3 and Figure 4).

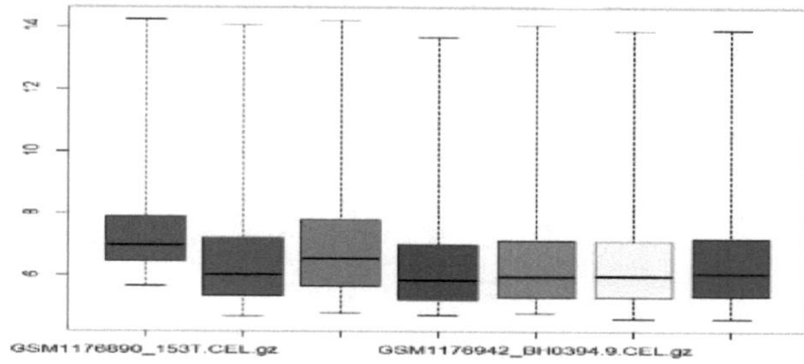

Fig. 3. Boxplot of unnormalized intensity values

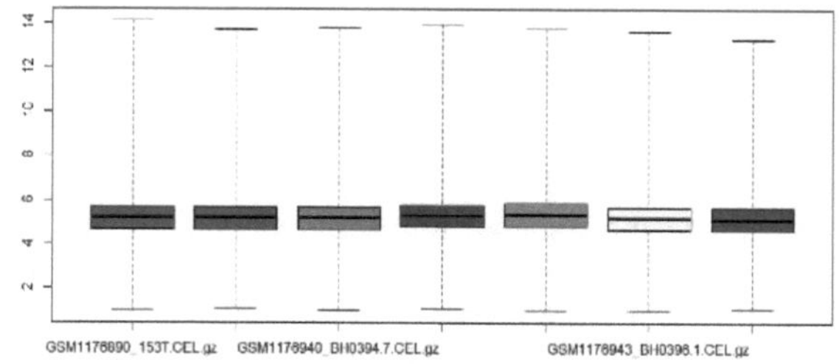

Fig. 4. Boxplot of normalized intensity values

From the plots in Figure 5 and Figure 6, we can conclude that normalization has brought the intensities from all of the chips into distributions with similar characteristics.

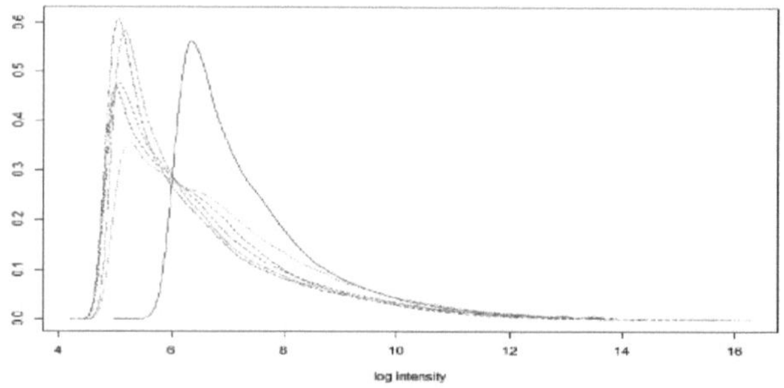

Fig. 5. Density vs. log intensity histogram for the unnormalized data

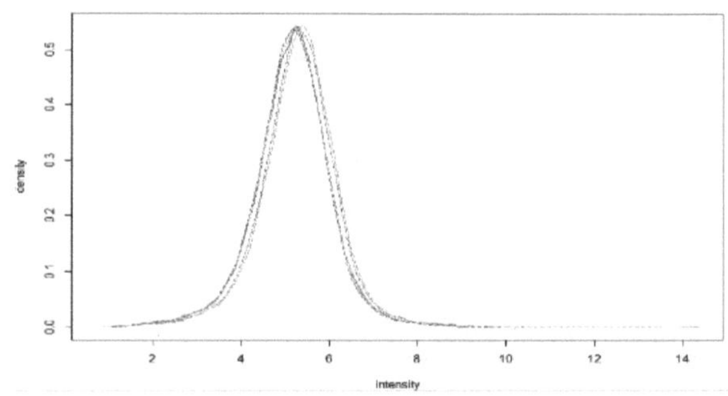

Fig. 6. Density vs. log intensity histogram for the normalized data

Using the Bioconductor package *affyPLM*, we can compute Relative Log Expression (RLE) and Normalized Unscaled Standard Error (NUSE) scores using our normalized data and visualize statistical characteristics of the CEL files (Figure 7).

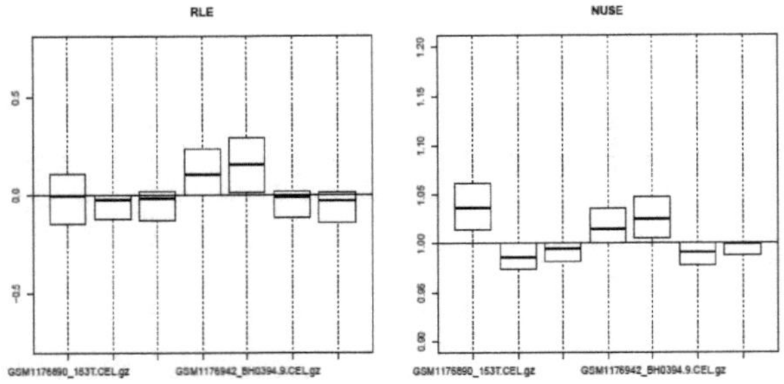

Fig. 7. RLE vs NUSE plots of the CEL files

Microarray analysis is commonly characterized in a number of genes much larger than the number of samples, thus leading to the issue of high dimensionality. Not all of the thousands of genes are relevant and needed for classification. Moreover, they lead to computational burden and presents unnecessary noise in the classification process, therefore it is essential to arrive at a reduced set of features/genes, suffice for good classification [8].

For the **noise filtering and dimensionality reduction part,** we choose a basic method based on three well defined metrics [9]. Other methods that reduce dimensionality by replacing a large number of predictors (genes) with just a few significant, beside the one we used are PLS or PCA. In this paper, we select genes that pass each of the three following criteria:

- genes expressed in at least 5% of samples;
- genes having a significantly different variance from the median variance of all probe sets using a threshold of p smaller than 0.01. In this way are removed probes with median intensity values below a pre-specified threshold considered to be the same as noise;
- genes having a coefficient of variation larger than 0.186;

We compute these metrics for our normalized data to arrive at a reduced set of features.

A powerful analytical tool to leverage with large sample sizes is **clustering**. Clustering is an unsupervised method for grouping sets of similar objects based on some criterion, usually a series of features whose similarity is defined by some distance function.

For this step, we choose hierarchical method because it is used on a large scale due to its intuitive appeal and visualization properties. Also, it does not require no apriori information about the number of clusters required, so can be extremely useful in exploratory data analysis.

We perform **hierarchical clustering** on the data matrix and cut the dendogram such that the samples are divided into clusters (Figure 8).

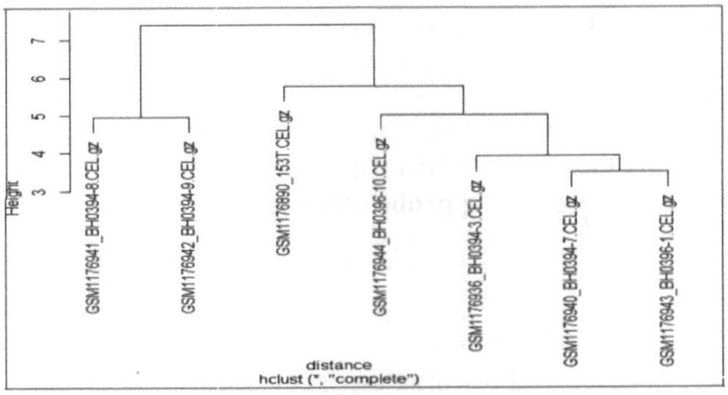

Fig. 8. Dendogram

We also display filtered data as a heat map with clustered columns. In Figure 9 we can see colored increasing intensity values of genes from the seven CEL files.

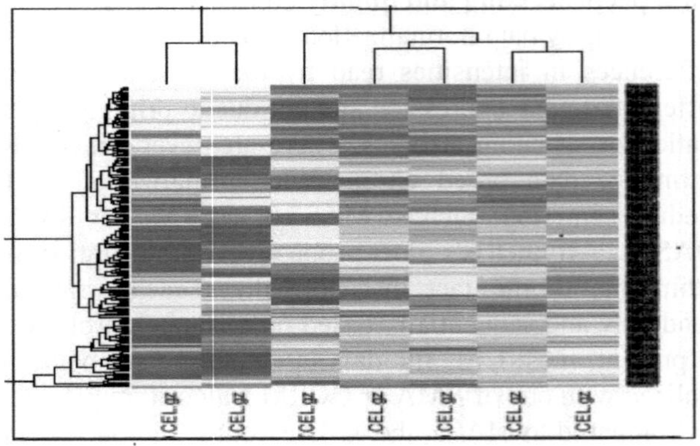

Fig. 9. Heat map

Using the data matrix and the cluster memberships, we identify genes differentially expressed between a given cluster and all other clusters (Figure 10.) using a t-test, an univariate statistical method unaffected by the ratio of features to samples (e.g. number of genes differentially expressed, p-val smaller than 0.05).

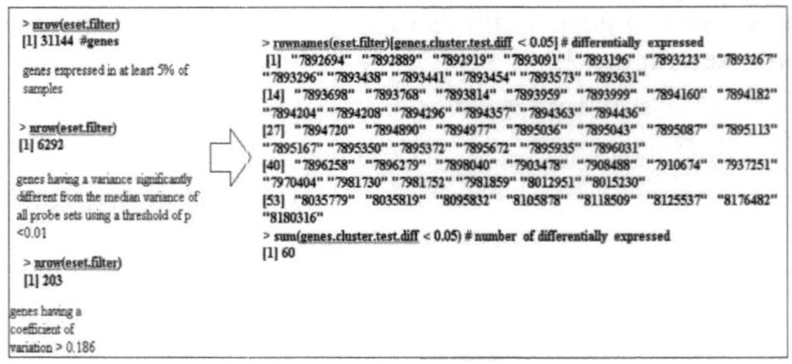

Fig. 10. Steps to genes differentially expressed

Each found cluster or molecular subtype has various pathological features, different molecular alterations, gene expressions at different level or deregulated signaling pathways.

For **future prospects**, we need to identify, interpret and validate the generated data (clustered gene) using GO (Gene Ontology), then build a model which can characterize cancer subtypes based on gene expression and the defining genes class in the system and predict changes of genes from a subset of cancer to another [10].

IV. CONCLUSIONS

While the large datasets generated by microarrays are a potential goldmine of information, their large size makes analysis a cumbersome task. Extracting the right information from microarray data sets can have a great significance and importance in understanding molecular basis of different diseases, which can lead to prevention and treatment. Molecular subtypes help us to identify specific markers for a particular type of cancer or profile gene, markers that will be targets for future drug development and prognostic prediction.

A substantial challenge of this approach, using R and the methods mentioned above, is to obtain new biological information which we hope that will contribute to the biological field.

The main goal of this microarray analysis is to be able to identify relevant genes and specific biological pathways that had a strong correlation with a phenotype of interest (cell growth or cancer).

Scientists anticipate that molecular mutations analysis will lead to new stages of detection and treatment multifactorial diseases, such as cancer, thus this project of finding differentially expressed probe sets comes to help them by continuing finding new approaches in understanding and controlling tumoral cell signals.

CONFLICT OF INTEREST

The authors declare that they have no conflict of interest.

REFERENCES

1. Cancer info at http://www.who.int/mediacentre/factsheets/fs297/en/
2. Alberts B et al. (2002) Molecular Biology of The cell. Fourth ed., New York: Garland Science
3. Lodish H, Kaiser A, Baltimore D et al. (2000) Molecular Cell Biology. Fourth Edi., New York: W.H.Freeman
4. Chen S C, Tsai T H, Chung C H et al. (2015) Dynamic association rules for gene expression data analysis. BMC Genomics, vol. 16, no. 1, p. 786
5. Ernst J (2008) Computational Methods for Analyzing and Modeling Gene Regulation Dynamics. Sch. Comput. Sci. Mach. Learn. Dep.
6. Information about GEO at http://www.ncbi.nlm.nih.gov/books/NBK159736/
7. Cope L, Irizarry R, Jafee H W, Speed TP (2003) A benchmark for Affymetrix Gene Chip expression measures. Bioinformatics 1:1–13
8. Li Y, Chen L (2014) "Big Biological Data: Challenges and Opportunities. Genomics. Proteomics Bioinformatics, vol. 12, pp. 187–189
9. Marisa L et al. (2013) Gene expression classification of Colon Cancer into Molecular Subtypes: Characterization, Validation and Prognostic Value. PLOS Medicine, Volume 10
10. Chassagnole C. (2009). Making better Cancer Therapies with Modelling", COO Epic London

Author Index

Keyword Index

MIX
Papier aus verantwortungsvollen Quellen
Paper from responsible sources
FSC® C105338

If you have any concerns about our products,
you can contact us on
ProductSafety@springernature.com

In case Publisher is established outside the EU,
the EU authorized representative is:
Springer Nature Customer Service Center GmbH
Europaplatz 3, 69115 Heidelberg, Germany

Printed by Libri Plureos GmbH
in Hamburg, Germany